LGBT HEALTH

K. Bryant Smalley, PhD, PsyD, MBA, is a licensed clinical psychologist focused on health disparities research. He cofounded and serves as the executive director of the Rural Health Research Institute at Georgia Southern University. The Rural Health Research Institute is an innovative, interdisciplinary hub of research and outreach dedicated to improving health outcomes and reducing health disparities in rural and minority populations. In addition, he is an associate professor of psychology and has served in multiple leadership roles (including director of clinical training) for the PsyD program at Georgia Southern University, a clinical psychology program focused on preparing mental health practitioners for practice in underserved areas. Dr. Smalley currently serves on the American Psychological Association's Committee on Rural Health, is a Health Equity Ambassador for the American Psychological Association, and has previously been invited to discuss health disparity issues with the White House Rural Council. Dr. Smalley's work has been funded by organizations including the National Institutes of Health, the Health Resources and Services Administration (HRSA), and the federal Corporation for National and Community Service (CNCS), including Center of Excellence funding through the National Institute on Minority Health and Health Disparities. His research has been published in more than 50 journal articles, books, and book chapters, including publications in *LGBT Health, Health Psychology, Journal of Gay and Lesbian Mental Health, International Journal of Transgenderism, Journal of Bisexuality,* and *Psychology of Men and Masculinity.*

Jacob C. Warren, PhD, MBA, is a behavioral epidemiologist specializing in health disparities research. He is the Rufus C. Harris Endowed Chair, director of the Center for Rural Health and Health Disparities, and associate professor of community medicine at the Mercer University School of Medicine, which is dedicated to meeting the health needs of rural and underserved populations. He has served in a variety of academic and research leadership positions, including as a Medical Care section councilor within the American Public Health Association, and has been principal investigator on numerous federally funded research and service grants focused on the study and elimination of health disparities in various groups. His work has been supported by the Centers for Disease Control and Prevention, the National Institutes of Health, CNCS, and HRSA, including Center of Excellence funding through the National Institute on Minority Health and Health Disparities. Dr. Warren has published over 50 journal articles, books, and book chapters, including publications in *LGBT Health, International Journal of Transgenderism, Journal of Bisexuality, AIDS Care, AIDS Education and Prevention,* and *AIDS and Behavior.*

K. Nikki Barefoot, PsyD, is a licensed clinical psychologist and assistant director of the Rural Health Research Institute at Georgia Southern University, which is focused on meeting the physical health, mental health, and prevention needs of diverse communities. Her work focuses on health disparities in LGBT and rural populations, including extensive clinical experience in working with the needs of LGBT and other underserved youth. Her work has been published in journals including *Rural and Remote Health, Stigma and Health, International Journal of Transgenderism, LGBT Health, Journal of Bisexuality,* and *Journal of Gay and Lesbian Mental Health.*

LGBT HEALTH

Meeting the Needs of Gender and Sexual Minorities

K. Bryant Smalley, PhD, PsyD, MBA

Jacob C. Warren, PhD, MBA

K. Nikki Barefoot, PsyD

Editors

SPRINGER PUBLISHING COMPANY

Springer Publishing Company, LLC
11 West 42nd Street
New York, NY 10036
www.springerpub.com

Acquisitions Editor: Sheri W. Sussman
Compositor: Newgen KnowledgeWorks

ISBN: 978-0-8261-3377-9
ebook ISBN: 978-0-8261-3378-6

Instructor's Materials: Qualified instructors may request supplements by emailing textbook@ springerpub.com:
Instructor's PowerPoints: 978-0-8261-3518-6

17 18 19 20 21 / 5 4 3 2 1

The author and the publisher of this Work have made every effort to use sources believed to be reliable to provide information that is accurate and compatible with the standards generally accepted at the time of publication. The author and publisher shall not be liable for any special, consequential, or exemplary damages resulting, in whole or in part, from the readers' use of, or reliance on, the information contained in this book. The publisher has no responsibility for the persistence or accuracy of URLs for external or third-party Internet websites referred to in this publication and does not guarantee that any content on such websites is, or will remain, accurate or appropriate.

Library of Congress Cataloging-in-Publication Data
Names: Smalley, K. Bryant, editor. | Warren, Jacob C., editor | Barefoot, K. Nikki, editor.
Title: LGBT health : meeting the needs of gender and sexual minorities /
 [edited by] K. Bryant Smalley, Jacob C. Warren, K. Nikki Barefoot.
Other titles: LGBT health (Smalley)
Description: New York : Springer Publishing Company, [2017] |
 Includes bibliographical references.
Identifiers: LCCN 2017030258| ISBN 9780826133779 (paper back) |
 ISBN 9780826133786 (e-book)
Subjects: | MESH: Sexual Minorities | Health Equity | Minority Health |
 Delivery of Health Care | United States
Classification: LCC RA564.9.H65 | NLM WA 300 AA1 | DDC 362.1086/6—dc23
LC record available at https://lccn.loc.gov/2017030258

Contact us to receive discount rates on bulk purchases.
We can also customize our books to meet your needs.
For more information please contact: sales@springerpub.com

Printed in the United States of America by Gasch Printing.

To all the gender and sexual minority trailblazers, current and past.
Thank you.
—Bryant, Jacob, and Nikki

CONTENTS

SECTION III. SPECIAL CONSIDERATIONS FOR SPECIFIC GROUPS

SECTION IV. RECOMMENDATIONS AND FUTURE DIRECTIONS

CONTRIBUTORS

Laika D. Aguinaldo, LICSW
Research Social Worker
Boston Children's Hospital
Boston, Massachusetts

Michelle T. Aihe, MS
Research Intern
Department of Health Outcomes and
Behavior
H. Lee Moffitt Cancer Center and
Research Institute
Tampa, Florida

K. Nikki Barefoot, PsyD
Assistant Director
Rural Health Research Institute
Georgia Southern University
Statesboro, Georgia

Maria T. Brown, LMSW, PhD
Assistant Research Professor, Aging
Studies Institute
David B. Falk College of Sport and
Human Dynamics
Syracuse University
Syracuse, New York

Taylor A. Burke, MA
Doctoral Student in Clinical Psychology
Temple University
Philadelphia, Pennsylvania

Matthew R. Capriotti, PhD
Assistant Professor of Psychology
San José State University
San José, California; and
Research Associate
Department of Medicine
University of California San Francisco
San Francisco, California

Stephen P. Casazza, MS
Doctoral Student in Counseling
Psychology
Radford University
Radford, Virginia

Tracy J. Cohn, PhD, LCP
Associate Professor
of Psychology
Radford University
Radford, Virginia

Elizabeth M. Cottrell, MA
Doctoral Student in Counseling
Psychology
Radford University
Radford, Virginia

lore m. dickey, PhD
Assistant Professor and Doctoral Training
Director
Combined Counseling/School Psychology
PhD Program
Department of Educational
Psychology
Northern Arizona University
Flagstaff, Arizona

Franco Dispenza, PhD, CRC
Assistant Professor of Clinical
Rehabilitation Counseling and
Counselor Education
Georgia State University
Atlanta, Georgia

Ashby Dodge, LCSW
Clinical Director
The Trevor Project
New York, New York

Lake Dziengel, PhD
Associate Professor of Social Work
University of Minnesota Duluth
Duluth, Minnesota

Annesa Flentje, PhD
Assistant Professor of Community
  Health Systems
University of California San Francisco
San Francisco, California

Nicholas Grant, PhD
Congressional Fellow
American Psychological Association
Washington, DC

Melvin C. Hampton, PhD, MDiv
Post-Doctoral Research Fellow
Center for Interdisciplinary Research
  on AIDS
Yale School of Public Health
New Haven, Connecticut

Nicholas C. Heck, PhD
Assistant Professor of Psychology
Marquette University
Milwaukee, Wisconsin

Kristin E. Heron, PhD
Assistant Professor of Psychology
Old Dominion University
Norfolk, Virginia

Keith J. Horvath, PhD
Associate Professor of Epidemiology
  and Community Health
University of Minnesota
Minneapolis, Minnesota

Janella N. Hudson, PhD
Postdoctoral Fellow
Department of Health Outcomes
  and Behavior
H. Lee Moffitt Cancer Center and
  Research Institute
Tampa, Florida

Tameeka L. Hunter, MS, CRC
Director of Disability Resource Center
Clayton State University
Morrow, Georgia

Colt Keo-Meier, PhD
Clinical Psychologist
Psychology Lecturer, University of
  Houston; and
Medical Student, University of Texas
  Medical Branch; and
Assistant Professor of Psychiatry and
  Behavioral Sciences, Baylor College of
  Medicine
Houston, Texas

K. Abel Knochel, PhD
Assistant Professor of Social Work
University of Minnesota Duluth
Duluth, Minnesota

Nathaniel Kralik, BA
Osteopathic Medical Student
Heritage College of Osteopathic Medicine
Ohio University
Dublin, Ohio

Shalini Kulasingam, MPH, PhD
Associate Professor of Epidemiology and
  Community Health
University of Minnesota
Minneapolis, Minnesota

Asha Kumar, MS
Clinical Rehabilitation Counselor
Atlanta, Georgia

Sara Lammert, MPH
Graduate Research Assistant
Division of Epidemiology and
  Community Health
University of Minnesota
Minneapolis, Minnesota

Robin J. Lewis, PhD
Professor of Psychology
Old Dominion University
Norfolk, Virginia

Alan R. Lifson, MD, MPH
Professor of Epidemiology and
    Community Health
University of Minnesota
Minneapolis, Minnesota

Richard T. Liu, PhD
Assistant Professor of Psychiatry
    and Human Behavior
Alpert Medical School
Brown University
East Providence, Rhode Island

Tyler B. Mason, PhD
Assistant Professor of Clinical
    Preventative Medicine
University of Southern California
Los Angeles, California

Zachary McClain, MD
Assistant Professor of Clinical Pediatrics
Perelman School of Medicine,
    University of Pennsylvania
Craig-Dalsimer Division of Adolescent
    Medicine, The Children's Hospital
    of Philadelphia
Philadelphia, Pennsylvania

Jane A. McElroy, PhD
Associate Professor of Family and
    Community Medicine
School of Medicine
University of Missouri
Columbia, Missouri

**Kimberly H. McManama O'Brien,
PhD, LICSW**
Research Scientist
Education Development Center
Boston Children's Hospital
Harvard Medical School
Boston, Massachusetts

Lucas A. Mirabito, MA
Psychology Graduate Student
Marquette University
Milwaukee, Wisconsin

Rita M. Melendez, PhD
Associate Professor of Sexuality Studies
    and Sociology
San Francisco State University
San Francisco, California

Jeri Muse, PhD, DAAPM
Clinical Psychologist, VA San Diego
    Healthcare System; and
Assistant Professor, University of
    California, San Diego School of
    Medicine
San Diego, California

John E. Pachankis, PhD
Associate Professor of Epidemiology
Yale School of Public Health
New Haven, Connecticut

Jennifer M. Putney, PhD, LICSW
Assistant Professor of Social Work
Simmons College
The Fenway Institute
Boston, Massachusetts

Gwendolyn P. Quinn, PhD
Senior Member and Director of Survey
    Methods Core
H. Lee Moffitt Cancer Center and
    Research Institute
Professor of Oncologic Sciences
Morsani College of Medicine
University of South Florida
Tampa, Florida

Amanda Rickard, PsyD, NCSP
Clinical Psychologist
Regents Center for Learning Disorders
Georgia Southern University
Statesboro, Georgia

Jillian Crystal Salazar
MA Candidate
Department of Sexuality Studies and
    Sociology
San Francisco State University
San Francisco, California

Matthew B. Schabath, PhD
Associate Member
Department of Cancer Epidemiology
H. Lee Moffitt Cancer Center & Research
  Institute
Associate Professor of Oncologic Sciences
Morsani College of Medicine
University of South Florida
Tampa, Florida

Daniel Skinner, PhD
Assistant Professor of Health Policy
Heritage College of Osteopathic Medicine
Ohio University
Dublin, Ohio

K. Bryant Smalley, PhD, PsyD, MBA
Executive Director
Rural Health Research Institute
Associate Professor of Psychology
Georgia Southern University
Statesboro, Georgia

Rosemary Thomas, MPH, CHES
Program Coordinator
Penn Medicine Program for LGBT Health
Perelman School of Medicine, University
  of Pennsylvania
Philadelphia, Pennsylvania

Jacob C. Warren, PhD, MBA
Rufus C. Harris Endowed Chair
Director, Center for Rural Health and
  Health Disparities
Associate Professor of Community Medicine
Mercer University School of Medicine
Macon, Georgia

Genevieve Weber, PhD, LMHC
Associate Professor of Counseling and
  Mental Health Professions
Hofstra University
Hempstead, New York

Lauren E. Wilson, BS
Research Coordinator
Department of Health Outcomes and
  Behavior
H. Lee Moffitt Cancer Center and
  Research Institute
Tampa, Florida

Nicholas Yared, MD
Infectious Disease Fellow
Department of Medicine and
  Division of Epidemiology and
  Community Health
University of Minnesota
Minneapolis, Minnesota

Baligh R. Yehia, MD, MPP, MSc
Adjunct Assistant Professor
  of Medicine
Perelman School of Medicine,
  University of Pennsylvania
Philadelphia, Pennsylvania

Juan P. Zapata, BA
Psychology Graduate Student
Marquette University
Milwaukee, Wisconsin

PREFACE

Few would disagree that the past 25 years have been transformative in the lives of gender and sexual minority (GSM) people living in the United States. In that time, we have progressed from a society with virtually no visibility given to the lesbian, gay, bisexual, and transgender (LGBT) community to one in which our gender and sexual minority celebrities are not only increasingly prominent but also are counted among some of the most successful in their fields. Recent years have also seen landmark events such as the federal protection of same-sex marriage that will shape the future in profound ways. It is clear that we are in the midst of the naissance of the most LGBT-inclusive period in history.

With all of these advancements, it is easy for many to overlook the persistence of substantial challenges faced by members of the LGBT community. For example, the ability to marry has not been paired with legal protections for those individuals once wed, and the "married today, fired tomorrow" phenomenon is still a real and present threat for same-sex couples because of a lack of federal nondiscrimination protections in employment. More relevant to this book, legal reform does not sweep away generations of stigma, discrimination, and hostility that have manifested in a shocking array of health disparities and related inequalities. Although we may be in the emergence of a golden age of LGBT rights, we are still under the shadow of hundreds of years of conflict and oppression. With researchers only recently able to begin investigating these dynamics because of an earlier lack of interest, funding, and venues for gender and sexual minority health research, we are only now beginning to realize the magnitude of the challenges that exist.

At the same time, however, we are also learning more about the remarkable levels of resiliency, innovation, and determination that those years of struggle have forged. The LGBT community is diverse yet united, in need yet strong, and oppressed yet resilient. As the field of gender and sexual minority health advances, we are simultaneously learning about the threats and the potential solutions, and combining those two bodies of knowledge is essential to achieving true change.

As such, it is our hope that this book will serve simultaneously as a reference, a call to action, and a guide for change in addressing the multitude of health challenges described in its pages. At all times, we attempt to balance the often troubling reality of the topic being discussed with specific, applied knowledge that can be translated into action and change. We begin the book with an overview of the history, current status, and terminology associated with the health of gender and sexual minority groups, as well as discussion of some overarching themes that are relevant to health topics (e.g., barriers to care and general health risks). We then explore a multitude of individual health outcomes ranging from chronic disease to intimate partner violence, describing what is currently known, what remains to be discovered, and what avenues there are to improve the outcome. Subsequently, we examine the specific factors impacting the health of particular GSM groups, such as gender minority populations and GSM veterans. We then conclude with a discussion of evidence-based interventions, recommendations for health care providers, and future directions for the field.

The field of gender and sexual minority health may be full of areas of need documented throughout this book that at times can seem overwhelming, but this presents countless areas of opportunity for dedicated professionals and community members to make a true difference. We hope this book inspires you to begin or to continue such work.

—Bryant, Jacob, and Nikki

As an aid for instructors using this text in their course work, an ancillary PowerPoint deck with discussion questions is available for download. To access this PowerPoint deck, qualified instructors should send an email to textbook@springerpub.com.

SECTION I

INTRODUCTION AND OVERVIEW

CHAPTER 1

Gender and Sexual Minority Health: History, Current State, and Terminology

K. Bryant Smalley, Jacob C. Warren, and K. Nikki Barefoot

The past several years have been ones of unprecedented expansion of social awareness and acceptance of individuals who identify as lesbian, gay, bisexual, transgender, and other gender and sexual minority (GSM) groups. The historic Supreme Court cases of *United States v. Windsor* (2013) and *Obergefell v. Hodges* (2015) thrust the civil rights of GSM groups into the forefront of American culture in a way never seen before, and one that is unlikely to be repeated. Although many outside of the lesbian, gay, bisexual, and transgender (LGBT) community may perceive these marriage-related victories as the end of the struggle for equal rights and opportunity, such a view ignores the fact that GSM individuals face stark challenges in achieving and maintaining health. The reasons for these challenges are diverse and discussed throughout this book, but many relate back to ongoing issues ranging from social and systemic effects of oppression and discrimination to sometimes surprising levels of inter- and even intra-personal barriers to healthy decision making.

Traditionally, and for legitimate historical reasons discussed in more detail subsequently, the health of GSM individuals has been focused primarily on risk, that is, higher levels of engagement in risk-taking behaviors and disparities in health outcomes when compared to non-GSM populations. This line of inquiry has shown that stark differences exist in behaviors such as consumption of alcohol

(Cabaj, 2014; Green & Feinstein, 2012; Kann et al., 2011), cigarette smoking (Balsam, Beadnell, & Riggs, 2012), sexual risk taking (Herbst et al., 2008; Jones and Hoyler, 2006; Liau, Millett, and Marks, 2006), self-injurious behavior (Batejan, Jarvi, & Swenson, 2015; Davey, Arcelus, Meyer, & Bouman, 2016), and poor nutrition habits (Diemer, Grant, Munn-Chernoff, Patterson, & Duncan, 2015; Feldman & Meyer, 2007; Gay and Lesbian Medical Association [GLMA], 2001). The prevailing model explaining these differences is that of minority stress; specifically, the discrimination, victimization, and harassment that result from heterosexism (the assumption that all individuals are heterosexual) and homophobia/transphobia (fear and/or dislike of GSM individuals) negatively impact the ability to maintain both mental and physical health at the same levels seen in non-GSM groups (Hendricks & Testa, 2012; Meyer, 1995, 2003, 2013).

More recently, researchers have begun to focus on the actual experience of GSM individuals within the health care system. As such, minority stress theory can also be applied to findings that GSM groups are less likely to seek out needed and ongoing health care (Lick, Durson, & Johnson, 2014; Meyer & Frost, 2013), a factor so impactful that it has been named as the most significant health risk factor for GSM health (Johnson, Mimiaga, & Bradford, 2008). This can largely be tied to an experience-based fear and mistrust of the medical community. While many point to the fact that homosexuality was considered a diagnosable illness in the United States until the late 1970s as the source of this mistrust (Bayer, 1987; Minton, 2002), fears are not simply historical. The "right" of physicians to refuse medical services to a GSM individual remains the law in more than half of states—only 21 states have antidiscrimination laws protecting the provision of public services (including health care) regardless of sexual orientation, and only 19 states have laws protecting gender identity (Lambda Legal, 2017). While federal protection against discrimination based on gender identity was included in the Affordable Care Act (Section 1557), this protection applies only to providers and organizations receiving federal funding. This leaves GSM groups with patchwork protection against medical discrimination (making it a real and present threat). This has resulted in heterosexism/homophobia and cisgenderism/transphobia being some of the most common forms of discrimination experienced in the health care system (Alencar Albuquerque et al., 2016; Brotman, Ryan, Jalbert, & Rowe, 2002; Dodds, Keogh, & Hickson, 2005; Fish & Bewley, 2010; Grant et al., 2011; Institute of Medicine [IOM], 2011; Kosenko, Rintamaki, Raney, & Maness, 2013; Sinding, Barnhoff, & Grassu, 2004). The persistent impact discrimination experiences can have is profound, as negative experiences with providers can result in even further avoidance of care, which only exacerbates existing problems (Facione & Facione, 2007; Li, Matthews, Aranda, Patel, & Patel, 2015; Lick et al., 2014).

Most recently, researchers have begun to look beyond areas of traditional focus to a more holistic view of GSM health, that is, while still recognizing the profound impact of health behavior differences and resulting disparities, also recognizing that GSM individuals simultaneously operate within the larger health context that impacts all individuals, regardless of sexual orientation and gender identity. Specifically, researchers are now looking beyond the sexually transmitted disease (STD), substance use, and mental health outcomes of the traditional GSM health literature to also recognize the many other pressing health outcomes within the population (which, on the whole, is much more likely to face a diagnosis of cancer, depression, diabetes, or heart disease than HIV/AIDS, overdose, or suicide).

Given this expanding perspective on GSM health, there is a need for a centralized resource that synthesizes epidemiological, medical, psychological, sociological, and public health research related to not only its current state, but also ways to improve health within the LGBT community. This text is designed to that end. Within this introductory chapter, we first discuss the evolution of terminology used within GSM research and justify the selection of terms used within this text. Then, we discuss some of the methodological challenges that the field faces in producing research results that sometimes yield contradictory or difficult-to-interpret findings. Finally, we conclude with an overall introduction to the remainder of the text.

■ TERMINOLOGY

To preface both the remainder of this chapter and the chapters that follow, it is helpful to review the terminology used to refer to people who identify as a gender and/or sexual minority, and the remarkable evolution in terminology that has occurred during the past 30 years. We acknowledge that preferences in terminology differ between generations and even from person to person; however, we have attempted to summarize the general understanding regarding both current and previous terminology, discussing their appropriate use, and identifying terms that may now be considered outdated or offensive. We conclude with a discussion of the terminology selected for use within the text, and the justification for its selection.

Defining Sexual Orientation and Gender Identity

As the formative concept for this text, we would be remiss not to discuss the underlying definitions of both sexual orientation and gender identity. Although these two concepts are frequently discussed in tandem, as in this book, it is crucial to understand the difference between the two, and recognize them as distinct concepts that each can have a unique impact on health. Fenway Health (2010) defines sexual orientation as "a person's enduring physical, romantic, emotional, and/or spiritual attraction to another person." For the most part, the general public is fairly aware of the concept of sexual orientation, particularly heterosexual/straight, gay, lesbian, and bisexual. Less well-known orientations include queer, pansexual, omnisexual, asexual, and demisexual. While the terms *queer, pansexual*, and *omnisexual* are relatively new with regard to sexual orientation and do not have precise definitions, people who identify as queer typically reject traditional binary sexual orientation labels, instead preferring to use *queer* as a fluid, umbrella term for all sexual identities outside of the cis/heteronormative majority (Owen, 2014). Often used interchangeably, the terms *omnisexual* and *pansexual* are typically used to describe individuals who have attraction that crosses all gender lines, as contrasted, for instance, with a bisexual man who may not feel attraction to transgender men.

For example, a pansexual individual may be attracted to individuals who identify as female gender, regardless of the sex assigned at birth, or to individuals of all genders, also regardless of the sex assigned at birth. Persons identifying as asexual report not having sexual attraction to any gender, and those identifying as demisexual report that they feel sexual attraction only to those with whom they have an emotional connection (typically regardless of gender).

Although often conflated with sexual orientation, gender identity is a completely separate concept. Gender identity describes an individual's "innate, deeply felt psychological identification as a man, woman, or something else, which may or may not correspond to the person's external body or assigned sex at birth" (Fenway Health, 2010). The most frequently recognized gender minority identity is transgender, which describes an individual whose assigned sex (typically based on external genitalia at birth) and true gender do not align (e.g., an individual who was assigned female sex at birth, but identifies as male). In contrast, individuals who do identify with their external body and the sex they were assigned at birth are referred to as *cisgender*, a term not in common use outside the LGBT community, which is used to describe individuals who do not identify as a gender minority. Other gender identities include *genderqueer, non-binary, androgynous,* and *two-spirit*. While these terms tend to lack precise definitions, individuals identifying with these gender identities typically fall on a spectrum of not identifying exclusively with either the male or female gender (potentially identifying as both or neither), with two-spirit identification typically associated with persons of Native American heritage. One of the most important aspects of gender identity is that it is completely independent of sexual orientation; information about one's sexual orientation or gender identity does not provide any information regarding the other. For instance, a transgender woman may be straight (attracted to men), lesbian (attracted to women), or any other sexual orientation. Thus, both sexual orientation and gender identity must be considered for any individual as a person can be a gender minority without being a sexual minority (and vice versa).

Evolution of Terminology

Before presenting the terminology selected for use throughout this book, we thought it helpful to discuss how current terminology has evolved and describe some terms that, although previously in common use, may now be considered outdated or even offensive. Similarly, we discuss terms that were previously considered offensive that have been "reclaimed" and are now in common use within the LGBT community, even if not considered acceptable outside of the LGBT community.

Perhaps the most technical term used to describe sexual orientation is *homosexual*, purportedly coined in the late 19th century (Herek, 2010); interestingly, the term *lesbian* is also believed to have gained its current usage around the same time (Enszer, 2015). Although in common use before the time, in 1952, homosexuality was used in the first edition of the *Diagnostic and Statistical Manual of Mental Disorders* (*DSM-I*; American Psychiatric Association, 1952), clearly indicating the view of same-sex attraction as both deviant and pathological. Incidentally, this inclusion may underlie many individuals' aversion to the term, as it was included within the *DSM* under the umbrella diagnosis of "sexual deviation" alongside pedophilia, rape, sexual assault, and sexual mutilation. Around the time of the publication of the *DSM*, the term *gay* in its current sense appears to have entered common use within the LGBT community as a term preferred to the more clinical *homosexual* (Norton, 2005). In its most literal definition, "homosexual" was intended to describe individuals sexually attracted to members of the same sex, regardless of actual action on that attraction. In addition, the term lacked a recognition of the role of emotional and relational connection.

The focus of the term *homosexual* on sexual attraction and not action became important with the emergence of the AIDS pandemic. During this period, terminology underwent a major overhaul, potentially due to the previously unprecedented degree of external focus on the LGBT community. While the potential for attraction to both men and women was recognized with the coining of the term *bisexual* in the early 20th century (Angelides, 2001), as research into the AIDS pandemic began, the need for a term that was more descriptive of behavior than attraction emerged. As a result, the term *men who have sex with men*, abbreviated as MSM, became widely used. The goal was to describe men who, regardless of their professed sexual orientation, had sex with other men. Thus, the term included not only men who identified as gay or bisexual, but also men who did not identify as members of the LGBT community but still engaged in same-sex sexual activity. While this shift in terminology is understandable as sex between men emerged as a dominant risk factor for the transmission of HIV, it unfortunately had the effect of focusing the terminology onto sexual activity, again neglecting the importance of emotional and relational attraction. The term *MSM* is still frequently used within the research literature, and while technically accurate, may be viewed by some as reductionistic and reinforcing of the centrality of sexual activity in nomenclature. Furthermore, the suitability of the term *MSM* to describe youth before sexual debut or adult men who have never acted upon same-sex attraction is questionable. Thus, the terms *gay*, *lesbian*, and *bisexual* are currently preferred, as they have come to represent the broader sexual, emotional, and relational attraction under consideration. The expansion of terminology beyond these terms—including those defined earlier—has continued the evolution of terminology regarding sexual orientation, and as our understanding grows, it is likely that new terms will enter use.

One term that merits specific examination is *queer*. Viewed by many as a strongly pejorative noun used to refer to a gay man, the word has been reclaimed by the LGBT community, particularly as a global adjective referring to someone who is a gender and/or sexual minority. Increasingly, the term is even coming to represent its own designation as a sexual orientation that rejects prior labels in favor of simply labeling oneself as nonheterosexual. There is ongoing disagreement regarding the acceptability of the word, with many within the LGBT community still finding the word to be offensive, and a prevailing intolerance of the use of the word by someone outside the LGBT community (Fenway Health, 2010; Human Rights Campaign, 2016; Owen, 2014). However, many individuals strongly identify with the descriptor *queer*, and it is clear that the term will become increasingly important when describing GSM individuals.

Terminology regarding gender minority individuals has similarly evolved over time. While not representative of gender minority status, one of the earliest terms proximal to the gender minority community was that of *transvestite*, used to refer to a person who dressed in clothing other than what the gender society would expect of them. The term has long been associated with a sexual aspect, most recently as a fetishism, and thus is not viewed as an appropriate or acceptable term for a gender minority individual. In fact, according to the current edition of the *Diagnostic and Statistical Manual of Mental Disorders* (5th ed.; *DSM-5*; American Psychiatric Association, 2013), the majority of adults who meet criteria for the official "diagnosis" of transvestic fetishism are heterosexual-identified cisgender men; therefore, this term is not appropriate for describing gender minority individuals. The first term designed to specifically describe the experiences of gender minority groups appears to be *transsexual*, intended to designate an individual who wished—through surgical intervention—to modify their* current body to that of a different sex. The limitations of this term center on this aspect of surgical transition, which represents only a subset of individuals who identify as a gender minority. Further, the term has come to have a negative connotation due to its history of use as a clinical diagnosis, perpetuating the pathologization of non-cisgender identities (Fenway Health, 2010). The currently acceptable term of *transgender* that entered common use in the 1970s (Stryker, 2008) intended to focus more on gender (e.g., the psychological and external expression of identity) than sex (e.g., the physical/biological characteristics).

Early on, the word tended to be used as both a verb and a noun rather than its current usage as an adjective; that is, a person was described as "transgendered" or as "a transgender." The use of either—particularly "a transgender"—is now largely considered inappropriate and offensive. The abbreviation *trans* has now entered common usage (e.g., trans woman or describing oneself as trans). Reflecting this shift from a focus on sex (i.e., transsexual) to a focus on gender (i.e., transgender), the phrase *gender confirmation surgery* is now preferred to "sex change" or "sex reassignment" surgery. Other now outdated terms previously in common use include the distinction of "pre-op" and "post-op." These terms were intended to distinguish between individuals who had not undergone gender confirmation surgeries versus those who had; however, the terms harken back to the use of the term "transsexual" by focusing on the external physical makeup (i.e., sex) of the individual rather than the person's lived identity (i.e., gender). While it can be very important to assess a transgender person's surgical history to provide adequate medical care, the use of a specific identifier when referring to a person (e.g., labeling someone a "pre-op transgender man") is considered non-affirming and perpetuates an assumption that all transgender individuals desire surgery.

Similarly, the terms *male-to-female transgender* (MtF) and *female-to-male transgender* (FtM) are increasingly falling out of favor. The terms were intended to acknowledge the gender differences within the transgender community (i.e., to allow linguistic separation of transgender men and transgender women), but retained

---

* Throughout this text, we utilize "they" and "their" as genderless third-person pronouns in both the singular and plural. See discussion of this choice of terminology later in this chapter.

the focus on gender assigned at birth rather than the individual's true gender identity. The terms have been replaced with the simpler and more affirming *transgender woman* (or transgender female) for an individual assigned male at birth but whose true gender identity is female, and *transgender man* (or transgender male) for an individual assigned female at birth but whose true gender identity is male. Correspondingly, an additional recent shift has been away from phrases such as "the sex a person was born"—that is, stating that a transgender woman was "born a man" or "born a male"— to the use of the more affirming phrase of *sex assigned at birth* (or gender assigned at birth). Thus, the appropriate phrasing would be to say that a transgender woman was "assigned male at birth." As with sexual orientation, as our understanding of diverse gender identities has evolved, additional terms defined earlier, such as genderqueer, non-binary, and others, have also entered use, but remain largely unknown outside the LGBT community.

As terminology regarding individual sexual orientations and gender identities evolved, so did the terminology regarding the community of individuals united by the commonality of being a gender and/or sexual minority individual. As the AIDS pandemic grew in the United States, the notion of what had previously been referred to as the "gay community" began to expand and become more inclusive. To acknowledge the growing social interconnections of lesbians, gay men, and bisexual men and women, the term *LGB* began gaining traction, and eventually expanded into the now well-known *LGBT* (Fenway Health, 2010; Parent, DeBlaere, & Moradi, 2013) to recognize the similarity in community between those of minority sexual orientations and minority gender identities. To acknowledge the other gender identities that exist, the term *LGBT** was in use for a time. In recent years, additional letters have been added to represent a variety of other sexual orientations and gender identity groups, including questioning, queer, intersex, allies, and many others (e.g., *LGBTQ* and *LGBTQIQ*). While the goal of increasing the initialism to be more inclusive is admirable, it has led to confusion and the inevitability of leaving out certain groups. Thus, most recently, a more global terminology has emerged, and has been selected to be utilized in this text.

Terminology in This Text

For the purposes of this text, we have elected to use the phrase, *gender and sexual minority*, or GSM, as our global term to refer to individuals who identify with a gender identity other than cisgender and/or a sexual orientation other than heterosexual. This term is increasingly preferred over LGBT as it is more inclusive by inherently acknowledging all individuals of diverse sexual orientations and gender identities, including ones that have yet to reach common knowledge (e.g., use of "T" can be seen as disenfranchising by individuals who identify as genderqueer rather than transgender). There is disagreement within the field regarding the order of "gender" and "sexual;" for instance, the National Institutes of Health (NIH) has recently begun to use the phrase "sexual and gender minority." At the time of publication of this text, the more frequently used order is *GSM*; therefore, throughout this text, we elected to use the phrase in that order. Accordingly, in general, the phrase *sexual minority* is used by itself in preference to LGB. With regard to *gender minority*, a challenge occurs with regard to precision, as the more commonly used umbrella term *transgender* actually represents a subgroup of the gender minority community. Thus, for the purposes of this text, the term *transgender* is used when referring solely to individuals identifying as transgender, whereas the term *gender minority* is used when referring to individuals of diverse gender identities (inclusive of transgender). Another common term when describing gender identity is "gender non-conforming." Although this term has gained traction within the research community, we avoid its use within this text as many feel that the term implies a judgment that individuals should "conform" to a certain gender identity. Further, we avoid the use of any descriptor as a noun, as this is largely considered offensive (e.g., referring to a gay man as "a gay" or a transgender man as "a transgender")— the major exception is the use of lesbian as a noun, as this is the prevailing use of the term (e.g., lesbians and bisexual women). In addition, we have utilized *they* and *their* as third-person pronouns throughout the text in both the singular and plural sense. *Utilizing their rather than the more traditional his or her avoids reifying the gender binary and is thus more affirming of nonbinary individuals.*

The main exception in this text to the use of GSM is the use of the phrase *LGBT community* when referring to the broader social network of individuals who identify as a gender or sexual minority. This was largely a matter of deference to predominant language, as the phrase *LGBT community* is used in common parlance and is by far the most frequently used phrase to encapsulate the community. We acknowledge that this term can be seen as less inclusive than GSM; however, the phrase *GSM community* is not currently in common use. Similarly, we use the phrase *LGBT-affirming* when describing the provision of culturally competent care, given its widespread use in the literature.

■ CHALLENGES IN GSM HEALTH RESEARCH

As can be seen even through the continued evolution of terminology, the field of GSM health research is still in its infancy. There was virtually no focus on the unique needs of the LGBT community until the emergence of the AIDS pandemic, and it is only recently that researchers have begun to look at the broader health needs of the LGBT community beyond STDs, substance use, and mental health. As researchers explore this new line of inquiry, however, there are a number of realities that must be considered that present challenges to conducting and/or interpreting research within the LGBT community.

One persistent challenge reflected in the preceding discussion of this chapter is the inherent complication of evolving definitions and terminology that result from an expanding understanding of the dynamics of both sexual orientation and gender identity. In research circles, terms and associated definitions are largely dictated by the line of inquiry. When considering STDs, it is logical to focus on sexual behavior as a defining characteristic, and thus utilize terms such as MSM. In this sense, despite clearly being a member of the LGBT community, a bisexual man may be entirely excluded from a study if he has not engaged in same-sex sexual activity. When focusing on the psychological risk factors for suicidality, however, the larger societal impact of being a self-identified member of the LGBT community would indicate the need to focus on self-defined identity regardless of sexual behavior (e.g., internally identifying as a member of the LGBT community), resulting in the use of broader terms such as gay or bisexual. Therein lies one of the most challenging aspects of GSM health research—the differences in intent of the study and resulting definitions/terminologies must be kept in mind when interpreting findings. Even if accurate and representative, findings built on research focused on women who have sex with women, for example, may be different from findings built on research focused on women who identify as lesbian or bisexual. The distinction is not simply academic when designing research; it is important to deliberately consider the operational definition utilized. Is sexual attraction, sexual behavior, romantic attraction, current relationship, prior relationships, or self-definition the most appropriate way to delineate the population of interest? The reality is that it depends on the study, which, while being more precise, does serve to somewhat muddy the field.

The other major complication in GSM health research is that while the number of GSM individuals nationwide is substantial (Gates, 2011), their broad geographic dispersion within a context that is historically unaccepting of their identity greatly complicates recruitment into studies. As a result, GSM health research has tended to be highly localized in its execution. This results from the fact that the LGBT community is a "hidden population"—in technical terms, there is no traditional sampling method by which to draw a representative sample of GSM individuals. Furthermore, the still-present factors of discrimination and victimization can significantly impact the willingness of individuals to not only self-identify, but also to participate in health research (Institute of Medicine [IOM], 2011; Meyer & Wilson, 2009).

As a result of these two challenges, and the historical prejudice that discouraged lines of inquiry surrounding the LGBT community (Coulter, Kenst, Bowen, & Scout, 2014; GLMA, 2001; Institute of Medicine [IOM], 2011), there are many critical unanswered questions regarding the health of GSM groups. However, there has been an explosion of research in the area—particularly in the past 10 years—that has begun to shed light on both the nature of the challenges faced by the LGBT community and the potential ways in which to best meet the health needs—physical and mental, treatment and prevention—of GSM individuals. The remainder of this text is intended to serve as a guide to that existing knowledge base, and as a call for additional work to fill the many remaining gaps in understanding.

■ INTRODUCTION TO THE TEXT

We hope that the preceding discussion of terminology and research challenges has laid a groundwork for the remaining content of the book. The text itself is divided into four main sections. Section I contains the introductory materials that lay the foundation needed to better understand the remaining sections, discussing issues of terminology, systematic barriers to health, and overall health risks experienced across the LGBT community. Section II presents current knowledge regarding specific health outcomes ranging from mental health to cancer, exploring what is known regarding disease burden and prevention/intervention. Section III examines specific populations within the LGBT community to describe what is known regarding their health needs and methods to improve health outcomes (e.g., youth, gender minority individuals, veterans). Section IV concludes the text with a survey of the evidence base for GSM health programs and interventions, recommendations for clinical practitioners and community members, and a discussion of future directions within the field.

The field of GSM health is new and rapidly evolving, with many exciting lines of inquiry now bearing their first fruit. By more fully understanding and appreciating not only the challenges that GSM individuals face in achieving and maintaining health, but also the unique opportunities for innovative approaches to promoting cultural competency and implementing interventional programming, we hope that readers of this book will gain useful knowledge in their own GSM health-related work, or become part of the growing movement to understand and improve the lives of GSM individuals.

◼ REFERENCES

Alencar Albuquerque, G., de Lima Garcia, C., da Silva Quirino, G., Alves, M. J., Belém, J. M., dos Santos Figueiredo, F. W.,… Adami, F. (2016). Access to health services by lesbian, gay, bisexual, and transgender persons: Systematic literature review. *BMC International Health and Human Rights, 16,* 2. doi:10.1186/s12914-015-0072-9

American Psychiatric Association. (1952). *Diagnostic and statistical manual of mental disorders.* Washington, DC: Author.

American Psychiatric Association. (2013). *Diagnostic and statistical manual of mental disorders* (5th ed.). Arlington, VA: American Psychiatric Publishing.

Angelides, S. (2001). *A history of bisexuality,* Chicago, IL: University of Chicago Press.

Balsam, K. F., Beadnell, B., & Riggs, K. R. (2012). Understanding sexual orientation health disparities in smoking: A population-based analysis. *American Journal of Orthopsychiatry, 82*(4), 482–493. doi:10.1111/j.1939-0025.2012.01186.x

Batejan, K. L., Jarvi, S. M., & Swenson, L. P. (2015). Sexual orientation and non-suicidal self-injury: A meta-analytic review. *Archives of Suicide Research, 19*(2), 131–150. doi:10.1080/13811118.2014.957450

Bayer, R. (1987). *Homosexuality and American psychiatry: The politics of diagnosis.* Revised. Princeton, NJ: Princeton University Press.

Brotman, S., Ryan, B., Jalbert, Y., & Rowe, B. (2002). The impact of coming out on health and health care access: The experiences of gay, lesbian, bisexual and two-spirit people. *Journal of Health & Social Policy, 15*(1), 1–29.

Cabaj, R. P. (2014). Substance use issues among gay, lesbian, bisexual, and transgender people. In M. Galanter, H. D. Kleber, & K. T. Brady (Eds.), *Textbook of substance abuse treatment* (pp. 707–721). Washington, DC: American Psychiatric Association.

Coulter, R. W., Kenst, K. S., Bowen, D. J., & Scout (2014). Research funded by the National Institutes of Health on the health of lesbian, gay, bisexual, and transgender populations. *American Journal of Public Health, 104*(2), e105–e112. doi:10.2105/AJPH.2013.301501

Davey, A., Arcelus, J., Meyer, C., & Bouman, W. P. (2016). Self-injury among trans individuals and matched controls: Prevalence and associated factors. *Health & Social Care in the Community, 24*(4), 485–494. doi:10.1111/hsc.12239

Diemer, E. W., Grant, J. D., Munn-Chernoff, M. A., Patterson, D. A., & Duncan, A. E. (2015). Gender identity, sexual orientation, and eating-related pathology in a national sample of college students. *Journal of Adolescent Health, 57*(2), 144–149.

Dodds, C., Keogh, P., & Hickson, F. (2005). *It makes me sick: Heterosexism, homophobia and the health of gay and bisexual men.* London, UK: Sigma Research. Retrieved from http://sigmaresearch.org.uk/files/report2005a.pdf

Enszer, J. R. (2015). Lesbian. *International Encyclopedia of Human Sexuality.* Retrieved from http://onlinelibrary.wiley.com/doi/10.1002/9781118896877.wbiehs264/abstract

Facione, N. C., & Facione, P. A. (2007). Perceived prejudice in healthcare and women's health protective behavior. *Nursing Research, 56*(3), 175–184.

Feldman, M. B., & Meyer, I. H. (2007). Eating disorders in diverse lesbian, gay, and bisexual populations. *International Journal of Eating Disorders, 40*(3), 218–226. doi:10.1002/eat.20360

Fenway Health (2010). Glossary of gender and transgender terms. Retrieved from http://fenwayhealth.org/documents/the-fenway-institute/handouts/Handout_7-C_Glossary_of_Gender_and_Transgender_Terms__fi.pdf

Fish, J., & Bewley, S. (2010). Using human rights-based approaches to conceptualise lesbian and bisexual women's health inequalities. *Health & Social Care in the Community, 18*(4), 355–362. doi:10.1111/j.1365-2524.2009.00902.x

Gates, G. J. (2011). *How many people are lesbian, gay, bisexual, and transgender?* Los Angeles: The Williams Institute, University of California, Los Angeles School of Law. Retrieved from http://williamsinstitute.law.ucla.edu/wp-content/uploads/Gates-How-Many-People-LGBT-Apr-2011.pdf

Gay and Lesbian Medical Association. (2001). *Healthy People 2010: Companion document for lesbian, gay, bisexual, and transgender (LGBT) health.* San Francisco, CA: Author. Retrieved from http://glma.org/_data/n_0001/resources/live/HealthyCompanionDoc3.pdf

Grant, J. M., Mottet, L. A., Tanis, J., Harrison, J., Herman, J. L., & Keisling, M. (2011). *Injustice at every turn: A report of the national transgender discrimination survey.* Retrieved from http://endtransdiscrimination.org/PDFs/NTDS_Report.pdf

Green, K. E., & Feinstein, B. A. (2012). Substance use in lesbian, gay, and bisexual populations: An update on empirical research and implications for treatment. *Psychology of Addictive Behaviors, 26*(2), 265–278. doi:10.1037/a0025424

Hendricks, M. L., & Testa, R. J. (2012). A conceptual framework for clinical work with transgender and gender nonconforming clients: An adaptation of the Minority Stress Model. *Professional Psychology: Research and Practice, 43*, 460–487. doi:10.1037/a0029597

Herbst, J. H., Jacobs, E. D., Finlayson, T. J., McKleroy, V. S., Neumann, M. S., & Crepaz, N.; HIV/AIDS Prevention Research Synthesis Team. (2008). Estimating HIV prevalence and risk behaviors of transgender persons in the United States: A systematic review. *AIDS and Behavior, 12*(1), 1–17.

Herek, G. M. (2010). Sexual orientation differences as deficits: Science and stigma in the history of American psychology. *Perspectives on Psychological Science, 5*(6), 693–699. doi:10.1177/1745691610388770

Human Rights Campaign. (2016, June). HRC officially adopts the use of "LGBTQ" to reflect diversity of own community. Retrieved from http://www.hrc.org/blog/hrc-officially-adopts-use-of-lgbtq-to-reflect-diversity-of-own-community

Institute of Medicine, Gay, Bisexual, and Transgender Health Issues and Research Gaps and Opportunities. (2011). *The health of lesbian, gay, bisexual, and transgender people: Building a foundation for better understanding.* Washington, DC: National Academies Press.

Johnson, C. V., Mimiaga, M. J., & Bradford, J. (2008). Health care issues among lesbian, gay, bisexual, transgender and intersex (LGBTI) populations in the United States: Introduction. *Journal of Homosexuality, 54*(3), 213–224.

Jones, A. R., & Hoyler, C. L. (2006). HIV/AIDS among women who have sex with women. In F. Fernandez & P. Ruiz (Eds.), *Psychiatric aspects of HIV/AIDS* (pp. 299–307). Philadelphia, PA: Lippincott Williams & Wilkins.

Kann, L., Olsen, E. O., McManus, T., Kinchen, S., Chyen, D., Harris, W. A., & Wechsler, H. (2011). Sexual identity, sex of sexual contacts, and health-risk behaviors among students in grades 9–12: Youth Risk Behavior Surveillance, selected sites United States, 2001–2009. *MMWR Surveillance Summary, 60*(SS07), 1–133.

Kosenko, K., Rintamaki, L., Raney, S., & Maness, K. (2013). Transgender patient perceptions of stigma in health care contexts. *Medical Care, 51*(9), 819–822. doi:10.1097/MLR.0b013e31829fa90d

Lambda Legal (2007). In your state: Public accommodations. Retrieved from http://www.lambdalegal.org/states-regions/in-your-state

Li, C. C., Matthews, A. K., Aranda, F., Patel, C., & Patel, M. (2015). Predictors and consequences of negative patient-provider interactions among a sample of African American sexual minority women. *LGBT Health, 2*(2), 140–146.

Liau, A., Millett, G., & Marks, G. (2006). Meta-analytic examination of online sex-seeking and sexual risk behavior among men who have sex with men. *Sexually Transmitted Diseases, 33*(9), 576–584.

Lick, D. J., Durson, L. E., & Johnson, K. L. (2014). Minority stress and physical health among sexual minorities. *Perspectives on Psychological Science, 8*, 521–548. doi:10.1177/1745691613497965

McKay, B. (2011). Lesbian, gay, bisexual, and transgender health issues, disparities, and information resources. *Medical Reference Services Quarterly, 30*(4), 393–401. doi:10.1080/02763869.2011.608971

Meyer, I. H. (1995). Minority stress and mental health in gay men. *Journal of Health and Social Behavior, 36*, 38–56. doi:10.2307/2137286

Meyer, I. H. (2003). Prejudice, social stress, and mental health in lesbian, gay, and bisexual populations: Conceptual issues and research evidence. *Psychological Bulletin, 129*(5), 674–697. doi:10.1037/0033-2909.129.5.674

Meyer, I. H. (2013). Prejudice, social stress, and mental health in lesbian, gay, and bisexual populations: Conceptual issues and research evidence. *Psychology of Sexual Orientation and Gender Diversity, 1*(Suppl.), 3–26. doi:10.1037/2329-0382.1.S.3

Meyer, I. H., & Frost, D. M. (2013). Minority stress and the health of sexual minorities. In C. J. Patterson & A. R. D'Augelli (Eds.), *Handbook of psychology and sexual orientation* (pp. 252–266). New York, NY: Oxford University Press.

Meyer, I. H., & Wilson, P. A. (2009). Sampling lesbian, gay, and bisexual populations. *Journal of Counseling Psychology, 56*(1), 23–31. doi:10.1037/a0014587

Minton, H. L. (2002). *Departing from deviance: A history of homosexual rights and emancipatory science in America.* Chicago, IL: University of Chicago Press.

Norton, R. (2005). The history of the word "gay" and other queerwords. Retrieved from http://rictornorton.co.uk/though23.htm

Obergefell v. Hodges, 135 S.Ct. 2071 (2015).

Owen, L. (2014, October) About the Q. PFLAG. Retrieved from https://www.pflag.org/blog/about-q

Parent, M. C., DeBlaere, C., & Moradi, B. (2013). Approaches to research on intersectionality: Perspectives on gender, LGBT, and racial/ethnic identities. *Sex Roles, 68*(11–12), 639–645.

Sinding, C., Barnhoff, L., & Grassu, P. (2004). Homophobia and heterosexism in cancer care: The experiences of lesbians. *Canadian Journal of Nursing Research, 36*(4), 170–188.

Stryker, S. (2008). Transgender history, homonormativity, and disciplinarity. *Radical History Review, 2008*(100), 145–157. doi:10.1215/01636545-2007-026

United States v. Windsor, 133 S.Ct. 2675 (2013).

CHAPTER **2**

Sociocultural and Systemic Barriers to Health for Gender and Sexual Minority Populations

Zachary McClain, Rosemary Thomas, and Baligh R. Yehia

As discussed throughout this book, the lesbian, gay, bisexual, and transgender (LGBT) community has recently gained more visibility and social acceptance than ever before. Some of the progress the LGBT community has made in regard to civil liberties includes the 2010 repeal of "Don't Ask, Don't Tell," and the 2013 United States Supreme Court ruling that Section 3 of the Defense of Marriage Act was unconstitutional. Additionally, reports from the Institute of Medicine (IOM), the Department of Health and Human Services (HHS), and the Joint Commission have highlighted the need for increased attention to the health needs of the LGBT community. However, cultural, structural, and other barriers still exist to achieving true social and health equity for gender and sexual minority (GSM) populations, and many protections remain at the mercy of shifts in political power. Ongoing challenges include the lack of federal anti-discrimination laws, inequalities in access to appropriate and affirming health care, and systemic social factors that predispose gender and sexual minorities to poorer health outcomes ranging from cancer to violence (Valanis et al., 2000; Walters, Chen, & Brieding, 2013). The magnitude of these health disparities is discussed in detail throughout this book. This chapter aims to provide an overview of: (a) the current social and cultural climate for GSM populations; (b) the individual, systemic, and environmental barriers to health for GSM populations; and (c) recommendations for addressing these barriers. For a summary of these barriers, and recommendations for addressing them, see Table 2.1. Additional recommendations for practitioners can be found in Chapter 22.

■ SOCIAL AND CULTURAL CLIMATE FOR GSM POPULATIONS

Social acceptance of the LGBT community has increased dramatically over the past decade. In fact, 92% of GSM adults report that society is more accepting than it was 10 years ago, and attribute this to increased visibility of GSM people (Pew Research Center, 2013). However, as a population, GSM individuals lack key nondiscrimination protections related to their sexual orientation and/or gender identity. As of June 2016, only 18 states have specific, inclusive, nondiscrimination protections for the LGBT community (Human Rights Campaign, 2015). Moreover, numerous states have introduced bills to bar transgender individuals from gender-affirming use of public restrooms and to limit transgender youth from fully participating in school (Human Rights Campaign, 2015), and as of the publication of this text the fate of transgender military servicemembers remains undecided. In addition to the lack of formal protections, GSM individuals and families are more likely to experience poverty, homelessness, obstacles to quality education, and family disruption than their non-GSM peers (Burwick, Gates, Baumgartner, & Friend, 2015).

Discrimination and the LGBT Community

Over two-thirds of sexual minority people report discrimination in their personal lives and between 15% and 43% of sexual minority individuals have experienced some form of discrimination at work (Sears & Mallory, 2011). More disturbing is the prevalence of hate-motivated violence affecting the LGBT community. Research demonstrates that gay men face higher rates of hate crime violence than lesbians, bisexuals, African Americans, or Jewish Americans (Stotzer, 2012). Rates of discrimination and hate-motivated violence are even higher among the transgender community (Grant et al., 2011). The National Transgender Discrimination Survey (NTDS) reports that 90% of transgender respondents report harassment, mistreatment, or discrimination on the job (Grant et al., 2011).

In 2015, 67% of GSM homicide victims of hate crimes were transgender women, and 54% of those victims were transgender women of color (Walters et al., 2013). High rates of violence and victimization in the transgender community led to the 2015 formation of a Congressional task force on Transgender Equality in response to the "epidemic of violence against the transgender community" (Human Rights Campaign, 2015). However, transgender individuals, especially transgender women of color, continue to bear an elevated burden of hate-motivated violence and discrimination even beyond that faced by the rest of the LGBT community.

GSM youth are greatly impacted by discrimination and harassment, and are at higher risk of childhood maltreatment compared to heterosexual youth (Burwick et al., 2015). Over 50% of GSM students have personally experienced discriminatory policies and practices at school. Moreover, 56% and 38% of GSM youth report feeling unsafe at school because of their sexual orientation and gender identity, respectively

TABLE 2.1: Individual, System, and Environmental Barriers to GSM Health and Associated Recommendations

BARRIERS	RECOMMENDATIONS
Individual	
Discrimination in health care	• Providers and health care staff should receive LGBT cultural competence training. • Health systems should adopt inclusive and affirming policies. • Sexual Orientation and Gender Identity/Expression should be included in health system nondiscrimination policies.
Lack of health coverage for GSM individuals	• Advocating for inclusion of GSM health needs as part of basic health plan coverage should continue.
System	
Lack of provider competency and lack of resources	• LGBT competent providers should be identified and promoted. • LGBT clinical and cultural competency should be included in medical and health professional education. • LGBT cultural competency should be included in all health care staff training and continuing education.
Lack of research and data	• Medical records should be updated to collect data on LGBT populations.
Environmental	
Lack of federal or state nondiscrimination protections	• Advocacy to improve GSM equality should continue.
Physical and clinical spaces	• Materials showing diverse GSM people should be on display in clinical settings. • Bathrooms should be gender neutral or single use. • LGBT symbols can be displayed either in the clinical space or worn by staff. • The electronic medical record should collect information on name in use, gender identity, sexual orientation and relationship status beyond "married or single."

GSM, gender and sexual minority; LGBT, lesbian, gay, bisexual, and transgender.

(Kosciw, Greytak, Palmer, & Boesen, 2014). GSM youth also face disproportionate rates of homelessness. Approximately 40% of homeless youth identify as GSM and 68% attribute their homeless status to family rejection due to their sexual orientation and/or gender identity (Durso & Gates, 2012). Taken together, these systemic and persistent societal factors limit the ability of GSM individuals to achieve ideal health.

■ BARRIERS TO HEALTH CARE FOR GSM POPULATIONS

Although the previous barriers impact health in ways related more to social standing and lived experiences, other barriers to health are more direct. Such barriers to care for GSM individuals are multifactorial and can be divided into individual, system-based, and environmental factors. Individual barriers are those that exist on a personal level, such as resource limitations, lack of insurance, and transportation challenges. System-based barriers relate to health system policies, health care practices and guidelines, and availability of LGBT-competent providers. Environmental barriers refer to the context in which care is delivered, including the physical and sociocultural environment.

Individual Level Barriers: Health Coverage for GSM Populations

The Affordable Care Act (ACA) expanded health care access for millions of Americans, including the LGBT community. Expanded insurance coverage, non-discrimination provisions, and recommendations for routine data collection on health disparities in the LGBT community are key components of the ACA important to improving the health of GSM individuals (Ranji, Beamesderfer, Kates, & Salganicoff, 2014). Additionally, the Department of Health and Human Services issued regulations barring discrimination based on sexual orientation and gender identity in health insurance marketplaces and health plans (HHS, 2016), one of the first times such provisions have been federalized.

Since the implementation of the ACA, the Health Reform Monitoring Survey found decreases in the number of uninsured sexual minority adults (22% in 2013 to 11% in 2015; Karpman, Skopec, & Long, 2016). However, additional data on rates of insurance for GSM populations is limited. Moreover, despite the progress made by health reform, 19 states have not expanded Medicaid coverage to reach those who fall into a "coverage gap," potentially leaving many in the GSM population without health insurance. Expansion of the Medicaid program (i.e., inclusion of poverty in adult eligibility for Medicaid benefits) is particularly important because GSM adults experience rates of poverty as high or higher than cisgender heterosexual adults (Albelda, Badgett, Schneebaum, & Gates, 2009). Additionally, the National Transgender Discrimination Survey (NTDS) found that transgender individuals are four times more likely than the general population to live in extreme poverty (i.e., household income less than $10,000 per year), placing transgender adults at even higher risk for being uninsured in states that did not expand Medicaid (Grant et al., 2011).

System Level Barriers: Provider Competency and Availability of LGBT Health Care Resources

Given that 56% of sexual minority adults and 70% of transgender individuals report experiencing discrimination in health care settings, it is paramount that providers create a safe, healing space for their GSM patients (Snowdon, 2013). Although many GSM patients have safe, comforting interactions with their medical providers, some delay or do not seek care because of the discrimination, stigma, social isolation, and violence associated with their sexual orientation and/or gender identity (IOM, 2011). GSM patients often seek out providers who are comfortable working with the LGBT community because they are nervous about their health care provider's reactions to their sexual orientation and/or gender identity (Neville & Henrickson, 2006). In fact, 29% of sexual minority individuals and 73% of transgender individuals perceived that they would be treated differently (i.e., negatively) by medical personnel if they were open about their sexual orientation and/or gender identity (Neville & Henrickson, 2006). Furthermore, many GSM individuals believe that they may even be denied health services due to their sexual orientation and/or gender identity (Lambda Legal, 2010).

Identifying providers and health organizations that understand the unique health care needs of GSM populations is challenging. One study found that only 15% of academic medical institutions in the United States had an available list of LGBT-competent physicians associated with their institution. Furthermore, in terms of LGBT-competency training, the majority of institutions did not have any at all (52%), 32% had some training available, and only 16% reported comprehensive LGBT-competency training (Khalili, Leung, & Diamant, 2015). The American College of Physicians recommends that future physicians be trained in culturally and clinically competent GSM health care, and call for increased understanding of the health needs of the GSM population by practicing physicians (Daniel, Butkus, & Health and Public Policy Committee of American College of Physicians, 2015), but it is unclear to what extent this recommendation is translated into curricular change.

Many studies have examined what GSM patients want from a provider. A study of GSM adolescents found that sexual minority youth want to be treated with respect and have a provider who is well educated and a good listener (Ginsburg et al., 2002). Further, research with gender minority youth identified additional needs from providers, such as the following: time to speak with them privately, patience to hear their concerns, flexibility to appreciate their individual identity, and validation that they know who they are (Hawkins, 2009). Similar needs have been identified by GSM adults. For example, transgender adult patients have identified that they want providers to be easy to talk to, nonjudgmental, fair, and respectful (Bockting, Robinson, Benner, & Scheltema, 2004). These findings highlight the need to ensure that providers are trained to ask culturally sensitive questions about sexual orientation and gender identity, and that health organizations increase visibility of LGBT-competent providers.

System Level Barriers: Lack of Research and Data

The IOM's (2011) report on improving the health of GSM people identified that one of the main challenges in understanding their health needs is the lack of data. Questions about sexual orientation and gender identity are often overlooked in demographic surveys conducted in research. Given the discrimination and stigmatization that GSM individuals face, questions about sexual orientation and gender identity must be carefully and competently asked. Depending on how sensitively the questions are asked, GSM individuals may not disclose and thus accurate data may not be captured. Over the past few years, however, more reliable data collection, research, and a better understanding of barriers to health care access for GSM individuals have emerged (Daniel et al., 2015).

Electronic health records (EHRs) hold great potential as a source of data collection for GSM populations and the IOM (2011) recommends routine sexual orientation and gender identity data collection on all patients. Many health system EHRs do not yet have explicit fields to collect this data but do provide options to record the gender of sexual partners. However, research has shown that documentation of the gender of sexual partners in EHRs is low (45%) (Nguyen & Yehia, 2015). Recent changes in mandates for health care professionals require the inclusion of both sexual orientation and gender identity in EHRs in order to reach higher designations of meaningful use (and thus enhanced reimbursement; Cahill, Baker, Deutsch, Keatley, & Makadon, 2016); however, the benefits of this enhanced data collection are likely many years away and there is a lack of cultural competency training regarding affirming methods of collecting such information. Furthermore, such data collection requirements are subject to changing political climates (e.g., following the 2016 US Presidential election federal requests for the inclusion of sexual orientation and gender identity questions to be added to Census surveys were rescinded).

Environmental Level Barriers: Discrimination of GSM Populations Within Health care

As discussed previously, the LGBT community faces many barriers to accessing and receiving health care, including discrimination within the health care system, heterosexism, fear of disclosing sexual orientation and/or gender identity, and lack of insurance. Compared to heterosexual individuals, sexual minority individuals are more likely to delay or avoid necessary medical care (29% vs. 17%; Khalili et al., 2015). This may be secondary to prior negative health care experiences, concerns about confidentiality, and/or fears of homophobic or stigmatizing reactions (Mayer et al., 2008). A survey by Lambda Legal (2010) found that 8% of sexual minority and 27% of transgender individuals have been refused needed health care, and almost 11% of sexual minority and 21% of transgender people reported health care professionals using harsh or abusive language toward them. Likely as a result, many GSM individuals continue to be reluctant to disclose their sexual orientation or gender identity when receiving medical care (Mayer et al., 2008). All of these findings may lead GSM patients to avoid needed medical care or withhold information important to their medical treatment.

Research around discrimination in health care has focused primarily on GSM adults; however, GSM youth are also affected. Sexual orientation and gender identity typically emerge during adolescence, making this developmental period particularly vulnerable to discrimination and stigmatization. In order to address these barriers, key stakeholders in the health of GSM youth have weighed in on the barriers and provided recommendations to help those in the health care field to be cognizant of what may be preventing these youth from seeking the affirming care they deserve. In a policy statement on office-based care for GSM youth, the American Academy of Pediatrics acknowledged that the effects of homophobia and heterosexism can contribute to health disparities, particularly mental health disparities (Levine et al., 2013). Additionally, the Society for Adolescent Health and Medicine released a position paper that clearly stated that GSM youth face added challenges because of the difficulties of the coming out process, as well as societal discrimination and bias against GSM individuals (Reitman et al., 2013). Finding ways to provide affirming care to all GSM individuals, and especially to children and youth, will be critical in curbing the ongoing problems of discrimination and alienation from health care.

Environmental Level Barriers: Physical and Clinical Spaces

The physical environment of a clinical space is important to many patients. A systematic review to determine the effects of physical environment stimuli on health determined that sunlight, presence of windows, and pleasing aromas positively affected patient satisfaction and well-being (Dijkstra, Pieterse, & Pruyn, 2006). Along these lines, studies have shown that patients treated in single bedrooms are more likely to be satisfied with their care than those in multiple bedrooms, while health care settings that are noisy are associated with reduced patient satisfaction. Additionally, windowless hospital rooms are linked to anxiety and depression, and, conversely, art in patient rooms is associated with reduced anxiety and pain levels (Schweitzer, Gilpin, & Frampton, 2004). These results demonstrate the critical role the health care environment has in improving health outcomes and creating satisfying experiences with health care.

GSM individuals face barriers when interacting with the physical space of the health care environment as well as the procedural environment. Most health care spaces do not signal that they are safe spaces for GSM individuals. The majority of posters, pamphlets, and materials from the clinical space show heterosexual individuals or couples. Additionally, rainbow pride flags for the LGBT social movement are rarely visible. Gender affirming and inclusive bathrooms are not commonplace. On a more individual level, barriers for GSM individuals permeate into the medical record, where incorrect names and pronouns are used, and intake forms frequently lack affirming language regarding relationship status (Deutsch & Feldman, 2013). Taken together, these can lead to unwelcoming or poor experiences for GSM individuals that may discourage them from interacting with the health care system itself.

A study of GSM adolescents explored factors that make them feel safe in a health care setting and found that the top factors identified as important were not related to their sexual orientation, but instead, the clinical environment: the cleanliness of the health care space, instruments, and provider (Ginsburg et al., 2002). However, GSM adults would like staff to be friendly, courteous, and respectful of appropriate name and pronoun use, specifically when handling phone calls and appointments (Bockting et al., 2004). Lastly, both GSM adults and adolescents are concerned with discussions around confidentiality and access to medical records. Therefore, providers should be explicit that the care they receive is confidential and protected (Ginsburg et al., 2002; St. Pierre, 2012).

■ RECOMMENDATIONS

Every health care institution should strive to create a caring, honest, clean, and confidential system that provides a welcoming and competent environment for all patients, including GSM patients. These systems should take into consideration the significant barriers GSM individuals face to get the care they deserve. In order to do so, systems should focus on addressing the barriers on the levels of the providers, clinical environment, and policy. Research and programming to address health disparities, improve health outcomes, and ensure quality care for GSM populations are also needed to achieve true health equity.

The health care space for GSM individuals is greatly influenced by those who inhabit it—the providers and staff. First and foremost, LGBT-competent providers should be easily identified. This awareness, or "outing," of competent clinicians can very quickly put GSM patients at ease. LGBT-competent providers can be identified with cyber outings (i.e., a list of LGBT-friendly providers on an institution's website) and/or buttons, pins, or stickers on a provider's identification badge or white coat. Clinical providers should work to be comforting, nonjudgmental, and open to all patients, especially GSM patients. Providers should ask open-ended questions and not assume that the individual seeking care is cisgender and/or heterosexual. Furthermore, the use of gender-neutral pronouns and asking, not assuming, how the individual identifies in terms of gender and sexual orientation should be encouraged when working with all patients. Medical providers should be keenly aware of the unique health needs of sexual and gender minority individuals, and the profound discrimination, stigma, social isolation, and violence they may experience on a daily basis. From the front desk to the examination room, clinical staff should be knowledgeable in how to interact and communicate with GSM individuals (McClain, Hawkins, & Yehia, 2016).

In order to create providers who are competent in the care of GSM individuals, medical centers need to provide training in their unique health care needs. In particular, for physicians, LGBT-competency training should be part of their medical education curriculum from the very first year. Similar curricula should be in place for nurse practitioners, nurses, physician assistants, and medical assistants. Hospitals and medical centers should provide LGBT-competency training for all medical staff, and support continuing education focused on ongoing cultural competency.

The environment or physical, clinical space of an institution should be LGBT-friendly. This can be achieved by placing health information materials that are inclusive of the GSM diversity in our society, such as pamphlets that show GSM individuals or couples. Clinical spaces should display posters that also are LGBT-inclusive. Furthermore, the microenvironment of the clinical space (e.g., the health record) should also be LGBT-inclusive, and in particular, sensitive to gender minority patients. Medical providers should urge their institution to make certain that a patient's medical record uses their preferred name and pronoun. An LGBT-friendly and competent environment can enhance the care for the LGBT community and create clinical spaces that are free from discrimination (McClain et al., 2016).

■ CONCLUSION

Social and cultural acceptance of the LGBT community has improved dramatically over the past decade. However, significant discrimination, stigmatization, and violence still occur for GSM individuals. This discrimination has even permeated the health system and the individuals who constitute it, leading to multiple disparities in health outcomes for GSM individuals. GSM individuals may not even seek care out of fear of a negative outcome or a previous experience of discrimination or homophobia. Furthermore, even when GSM individuals decide to seek care, they may encounter an environment that is not equipped to provide LGBT-competent care. The awareness of these barriers, and the research that surrounds them, has created an environment of inquiry and provided researchers, institutions, and policy makers the opportunity to make improvements. Key stakeholders in the care of GSM individuals, such as the American College of Physicians and the American Academy of Pediatrics, have made recommendations and policy statements advocating for equal, competent, and sensitive care for the GSM population. We now know that identifying and breaking down barriers to health care for GSM individuals not only improves health outcomes for these individuals, but also reduces the discrimination and violence this community faces on a daily basis.

■ REFERENCES

Albelda, R., Badgett, M. V. L., Schneebaum, A., & Gates, G. J. (2009). *Poverty in the lesbian, gay, and bisexual community*. Los Angeles, CA: Williams Institute. Retrieved from https://williamsinstitute.law.ucla.edu/wp-content/uploads/Albelda-Badgett-Schneebaum-Gates-LGB-Poverty-Report-March-2009.pdf

Bockting, W., Robinson, B., Benner, A., & Scheltema, K. (2004). Patient satisfaction with transgender health services. *Journal of Sex & Marital Therapy, 30*(4), 277–294. doi:10.1080/00926230490422467

Burwick, A., Gates, G., Baumgartner, S., & Friend, D. (2015). *Human services for low-income and at-risk LGBT populations: An assessment of the knowledge base and research needs*. Princeton, NJ: Mathematica Policy Research. Retrieved from http://www.acf.hhs.gov/sites/default/file s/opre/lgbt_hsneeds_assessment_reportf inal1_12_15.pdf

Cahill, S. R., Baker, K., Deutsch, M. B., Keatley, J., & Makadon, H. J. (2016). Inclusion of sexual orientation and gender identity in Stage 3 Meaningful Use guidelines: A huge step forward for LGBT health. *LGBT Health, 3*(2), 100–102. doi:10.1089/lgbt.2015.0136

Daniel, H., Butkus, R.; Health and Public Policy Committee of American College of Physicians. (2015). Lesbian, gay, bisexual, and transgender health disparities: Executive summary of a policy position paper from the American College of Physicians. *Annals of Internal Medicine, 163*(2), 135–137. doi:10.7326/M14-2482

Deutsch, M. B., & Feldman, J. L. (2013). Updated recommendations from the world professional association for transgender health standards of care. *American Family Physician, 87*(2), 89–93. PMID: 23317072.

Dijkstra, K., Pieterse, M., & Pruyn, A. (2006). Physical environmental stimuli that turn healthcare facilities into healing environments through psychologically mediated effects: Systematic review. *Journal of Advanced Nursing, 56*(2), 166–181. doi:10.1111/j.1365-2648.2006.03990.x

Durso, L. E., & Gates, G. J. (2012). *Serving our youth: Findings from a national survey of service providers working with lesbian, gay, bisexual, and transgender youth who are homeless or at risk of becoming homeless*. Los Angeles, CA: The Williams Institute with True Colors Fund and The Palette Fund. Retrieved from http://williamsinstitute.law.ucla.edu/wp-content/uploads/Durso-Gates-LGBT-Homeless-Youth-Survey-July-2012.pdf

Ginsburg, K. R., Winn, R. J., Rudy, B. J., Crawford, J., Zhao, H., & Schwarz, D. F. (2002). How to reach sexual minority youth in the health care setting: The teens offer guidance. *Journal of Adolescent Health, 31*(5), 407–416.

Grant, J. M., Mottett, L. A., Tanis, J., Harrison, J., Herman, J. L., & Keislling, M. (2011). *Injustice at every turn: A report of the National Transgender Discrimination Survey.* Washington, DC: National Center for Transgender Equality and National Gay and Lesbian Task Force. Retrieved from http://www.thetaskforce.org/static_html/downloads/reports/reports/ntds_full.pdf

Hawkins, L. A. (2009). *Gender identity development among transgender youth: A qualitative analysis of contributing factors* (Doctoral dissertation). Retrieved from ProQuest Dissertations and Theses (305248568).

Human Rights Campaign. (2015). *Beyond marriage equality: A blueprint for federal non-discrimination protections.* Washington, DC: Author. Retrieved from http://www.hrc.org/campaigns/beyond-marriage-equality-a-blueprint-for-federal-non-discrimination-protect

Institute of Medicine, Committee on Lesbian, Gay, Bisexual, and Transgender Health Issues and Research Gaps and Opportunities (2011). *The health of lesbian, gay, bisexual, and transgender people: Building a foundation for better understanding.* Washington, DC: National Academies Press.

Karpman, M., Skopec, L., & Long, S. K. (2016). Quicktake: Uninsurance rate nearly halved for lesbian, gay, and bisexual adults since mid-2013. Retrieved from http://hrms.urban.org/quicktakes/Uninsurance-Rate-Nearly-Halved-for-Lesbian-Gay-and-Bisexual-Adults-since-Mid-2013.html

Khalili, J., Leung, L. B., & Diamant, A. L. (2015). Finding the perfect doctor: Identifying lesbian, gay, bisexual, and transgender-competent physicians. *American Journal of Public Health, 105*(6), 1114–1119. doi:10.2105/AJPH.2014.302448

Kosciw, J. G., Greytak, E. A., Palmer, N. A., & Boesen, M. J. (2014). *2013 National School Climate Survey: The experiences of lesbian, gay, bisexual and transgender youth in our nation's schools.* New York, NY: Gay, Lesbian and Straight Education Network (GLSEN). Retrieved from https://www.glsen.org/sites/default/files/2013%20National%20School%20Climate%20Survey%20Full%20Report_0.pdf

Lambda Legal (2010). When health care isn't caring: Lambda legal's survey of discrimination against LGBT people and people with HIV. New York, NY: Lambda Legal.

Levine, D. A., Braverman, P. K., Adelman, W. P., Breuner, C. C., Marcell, A. V., Murray, P. J., & O'Brien, R. F. (2013). Office-based care for lesbian, gay, bisexual, transgender, and questioning youth. *Pediatrics, 132*(1), e297–e313.

Mayer, K. H., Bradford, J. B., Makadon, H. J., Stall, R., Goldhammer, H., & Landers, S. (2008). Sexual and gender minority health: What we know and what needs to be done. *American Journal of Public Health, 98*(6), 989–995. doi:10.2105/AJPH.2007.127811

McClain, Z., Hawkins, L. A., & Yehia, B. R. (2016). Creating welcoming spaces for lesbian, gay, bisexual, and transgender (LGBT) patients: An evaluation of the health care environment. *Journal of Homosexuality, 63*(3), 387–393. doi:10.1080/00918369.2016.1124694

Neville, S., & Henrickson, M. (2006). Perceptions of lesbian, gay and bisexual people of primary healthcare services. *Journal of Advanced Nursing, 55*(4), 407–415. doi:10.1111/j.1365-2648.2006.03944.x

Nguyen, G. T., & Yehia, B. R. (2015). Documentation of sexual partner gender is low in electronic health records: Observations, predictors, and recommendations to improve population health management in primary care. *Population Health Management, 18*(3), 217–222.

Pew Research Center (2013). *A survey of LGBT Americans: Attitudes, experiences, and values in changing times.* Washington, DC: Author. Retrieved from http://www.pewsocialtrends.org/files/2013/06/SDT_LGBT-Americans_06-2013.pdf

Ranji, U., Beamesderfer, A., Kates, J., & Salganicoff, A. (2014). *Health and access to care and coverage for lesbian, gay, bisexual, and transgender individuals in the US (issue brief)*. Menlo Park, CA: Henry J. Kaiser Family Foundation.

Reitman, D. S., Austin, B., Belkind, U., Chaffee, T., Hoffman, N. D., Moore, E.,... Ryan, C. (2013). Recommendations for promoting the health and well-being of lesbian, gay, bisexual, and transgender adolescents: A position paper of the Society for Adolescent Health and Medicine. *Journal of Adolescent Health, 52*(4), 506–510. doi:10.1016/j.jadohealth.2013.01.015

Schweitzer, M., Gilpin, L., & Frampton, S. (2004). Healing spaces: Elements of environmental design that make an impact on health. *Journal of Alternative & Complementary Medicine, 10*(Suppl. 1), S71–S83.

Sears, B., & Mallory, C. (2011). *Documented evidence of employment discrimination & its effects on LGBT people*. Los Angeles, CA: The Williams Institute. Retrieved from http://williams institute.law.ucla.edu/wp-content/uploads/Sears-Mallory-Discrimination-July-20111.pdf

Snowdon. (2013). *Healthcare Equality Index 2013: Promoting equitable & inclusive care for lesbian, gay, bisexual and transgender patients and their families*. Washington, DC: Human Rights Campaign. Retrieved from http://www.paloalto.va.gov/docs/HEI_2013_final.pdfs

St. Pierre, M. (2012). Under what conditions do lesbians disclose their sexual orientation to primary healthcare providers? A review of the literature. *Journal of Lesbian Studies, 16*(2), 199–219. doi:10.1080/10894160.2011.604837

Stotzer, R. (2012). *Comparison of hate crime rates across protected and unprotected groups: An update*. Los Angeles, CA: The Williams Institute. Retrieved from http://williams institute.law.ucla.edu/wp-content/uploads/Stotzer-Hate-Crime-Update-Jan-2012.pdf

U.S. Department of Health and Human Services (HHS). (2016, May) Nondiscrimination in health programs and activities. Federal Register. Retrieved from https://www.federalregister.gov/articles/2016/05/18/2016-11458/nondiscrimination-in-healthprograms-and-activities

Valanis, B. G., Bowen, D. J., Bassford, T., Whitlock, E., Charney, P., & Carter, R. A. (2000). Sexual orientation and health: Comparisons in the women's health initiative sample. *Archives of Family Medicine, 9*(9), 843–853.

Walters, M. L., Chen, J., & Breiding, M. (2013). *The National Intimate Partner and Sexual Violence Survey (NISVS): 2010 Findings on victimization by sexual orientation*. Atlanta, GA: National Center for Injury Prevention and Control, Centers for Disease Control and Prevention.

CHAPTER 3

Health Risk Behaviors in the Gender and Sexual Minority Population

Nathaniel Kralik and Daniel Skinner

The concept of risk behaviors became a model for public health interventions in the late 1970s and 1980s (Institute of Medicine [IOM], 2001). To address the growing prevalence of chronic illnesses and other causes of morbidity and mortality, researchers conducted large-scale analyses of individual behavioral choices to understand their role in community health. Initial areas of study included seatbelt use and cigarette smoking, but the growing HIV/AIDS epidemic in the 1980s became central to risk-behavior research and intervention (IOM, 2001). Initial research was initiated outside of academia in grassroots efforts by gay and lesbian groups affected by AIDS who released pamphlets encouraging community members to engage in safe sex in 1982 (Merson, O'Malley, Serwadda, & Apisuk, 2008). By 1984, academic studies emerged investigating the roles of unprotected anal intercourse and alcohol and drug use in HIV transmission among sexual minority men (Stall, Coates, & Hoff, 1988). These publications marked the beginning of HIV risk-behavior research on sexual minorities, which would later grow into the broader field of study on gender and sexual minority (GSM) persons and the variety of risk behaviors that affect their health.

This chapter describes contemporary knowledge on the risk behaviors of GSM persons. Section I highlights research findings, with particular attention paid to studies of different GSM subgroups, and evaluates interventions that have sought to modify behaviors in the pursuit of better health outcomes. Section II focuses on the potential contributions of other theoretical frameworks to the study of GSM risk behaviors, including opportunities to incorporate disclosure, resilience, intersectionality, and minority stress theories. Section III presents recommendations for future directions for researching health risk behaviors among GSM persons, addressing the risk of harming GSM populations, and diverting attention and resources from addressing justice and social determinants of GSM health. We conclude with suggestions for future research and interventions in support of more equitable health outcomes.

■ SPECIFIC RISK BEHAVIORS AND GSM HEALTH DISPARITIES

Sex and Sex-Related Behaviors

Much research on GSM risk behaviors has focused on HIV and other sexually transmitted infections (STI) among sexual minority men. Sexual risk-behavior research has aimed primarily to curb the spread of STIs and prevent new infections. Although vaginal sex carries some risk of HIV infection, anal sex is understood to pose the highest risk of HIV infection, especially for receptive partners; therefore, populations who report high rates of receptive anal sex are particularly at risk (Centers for Disease Control and Prevention [CDC], 2016). In the United States, gay and bisexual men accounted for 81% of new HIV diagnoses in 2013 (CDC, 2014). There is a dearth of health data on transgender persons, but studies estimate that 19% of transgender women in high-income countries live with HIV, making them 46 times more likely to be HIV positive than all reproductive-age adults in the general population (Baral et al., 2013). Research on other gender minorities is even more limited, but studies suggest their risk of HIV acquisition is more dependent on other risk factors, such as mental health, substance abuse, and social stigma (Herbst et al., 2008). There is a need for further research to adequately assess HIV risk and prevalence among transgender and queer populations.

Other sex-related behaviors play a role in high rates of STI infection. Key areas of study include anal sex without consistent condom use, sex with multiple partners, drug and alcohol intoxication during intercourse, and commercial sex work, with prevalence of these behaviors varying between the GSM subgroups at risk (Bowers, Branson, Fletcher, & Reback, 2012). Combined data from studies looking at predicting factors of HIV sexual risk behavior are not conclusive (Huebner & Perry, 2015), and although behavioral interventions have shown success in reducing sexual risk behaviors, the literature could be improved by increasing rigor and standardizations in studies (Hergenrather, Emmanuel, Durant, & Rhodes, 2016).

As increased awareness about safer sexual practices has arisen—supported by decreasing stigmatization of GSM people—certain GSM communities have adjusted their behavior to modulate their risk outside the traditional risk framework (Hart, Boulton, Fitzpatrick, McLean, & Dawson, 1992). Some men may report higher rates of unprotected sex when engaged in mutually monogamous sexual relationships, showing that they negotiate their risk while engaging in "risk behavior" (Hart, et al., 1992). Moreover, some HIV positive men seek out sexual partners who are also HIV positive as an attempt at sexual risk reduction. For example, Frost, Stirratt, and Ouellette (2008) found "seroconcordant" partner selection to be motivated by a goal of reducing risk while accommodating multiple forms of intimacy, which suggests that "serosorting" is not only motivated by risk reduction, but also more complex and richer social connections. For a detailed discussion of other HIV-related risk factors, and the dynamics that underscore them, see Chapter 13.

Smoking

High rates of cigarette smoking, historically attributed to socially gathering at bars and nightclubs, continue to affect GSM persons. Boehmer, Miao, and Ozonoff (2012) report that sexual minority women and gay men are more likely to smoke than their heterosexual counterparts. In an extension of these findings, sexual minority women also reported higher frequency and regularity of smoking. Other studies report similar findings. For example, a study conducted by Tang et al. (2004) found that the smoking rate among lesbians (25%) was about 70% higher than that of cisgender heterosexual women (15%). Similarly, Tang et al. found that gay men smoked at a rate of 33% and cisgender heterosexual men at 21%. Building on a focus on the intersections of GSM identity and smoking, a more recent study found that levels of smoking among lesbian and bisexual adolescents were six times that of cisgender heterosexual populations (Lee, Griffin, & Melvin, 2009). Transgender individuals have also been found to have elevated smoking rates, especially those who identify their sexual orientation as straight/heterosexual, who report smoking at a rate more than twice that of U.S. adults at large (Smalley, Warren, & Barefoot, 2016).

Finally, a study by Bennett, Ricks, and Howell (2014), appropriately titled "It's Just a Way of Fitting In," found that sexual minority residents of Appalachia link both stress and culture to use of tobacco, but do not typically recognize the link between concealment and the stress that may underlie their smoking. As is well documented, smoking that begins early and thus forms a cornerstone of one's identity tends to persist (Lantz et al., 2000). This social dynamic is compounded by exposure to tobacco industry advertising, as Dilley, Spigner, Boysun, Dent, and Pizacani (2008) found that sexual minority women report more exposure to tobacco industry marketing than their cisgender heterosexual counterparts. The relationship between the tobacco industry advertising and GSM risk behavior becomes even more disconcerting when one considers a study of tobacco industry funding of LGBT organizations, which centered on asking the groups' leaders about important issues facing their communities. The study found that 22% of the 74 leaders interviewed reported accepting funding from the tobacco industry although only 24% identified tobacco as a priority (Offen, Smith, & Malone, 2008). Addressing these community factors could play an important role in future interventions.

Alcohol

The literature on alcohol use among GSM populations is extensive and growing. In an early study, McKirnan and Peterson (1989) found that while rates of heavy drinking were consistent across populations, gay men and lesbians experienced higher rates of alcohol and other substance abuse due to psychosocial vulnerability. Bloomfield (1993) compared alcohol consumption among sexual minority women and cisgender heterosexual women in urban populations, and found that sexual minority women consumed alcohol at approximately the same rate as cisgender heterosexual women. A few years later, Bux (1996) found drinking among 25% of lesbians to be excessive while an additional 10% were alcoholics, compared to 5% and 0%, respectively, for heterosexual women. For men, the study found "excessive" drinking among 19% of gay men, and characterized an additional 11% as alcoholics, with comparable figures of 11% and 9% for heterosexual men.

Though Bux's (1996) study is now 20 years old, these findings have been continually confirmed, and more specific inquiries have led to more complex data on sexuality and alcohol use. For example, Drabble and Trocki (2005) found that, while overall rates of alcohol consumption were similar across groups, lesbian and bisexual women were more likely to be affected by dependence and abuse than their heterosexual-identified counterparts. Newcomb, Heinz, and Mustanski (2012) found similar results, noting that earlier initiation and steeper drinking trajectories for GSM youth tend to exceed those of heterosexual youth. Though Newcomb and colleagues' (2012) study signals an increased focus on transgender individuals, recent studies have begun to produce a more nuanced understanding of risk behaviors among transgender populations. However, research on drinking among transgender populations is still emerging, and is usually embedded in broader GSM research. Accordingly, as we discuss more subsequently, it will be important in the future to disambiguate GSM studies to better understand the specific needs of unique populations within the umbrella of GSM identities.

Other Substance Use

The use of other substances has a similarly high prevalence among GSM persons, and there is a large literature discussing a variety of substances with elevated rates of use among GSM adults (see Chapter 12). For example, population-based data reveals that, when compared to their heterosexual counterparts, sexual minority individuals are significantly more likely to report recent illicit drug use, with prevalence rates varying substantially between subgroups (i.e., lesbians: 9.7%; gay men: 23.5%; bisexual men: 19.9%; and bisexual women: 39.4%; Conron, Mimiaga, & Landers, 2010). Rates of illicit drug use are also higher among gender minority individuals when compared to the general population and/or their cisgender counterparts, with estimated rates of recent use as follows: prescription drugs (non-medical use), 26.5% (Benotsch et al., 2013); marijuana, 39.6%; and non-marijuana illicit drug use, 19.0% (Keuroghlian, Reisner, White, & Weiss, 2015). Rates of recent polysubstance use (i.e., using illicit drugs while drinking or combining different drugs) are also alarmingly high among GSM groups (e.g., Bauer, Flanders, MacLeod, & Ross, 2016; Benotsch et al., 2013; Halkitis, Palamar, Mukherjee, 2007;

Keuroghlian et al., 2015). These differences should be interpreted responsibly, however. They do not suggest that being a gender and/or sexual minority person is itself associated with substance use, or that identification and involvement with the LGBT community is a "risk factor" for substance use. Rather, these studies indicate that a broader examination is needed that investigates the specific subfactors related to elevated rates of substance use (e.g., minority stress).

Drug use among GSM youth and adolescents is necessarily and inextricably intertwined with a corollary problem, namely the GSM homelessness epidemic (Keuroghlian, Shtasel, & Bassuk, 2014). Though the exact role of homelessness is unclear, a meta-analysis undertaken by Marshal and colleagues (2008) found substance use among sexual minority youth to be a staggering 190% higher than for cisgender heterosexuals. Rates of use were markedly higher for bisexual youth (340%) and sexual minority females (400%). Studies have also shown how the severity of substance abuse among GSM persons poses additional challenges in recovery in part due to the lack of culturally-tailored intervention and prevention programs focused on GSM health (Cochran & Cauce, 2006).

Diet

Diet is an important element of individual health, as poor diet contributes to negative health outcomes such as high blood pressure, poor cholesterol, diabetes, and even heart disease (National Heart, Lung, and Blood Institute, 2016). Equally as damaging to individual health as poor diet is the presence of an eating disorder, and a recent report from the National Eating Disorder Association (2016) found that GSM individuals, especially youth, may be at a higher risk of developing eating disorders. According to the report, GSM populations experience stress stemming from experiences of discrimination; emotional, verbal, physical or sexual abuse; and issues with social and/or familial acceptance. The report also found that sexual minorities reported elevated rates of binge eating and purging by vomiting or laxative use than their cisgender heterosexual peers.

Research consistently demonstrates that, in comparison to their cisgender heterosexual counterparts, sexual minority men are more likely to report a pattern of disordered eating (i.e., subclinical) and/or a lifetime history of at least one clinical eating disorder (e.g., Feldman & Meyer, 2007; Gigi, Bachner-Melman, & Lev-Ari, 2016; Mathews-Ewald, Zullig, & Ward, 2014; Shearer et al., 2015). For example, Feldman and Meyer (2007) found that 8.8% of a sample of sexual minority men reported a lifetime history of a full-syndrome eating disorder, with 15.5% reporting a history of a subclinical eating disorder. This heightened risk for disordered eating among sexual minority men appears to be largely related to the greater emphasis on physical appearance (including being thin and muscular) within the gay community (Drummond, 2005; Kaminski, Chapman, Haynes, & Own, 2005; Levesque & Vichesky, 2006). Siconolfi, Halkitis, Allomong, and Burton (2009) found that higher body dissatisfaction scores among gay men were associated with external motivations for working out and older age, while higher eating disorder scores were correlated with negative experiences and attitudes regarding sexual orientation. Brennan, Crath, Hart, Gadalla, and Gillis (2011) garnered similar findings of their study of body dissatisfaction and disordered eating among sexual minority men in Canada. Utilizing data from the American College Health Association-National College Health Assessment II, Diemer, Grant, Munn-Chernoff, Patterson, and Duncan (2015) found that, compared to both their cisgender sexual minority and heterosexual counterparts, transgender college students had significantly higher self-reported rates of being diagnosed and/or treated for an eating disorder (i.e., anorexia or bulimia) in the past year (15.8% vs. 0.6–3.7%) and were also more likely to report the use of diet pills (13.5% vs. 1.9–5.1%) and/or vomiting or laxative use (15.0% vs. 0.7–5.4%) to control their weight in the past month. Overall, GSM persons experience higher rates of body dissatisfaction, weight control issues, and eating disorders. These issues may be related to the discrimination and stigma that they face daily or to the barriers they face in their search for adequate health care.

Physical Activity

Regular physical activity reduces the risk of cardiovascular disease, type II diabetes, and certain kinds of cancers while strengthening bones, muscles, and mental well being (CDC, 2015). According to Calzo et al. (2014), sexual minorities report significantly fewer hours of physical activity than their cisgender heterosexual counterparts. They are 46% to 76% less likely to participate in team sports than their heterosexual same-gender peers. The disparity is particularly pronounced for sexual minority women, who participate in physical activity and team sports at a rate far less than cisgender heterosexual women.

A National LGB&T Partnership (2016) report found similar results; only 42% of GSM people met a level of physical activity required for good health, compared to 59% from the non-GSM population. Fifty-five percent of GSM men were not active enough to maintain the standard of good health, compared to 33% of non-GSM men, while 56% of GSM women were not active enough to maintain good health compared to 45% of non-GSM women. Sixty-four percent of genderfluid or genderqueer individuals did not meet standards of physical activity necessary to maintain good health (National LGB&T Partnership, 2016). When looking across GSM groups, transgender women have been found to be least likely to engage in 3 or more days per week of physical activity (24.3%), with all other groups demonstrating at least 35% (Smalley et al., 2016).

A recent "Call to Action" from the *American Journal of Preventive Medicine* highlighted the lack of continuity between documented inadequacies in physical activity for GSM individuals and the lack of GSM-specific resources to address the issue (Gorczynski & Brittain, 2016). The report included a brief analysis of the barriers that GSM individuals experience in their engagement with physical activity, and the proposed barriers included social exclusion and bullying by heterosexual and cisgender peers. It also highlighted the need for additional research in the area in order to improve understanding of variables that influence physical activity levels among GSM people (Gorczynski & Brittain, 2016).

Engagement with the Health Care System

Access to health care remains a significant challenge in the United States, even with the passage of the Affordable Care Act in 2010. On its face, impediments to accessing health care services might not seem to qualify as a risk behavior. However, the failure to insure a significant portion of Americans constitutes a policy level risk behavior that puts certain populations, including GSM persons, at disproportionate risk. This is because poor health and insufficient access to health care are interrelated with individuals' socioeconomic status, which correlates with risk behavior (Griskevicius, Tybur, Delton, & Robertson, 2011). GSM individuals receive fewer opportunities to access quality health care than do their cisgender heterosexual counterparts. As a result of their limited access to health care, members of the LGBT community often experience an increased risk of certain types of cancers, STIs, and often struggle with unhealthy weight and body image, among many other issues (Gay and Lesbian Medical Association [GLMA], 2001).

The increased presence of free clinics offers potential sources of health care for many members of the LGBT community who reside in underserved communities (McWayne et al., 2010). At the same time, formal access does not equal actual access; in fact, stigma and judgment by health care providers serves as a palpable barrier to true access to care (see Chapters 2 and 22 for a more thorough discussion of challenges in finding affirming care). Many recommendations in the *Healthy People 2010* LGBT Companion Document offer insight for improved health care, such as GSM-sensitive support of patients, GSM-specific cultural competency training for health care professionals, and new standards to ensure that all discriminatory language related to sexual orientation and gender identity is eliminated in literature supporting publicly funded health programs (GLMA, 2001). This body of emerging evidence supports the conclusion that non-affirming care, and the resulting avoidance of care, is more significant than actual physical access to health care. After all, increased access points created by recent health care reform initiatives are only as meaningful as the impact of cultural sensitivity and training of the workforce on making clinical spaces more welcoming and competent to GSM needs.

Suicidal Ideation, Depression, and Bullying

While a more comprehensive summary of literature regarding suicidal behavior can be found in Chapter 11, we present a brief summary here. The lack of psychosocial supports for and the systematic discrimination against GSM persons have particular relevance for risk behaviors such as suicide (Hatzenbuehler, Keyes, & Hasin, 2009; Hatzenbuehler, McLaughlin, Keyes, & Hasin, 2010). Garofalo, Wolf, Kessel, Palfrey, and DuRant (1998) examined the association between sexual orientation and health risk behaviors among 4,159 high school students, finding that GSM youth were more likely to be victimized, threatened, and to have engaged in suicidal thoughts than their heterosexual schoolmates, leading to suicide attempts, substance abuse, and risky sexual behaviors. A study by Haas and colleagues (2011) assessed the risk of suicide among GSM persons, and the resulting elevated levels of risk led to a call for a national effort to fund research, raise awareness, and develop interventions. Specifically addressing the needs of transgender persons, a study by Clements-Nolle, Marx, Guzman, and Katz (2001) examined links between HIV prevalence, risk behaviors, health care use, and mental health status of transgender persons. More than half of transgender men and women reported being depressed, and a third of each group reported attempting suicide.

When broadening beyond suicide, Bontempo and D'Augelli (2002) compared victimization at school as linked to health risk behaviors among heterosexual and GSM adolescents. The combined effect of sexual minority status and high victimization in school was strongly correlated with health risk behaviors. Accordingly, the combined effect of heterosexual status and low incidence of victimization at school yielded lower levels of health risk behaviors. Robin and colleagues (2002) found that GSM high school students were significantly more likely to report health risk behaviors, including engaging in violence, binge drinking, drug use, and weight problems. It is unsurprising that the CDC found that "going to a school that creates a safe and supportive learning environment for all students and having caring and accepting parents are especially important" (CDC, 2014).

■ POSSIBLE THEORETICAL CONTRIBUTIONS

Disclosure and Resilience

The response by family members regarding the gender and sexual identities of GSM youth plays an important role in shaping future risk behaviors. In a study measuring the effects of increasing levels of rejection by caregivers, adolescents who felt rejected for their sexual minority identity engaged in unprotected sex and illicit substance use at higher rates than those who experienced less or no rejection (Ryan, Huebner, Diaz, & Sanchez, 2009). In contrast, high levels of acceptance were associated with fewer risk behaviors among GSM adolescents, such as substance abuse and suicide attempts (Ryan, Russell, Huebner, Diaz, & Sanchez, 2010). These findings suggest the need for working with the parents and caregivers of GSM youth to help families understand the relationship between social supports and the well-being of these youth.

In the absence of such supports, resilience—or the strengths and assets people use to avoid negative behaviors or outcomes—becomes a default measure of how GSM persons survive social disapproval and thrive in a way that does not yield comparatively high levels of risk behavior. In response, researchers in adolescent health have developed frameworks to represent how certain types of resilience can positively affect youth through reducing their engagement in risk behaviors and protecting youth who are engaging in risk behaviors from reaching poor outcomes (Fergus & Zimmerman, 2005). Future research is needed to determine how resilience can be supported and elicited among both GSM youth and adults.

Intersectionality and Minority Stress

It is important to note that the intersections of gender and sexual identity, race, class, disability, and other identities create important differences that must be considered when describing and identifying ways to address GSM risk behaviors. For example, when researchers examined smoking behaviors of women in three metropolitan areas in the United States, they found that although lesbians as a group were not more likely to smoke than their cisgender heterosexual peers,

African American lesbians smoked at higher rates than White lesbians or heterosexual African American women, suggesting that the discrimination and stressors experienced by African American lesbians puts them at higher comparative risk (Hughes, Johnson, & Matthews, 2008). A study of young Latino sexual minority men in New York City found that connection to ethnic communities, and not a connection to gay communities, was significantly associated with lower rates of reported unprotected anal intercourse, suggesting that ethnically based community organizations could play an important role in HIV risk reduction strategies (O'Donnell et al., 2002). A study investigating use of crystal methamphetamines among Latino sexual minority men in Miami found a similar protective effect of identification with one's ethnic identity (Fernández et al., 2007). Thus, examining intersectional identities can reveal important disparities in health risk behaviors and provide an important framework for building new interventions.

Further research has been done to study the specific ways in which microaggressions, or repeated experiences of discrimination faced by members of oppressed minorities, affect GSM people of color. For example, microaggressions based on sexual identity by peers in one's racial or ethnic group have been associated with increased stress (Balsam, Molina, Beadnell, Simoni, & Walters, 2011). These studies provide an important foundation for understanding the racial disparities affecting GSM risk behaviors and health outcomes. Future research should become increasingly intersectional to understand how GSM identification interacts with social positions owing to race, class, and disability status. A more thorough discussion of the intersection of race/ethnicity and GSM status can be found in Chapter 15.

RECOMMENDATIONS

Responsibility of Researchers

Even culturally sensitive research can carry risks for GSM persons when results are interpreted as reinforcing negative stereotypes and lead to blaming (Molyneux et al., 2016). Although the literature on risk behaviors among GSM persons is growing and advancing in its sensitivity, safeguards are still required to ensure that new information is constructive rather than stigmatizing. This is particularly important in studying risk behavior because GSM identity itself often appears to be socially constructed precisely in terms of supposedly risky behaviors—perhaps even to the extent to which being GSM signifies risk (Breakwell & Millward, 1997). A sufficiently critical analysis of risk-taking must start from a fundamental analysis of the term itself.

A larger question concerns whether risk-taking is a critical enough concept to do the work that 21st-century public health requires. A study of risk behavior and perceptions of risk among students found that while communicating risk is an important goal of public health, awareness about risk fails to explain differences in behavior (Cook & Bellis, 2001). The lack of a rational basis for risk-taking behavior makes sense considering the powerful social forces that condition such behavior. It has long been known, for example, that risk-taking behavior among youth is largely driven by peer pressure (Lewis & Lewis, 1984). Because of the isolating effect of focusing risk-taking on the level of individual actions, what is needed is a model that allows for attention to individual actions while casting individual actions as functions of larger social forces (e.g., Bronfenbrenner's Ecological Systems Theory, 1979). Accordingly, some have sought to recast risk-taking as a public health phenomenon. Such an approach contextualizes analyses of the rational deliberations of individuals within the broader context of power relations, marginalization, behavioral health, and beyond.

Directions for Future Research, Programming, and Education

A recent report by the Institute of Medicine (2011), *The Health of Lesbian, Gay, Bisexual, and Transgender People: Building a Foundation for Better Understanding*, calls attention to a number of areas in which adequate research is lacking to understand GSM health needs, with significant consequences for understanding the relationship between risk-taking and health. When studying LGBT community members, it is important to note that many individuals who may place themselves under the larger umbrella of GSM have distinct gender and/or sexual identities outside of being lesbian, gay, bisexual, or transgender (e.g., queer, pansexual, non-binary). While the vast majority of studies either exclude these smaller groups from data analysis or combine their data with that of other similar identities, a landmark study by Smalley et al. (2016) evaluated the health risk behaviors of gender and sexual minorities with particular attention to rarely studied GSM subgroups, such as those identifying as genderqueer, nonbinary, queer, or noncisgender straight. Their findings indicate that health risk behaviors across a wide variety of behaviors ranging from diet to engagement with health care vary substantially not only across sexual orientations, but also across gender identities.

Strategies for improving health risk-taking behavior include intensive, skill-based programs to train participants to avoid risk behaviors. For example, Canadian researchers developed Project PRIDE, a small group counseling program designed to reduce participants' HIV risk by training young sexual minority men to build effective coping skills when dealing with triggers for unprotected sex (Smith et al., 2016). Programs like these that work on building resilience and adaptive skills may be a successful way for some GSM individuals to manage their health by reducing risk behaviors, possibly in several different areas. Effective programming to reduce risk behaviors should reflect cultural groups' different needs. A study of Guatemalan sexual minority men and transgender persons found that participants reported needing basic information about preventing and treating HIV and STIs, avoiding triggers leading to unprotected sex, and accessing available services. The researchers found that tailoring programming to informal social networks and reflecting Mayan descent increased programmatic effectiveness (Rhodes et al., 2014).

The existing literature as well as a need for more critical approaches to GSM health needs in areas intersecting with risk-taking behaviors also suggest the need for changes in medical education, where some ground has been made in cultural competency training but considerable problems persist (Corliss, Shankle, & Moyer, 2007; Sanchez, Rabatin, Sanchez, Hubbard, & Kalet, 2006; Tesar & Rovi,

1998). Indeed, existing studies suggest the need for focused attention on physician attitudes about GSM patients. Results have shown that practitioner comfort is significantly associated with the ability to provide effective, supportive care that leaves providers feeling more empowered to help their patients meet their health behavior goals (Khan, Plummer, Hussain, & Minichiello, 2008).

CONCLUSION

In this chapter, we have reviewed important scholarly data and perspectives on GSM risk-taking behavior. While warning against defining GSM people as people who engage in disproportionately risky behavior, we also sought to highlight the degree to which the social marginalization and mistreatment of GSM people creates conditions that are axiomatically related to risk-taking. To the extent to which this vicious cycle characterizes some, if not all, of the key challenges facing public health approaches to GSM health, it is clear that the focus must not be limited only to reducing risk-taking among individuals, or even groups, but instead engaging in a longer-term project of removing the social forms of discrimination that drive much of GSM risk-taking.

At the same time, there is a danger that, in focusing on GSM risk-taking, we simultaneously exculpate or simply miss widespread risk-taking behaviors among cisgender heterosexual persons. This contrast makes clear that a focus of GSM risk-taking often arises against what is presumed to be healthier, less risky heterosexual behaviors that, on closer inspection, do not always hold up (Bancroft et al., 2004; McCoul & Haslam, 2001). Greater care in developing research questions and designing behavioral risk interventions will ensure that the diverse needs of GSM populations are addressed in a way that marks progress toward health equity for all.

ACKNOWLEDGMENT

The authors wish to thank Abigail Stephens for helpful research assistance in drafting this chapter.

REFERENCES

Balsam, K. F., Molina, Y., Beadnell, B., Simoni, J., & Walters, K. (2011). Measuring multiple minority stress: The LGBT People of Color Microaggressions Scale. *Cultural Diversity & Ethnic Minority Psychology, 17*(2), 163–174. doi:10.1037/a0023244

Bancroft, J., Janssen, E., Carnes, L., Goodrich, D., Strong, D., & Long, J. S. (2004). Sexual activity and risk taking in young heterosexual men: The relevance of sexual arousability, mood, and sensation seeking. *The Journal of Sex Research, 41*(2), 181–192.

Baral, S., Poteat, T., Stromdahl, S., Wirtz, A., Guadamuz, T., & Beyrer, C. (2013). Worldwide burden of HIV in transgender women: A systematic review and meta-analysis. *The Lancet: Infectious Diseases, 13*(3), 214–222. doi:10.1016/S1473-3099(12)70315-8

Bauer, G. R., Flanders, C., MacLeod, M. A., & Ross, L. E. (2016). Occurrence of multiple mental health or substance use outcomes among bisexuals: A respondent-driven sampling study. *BMC Public Health, 16*, 497. doi:10.1186/s12889-016-3173-z

Bennett, K., Ricks, J. M., & Howell, B. M. (2014). "It's just a way of fitting in": Tobacco use and the lived experience of lesbian, gay, and bisexual Appalachians. *Journal of Health Care for the Poor and Underserved, 25*(4), 1646–1666. doi:10.1353/hpu.2014.0186

Benotsch, E. G., Zimmerman, R., Cathers, L., McNulty, S., Pierce, J., Heck, T.,…Snipes, D. (2013). Non-medical use of prescription drugs, polysubstance use, and mental health in transgender adults. *Drug and Alcohol Dependence, 132*, 391–394. doi:10.1016/j.drugalcdep.2013.02.027

Bloomfield, K. (1993). A comparison of alcohol consumption between lesbians and heterosexual women in an urban population. *Drug and Alcohol Dependence, 33*(3), 257–269.

Boehmer, U., Miao, X., & Ozonoff, A. (2012). Health behaviors of cancer survivors of different sexual orientations. *Cancer Causes & Control, 23*(9), 1489–1496. doi:10.1007/s10552-012-0023-x

Bontempo, D., & D'Augelli, A. (2002). Effects of at-school victimization and sexual orientation on lesbian, gay, or bisexual youths' health risk behavior. *Journal of Adolescent Health, 30*(5), 364–374.

Bowers, J. R., Branson, C. M., Fletcher, J. B., & Reback, C. J. (2012). Predictors of HIV sexual risk behavior among men who have sex with men, men who have sex with men and women, and transgender women. *International Journal of Sexual Health, 24*(4), 290–302.

Breakwell, G. M., & Millward, L. J. (1997) Sexual self-concept and sexual risk-taking. *Journal of Adolescence, 20*(1), 29–41.

Brennan, D. J., Crath, R., Hart, T. A., Gadalla, T., & Gillis, L. (2011). Body dissatisfaction and disordered eating among men who have sex with men in Canada. *International Journal of Men's Health, 10*(3), 253–268.

Bronfenbrenner, U. (1979). *The ecology of human development: Experiments by nature and design.* Cambridge, MA: Harvard University Press.

Bux, D., Jr. (1996). The epidemiology of problem drinking in gay men and lesbians: A critical review. *Clinical Psychology Review, 16*(4), 277–298.

Calzo, J., Roberts, A., Corliss, H., Blood, E., Kroshus, E., & Austin, S. B. (2014). Physical activity disparities in heterosexual and sexual minority youth ages 12–22 years old: Roles of childhood gender nonconformity and athletic self-esteem. *Annals of Behavioral Medicine, 47*(1), 17–27. doi:10.1007/s12160-013-9570-y

Centers for Disease Control and Prevention. (2014). LGBT youth. Retrieved from http://www.cdc.gov/lgbthealth/youth.htm

Centers for Disease Control and Prevention. (2015). The benefits of physical activity. Retrieved from https://www.cdc.gov/physicalactivity/basics/pa-health

Centers for Disease Control and Prevention. (2016). Anal sex. Retrieved from https://wwwn.cdc.gov/hivrisk/transmit/activities/anal_sex.html

Clements-Nolle, K., Marx, R., Guzman, R., & Katz, M. (2001). HIV prevalence, risk behaviors, health care use, and mental health status of transgender persons: Implications for public health intervention. *American Journal of Public Health, 91*(6), 915–921.

Cochran, B., & Cauce, A. (2006). Characteristics of lesbian, gay, bisexual, and transgender individuals entering substance abuse treatment. *Journal of Substance Abuse Treatment, 30*(2), 135–146.

Conron, K. J., Mimiaga, M. J., & Landers, S. J. (2010). A population-based study of sexual orientation identity and gender differences in adult health. *American Journal of Public Health, 100*(10), 1953–1960. doi:10.2105/AJPH.2009.174169

Cook, P., & Bellis, M. (2001). Knowing the risk: Relationships between risk behaviour and health knowledge. *Public Health, 115*(1), 54–61.

Corliss, H., Shankle, M., & Moyer, M. (2007). Research, curricula, and resources related to lesbian, gay, bisexual, and transgender health in US schools of public health. *American Journal of Public Health, 97*(6), 1023–1027.

Diemer, E. W., Grant, J. D., Munn-Chernoff, M. A., Patterson, D. A. & Duncan, A. E. (2015). Gender identity, sexual orientation, and eating-related pathology in a national sample of college students. *Journal of Adolescent Health, 57*(2), 144–149. doi:10.1016/j.jadohealth.2015.03.003

Dilley, J. A., Spigner, C., Boysun, M. J., Dent, C. W., & Pizacani, B. A. (2008). Does tobacco industry marketing excessively impact lesbian, gay and bisexual communities? *Tobacco Control, 17*(6), 385–390. doi:10.1136/tc.2007.024216

Drabble, L., & Trocki, K. (2005). Alcohol consumption, alcohol-related problems, and other substance use among lesbian and bisexual women. *Journal of Lesbian Studies, 9*(3), 19–30.

Drummond, M. J. (2005). Men's bodies listening to the voices of young gay men. *Men and Masculinities, 7*(3), 270–290. doi:10.1177/1097184X04271357

Feldman, M. B., & Meyer, I. H. (2007). Eating disorders in diverse lesbian, gay, and bisexual populations. *International Journal of Eating Disorders, 40*(3), 218–226. doi:10.1002/eat.20360

Fergus, S., & Zimmerman, M. (2005). Adolescent resilience: A framework for understanding healthy development in the face of risk. *Annual Reviews of Public Health, 26,* 399–419. doi:10.1146/annurev.publhealth.26.021304.144357

Fernández, M. I., Bowen, G. S., Warren, J. C., Ibañez, G. E., Hernandez, N., Harper, G. W., & Prado, G. (2007). Crystal methamphetamine: A source of added sexual risk for Hispanic men who have sex with men? *Drug and Alcohol Dependence, 86*(2–3), 245–252.

Frost, D., Stirratt, M., & Ouellette, S. (2008). Understanding why gay men seek HIV-seroconcordant partners: Intimacy and risk reduction motivations. *Culture, Health & Sexuality, 10*(5), 513–527. doi:10.1080/13691050801905631

Garofalo, R., Wolf, R. C., Kessel, S., Palfrey, J., & DuRant, R. (1998). The association between health risk behaviors and sexual orientation among a school-based sample of adolescents. *Pediatrics, 101*(5), 895–902.

Gay and Lesbian Medical Association. (2001). *Healthy People 2010: Companion document for lesbian, gay, bisexual, and transgender health.* San Francisco, CA: Author. Retrieved from https://www.nalgap.org/PDF/Resources/HP2010CDLGBTHealth.pdf

Gigi, I., Bachner-Melman, R., & Lev-Ari, L. (2016). The association between sexual orientation, susceptibility to social messages and disordered eating in men. *Appetite, 99,* 25–33. doi:10.1016/j.appet.2015.12.027

Gorczynski, P., & Brittain, D. (2016). Call to action: The need for an LGBT-focused physical activity research strategy. *American Journal of Preventive Medicine, 51*(4), 527–530. doi:10.1016/j.amepre.2016.03.022

Griskevicius, V., Tybur, J., Delton, A., & Robertson, T. (2011). The influence of mortality and socioeconomic status on risk and delayed rewards: A life history theory approach. *Journal of Personality and Social Psychology, 100*(6), 1015–1026. doi:10.1037/a0022403

Haas, A. P., Eliason, M., Mays, V. M., Mathy, R. M., Cochran, S. D., D'augelli, A. R., & Clayton, P. J. (2011). Suicide and suicide risk in lesbian, gay, bisexual, and transgender populations: Review and recommendations. *Journal of Homosexuality, 58*(1), 10–51. doi:10.1080/00918369.2011.534038

Halkitis, P. N., Palamar, J. J., & Mukherjee, P. P. (2007). Poly-club-drug use among gay and bisexual men: A longitudinal analysis. *Drug and Alcohol Dependence, 89*(2), 153–160. doi:10.1016/j.drugalcdep.2006.12.028

Hart, G., Boulton, M., Fitzpatrick, R., McLean, J. & Dawson, J. (1992). 'Relapse' to unsafe sexual behaviour among gay men: A critique of recent behavioural HIV/AIDS research. *Sociology of Health & Illness, 14*(2), 216–232.

Hatzenbuehler, M., Keyes, K., & Hasin, D. (2009). State-level policies and psychiatric morbidity in lesbian, gay, and bisexual populations. *American Journal of Public Health, 99*(12), 2275–2281. doi:10.2105/AJPH.2008.153510

Hatzenbuehler, M., McLaughlin, K., Keyes, K., & Hasin, D. (2010). The impact of institutional discrimination on psychiatric disorders in lesbian, gay, and bisexual populations: A prospective study. *American Journal of Public Health, 100*(3), 452–459. doi:10.2105/AJPH.2009.168815

Herbst, J. H., Jacobs, E. D., Finlayson, T. J., McKleroy, V. S., Neumann, M. S., Crepaz, N., & HIV/AIDS Prevention Research Synthesis Team. (2008). Estimating HIV prevalence and risk behaviors of transgender persons in the United States: A systematic review. *AIDS Behavior, 12*(1), 1–17.

Hergenrather, K. C., Emmanuel, D., Durant, S., & Rhodes, S. D. (2016). Enhancing HIV prevention among young men who have sex with men: A systematic review of HIV behavioral interventions for young gay and bisexual men. *AIDS Education and Prevention, 28*(3), 252–271. doi:10.1521/aeap.2016.28.3.252.

Huebner, D. M., & Perry, N. S. (2015). Do behavioral scientists really understand HIV-related sexual risk behavior? A systematic review of longitudinal and experimental studies predicting sexual behavior. *Archives of Sexual Behavior, 44*(7), 1915–1936. doi:10.1007/s10508-015-0482-8

Hughes, T. L., Johnson, T. P., & Matthews, A. K. (2008). Sexual orientation and smoking: Results from a multisite women's health study. *Substance Use & Misuse, 43*(8–9) 1218–1239. doi:10.1080/10826080801914170

Institute of Medicine, Committee on Health and Behavior: Research, Practice, and Policy. (2001). *Health and behavior: The interplay of biological, behavioral, and societal influences.* Washington, DC: National Academies Press. Retrieved from https://www.ncbi.nlm.nih.gov/books/NBK43749/

Institute of Medicine, Committee on Lesbian, Gay, Bisexual, and Transgender Health Issues and Research Gaps and Opportunities. (2011). *The health of lesbian, gay, bisexual, and transgender people: Building a foundation for better understanding.* Washington, DC: National Academies Press. Retrieved from https://www.ncbi.nlm.nih.gov/books/NBK64806/

Kaminski, P. L., Chapman, B. P., Haynes, S. D., & Own, L. (2005). Body image, eating behaviors, and attitudes toward exercise among gay and straight men. *Eating Behaviors, 6*(3), 179–187. doi:10.1016/j.eatbeh.2004.11.003

Keuroghlian, A. S., Reisner, S. L., White, J. M., & Weiss, R. D. (2015). Substance use and treatment of substance use disorders in a community sample of transgender adults. *Drug and Alcohol Dependence, 152*, 139–146. doi:10.1016/j.drugalcdep.2015.04.008

Keuroghlian, A. S., Shtasel, D., & Bassuk, E. L. (2014). Out on the street: A public health and policy agenda for lesbian, gay, bisexual, and transgender youth who are homeless. *The American Journal of Orthopsychiatry, 84*(1), 66–72. doi:10.1037/h0098852

Khan, A., Plummer, D., Hussain, R., & Minichiello, V. (2008). Does physician bias affect the quality of care they deliver? Evidence in the care of sexually transmitted infections. *Sexually Transmitted Infections, 84*(2), 150–151.

Lantz, P., Jacobson, P., Warner, K., Wasserman, J., Pollack, H., Berson, J., & Ahlstrom, A. (2000). Investing in youth tobacco control: A review of smoking prevention and control strategies. *Tobacco Control, 9*(1), 47–63.

Lee, J., Griffin, G., & Melvin, C. (2009). Tobacco use among sexual minorities in the USA, 1987 to May 2007: A systematic review. *Tobacco Control, 18*(4), 275–282.

Levesque, M. J., & Vichesky, D. R. (2006). Raising the bar on the body beautiful: An analysis of the body image concerns of homosexual men. *Body Image, 3*(1), 45–55. doi:10.1016/j.bodyim.2005.10.007

Lewis, C. E., & Lewis, M. A. (1984) Peer pressure and risk-taking behaviors in children. *American Journal of Public Health, 74*(6), 580–584.

Marshal, M., Friedman, M., Stall, R., King, K., Miles, J., Gold, M.,…Morse, J. Q. (2008). Sexual orientation and adolescent substance use: A meta-analysis and methodological review. *Addiction, 103*(4), 546–556. doi:10.1111/j.1360-0443.2008.02149.x

Matthews-Ewald, M. R., Zullig, K. H., & Ward, R. M. (2014). Sexual orientation and disordered eating behaviors among self-identified male and female college students. *Eating Behaviors, 15*(3), 441–444. doi:10.1016/j.eatbeh.2014.05.002

McCoul, M., & Haslam, N. (2001). Predicting high risk sexual behaviour in heterosexual and homosexual men: The roles of impulsivity and sensation seeking. *Personality and Individual Differences, 31*(8), 1303–1310.

McKirnan, D. J., & Peterson, P. (1989). Alcohol and drug use among homosexual men and women: Epidemiology and population characteristics. *Addictive Behaviors, 14*(5), 545–553.

McWayne, J., Green, J., Miller, B., Porter, M., Poston, C., Sanchez, G.,... Rivers, J. (2010). Lesbian, gay, bisexual, and transgender health disparities, and President Obama's commitment for change in health care. *Race, Gender & Class, 17*(3/4), 272–287.

Merson, M., O'Malley, J., Serwadda, D., & Apisuk, C. (2008). The history and challenge of HIV prevention. *The Lancet, 372*(9637), 475–488. doi:10.1016/S0140-6736(08)60884-3

Molyneux S., Sariola S., Allman D., Dijkstra, M., Gichuru, E., Graham, S., ... Sanders, E. (2016). Public/community engagement in health research with men who have sex with men in sub-Saharan Africa: Challenges and opportunities. *Health Research Policy and Systems, 14*(1), 40. doi:10.1186/s12961-016-0106-3

National Eating Disorders Association. (2016). Eating disorders in LGBT populations. Retrieved from https://www.nationaleatingdisorders.org/eating-disorders-lgbt-populations

National Heart, Lung, and Blood Institute. (2016). Assessing your weight and health risk. Retrieved from http://www.nhlbi.nih.gov/health/educational/lose_wt/risk.htm

National LGB&T Partnership. (2016). Lesbian, gay, bisexual & trans people and physical activity: What you need to know. Retrieved from https://nationallgbtpartnership dotorg.files.wordpress.com/2016/02/lgbt-people-and-physical-activity-what-you-need-to-know.pdf

Newcomb, M., Heinz, A., & Mustanski, B. (2012). Examining risk and protective factors for alcohol use in lesbian, gay, bisexual, and transgender youth: A longitudinal multilevel analysis. *Journal of Studies on Alcohol and Drugs, 73*(5), 783–793.

O'Donnell, L., Agronick, G., San Doval, A., Duran, R., Myint, U. A., & Stueve, A. (2002). Ethnic and gay community attachments and sexual risk behaviors among urban Latino young men who have sex with men. *AIDS Education and Prevention, 14*(6), 457–471.

Offen, N., Smith, E., & Malone, R. (2008). Is tobacco a gay issue? Interviews with leaders of the lesbian, gay, bisexual and transgender community. *Culture, Health & Sexuality, 10*(2), 143–157. doi:10.1080/13691050701656284

Rhodes, S. D., Alonzo, J., Mann, L., Downs, M., Simán, F. M., Andrade, M.,...Bachmann L. H. (2014). Novel approaches to HIV prevention and sexual health promotion among Guatemalan gay and bisexual men, MSM, and transgender persons. *AIDS Education and Prevention, 26*(4), 345–361. doi:10.1521/aeap.2014.26.4.345

Robin, L., Brener, N., Donahue, S., Hack, T., Hale, K., & Goodenow, C. (2002). Associations between health risk behaviors and opposite-, same-, and both-sex sexual partners in representative samples of Vermont and Massachusetts high school students. *Archives of Pediatrics & Adolescent Medicine, 156*(4), 349–355.

Ryan, C., Huebner, D., Diaz, R., & Sanchez, J. (2009). Family rejection as a predictor of negative health outcomes in White and Latino lesbian, gay, and bisexual young adults. *Pediatrics, 123*(1), 346–352. doi:10.1542/peds.2007-3524.

Ryan, C., Russell, S., Huebner, D., Diaz, R., & Sanchez, J. (2010). Family acceptance in adolescence and the health of LGBT young adults. *Journal of Child and Adolescent Psychiatric Nursing, 23*(4), 205–213. doi:10.1111/j.1744-6171.2010.00246.x.

Sanchez, N., Rabatin, J., Sanchez, J., Hubbard, S., & Kalet, A. (2006). Medical students' ability to care for lesbian, gay, bisexual, and transgendered patients. *Family Medicine, 38*(1), 21–27.

Shearer, A., Russon, J., Herres, J., Atte, T., Kodish, T., & Diamond, D. (2015). The relationship between disordered eating and sexuality amongst adolescents and young adults. *Eating Behaviors, 19*, 115–119. doi:10.106/j.eatbeh.2015.08.001

Siconolfi, D., Halkitis, P., Allomong, T., & Burton, C. (2009). Body dissatisfaction and eating disorders in a sample of gay and bisexual men. *International Journal of Men's Health, 8*(3), 254–264. doi:10.3149/jmh.0803.254

Smalley, K. B., Warren, J., & Barefoot, N. (2016). Differences in health risk behaviors across understudied LGBT subgroups. *Health Psychology, 35*(2), 103–114. doi:10.1037/hea0000231

Smith, N. G., Hart, T. A., Moody, C., Wills, A., Andersen, M. F., Blais M., & Adam, B. (2016). Project PRIDE: A cognitive-behavioral group intervention to reduce HIV risk behaviors among HIV-negative young gay and bisexual men. *Cognitive and Behavioral Practice, 23*(3), 398–411. doi:10.1016/j.cbpra.2015.08.006

Stall, R., Coates, T., & Hoff, C. (1988). Behavioral risk reduction for HIV infection among gay and bisexual men: A review of results from the United States. *American Psychologist, 43*(11), 878–885.

Tang, H., Greenwood, G., Cowling, D., Lloyd, J., Roeseler, A., & Bal, D. (2004). Cigarette smoking among lesbians, gays, and bisexuals: How serious a problem? *Cancer Causes & Control, 15*(8), 797–803.

Tesar, C., & Rovi, S. (1998). Survey of curriculum on homosexuality/bisexuality in departments of family medicine. *Family Medicine, 30*(4), 283–287.

SECTION **II**

OUTCOMES AND CONDITIONS

CHAPTER 4

Obesity in Gender and Sexual Minority Groups

Tyler B. Mason, Robin J. Lewis, and Kristin E. Heron

Obesity is a tremendous public health problem in the United States and is associated with increased mortality as well as a constellation of diseases including diabetes, heart disease, and cancer (Cecchini et al., 2010; Flegal, Graubard, Williamson, & Gail, 2005). In addition, obesity is associated with greater health care utilization and spending (Sturm, 2002), and reduced quality of life (Kushner & Foster, 2000). Overweight and obesity are defined as having too much excess body fat and are typically assessed with body mass index (BMI). The criterion for being overweight is having a BMI greater than or equal to 25 and less than 30 and the criterion for being obese is having a BMI greater than or equal to 30 (Flegal et al., 2005). Using data from the 2011 to 2014 National Health and Nutrition Examination Survey, the prevalence of obesity in the general population of U.S. adults was approximately 36% (Ogden, Carroll, Fryar, & Flegal, 2015).

The Institute of Medicine (IOM, 2011) has specifically identified obesity as an important health problem among gender and sexual minority (GSM) individuals, especially among lesbian and bisexual women. Despite the serious health ramifications of being overweight and obese, relatively little is known about these phenomena among GSM individuals. This chapter will focus on the prevalence, etiology, and treatment of obesity among GSM populations.

A useful framework that has been applied to understanding negative health outcomes and health disparities among GSM individuals was proposed by Hatzenbuehler (2009). Hatzenbuehler argued that both general psychological processes (e.g., affective, cognitive, and social factors) and group-specific processes (e.g., factors related to GSM status such as internalization of negative societal attitudes, concealment) contribute to elevated risk among GSM groups for anxiety, depression, and substance use. Meyer (2003) also argued unique stressors related to marginalized and stigmatized status (e.g., discrimination, violence, harassment) are associated with negative health outcomes. In this chapter, we begin with a discussion of obesity prevalence and health disparities. Then, consistent with Hatzenbuehler (2009) and Meyer (2003), we discuss risk and maintenance factors and intervention for obesity in terms of general processes (based on a review of the literature among the general population) as well as GSM-specific processes.

OBESITY DISPARITIES AND PREVALENCE RATES IN GSM INDIVIDUALS

Health disparities are potentially avoidable differences in health that affect marginalized individuals and carry both economic and moral burden (Braveman et al., 2011; LaVeist, Gaskin, & Richard, 2011). Health disparities in obesity have been identified for a number of GSM subgroups, notably lesbians, bisexual women, and transgender individuals, and these disparities may contribute to physical and mental disease, early mortality, and reduced quality of life (Cecchini et al., 2010). Several recent reviews concluded that lesbians are more likely to be obese compared to cisgender heterosexual women (Bowen, Balsam, & Ender, 2008; Eliason et al., 2015; Mason & Lewis, 2014). Some, but not all, studies also report greater obesity among bisexual women compared to cisgender heterosexual women (Austin, Ziyadeh, Corliss, Haines, et al., 2009; Struble, Lindley, Montgomery, Hardin, & Burcin, 2010). Further, risk for obesity for sexual minority women appears to be elevated across the lifespan with increased risk for obesity among both sexual minority adolescent girls (Austin, Nelson, Birkett, Calzo, & Everett, 2013; Mereish & Poteat, 2015) and older adults who are lesbians (Fredriksen-Goldsen et al., 2013). Overall, research among sexual minority women converges to show increased disparities in obesity compared to cisgender heterosexual women.

Sexual minority men, especially gay men, are at lower risk for obesity compared to cisgender heterosexual men (Austin, Ziyadeh, Corliss, Haines, et al., 2009; Conron, Mimiaga, & Landers, 2010; Deputy & Boehmer, 2010; Fredriksen-Goldsen et al., 2013; Kipke et al., 2007). Further, one study suggests gay and bisexual men are still less likely to be obese compared to cisgender heterosexual men even after accounting for differences in diet and physical activity (Deputy & Boehmer, 2010). However, other studies have found increased risk for obesity among bisexual male adolescents (Austin et al., 2013) and bisexual college men (Laska et al., 2015). Notably, Richmond, Walls, and Austin (2012) reported that gay men were more likely than heterosexual men to under-report their weight, which may exaggerate findings of lower risk at least among gay men. Altogether, current research suggests that gay men are less likely to be obese, whereas there are more conflicting findings regarding bisexual men, with some studies showing an increased risk for obesity (particularly among younger men), and others finding a lower obesity risk more similar to gay men.

Regarding transgender individuals, studies have found greater obesity among combined samples of both transgender female and transgender male college students (VanKim et al., 2014) and older adults (Fredriksen-Goldsen et al., 2014) compared to cisgender individuals. Further, Warren, Smalley, and Barefoot (2016) found that transgender men had the highest prevalence of obesity compared to cisgender sexual minority individuals and transgender women. Also, in a separate study, greater gender nonconformity in female adolescents was associated with higher BMI whereas greater gender nonconformity in male adolescents was associated with lower BMI and lower gains in BMI (Austin et al., 2016). However, it should be noted that there are relatively few studies of obesity in transgender individuals, and among those, few consider gender identity or examine transgender men and women separately. There is even less focus in the existing literature regarding weight status among gender minority groups beyond transgender. Clearly, more research is needed before conclusions regarding prevalence rates in gender minority populations can be made.

Although health disparities in obesity have been identified among GSM individuals, the IOM (2011) report determined there was a paucity of research examining risk and maintenance factors of obesity in GSM individuals. In order to inform intervention and prevention to reduce obesity in GSM individuals, it is important to understand both risk and maintenance factors in the general population as well as the current state of knowledge regarding risk and maintenance factors specifically among GSM groups. Based on the extant literature, most of the information we provide relates to sexual minority women. We present material on gay and bisexual men as well as transgender individuals where information is available.

◼ RISK AND MAINTENANCE FACTORS FOR OBESITY

A multitude of biopsychosocial and behavioral risk and maintenance factors for obesity have been investigated in the general population (i.e., those who report a heterosexual identity or for whom sexual identity was not assessed). Associations between many of these factors and obesity likely involve complex, interconnected processes including bi- and multi-directional causal pathways. To keep the focus of this review on obesity among GSM individuals, risk and maintenance factors for obesity in the general population are only briefly reviewed (see Hu, 2008 for an in-depth review of obesity risk and maintenance factors). It is important to recognize, however, that many risk and maintenance factors associated with obesity are likely relevant regardless of sexual orientation and/or gender identity. For example, in their qualitative review of the literature, Eliason and Fogel (2015) note few differences in individual-level risk and maintenance factors for obesity between sexual minority women and cisgender heterosexual women. In the following section, we briefly describe the demographic, behavioral, social, psychological, and biological factors that may influence the onset and maintenance of obesity in the general population as well as specific risk and maintenance factors for obesity for GSM individuals. Identifying both general and GSM-specific risk and maintenance factors is important to inform treatment and prevention research.

Demographic Factors

A number of demographic variables are related to greater obesity rates in the general population including older age, living in a rural area, being a racial/ethnic minority, and lower socioeconomic status (Van Lenthe, Droomers, Schrijvers, & Mackenbach, 2000). Interestingly, the same demographic trends in obesity seen in general samples have also been found in sexual minority individuals, including older age, living in a rural location, being of a non-White race, and having lower socioeconomic status. For example, in samples of sexual minority men and women, non-White race, older age, and lower socioeconomic status were associated with obesity (Aaron & Hughes, 2007; Guadamuz, Lim, Marshal, Friedman, Stall, & Silvestre, 2012; Mason, 2016; Mason & Lewis, 2015; Warren et al., 2016; Yancey, Cochran, Corliss, & Mays, 2003). Living in a rural location also has been associated with obesity in lesbians (Barefoot, Warren, & Smalley, 2015; Mason, 2016). In a study that included transgender women and men, no demographic factors were identified as specific risk or maintenance factors for obesity for these groups (Warren et al., 2016). Future research on demographic risk or maintenance factors may identify unique demographic factors for obesity among GSM individuals, but to date, it appears that demographic risk and maintenance factors for obesity are quite similar for GSM and non-GSM individuals.

Behavioral Factors

Numerous behavioral factors that place individuals at risk for becoming obese or maintaining obesity have been identified in general population samples, and to a lesser extent, in sexual minority samples. In the general population, obesity is related to poor diet (He et al., 2004; Malik, Pan, Willett, & Hu, 2013; Te Morenga, Mallard, & Mann, 2013), maladaptive eating behaviors and patterns (e.g., binge eating, grazing; Ma et al., 2003), less physical activity and more sedentary behavior (e.g., sitting, television viewing; Martinez, Kearney, Kafatos, Paquet, & Martínez-González, 1999), more dieting and extreme weight loss behaviors (Neumark-Sztainer et al., 2006; Stice, Presnell, Shaw, & Rohde, 2005), more alcohol use and heavy drinking (Arif & Rohrer, 2005), and less sleep (Di Milia, Vandelanotte, & Duncan, 2013). Not surprisingly, nearly all of these behavioral factors in some way contribute to the unbalanced energy intake and expenditure that is most commonly associated with being overweight or obese.

Similar behavioral correlates of obesity have been identified among sexual minority individuals as those that are seen with cisgender heterosexual individuals, including: (a) eating patterns, (b) physical activity, and (c) alcohol use. With respect to eating patterns, compared to cisgender heterosexual individuals, sexual minority individuals report poorer diet, unhealthy weight control behaviors, and maladaptive eating patterns (Austin, Ziyadeh, Corliss, Rosario, et al., 2009; Frederick & Essayli, 2016; Hadland, Austin, Goodenow, & Calzo, 2014; Laska et al., 2015; Mason, 2016; Matthews, Li, McConnell, Aranda, & Smith, 2016; Rosario et al., 2014; VanKim et al., 2016). Maladaptive eating patterns, such as binge eating, appear to be a fairly robust predictor of obesity in lesbians, as they are related to obesity even after controlling for demographic characteristics, physical activity, and diet (Mason, 2016; Matthews et al., 2016). In one study of African American sexual minority women, using food to cope with stress—arguably one example of a maladaptive eating pattern—was associated with obesity after controlling for perceived health, physical inactivity, and red meat consumption (Matthews et al., 2016).

In addition to eating behaviors, physical activity is another behavioral risk and maintenance factor associated with gaining and maintaining weight. Similar to findings in the general population, more physical activity, and specifically vigorous exercise, is related to lower likelihood of obesity in sexual minority women (Boehmer & Bowen, 2009; Brittain, Dinger, & Hutchinson, 2013; Mason, 2016; Matthews et al., 2016; Yancey et al., 2003), and reduced physical activity is associated with higher obesity rates in sexual minority samples (Calzo et al., 2014; Laska et al., 2015; Rosario et al., 2014). Finally, similar to cisgender heterosexual individuals, alcohol use (e.g., heavy/binge drinking) has also been linked to higher BMI and obesity rates in lesbians (Mason & Lewis, 2015). As is true in cisgender heterosexual persons, heavy drinking may be associated with obesity through excess calorie intake via alcohol or unplanned eating, and it may also disrupt physical activity efforts in the day following the drinking episode.

Taken together, a review of the available research on behavioral risk correlates among sexual minority men and women yields findings similar to research among the general population. This pattern is not particularly surprising given that behavioral factors related to energy intake (e.g., eating patterns, diet, alcohol use) and expenditure (e.g., physical activity) largely drive weight gain and maintenance. It should be noted, however, that much of the research on behavioral factors in this area is based on studies with sexual minority women, and there is much more limited (if any) research on gay men or gender minority individuals. As such, these behavioral risk and maintenance factors should be interpreted with caution for these groups.

Social and Relationship Factors

Social factors have also been implicated in the onset and maintenance of obesity, in particular factors related to interpersonal relationships and social norms regarding body shape and weight. In addition, studies of cisgender heterosexual samples have shown that obesity is linked to social networks (Christakis & Fowler, 2007) and is prominent in individuals who are in relationships (Martinez et al., 1999). Within different sexual minority subgroups, most notably lesbian and gay communities, differing social norms regarding body shape and weight have emerged. In lesbian communities and social networks, there is evidence that having a larger body size (including being overweight) is more socially acceptable than it is for cisgender heterosexual women (Bowen, Balsam, Diergaarde, Russo, & Escamilla, 2006; Thayer, 2010; VanKim, Porta, Eisenberg, Neumark–Sztainer, &Laska, 2016). While to our knowledge, there is no empirical evidence for this hypothesis, it is plausible that the acceptance of larger body sizes in lesbian communities could, in part, contribute to the higher overweight and obesity rates in lesbians as compared to cisgender heterosexual women (for whom thinness norms for women are likely more salient). In particular, because larger bodies may be more acceptable in the lesbian community and social networks, lesbians may have less desire to lose weight. This idea is partially supported by a study finding that sense of belonging in the lesbian community buffered the association between body dissatisfaction and depressive symptoms (Hanley & McLaren, 2015). Further, more public identification as a lesbian and outness have been associated with greater likelihood of being obese (Mason, 2016; Mason & Lewis, 2015). Bisexual women may not receive protective benefits of the lesbian community due to feelings of biphobia that are pervasive in the lesbian and gay communities (Hayfield, Clarke, & Halliwell, 2014; McLean, 2008); they may also feel pressure to conform to heterosexual men's typologies of beauty. In addition, lesbians who are less out or who are not involved in the lesbian community may not reap protective benefits and may be more likely to attempt to conform to mainstream thinness ideals seen for women.

In contrast to the weight-related norms in the lesbian community, gay male subculture places a strong importance on body consciousness and physical appearance (VanKim et al., 2016; Yelland & Tiggemann, 2003). In fact, compared to heterosexual men, the body-related social norms in gay communities may be more pronounced in their emphasis on both thinness and muscularity, as gay men report a greater desire for thinness and muscularly than their heterosexual counterparts (Frederick & Essayli, 2016; Morrison, Morrison, & Sager, 2004; Yelland & Tiggemann, 2003). These social norms in gay communities may in part explain the apparent lower rates of obesity in gay men, particularly given the documented elevated rates of eating disorders among gay men beginning in adolescence and continuing through adulthood (Austin et al., 2013; Bankoff, Richards, Bartlett, Wolf & Mitchell, 2016; Brown & Keel, 2015; Shearer et al., 2015).

In addition to social norms within the lesbian and gay communities, there are also social and relationship factors that serve as risk and maintenance factors. Several studies of lesbians have demonstrated that being partnered, having been in a longer relationship, and having a partner with a high BMI are all associated with being overweight or obese (Markey & Markey, 2014; Mason & Lewis, 2015; Thayer, 2010). Conversely, having support from an intimate partner and having higher relationship consensus (i.e., degree to which partners agree on decisions, values, and affection) may be protective, as they have been shown to be associated with a lower BMI in lesbians (Mason & Lewis, 2015; Thayer, 2010). Among sexual minority men, a higher BMI was associated with being less likely to reject potential sexual partners, having fewer sexual partners, and less condom use during anal intercourse (Moskowitz & Seal, 2010). In contrast, nonobese sexual minority men were more likely than obese sexual minority men to have had unsafe sex (controlling for body image and age; Kraft, Nordstrom, Bockting, & Rosser, 2006). Although not predictive of obesity per se, sexual minority men have been shown to exhibit fewer eating disorder symptoms when in relationships than when not (Brown & Keel, 2015). Taken together, it is evident that for both lesbians and sexual minority men, social and relationship factors are associated with obesity risk, or at minimum weight-related behaviors, although it is difficult to make strong conclusions based on the limited number of studies in this area.

Psychological Factors

Factors related to individuals' mental health, including psychological disorders or distress and body dissatisfaction, have been shown to be associated with obesity in general samples. Among cisgender heterosexual samples, indicators of poor psychological health such as mood disturbances and anxiety symptoms have been shown to be associated with obesity (Petry, Barry, Pietrzak, & Wagner, & 2008; Stice et al., 2005). In addition to general mental health symptoms, specific concerns regarding one's physical appearance are also associated with obesity. Body image dissatisfaction, which includes thoughts and feelings about physical appearance, body shape, and/or body weight, is so common among overweight and obese individuals that "some level of body dissatisfaction should be expected as the default" (Schwartz & Brownell, 2004, p. 53). This is important to note because research also suggests that poor body image can negatively affect psychosocial functioning and health behaviors (Davison & McCabe, 2006).

Although it is evident that there are psychological risk and maintenance factors for obesity in general samples, there is a small but growing literature in sexual minority populations. Similar to heterosexual individuals, poor mental health symptoms have been associated with obesity in sexual minority individuals. For example, depressive symptoms were associated with obesity among young adult lesbians (Mason & Lewis, 2015) and older sexual minority adults (Fredriksen-Goldsen et al., 2013). Similarly, among gay men, depression, anxiety, and stress symptoms were associated with obesity (Warren et al., 2016). As is the case with cisgender heterosexual individuals, among both sexual minority men and women, maladaptive body image concerns have been found to be related to higher BMI (Levesque & Vichesky, 2006; Mason & Lewis, 2016).

It is evident that at least among sexual minority individuals, psychological factors such as depression, anxiety, and stress are all associated with obesity. There is much more limited research on the role of body dissatisfaction in obesity among sexual minority groups; however, it is likely that, similar to cisgender individuals, among overweight and obese persons body dissatisfaction is a concern that can influence psychological well-being. Although, to our knowledge, there are no studies identifying psychological risk or maintenance factors for obesity in gender minority populations, very similar psychological factors identified in cisgender heterosexual samples have been found in sexual minority adults. Furthermore, bidirectional pathways likely exist between psychological factors and obesity whereby psychological factors can influence obesity, and being overweight or obese can also create psychological distress.

Biological Factors

Scientific advances in recent decades have also revealed biological and genetic factors associated with obesity risk. For instance, the hormones leptin and ghrelin influence eating behaviors and energy intake, and are commonly impaired in obese adults (Klok, Jakobsdottir, & Drent, 2007). In addition, a number of genetic variants and polymorphisms have been shown to be predisposing factors for obesity (Farooqi & O'Rahilly, 2007). Biological risk factors have not been investigated separately for GSM individuals. It is reasonable, however, to expect similar patterns among GSM individuals although there may be unique interactions between biological factors and other risk factors that may increase GSM individuals' risk for obesity and weight gain (e.g., the lived experiences of GSM individuals may result in epigenetic variations as they do in racial/ethnic minority individuals; Demerath et al., 2015).

GSM-Specific Risk Factors

GSM individuals face unique stressors and challenges related to their minority status such as experiences of harassment, victimization, discrimination, concealment of identity, and negative feelings about self as a minority. These minority stressors have been associated with negative health outcomes in a number of theories (Hatzenbuehler, 2009; Meyer, 2003) and empirically linked to maladaptive drug, alcohol, and tobacco use (Lewis, Milletich, Kelley, & Woody, 2012), and poor physical health (Frost, Lehavot, & Meyer, 2015). Minority stress is directly related to significant psychological distress (Hatzenbuehler, 2009; Meyer, 2003), unhealthy behaviors, and negative physical health conditions through both adverse psychological and physiological stress responses (Lick, Durso, & Johnson, 2013). These unique minority stressors may also be useful in explaining why GSM individuals appear to be more likely to be obese than heterosexual individuals. Distal stress (e.g., harassment and discrimination), structural barriers (e.g., not being eligible for partner benefits and health insurance), and proximal stress (e.g., internalized homophobia, stigma consciousness, and concerns related to disclosure of sexual orientation) may contribute to obesity disparities. Essentially, GSM individuals may engage in negative health behaviors to cope with minority stress, and these negative health behaviors may be associated with being overweight and obese via increased energy balance.

Although the association of minority stress and obesity itself has been examined almost exclusively among sexual minority women, this stress is experienced by individuals of all GSM identities. Minority stress and negative emotional symptoms have been directly and indirectly associated with unhealthy eating patterns in sexual minority individuals (e.g., binge eating, using food to cope; Katz-Wise et al., 2015; Mason & Lewis, 2015; 2016; Matthews et al., 2016; Roberts, Stuart–Shor, & Oppenheimer, 2010), and problem drinking among lesbians (Lewis, Mason, Winstead, & Kelley, 2016); it may also be associated with less exercising in lesbians (Roberts et al., 2010). Addressing the impact of minority stress on GSM individuals' health behaviors may assist with weight loss and obesity prevention and intervention and in promoting healthy lifestyles. Specifically, heterosexist discrimination (Mereish, 2014) and more openness and disclosure regarding sexual identity (Mason, 2016; Mason & Lewis, 2015) are related to greater likelihood of being obese in lesbians.

Summary of Risk Factors

In comparison to the general population, we know very little about risk and maintenance factors for obesity in GSM individuals and most of what is known relates to sexual minority women. Moreover, most of the limited research examining the risk and maintenance factors for obesity in GSM individuals comes from cross-sectional studies of convenience samples, which substantially limits the conclusions and generalizability of the findings. Studies have also been limited to examining demographic, psychosocial, and behavioral risk factors of obesity; biological research has not been conducted. However, the limited available research on obesity in GSM individuals is nonetheless critical for developing a more complete understanding of risk and maintenance factors for obesity among GSM individuals, and ultimately, is useful for developing culturally tailored intervention and prevention programs to improve GSM individuals' health and well-being, and to reduce disparities.

◼ TREATMENT APPROACHES FOR OBESITY

There are a multitude of treatment approaches that can be used to treat obesity. The primary goal of nearly all obesity interventions—and in particular, behavioral interventions—is to control one's energy balance, or the total amount of calories consumed (i.e., from food and beverages) versus energy expended (i.e., from physical activity). In the following section, we very briefly review the treatment options for obesity in general, as more comprehensive discussions of obesity treatment options are available elsewhere (see Glenny, O'Meara, Melville, Sheldon, & Wilson, 1997; Orzano, & Scott, 2004). Next, we discuss specific obesity treatment issues as they relate to GSM individuals.

Obesity Treatment in the General Population

There are several general methods of obesity intervention including bariatric surgery, behavioral approaches (e.g., diet and physical activity modification), and multifaceted lifestyle interventions. Bariatric surgery has proven very successful in producing large weight losses among those who are morbidly obese (i.e., BMI ≥ 40) or those with a BMI greater than or equal to 35 who have a serious health condition (e.g., diabetes or other obesity-related disease; Buchwald et al., 2004). However, surgery for obesity is never the first treatment option, and most weight loss approaches attempt to modify diet and/or physical activity and include other lifestyle changes and modifications. Behavioral interventions are successful at producing weight loss, with interventions that target both diet and exercise change being the most effective (Curioni & Lourenço, 2005). Lifestyle interventions, which combine diet and exercise change, behavior modification (e.g., self-monitoring, goal setting, and stimulus control), and psychosocial changes (e.g., social support; Hagobian & Phelan, 2013), also produce meaningful weight change, more so than behavioral changes alone. For example, the Health at Every Size (HAES) lifestyle intervention focuses on enhancing physical health without weight loss through taking the focus off of weight, discussing the ineffectiveness of diets, teaching intuitive eating, and encouraging physical activity (Robison, 2005). In sum, there are a number of viable treatment options that produce meaningful weight loss with larger losses associated with more invasive methods. Recent advancements have also integrated these standard behavioral and lifestyle interventions with pharmacological treatment as well as novel delivery modalities such as through the Internet, social media, or mobile phones (Thomas & Bond, 2014).

Obesity Treatment in GSM Individuals

Although there are efficacious intervention approaches for obese adults, there are no existing randomized trials to inform whether such interventions are also efficacious for GSM individuals. Moreover, standard obesity intervention and prevention programs do not address issues and concerns that are specifically relevant for successful weight loss for GSM individuals. At least among sexual minority women, there is evidence of more stress (including sexual minority stress) that must be considered in reducing obesity (Eliason & Fogle, 2015). Research shows that sexual minority individuals are interested in weight loss and health promotion interventions (Nyitray, Corran, Altman, Chikani, & Negrón, 2006). Specifically, sexual minority U.S. respondents indicated priority concern in the following health areas: fitness/exercise (67.4%), nutrition (64.6%), cancer (63.0%), depression/anxiety (58.7%), heart disease (56.5%), and weight control (56.1%; Nyitray et al., 2006). Also, among African American sexual minority women, 31% were interested in nutrition and exercise programs, and approximately 34% were interested in weight loss programs (Matthews et al., 2016). Based on minority stress theory, it is reasonable to assume that inclusion of GSM-specific components is a worthwhile endeavor. Research on GSM-specific risk and maintenance factors for obesity can offer guidance as to the most appropriate ways to develop tailored interventions to reduce obesity for gender and sexual minorities. Yet, with a plethora of treatment approaches, the question remains as to which treatment approaches would be most successful for treating obesity in GSM individuals.

When describing and evaluating obesity intervention approaches for GSM individuals, it is critical to consider whether the existing treatment programs or approaches could be tailored for this unique group and for subgroups (e.g., lesbians, gay men, bisexual women, transgender men), and if so, how. Known as culturally tailored interventions, this practice involves the modification of standard programs by integrating the unique culture, beliefs, attitudes, behaviors, and experiences of individuals of a minority group (including gender and sexual minorities) into intervention and practice. Studies have demonstrated the importance of culturally tailoring interventions for GSM individuals for several physical and mental health concerns, including smoking (Walls & Wisneski, 2011), depression (Ross, Doctor, Dimito, Kuehl, & Armstrong, 2008), and cancer screening (Bowen, Powers, & Greenlee, 2006). In obesity treatment specifically, standard obesity treatments have been culturally tailored for other minority groups, namely racial and ethnic minorities, and have been shown to be efficacious (Kong, Tussing-Humphreys, Odoms-Young, Stolley, & Fitzgibbon, 2014). Other than a lesbian weight loss support group (Fogel, Young, Dietrich, & Blakemore, 2012), we are not aware of any obesity interventions that have been tailored specifically for GSM individuals. Given the increased obesity rates in some GSM groups, developing novel intervention programs or adapting existing treatments for GSM individuals is an important next step in reducing disparate obesity rates between cisgender heterosexual individuals and gender and sexual minorities.

When designing culturally tailored interventions, researchers and clinicians should consider two essential components: surface structure elements and deep structure elements. Surface structure elements ensure that the intervention is acceptable to the target audience and is perceived as safe. Several ways to achieve an appropriate surface structure in interventions for GSM individuals may include having GSM staff members, using pictures of same-sex couples on program materials, or using gender-neutral, non-judgmental language when working with GSM individuals (Bauer & Wayne, 2005). Deep structure elements differ in that they are based on an understanding of cultural and social factors as well as health beliefs and behaviors of the target population and the effect these have on their health and ability to make changes in their behavior (Mason & Lewis, 2014; Resnicow, Baranowski, Ahluwalia, & Braithwaite, 1998). Incorporating deep structural elements into interventions and clinical practice with GSM individuals is the likely key to achieving successful outcomes for this population, which has received little previous attention in relation to obesity. For example, although stress management is often included in lifestyle interventions for obesity, adding content focused on techniques for handling minority stress and other GSM stressors may bolster intervention content (Pachankis, 2014). Surface elements (e.g., symbols, images, and unbiased language) and deep elements (e.g., educational materials on stress, body image, and social support) can be added into existing intervention and preventions materials, and by doing so, interventions may be more acceptable for GSM individuals. Finally, given disparities in obesity in other groups such as racial minorities and people with low socioeconomic status (Wang & Beydoun, 2007), being mindful of intersecting minority statuses (e.g., age, race, gender) and additional barriers that may exist (e.g., financial barriers; Rossen, 2014) is particularly important in obesity treatment and prevention.

■ CONCLUSION

This chapter highlighted the public health significance of obesity among GSM individuals. With over one-third of the U.S. adult population classified as obese, and research demonstrating that sexual minority women are more likely to be obese than cisgender heterosexual women, there is a clear call for research and intervention efforts to reduce obesity in this at-risk group. Some limited research also finds a pattern of obesity among gender minority individuals and young bisexual men. Less risk for obesity has been found among gay men; however, there is evidence that weight-related behavior is highly salient for this group. The various biopsychosocial risk and maintenance factors associated with obesity in the general population were briefly reviewed. Primarily stemming from research on sexual minority women, many similar risk and maintenance factors for obesity were identified among GSM individuals. Several unique variables related to being a gender and/or sexual minority are associated with obesity and health behaviors.

More longitudinal and population-based studies over the course of the lifespan are needed to determine causal and maintenance factors for obesity among LGBT individuals.

Our review appears to show that an individualized approach to addressing obesity in GSM individuals would be the most successful. As suggested by Eliason and Fogel's (2015) ecological approach, it is important to consider how individual factors (e.g., mental and physical health, health behaviors), relationship factors (e.g., partner, family, friends), the larger GSM and mainstream communities, institutional factors (e.g., health care, workplace, religion, education) and public policy/law may contribute to obesity among GSM individuals. For example, some individuals may need only a standard obesity intervention program while others may benefit from psychotherapeutic treatments for maladaptive behaviors (e.g., binge eating or substance use). In addition, focusing on the unique experiences of GSM individuals such as minority stress suggests that culturally tailoring interventions may also enhance compliance and effectiveness, although this remains an empirical question. Further, Rothblum (2014) suggested that the Health At Every Size approach should be used with sexual minority women as it focuses on health rather than weight, reduces stigma, and teaches body acceptance. Bariatric surgery may be a viable option of reducing weight for those meeting criteria. However, incorporating culturally tailored suggestions for weight maintenance and health promotion after surgery may be beneficial.

Finally, obesity research in gender and sexual minority individuals is an emerging area. Developing and testing obesity treatment and prevention programs for gender and sexual minority individuals is an important next step and is urgently needed. The benefits of culturally tailored interventions must also be examined. Additional resources related to obesity in gender and sexual minority individuals include reviews of obesity among sexual minority women (see Eliason Fogel, 2015; Eliason et al., 2015; Mason & Lewis, 2014), and the 2011 IOM report on gender and sexual minority health.

■ REFERENCES

Aaron, D. J., & Hughes, T. L. (2007). Association of childhood sexual abuse with obesity in a community sample of lesbians. *Obesity, 15,* 1023–1028. doi:10.1038/oby.2007.634

Arif, A. A., & Rohrer, J. E. (2005). Patterns of alcohol drinking and its association with obesity: Data from the Third National Health and Nutrition Examination Survey, 1988–1994. *BMC Public Health, 5,* 126. doi:10.1186/1471-2458-5-126

Austin, S. B., Nelson, L. A., Birkett, M. A., Calzo, J. P., & Everett, B. (2013). Eating disorder symptoms and obesity at the intersections of gender, ethnicity, and sexual orientation in US high school students. *American Journal of Public Health, 103,* e16–e22. doi:10.2105/AJPH.2012.301150

Austin, S. B., Ziyadeh, N. J., Calzo, J. P., Sonneville, K. R., Kennedy, G. A., Roberts, A. L.,...Scherer, E. A. (2016). Gender expression associated with BMI in a prospective cohort study of US adolescents. *Obesity, 24,* 506–515. doi:10.1002/oby.21338

Austin, S. B., Ziyadeh, N. J., Corliss, H. L., Haines, J., Rockett, H. R., Wypij, D., & Field, A. E. (2009). Sexual orientation disparities in weight status in adolescence: Findings from a prospective study. *Obesity, 17,* 1776–1782. doi:10.1038/oby.2009.72

Austin, S. B., Ziyadeh, N. J., Corliss, H. L., Rosario, M., Wypij, D., Haines, J.,... Field, A. E. (2009). Sexual orientation disparities in purging and binge eating from early to late adolescence. *Journal of Adolescent Health, 45*, 238–245. doi:10.1016/j.jadohealth.2009.02.001

Bankoff, S. M., Richards, L. K., Bartlett, B., Wolf, E. J., & Mitchell, K. S. (2016). Examining weight and eating behavior by sexual orientation in a sample of male veterans. *Comprehensive Psychiatry, 68*, 134–139. doi:10.106/j.comppsych.2016.03.007

Barefoot, K. N., Warren, J. C., & Smalley, K. B. (2015). An examination of past and current influences of rurality on lesbians' overweight/obesity risks. *LGBT Health, 2*, 154–161. doi:10.1089/lgbt.2014.0112

Bauer, G. R., & Wayne, L. D. (2005). Cultural sensitivity and research involving sexual minorities. *Perspectives on Sexual and Reproductive Health, 37*(1), 45–47.

Boehmer, U., & Bowen, D. J. (2009). Examining factors linked to overweight and obesity in women of different sexual orientations. *Preventive Medicine, 48*, 357–361. doi:10.1016/j.ypmed.2009.02.003

Bowen, D. J., Balsam, K. F., Diergaarde, B., Russo, M., & Escamilla, G. M. (2006). Healthy eating, exercise, and weight: Impressions of sexual minority women. *Women & Health, 44*, 79–93. doi:10.1300/J013v44n01_05

Bowen, D. J., Balsam, K. F., & Ender, S. R. (2008). A review of obesity issues in sexual minority women. *Obesity, 16*, 221–228. doi:10.1038/oby.2007.34

Bowen, D. J., Powers, D., & Greenlee, H. (2006). Effects of breast cancer risk counseling for sexual minority women. *Health Care for Women International, 27*, 59–74. doi:10.1080/07399330500377119

Braveman, P. A., Kumanyika, S., Fielding, J., LaVeist, T., Borrell, L. N., Manderscheid , R., & Troutman, A. (2011). Health disparities and health equity: The issue is justice. *American Journal of Public Health, 101*, S149–S155. doi:10.2105/AJPH.2010.300062

Brittain, D. R., Dinger, M. K., & Hutchinson, S. R. (2013). Sociodemographic and lesbian-specific factors associated with physical activity among adult lesbians. *Women's Health Issues, 23*, e103–e108. doi:10.1016/j.whi.2012.12.001

Brown, T. A. & Keel, P. K. (2015). Relationship status predicts lower restrictive eating pathology for bisexual and gay men across 10-year follow-up. *International Journal of Eating Disorders, 48*(6), 700–707. doi:10.1002/eat.22433

Buchwald, H., Avidor, Y., Braunwald, E., Jensen, M. D., Pories, W., Fahrbach, K., & Schoelles, K. (2004). Bariatric surgery: A systematic review and meta-analysis. *Journal of the American Medical Association, 292*, 1724–1737. doi:10.1001/jama.292.14.1724

Calzo, J. P., Roberts, A. L., Corliss, H. L., Blood, E. A., Kroshus, E., & Austin, S. B. (2014). Physical activity disparities in heterosexual and sexual minority youth ages 12–22 years old: Roles of childhood gender nonconformity and athletic self-esteem. *Annals of Behavioral Medicine, 47*, 17–27. doi:10.1007/s12160-013-9570-y

Cecchini, M., Sassi, F., Lauer, J. A., Lee, Y. Y., Guajardo-Barron, V., & Chisholm, D. (2010). Chronic diseases: Chronic diseases and development 3 tackling of unhealthy diets, physical inactivity, and obesity: Health effects and cost-effectiveness. *Lancet, 376*, 1775–1784. doi:10.1016/S0140-6736(10)61514-0

Christakis, N. A., & Fowler, J. H. (2007). The spread of obesity in a large social network over 32 years. *New England Journal of Medicine, 357*, 370–379. doi:10.1056/NEJMsa066082

Conron, K. J., Mimiaga, M. J., & Landers, S. J. (2010). A population-based study of sexual orientation identity and gender differences in adult health. *American Journal of Public Health, 100*, 1953–1960. doi:10.2105/AJPH.2009.174169

Curioni, C. C., & Lourenço, P. M. (2005). Long-term weight loss after diet and exercise: A systematic review. *International Journal of Obesity, 29*, 1168–1174. doi:10.1038/sj.ijo.0803015

Davison, T. E., & McCabe, M. P. (2006). Adolescent body image and psychosocial functioning. *The Journal of Social Psychology, 146*, 15–30. doi:10.3200/SOCP.146.1.15–30

Demerath, E. W., Guan, W., Grove, M. L., Aslibekyan, S., Mendelson, M., Zhou, Y. H.,…Boerwinkle, E. (2015). Epigenome-wide association study (EWAS) of BMI, BMI change and waist circumference in African American adults identifies multiple replicated loci. *Human Molecular Genetics, 24*(15), 4464–4479. doi:10.1093/hmg/ddv161

Deputy, N. P., & Boehmer, U. (2010). Determinants of body weight among men of different sexual orientation. *Preventive Medicine, 51*, 129–131. doi:10.1016/j.ypmed.2010.05.010

Di Milia, L., Vandelanotte, C., & Duncan, M. J. (2013). The association between short sleep and obesity after controlling for demographic, lifestyle, work and health-related factors. *Sleep Medicine, 14*, 319–323. doi:10.1016/j.sleep.2012.12.007

Eliason, M. J., & Fogel, S. C. (2015). An ecological framework for sexual minority women's health: Factors associated with greater body mass. *Journal of Homosexuality, 62*, 845–882. doi:10.1080/00918369.2014.1003007

Eliason, M. J., Ingraham, N., Fogel, S. C., McElroy, J. A., Lorvick, J., Mauery, D. R., & Haynes, S. (2015). A systematic review of the literature on weight in sexual minority women. *Women's Health Issues, 25*, 162–175. doi:10.1016/j.whi.2014.12.001

Farooqi, I. S., & O'Rahilly, S. (2007). Genetic factors in human obesity. *Obesity Reviews, 8*, 37–40. doi:10.1111/j.1467-789X.2007.00315.x

Flegal, K. M., Graubard, B. I., Williamson, D. F., & Gail, M. H. (2005). Excess deaths associated with underweight, overweight, and obesity. *Journal of the American Medical Association, 293*, 1861–1867. doi:10.1001/jama.293.15.1861

Fogel, S., Young, L., Dietrich, M., & Blakemore, D. (2012). Weight loss and related behavior changes among lesbians. *Journal of Homosexuality, 59*, 689–702. doi:10.1080/00918369.2012.673937

Frederick, D. A., & Essayli, J. H. (2016). Male body image: The roles of sexual orientation and body mass index across five national US studies. *Psychology of Men & Masculinity, 17*, 336–351. doi:10.1037/men0000031

Fredriksen-Goldsen, K. I., Cook-Daniels, L., Kim, H. J., Erosheva, E. A., Emlet, C. A., Hoy-Ellis, C. P.,… Muraco, A. (2014). Physical and mental health of transgender older adults: An at-risk and underserved population. *The Gerontologist, 54*, 488–500. doi:10.1093/geront/gnt021

Fredriksen-Goldsen, K. I., Emlet, C. A., Kim, H. J., Muraco, A., Erosheva, E. A., Goldsen, J., & Hoy-Ellis, C. P. (2013). The physical and mental health of lesbian, gay male, and bisexual (LGB) older adults: The role of key health indicators and risk and protective factors. *The Gerontologist, 53*, 664–675. doi:10.1093/geront/gns123

Frost, D., Lehavot, K., & Meyer, I. (2015). Minority stress and physical health among sexual minority individuals. *Journal of Behavioral Medicine, 38*, 1–8. doi:10.1007/s10865-013-9523-8.

Glenny, A. M., O'Meara, S., Melville, A., Sheldon, T. A., & Wilson, C. (1997). The treatment and prevention of obesity: A systematic review of the literature. *International Journal of Obesity, 21*(9), 715–737.

Guadamuz, T. E., Lim, S. H., Marshal, M. P., Friedman, M. S., Stall, R. D., & Silvestre, A. J. (2012). Sexual, behavioral, and quality of life characteristics of healthy weight, overweight, and obese gay and bisexual men: Findings from a prospective cohort study. *Archives of Sexual Behavior, 41*, 385–389. doi:10.1007/s10508-011-9859-5

Hadland, S. E., Austin, S. B., Goodenow, C. S., & Calzo, J. P. (2014). Weight misperception and unhealthy weight control behaviors among sexual minorities in the general adolescent population. *Journal of Adolescent Health, 54*, 296–303. doi:10.1016/j.jadohealth.2013.08.021

Hagobian, T. A., & Phelan, S. (2013). Lifestyle interventions to reduce obesity and diabetes. *American Journal of Lifestyle Modification, 7*, 84–98. doi:10.1177/1559827612449600

Hanley, S., & McLaren, S. (2015). Sense of belonging to layers of lesbian community weakens the link between body image dissatisfaction and depressive symptoms. *Psychology of Women Quarterly, 39*, 85–94. doi:10.1177/0361684314522420

Hatzenbuehler, M. L. (2009). How does sexual minority stigma "get under the skin"? A psychological mediation framework. *Psychological Bulletin, 135*, 707–730. doi:10.1037/a0016441

Hayfield, N., Clarke, V., & Halliwell, E. (2014). Bisexual women's understandings of social marginalisation: 'The heterosexuals don't understand us but nor do the lesbians'. *Feminism & Psychology, 24*, 352–372. doi:10.1177/0959353514539651

He, K., Hu, F. B., Colditz, G. A., Manson, J. E., Willett, W. C., & Liu, S. (2004). Changes in intake of fruits and vegetables in relation to risk of obesity and weight gain among middle-aged women. *International Journal of Obesity, 28*, 1569–1574. doi:10.1038/sj.ijo.0802795

Hu, F. (2008). *Obesity epidemiology.* New York, NY: Oxford University Press.

Institute of Medicine. (2011). *The health of lesbian, gay, bisexual, and transgender people: Building a foundation for better understanding.* Washington, DC: The National Academies Press.

Katz-Wise, S. L., Scherer, E. A., Calzo, J. P., Sarda, V., Jackson, B., Haines, J., & Austin, S. B. (2015). Sexual minority stressors, internalizing symptoms, and unhealthy eating behaviors in sexual minority youth. *Annals of Behavioral Medicine, 49*, 839–852. doi:10.1007/s12160-015-9718-z

Kipke, M. D., Kubicek, K., Weiss, G., Wong, C., Lopez, D., Iverson, E., & Ford, W. (2007). The health and health behaviors of young men who have sex with men. *Journal of Adolescent Health, 40*, 342–350. doi:10.1016/j.jadohealth.2006.10.019

Klok, M. D., Jakobsdottir, S., & Drent, M. L. (2007). The role of leptin and ghrelin in the regulation of food intake and body weight in humans: A review. *Obesity Reviews, 8*, 21–34. doi:10.1111/j.1467-789X.2006.00270.x

Kong, A., Tussing–Humphreys, L. M., Odoms–Young, A. M., Stolley, M. R., & Fitzgibbon, M. L. (2014). Systematic review of behavioural interventions with culturally adapted strategies to improve diet and weight outcomes in African American women. *Obesity Reviews, 15*, 62–92. doi:10.1111/obr.12203

Kraft, C., Nordstrom, D. L., Bockting, W. O., & Rosser, B. S. (2006). Obesity, body image, and unsafe sex in men who have sex with men. *Archives of Sexual Behavior, 35*, 587–595. doi:10.1007/s10508-006-9059-x

Kushner, R. F., & Foster, G. D. (2000). Obesity and quality of life. *Nutrition, 16*, 947–952. doi:10.1016/S0899-9007(00)00404-4

Laska, M. N., VanKim, N. A., Erickson, D. J., Lust, K., Eisenberg, M. E., & Rosser, B. S. (2015). Disparities in weight and weight behaviors by sexual orientation in college students. *American Journal of Public Health, 105*, 111–121. doi:10.2105/AJPH.2014.302094

LaVeist, T. A., Gaskin, D., & Richard, P. (2011). Estimating the economic burden of racial health inequalities in the United States. *International Journal of Health Services, 41*, 231–238. doi:10.2190/HS.41.2.c

Lewis, R. J., Mason, T. B., Winstead, B. A., & Kelley, M. L. (2016). Empirical investigation of a model of sexual minority specific and general risk factors for intimate partner violence among lesbian women. *Psychology of Violence, 7*(1), 110–119. doi:10.1037/vio0000036

Lewis, R. J., Milletich, R. J., Kelley, M. L., & Woody, A. (2012). Minority stress, substance use, and intimate partner violence among sexual minority women. *Aggression and Violent Behavior, 17*, 247–256. doi:10.1016/j.avb.2012.02.004

Levesque, M. J., & Vichesky, D. R. (2006). Raising the bar on the body beautiful: An analysis of the body image concerns of homosexual men. *Body Image, 3*, 45–55. doi:10.1016/j.bodyim.2005.10.007

Lick, D. J., Durso, L. E., & Johnson, K. L. (2013). Minority stress and physical health among sexual minorities. *Perspectives on Psychological Science, 8*, 521–548. doi:10.1177/1745691613497965

Ma, Y., Bertone, E. R., Stanek, E. J., Reed, G. W., Hebert, J. R., Cohen, N. L., … Ockene, I. S. (2003). Association between eating patterns and obesity in a free-living US adult population. *American Journal of Epidemiology, 158*, 85–92. doi:10.1093/aje/kwg117

Malik, V. S., Pan, A., Willett, W. C., & Hu, F. B. (2013). Sugar-sweetened beverages and weight gain in children and adults: A systematic review and meta-analysis. *The American Journal of Clinical Nutrition, 98*, 1084–1102. doi:10.3945/ajcn.113.058362

Markey, C. N., & Markey, P. M. (2014). Gender, sexual orientation, and romantic partner influence on body image: An examination of heterosexual and lesbian women and their partners. *Journal of Social and Personal Relationships, 31*, 162–177. doi:10.1177/0265407513489472

Martinez, J. A., Kearney, J. M., Kafatos, A., Paquet, S., & Martínez-Gonzélez, M. A. (1999). Variables independently associated with self-reported obesity in the European Union. *Public Health Nutrition, 2*, 125–133. doi:10.1017/S1368980099000178

Mason, T. B. (2016). Binge eating and overweight and obesity among young adult lesbians. *LGBT Health, 3*(6), 472–476. Advance online publication. doi:10.1089/lgbt.2015.0119

Mason, T. B., & Lewis, R. J. (2014). Reducing obesity among lesbian women: Recommendations for culturally tailored interventions. *Psychology of Sexual Orientation and Gender Diversity, 1*, 361–376. doi:10.1037/sgd0000074

Mason, T. B., & Lewis, R. J. (2015). Minority stress, depression, relationship quality, and alcohol use: Associations with overweight and obesity among partnered young adult lesbians. *LGBT Health, 2*, 333–340. doi:10.1089/lgbt.2014.0053

Mason, T. B., & Lewis, R. J. (2016). Minority stress, body shame, and binge eating among lesbian women: Social anxiety as a linking mechanism. *Psychology of Women Quarterly, 40*, 428–440.

Matthews, A. K., Li, C. C., McConnell, E., Aranda, F., & Smith, C. (2016). Rates and predictors of obesity among African American sexual minority women. *LGBT Health, 3*, 275–282. doi:10.1089/lgbt.2015.0026

McLean, K. (2008). Inside, outside, nowhere: Bisexual men and women in the gay and lesbian community. *Journal of Bisexuality, 8*, 63–80. doi:10.1080/15299710802143174

Mereish, E. H. (2014). The weight of discrimination: The relationship between heterosexist discrimination and obesity among lesbian women. *Psychology of Sexual Orientation and Gender Diversity, 1*, 356–360. doi:10.1037/sgd0000056

Mereish, E. H., & Poteat, V. P. (2015). Let's get physical: Sexual orientation disparities in physical activity, sports involvement, and obesity among a population-based sample of adolescents. *American Journal of Public Health, 105*, 1842–1848. doi:10.2105/AJPH.2015.302682

Meyer, I. H. (2003). Prejudice, social stress, and mental health in lesbian, gay, and bisexual populations: Conceptual issues and research evidence. *Psychological Bulletin, 129*, 674–697. doi:10.1037/0033-2909.129.5.674

Morrison, M. A., Morrison, T. G., & Sager, C. L. (2004). Does body satisfaction differ between gay men and lesbian women and heterosexual men and women? A meta-analytic review. *Body Image, 1*, 127–138. doi:10.1016/j.bodyim.2004.01.002

Moskowitz, D. A., & Seal, D. W. (2010). Revisiting obesity and condom use in men who have sex with men. *Archives of Sexual Behavior, 39*, 761–765. doi:10.1007/s10508-009-9478-6

Neumark-Sztainer, D., Wall, M., Guo, J., Story, M., Haines, J., & Eisenberg, M. (2006). Obesity, disordered eating, and eating disorders in a longitudinal study of adolescents: How do dieters fare 5 years later? *Journal of the American Dietetic Association, 106*, 559–568. doi:10.1016/j.jada.2006.01.003

Nyitray, A., Corran, R., Altman, K., Chikani, V., & Negrón, E. V. (2006). Tobacco use and interventions among Arizona lesbian, gay, bisexual, and transgender people. Retrieved from http://azmemory.azlibrary.gov/cdm/ref/collection/statepubs/id/3462

Ogden, C. L., Carroll, M. D., Fryar, C. D., & Flegal, K. M. (2015). *Prevalence of obesity among adults and youth: United States, 2011–2014.* NCHS Data Brief, 219.

Orzano, A. J., & Scott, J. G. (2004). Diagnosis and treatment of obesity in adults: An applied evidence-based review. *Journal of the American Board of Family Practice, 17*, 359–369. doi:10.3122/jabfm.17.5.359

Pachankis, J. E. (2014). Uncovering clinical principles and techniques to address minority stress, mental health, and related health risks among gay and bisexual men. *Clinical Psychology, 21*, 313–330. doi:10.1111/cpsp.12078

Petry, N. M., Barry, D., Pietrzak, R. H., & Wagner, J. A. (2008). Overweight and obesity are associated with psychiatric disorders: Results from the National Epidemiologic Survey on Alcohol and Related Conditions. *Psychosomatic Medicine, 70*, 288–297. doi:10.1097/PSY.0b013e3181651651

Resnicow, K., Baranowski, T., Ahluwalia, J. S., & Braithwaite, R. L. (1998). Cultural sensitivity in public health: Defined and demystified. *Ethnicity & Disease, 9*(1), 10–21.

Richmond, T. K., Walls, C. E., & Austin, S. B. (2012). Sexual orientation and bias in self-reported BMI. *Obesity, 20*, 1703–1709. doi:10.1038/oby.2012.9

Roberts, S. J., Stuart–Shor, E. M., & Oppenheimer, R. A. (2010). Lesbians' attitudes and beliefs regarding overweight and weight reduction. *Journal of Clinical Nursing, 19*, 1986–1994. doi:10.1111/j.1365-2702.2009.03182.x

Robison, J. (2005). Health at every size: Toward a new paradigm of weight and health. *Medscape General Medicine, 7*(3), 13.

Rosario, M., Corliss, H. L., Everett, B. G., Reisner, S. L., Austin, S. B., Buchting, F. O., & Birkett, M. (2014). Sexual orientation disparities in cancer-related risk behaviors of tobacco, alcohol, sexual behaviors, and diet and physical activity: Pooled Youth Risk Behavior Surveys. *American Journal of Public Health, 104*, 245–254. doi:10.2105/AJPH.2013.301506

Ross, L. E., Doctor, F., Dimito, A., Kuehl, D., & Armstrong, M. S. (2008). Can talking about oppression reduce depression? Modified CBT group treatment for LGBT people with depression. *Journal of Gay & Lesbian Social Services, 19*, 1–15. doi:10.1300/J041v19n01_01

Rossen, L. M. (2014). Neighbourhood economic deprivation explains racial/ethnic disparities in overweight and obesity among children and adolescents in the USA. *Journal of Epidemiology and Community Health, 68*, 123–129. doi:10.1136/jech-2012-202245

Rothblum, E. D. (2014). Commentary: Lesbians should take the lead in removing the stigma that has long been associated with body weight. *Psychology of Sexual Orientation and Gender Diversity, 1*, 377–382. doi:10.1037/sgd0000065

Schwartz, M. B., & Brownell, K. D. (2004). Obesity and body image. *Body Image, 1*, 43–56. doi:10.1016/S1740-1445(03)00007-X

Shearer, A., Russon, J., Herres, J., Atte, T., Kodish, T., & Diamond, D. (2015). The relationship between disordered eating and sexuality amongst adolescents and young adults. *Eating Behaviors, 19*, 115–119. doi:10.106/j.eatbeh.2015.08.001

Stice, E., Presnell, K., Shaw, H., & Rohde, P. (2005). Psychological and behavioral risk factors for obesity onset in adolescent girls: A prospective study. *Journal of Consulting and Clinical Psychology, 73*, 195–202. doi:10.1037/0022-006X.73.2.195

Struble, C. B., Lindley, L. L., Montgomery, K., Hardin, J., & Burcin, M. (2010). Overweight and obesity in lesbian and bisexual college women. *Journal of American College Health, 59*, 51–56. doi:10.1080/07448481.2010.483703

Sturm, R. (2002). The effects of obesity, smoking, and drinking on medical problems and costs. *Health Affairs, 21*, 245–253. doi:10.1377/hlthaff.21.2.245

Te Morenga, L., Mallard, S., & Mann, J. (2013). Dietary sugars and body weight: Systematic review and meta-analyses of randomised controlled trials and cohort studies. *The BMJ, 346*, e7492. doi:10.1136/bmj.e7492

Thayer, A. N. (2010). Community matters: The exploration of overweight and obesity within the lesbian population (Doctoral dissertation). Retrieved from Proquest. (Accession No. DP19730).

Thomas, J. G., & Bond, D. S. (2014). Review of innovations in digital health technology to promote weight control. *Current Diabetes Reports, 14*, 1–10. doi:10.1007/s11892-014-0485-1

Van Lenthe, F. J., Droomers, M., Schrijvers, C. T., & Mackenbach, J. P. (2000). Socio-demographic variables and 6-year change in body mass index: Longitudinal results from the GLOBE study. *International Journal of Obesity*, 24(8), 1077–1084.

VanKim, N. A., Erickson, D. J., Eisenberg, M. E., Lust, K., Rosser, B. S., & Laska, M. N. (2014). Weight-related disparities for transgender college students. *Health Behavior and Policy Review*, 1, 161–171. doi:10.14485/HBPR.1.2.8

VanKim, N. A., Erickson, D. J., Eisenberg, M. E., Lust, K., Rosser, B. R., & Laska, M. N. (2016). Relationship between weight-related behavioral profiles and health outcomes by sexual orientation and gender. *Obesity*, 24, 1572–1581. doi:10.1002/oby.21516

VanKim, N. A., Porta, C. M., Eisenberg, M. E., Neumark–Sztainer, D., & Laska, M. N. (2016). Lesbian, gay and bisexual college student perspectives on disparities in weight-related behaviours and body image: A qualitative analysis. *Journal of Clinical Nursing*, 25(23–24), 3676–3686. doi:10.1111/jocn.13106

Walls, N. E., & Wisneski, H. (2011). Evaluation of smoking cessation classes for the lesbian, gay, bisexual, and transgender community. *Journal of Social Service Research*, 37, 99–111. doi:10.1080/01488376.2011.524531

Wang, Y., & Beydoun, M. A. (2007). The obesity epidemic in the United States—gender, age, socioeconomic, racial/ethnic, and geographic characteristics: A systematic review and meta-regression analysis. *Epidemiologic Reviews*, 29, 6–28. doi:10.1093/epirev/mxm007

Warren, J. C., Smalley, K. B., & Barefoot, K. N. (2016). Differences in psychosocial predictors of obesity among LGBT subgroups. *LGBT Health*, 3, 283–291. doi:10.1089/lgbt.2015.0076

Yancey, A. K., Cochran, S. D., Corliss, H. L., & Mays, V. M. (2003). Correlates of overweight and obesity among lesbian and bisexual women. *Preventive Medicine*, 36, 676–683. doi:10.1016/S0091-7435(03)00020-3

Yelland, C., & Tiggemann, M. (2003). Muscularity and the gay ideal: Body dissatisfaction and disordered eating in homosexual men. *Eating Behaviors*, 4, 107–116. doi:10.1016/S1471-0153(03)00014-X

CHAPTER 5

Cancer in Gender and Sexual Minority Groups

Gwendolyn P. Quinn, Janella N. Hudson, Michelle T. Aihe,
Lauren E. Wilson, and Matthew B. Schabath

The gender and sexual minority (GSM) population reflects diverse experiences and represents a growing community spanning all races, ethnicities, ages, socioeconomic statuses, and regions of the United States (Boehmer, Miao, & Ozonoff, 2011). Previous surveys estimate approximately 3% to 12% of the adult U.S. population identify as a gender and/or sexual minority (Gates, 2011). The GSM population is at higher risk for multiple types of cancers (e.g., anal, penile, and oropharyngeal) compared to the cisgender heterosexual population. In this chapter, we review case studies that examine aspects of cancer prevention, treatment, psychosocial issues, and survivorship as they relate to the unique cancer health care needs of this underserved population (Quinn et al., 2015).

■ BARRIERS TO HEALTH CARE AND CANCER SCREENING FOR GSM GROUPS

Approximately 30% of GSM adults do not seek health care services and lack a regular health care provider (Buchmueller & Carpenter, 2010; Institute of Medicine [IOM], 2013; Kamen et al., 2014). The utilization of any health care service among GSM individuals may be adversely affected by a variety of factors including perceived stigma and intersectionality. Intersectionality relates to the construct that other "cultures" or sociodemographic groups may impact behaviors (Parent,

DeBlaere, & Moradi, 2013), including health behaviors. For example, a low-income lesbian who is African American and from a fundamental Christian religious family may experience stigmatization and marginalization from a variety of sources based on multiple factors, not just her sexual orientation.

In addition to stigma and intersectionality barriers, GSM individuals may experience structural and/or cognitive barriers to accessing health care. Despite the critical need for health care in the GSM population, structural and cognitive barriers to health care information and treatment significantly contribute to the avoidance or delay of seeking health care. For example, GSM cancer patients are more likely to remain silent about important health issues they fear may lead to additional stigmatization, a cognitive barrier (Boehmer et al., 2011). GSM populations may experience increased barriers to obtaining health insurance and forgo cancer screening or preventive care, a structural barrier (Eliason & Dibble, 2015). Cancer screening and early detection are particularly important for this population, but compared to cisgender and heterosexual individuals, previous studies have reported the GSM population is less likely to participate in cancer screening. This may be due to a variety of factors including the greater likelihood for GSM individuals to have lower incomes and reduced standard of living (IOM, 2011). Furthermore, many health care providers, including oncologists, lack knowledge of GSM health care needs and some have negative attitudes toward this population (Shetty et al., 2016). Other studies have reported a lack of trust and understanding in physician–patient relationships because patients fear substandard care or have concerns about confidentiality if they disclose their sexual orientation and/or gender identity (Barbara, Quandt, & Anderson, 2001; Boehmer & Case, 2004; Bonvicini & Perlin, 2003; Rounds, McGrath, & Walsh, 2013; Shetty et al., 2016).

An important theme in understanding the complexity of cancer care (both preventive and treatment) for GSM individuals is the multiple layers of experience and oppression they face. For example, women who are both a racial-ethnic minority and a sexual minority may have increased fears about disclosing GSM status to a health care provider. A recent study of African American women who identified as lesbian, bisexual, or queer and reported on experiences with cervical cancer screening stated they were concerned with being "treated differently" by health care providers (Agénor, Bailey, Krieger, Austin, & Gottlieb, 2015; Johnson, Nemeth, Mueller, Eliason, & Stuart, 2016). Many lesbian, bisexual, and queer women are concerned with finding GSM-friendly health care providers and some report negative experiences (e.g., with cervical cancer screening). Johnson et al. (2016) identified that peer support was a useful tool for increasing recommended cervical cancer screening among sexual minority women, but such approaches need further investigation, particularly in how to develop programs to counteract the intersecting layers of risk. When looking within the gender minority community, as an example, transgender men report a sense of "gender dissonance" with regard to cervical cancer screening and may avoid it as it not only increases stress but is also difficult for them to find a health care provider who is experienced with their health care needs (Johnson et al., 2016). Thus, the barriers to care are greater than just an individual's gender minority status; that status may directly impact engagement with care.

To illustrate the various types of challenges faced in achieving cancer health equity for GSM groups, we separately discuss different cancer sites, recognizing that many risks cut across cancer types. Each cancer is accompanied by fictional vignettes that help to reinforce the importance of keeping in mind the multilayered barriers to cancer screening and treatment that GSM groups face.

■ SITE-SPECIFIC CANCERS

Breast Cancer

Simone is a 53-year-old woman in a loving relationship with her wife, Cora, and together they have two daughters. Cora and Simone are both self-employed musicians. They utilize state-sponsored insurance for their daughters' health care needs, and have chosen to forgo purchasing a health care plan due to their highly variable and often inconsistent stream of income. Typically, Simone visits the doctor only if she is experiencing pain or a particularly acute issue that can't be managed with over-the-counter medications. She has had unpleasant interactions with previous providers who reacted negatively when she disclosed her sexual orientation or mentioned her wife. While showering one day, Simone feels pain under her arm. She initially dismisses the pain as a recreational hazard but notices that the pain continues to linger. The next week while having brunch with her parents, she casually mentions the annoying pain and her mother reacts very strongly: "Simone! You know that we have a strong family history of breast cancer. You're over 50. Have you had a mammogram?" Simone realizes that she has indeed forgotten to have a routine mammogram, but dreads having to go to the doctor. She is also unsure about where she can obtain a free mammogram.

Studies concerning the epidemiologic impact of breast cancer in cisgender heterosexual women compared to lesbian and bisexual women have produced mixed results. A study by Boehmer et al. (2011) reported that among cisgender heterosexual women, the weighted prevalence estimate of breast cancer was 20.6% and for lesbian and bisexual women, weighted prevalence estimates were 17.8% and 13.3%, respectively. However, other published reports have suggested lesbian and bisexual women are at higher risk of breast cancer compared to cisgender heterosexual women (Boehmer, Miao, Maxwell, & Ozonoff, 2014). In a separate study (Zaritsky & Dibble, 2010), breast cancer risk factors were compared between 370 lesbian and heterosexual sister pairs older than 40 years. Results showed lesbian sisters had significantly more education, fewer pregnancies, fewer total months pregnant, fewer children, fewer total months breastfeeding, higher body mass index (BMI), exercised fewer times per week, and performed fewer breast self-examinations (Zaritsky & Dibble, 2010). Thus, the authors suggest that lesbian women have a reproductive history (less childbearing and breastfeeding) and risk behaviors (high BMI, less exercise, and breast exams) that make them at increased risk of breast cancer. Pregnancy has been documented as a protective factor for breast cancer, and reduced pregnancy rates in lesbian and bisexual women equate to increased cancer risk (Clavelle, King, Bazzi, Fein-Zachary, & Potter, 2015). As discussed in Chapter 4, there are multiple recent studies that revealed lesbians have higher rates of obesity compared to cisgender heterosexual women (e.g., Boehmer & Bowen, 2009; Boehmer, Bowen, & Bauer, 2007; Russo, Moral, Balogh, Mailo, & Russo, 2005), an established risk factor for breast cancer. Despite limited published data over the last decade on breast cancer risk factors for lesbian and bisexual women (J. P. Brown & Tracy, 2008; Dibble, Roberts, & Nussey, 2004; Marrazzo & Stine, 2004; Zaritsky & Dibble, 2010), the IOM (2011) suggests a higher risk for breast cancer in this population because of higher prevalence of risk factors, such as nulliparity, alcohol use, smoking, and obesity. Further research is needed to formally address whether the elevated prevalence of these risks translates into actual higher rates of disease for lesbian and bisexual women, as well as explore culturally appropriate ways to modify risks among lesbians.

For women at average risk, breast cancer screening includes clinical breast exam and mammography (American Cancer Society, 2015). Results from studies on sexual minority women's participation in mammography screening have been inconsistent (J. P. Brown & Tracy, 2008; S. L. Hart & Bowen, 2009). Some studies reported sexual minority women were less likely than heterosexual women to have had a recent mammogram, while other studies reported lesbian women were more likely to get mammography than bisexual and cisgender heterosexual women, and still other studies observed no differences by sexual orientation (J. P. Brown & Tracy, 2008; S. L. Hart & Bowen, 2009). Many factors may contribute to lower screening rates including lower income and not having health care insurance (Burns, 2011; S. L. Hart & Bowen, 2009). Additionally, previous studies have shown the relationship between the health care provider and patient is crucial to the decision to obtain breast cancer screening and that sexual minority women often do not have positive relationships with their providers (S. L. Hart & Bowen, 2009; Hutchinson, Thompson, & Cederbaum, 2006). Thus, because of elevated prevalence of breast cancer risk behaviors and increased barriers to health care, sexual minority women may be an underserved population with regard to breast cancer screening and prevention.

Presently little is known about gender minorities and when transgender men and women participate (or need to participate) in mammography screening. A 2015 study on adherence to mammography screening among transgender persons suggests cisgender women are more likely to have had a recent mammogram (Bazzi, Whorms, King, & Potter, 2015); however, there is a strong need for additional research examining the cancer-specific risks that transgender men and women face.

To date, there are limited studies on breast cancer survivorship among sexual minority women. A study utilizing the National Health Interview Survey (NHIS) estimated age-adjusted relative risk (RR) for mortality attributed to breast cancer and found that lesbian women had greater disease-specific mortality (RR = 3.20, 95% confidence interval [CI] 1.01–10.21), but did not differ in their overall risk for mortality (Cochran & Mays, 2012). A study by Boehmer et al. (2011) reported that lesbian cancer survivors had nearly twice the odds (odds ratio [OR] = 1.98; 95% CI [1.15–3.42]) and bisexual women had over two-fold the odds (adjusted OR = 2.32; 95% CI [1.21–4.82]) of reporting fair or poor health compared to cisgender heterosexual women (Cochran & Mays, 2012). Although this study analyzed data across all cancers, breast cancer was the most frequently reported cancer site among cisgender women (20.6% among heterosexual, 17.8% among lesbian, and 13.3% among bisexual).

Quality of life (QoL) among cisgender heterosexual breast cancer survivors has been studied for several decades. Two studies comparing sexual minority and cisgender heterosexual breast cancer survivors found no differences in global QoL scores (Boehmer, Glickman, Milton, & Winter, 2012; Jabson, Donatelle, & Bowen, 2011). When specific treatment-related effects were examined, there were no differences between the groups regarding both morbidity of the arm (including lymphedema) and systemic side effects (Boehmer, Glickman, Winter, & Clark, 2013). Additionally, a study of lesbian and bisexual female breast cancer patients and healthy controls found no differences in overall sexual functioning between these groups, but did find that sexual minority breast cancer survivors were more likely to report lower sexual activity frequency, desire, and ability to reach orgasm, as well as higher levels of pain (Boehmer, Ozonoff, Timm, Winter, & Potter, 2014). However, a more recent study by Boehmer, Ozonoff, and Potter (2015) showed poorer QoL-related outcomes among sexual minority women cancer survivors compared to sexual minority women without cancer, including increased use of psychopharmacological drugs after treatment, worse eating habits, and less exercise.

Since many lesbians and bisexual women may delay seeking health care (Stevens, 1992), every clinical encounter, and not just preventive care visits, should be seen as an opportunity to promote cancer screening/early detection. It is also important for clinicians to be sensitive to the impact that breast disease and breast cancer treatment can have on relationships with sexual partners. Although there is limited research on the topic, several studies suggest decisions about breast-conserving therapies and requests for breast reconstruction are dissimilar between lesbians and cisgender heterosexual women. These studies suggest decisions about cancer treatment and survivorship are based on a value system and body image shaped at least in part by sexual orientation/identity (Boehmer, Freund, & Linde, 2005; Boehmer, Linde, & Freund, 2005; Scott & Kayser, 2009) that needs further investigation.

Anal Cancer

Anthony is a 33-year-old man in a new relationship with his live-in partner, John. Anthony noticed he had anal bleeding that accompanied his trips to the bathroom. He initially dismissed the bleeding as a symptom of his persistent hemorrhoids but started to develop pain and other gastrointestinal issues over time. Anthony considered seeking medical care but was uncomfortable consulting his female primary care provider. After a while, his partner John noticed that Anthony was increasingly uncomfortable and averse to sexual activity and strongly encouraged him to see a doctor for an assessment. Anthony consulted his primary care provider, and was sent for a biopsy of his anal lesions. Several weeks later, Anthony was stunned to learn that he had early stage anal cancer caused by a common strain of HPV.

Human papillomavirus (HPV), a sexually transmitted infection, is the most important causative factor in the development of several cancers, including anal cancer (Giuliano et al., 2015). Other factors significantly associated with anal cancer include number of lifetime sexual partners, coexistence of other sexually transmitted infections, cigarette smoking, and immunosuppression (Leonard, Beddy, & Dozois, 2011).

Epidemiologic studies have demonstrated that sexual risk factors, including male same-sex sexual intercourse, are strongly associated with anal cancer risk (Grulich et al., 2012). Due to sexual practices such as receptive anal intercourse, gay and bisexual men are at greater risk of anal cancer as a consequence of HPV infection than heterosexual men (Machalek et al., 2012), and HIV-positive men are at the highest risk—even when on antiretroviral therapy (Nadarzynski, Smith, Richardson, Jones, & Llewellyn, 2014).

To date, the best preventive measure of anal cancer is the HPV vaccine. As sexual minority men are at a higher risk of HPV-associated anal cancer compared to heterosexual men and women, they are an important target group for HPV vaccination (Hawkes & Lewis, 2014). A recent systematic review (Nadarzynski et al., 2014) and a single-site study (Hawkes & Lewis, 2014) on knowledge and beliefs about HPV and attitudes toward HPV vaccination among sexual minority men showed there is insufficient knowledge of HPV-related cancers and the availability of an HPV vaccine as a method of primary prevention (Koskan, LeBlanc, & Rosa-Cunha, 2016). However, despite poor knowledge about HPV, most sexual minority men are receptive to being vaccinated against HPV.

Two early detection approaches to identify anal lesions include anal Pap smears and high-resolution anoscopy (Hicks et al., 2015). Presently routine anal Pap smears are recommended only for HIV+ individuals. Randomized controlled trials conducted to date do not support effectiveness of anal cancer screening in the general population, and there are no formal guidelines for routine screening via anal Pap tests in non–HIV-infected individuals. However, a recent study of gay and bisexual men suggests the majority are willing and interested in self-administration of anal cancer screening through an anal swab kit (Thompson, Reiter, McRee, Moss, & Brewer, 2015).

Because anal cancer is a rare disease, limited studies have examined factors influencing patient survival or prognosis. There is evidence that patient factors such as sex, race/ethnicity, socioeconomic status, HPV positivity, and p16 protein expression status, which is a surrogate marker of HPV infection, play a role in disease prognosis (Bilimoria et al., 2009; Das, Crane, Eng, & Ajani, 2008; Serup-Hansen et al., 2014). To date, sexual orientation has not been addressed as a potential prognostic factor, and no study has evaluated differential effects of anal cancer outcomes by GSM status. No QoL studies have been done exclusively with anal cancer survivors and since few studies collect GSM status, specific outcomes for these patients are not known (Bouvier et al., 2008; Campos-Lobato, Alves-Ferreira, Lavery, & Kiran, 2011; Quach, Sanoff, Williams, Lyons, & Reeve, 2014).

Currently, HPV vaccination is recommended for all males from ages 9 to 21 and through age 26 specifically for sexual minority and HIV-infected males. This recommendation creates different practice guidelines for heterosexual and non-heterosexual males between the ages of 22 and 26 years (Petrosky et al., 2015). As published studies have reported that health care professionals do not routinely assess sexual orientation (Alexander et al., 2014; Sherman, Kauth, Shipherd, & Street Jr., 2014), this may result in a missed clinical opportunity to deliver the vaccine to groups most likely to benefit.

Cervical Cancer

Anastasia and her girlfriend have been together in a happy, monogamous relationship for 5 years. The two met during college, graduated together, and settled into an apartment as they searched for their first jobs. Anastasia settled into an unpaid internship for several years and used her parents' health insurance. However, when she turned 26 she had not yet found a job that offered health insurance and she went several years without a pap smear. Anastasia assumed that there was no need for frequent pelvic exams or pap smears given that she was in a monogamous relationship with a same-sex partner. When Anastasia had a pap smear several years later, she was devastated to learn that she had cervical cancer as the result of HPV. She subsequently learned that her partner also had HPV and had contracted it through previous contact with a male partner.

HPV, a sexually transmitted infection, is the most important and prevalent risk factor for cervical cancer. In fact, nearly all cervical cancers are caused by HPV infections, with two HPV types, 16 and 18, responsible for about 70% of all cases (Petrosky et al., 2015; Schiffman, Castle, Jeronimo, Rodriguez, & Wacholder, 2007). HPV transmission occurs through contact with infected genital skin, mucous membranes, or bodily fluids and skin-to-skin contact with the reproductive organs of an infected person. Therefore, women who have not had vaginal or anal intercourse with a male partner are still at risk for HPV infection and cervical cancer. Although previous studies have suggested sexually transmitted infections rarely occur between sexual minority women (Fethers, Marks, Mindel, & Estcourt, 2000; McNair, Power, & Carr, 2009), more recent studies (Gorgos & Marrazzo, 2011) found sexually transmitted infections are in fact common in this group and transmission does occur through sexual contact. Furthermore, as reviewed by Waterman and Voss (2015), research has demonstrated that many lesbians and their partners have had previous sexual contact with men. Additionally, lesbians may have higher rates of other cervical cancer risk factors and behaviors when compared to cisgender heterosexual women including higher BMI scores, increased alcohol consumption, and increased smoking history (Waterman & Voss, 2015). The cumulative impact of these risk factors, in combination with potential barriers to health care access, may require important changes to cervical screening guidelines for lesbians and bisexual women.

An important modality for the prevention of cervical cancer is HPV vaccination. Unfortunately, vaccination rates are low in the United States, and the HPV vaccine is currently not recommended to people 27 years of age or older. Some studies suggest lesbians erroneously perceive they are not at risk for HPV and do not need vaccination, which may explain why their uptake of HPV vaccine is likely lower than the general population (J. P. Brown & Tracy, 2008). To date, there are limited published data on HPV vaccination among sexual minority women. Using a web-based, respondent-driven sampling strategy, results from a study reported that 44.9% of lesbians and bisexual women aged 18 to 24 years received at least one dose of HPV vaccine compared to 51.1% of heterosexual women (Bernat, Gerend, Chevallier, Zimmerman, & Bauermeister, 2013). A more recent study that surveyed a national sample of young adults aged 18 to 26 years who self-identified as a gender or sexual minority found that 45% of respondents had initiated HPV vaccine and 70% of initiators reported completing the series (McRee, Katz, Paskett, & Reiter, 2014). Another recent study (Agénor, Peitzmeier, et al., 2015) examining awareness and initiation of HPV vaccine among women and girls found that 84% had heard of the HPV vaccine, whether they identified as a sexual minority or heterosexual. Eight percent of women who identified as lesbian reported initiating HPV vaccine compared to 32% of bisexual women and 28% of heterosexual women. Respondents with no lifetime or past-year sexual partners of either gender had significantly lower adjusted odds of HPV vaccine initiation compared to those with only male sexual partners. No differences were seen in participants with both male and female sexual partners compared to those with only male sexual partners in terms of vaccine initiation. Similar to studies conducted in majority populations (Centers for Disease Control and Prevention [CDC], 2012; Rimer, Harper, & Witte, 2014), programs designed to increase HPV vaccination should focus on improving health care provider recommendations, and disclosure of sexual orientation and gender identity by patients should be encouraged through the creation of welcoming and accepting environments.

Current cervical cancer screening guidelines do not include considerations for sexual minority women. The U.S. Preventive Services Task Force (USPSTF, 2012) recently changed the screening recommendations for Pap testing to every 3 years for all women aged 21 to 65 years who have a cervix, regardless of sexual history. However, because of potential misconceptions that sexual minority women are not at risk for cervical cancer, these women may not be screened at the same rates as the general population. A recent study (Reiter & McRee, 2014) analyzed a national sample of lesbians and bisexual women aged 21 to 26 years and found that Pap testing was more common among women who had disclosed their sexual orientation to their health care provider. However, Pap testing was less common among women who self-identified as lesbian but had not disclosed their orientation to a health care provider.

While barriers to health care, screening, and vaccination among transgender men and lesbian and bisexual women have received some attention in the published literature, there are no published data on patient outcomes in cervical cancer among these individuals (Agénor, Krieger, Austin, Haneuse, & Gottlieb, 2014). Also, no studies were identified that focused exclusively on QoL after cervical cancer for transgender men and sexual minority women. However, it is likely they would experience many of the same issues as cisgender heterosexual women, particularly those related to cancer treatment. A recent review indicates that the type of treatment(s) received by cervical cancer patients has the greatest impact on long-term QoL, with those who receive radiation at greatest risk of increased long-term bladder and bowel dysfunction, sexual dysfunction, and negative psychosocial consequences (Pfaendler, Wenzel, Mechanic, & Penner, 2015).

Standard recommendations for cervical cancer screening still apply for women who have never had sex with a male partner (Smith et al., 2015). Although no specific guidelines exist for the care of transgender men, health care providers should consider the psychological discomfort and gender dissonance that may be experienced by transgender men during a pelvic exam (Agénor et al., 2016).

Prostate Cancer

Wanda is a 55-year-old African American transgender woman who transitioned during her teenage years. Wanda takes gender-affirming hormones and has had no gender confirmation surgeries. She enjoys a successful career as a college professor and is happy with her dating life. Wanda begins to notice several troublesome symptoms, including blood in her urine, frequent urination at night, and discomfort when sitting. Wanda thought these changes were attributed to growing older and did not consult a physician for several years. When Wanda does see her physician and discloses that she is transgender, her physician suggests checking her prostate and reminds her that she must continue cancer screenings as needed for her natal sex. After subsequent tests, Wanda learns that she has prostate cancer and searches for additional information to make a decision concerning treatment.

Other than nonmelanoma skin cancer, prostate cancer is the most frequently diagnosed cancer in natal males and the second-leading cause of cancer death. Incidence rates for prostate cancer changed substantially due to widespread dissemination of the prostate-specific antigen (PSA) blood test for screening in the 1980s (Crawford, 2003). In 2015, the incidence rate in the United States was 146.6 per 100,000, the mortality was 23 per 100,000, and there were approximately 233,000 new cases of prostate cancer and nearly 25,000 prostate cancer–related deaths (American Cancer Society, 2016).

Although all natal males are at risk for prostate disease, there are limited data on the impact of prostate disease among sexual minority men. Based on a conservative estimate that 2% to 3% of the U.S. male population is gay or bisexual, a commentary in 2005 estimated at least 5,000 gay or bisexual men are diagnosed with prostate cancer each year, and 50,000 or more are survivors (Blank, 2005). Boehmer et al. (2011) utilized data on 51,233 men from the California Health Interview Survey and found gay men had a significantly lower weighted prevalence estimate for prostate cancer (5.3%) compared to heterosexual (16.5%) and bisexual men (14.3%). These data may reflect findings from the U.S. HIV/AIDS Cancer Match Study that HIV infection lowers rates of prostate cancer regardless of sexual orientation or gender identity (Shiels, Goedert, Moore, Platz, & Engels, 2010).

Advanced age, African ancestry, geographical location, and a family history of prostate cancer are well-established risk factors for prostate cancer (Cuzick et al., 2014). There are no published data comparing prostate cancer risk factors between heterosexual and sexual minority men. The American Cancer Society recommends annual PSA testing for men aged 50 years and over following shared decision making with a health care provider. While previous studies have shown that PSA-testing frequency differs by race/ethnicity, income, education, and other characteristics, there has been little published data on whether there are differences by sexual orientation (M. L. Brown, Potosky, Thompson, & Kessler, 1990; Gilligan, Wang, Levin, Kantoff, & Avorn, 2004). A cross-sectional analysis of 19,410 cisgender men in the California Health Interview Survey (Heslin, Gore, King, & Fox, 2008) found no overall differences in PSA testing comparing gay or bisexual men to heterosexual men. However, PSA testing among gay or bisexual African American men was 12% to 14% lower than that of heterosexual African American men and 15% to 28% lower than that of gay or bisexual White men.

Despite concerted efforts toward understanding treatment outcomes and QoL of cisgender men dealing with prostate cancer, there have been limited studies examining differences by sexual orientation. It has been suggested that effects of prostate cancer treatment on sexual function and QoL may differ by sexual orientation (Blank, 2005). Three studies (T. L. Hart et al., 2014; Lee, Breau, & Eapen, 2013; Motofei, Rowland, Popa, Kreienkamp, & Paunica, 2011) reported poorer physical outcomes and decreased QoL among gay men with prostate cancer compared to heterosexual men with prostate cancer. In contrast, a larger study among men with prostate cancer in the United States, Australia, Canada, United Kingdom, and other countries reported no significant differences in sexual function scores between heterosexual men and gay and bisexual men. However, another study found that gay and bisexual men reported significantly worse sexual bother, ejaculatory function, and ejaculatory bother after prostate cancer treatment (Wassersug, Lyons, Duncan, Dowsett, & Pitts, 2013).

The impact of prostate cancer cuts across multiple social and emotional domains that may impact QoL among survivors. Urinary and bowel treatment–related side effects have a significant and long-lasting effect on sexual functioning among the general population of prostate cancer patients (Chen et al., 2014; Davis et al., 2014; Ussher, Perz, Kellett, et al., 2016). This finding is mirrored in primarily qualitative studies that include gay prostate cancer survivors. However, the impact of poorer sexual functioning for gay men should be considered in light of sexual activity characteristics such as anal intercourse (which may require a firmer erection compared to vaginal sex) or may exacerbate concerns of anal discomfort (Blank, 2005). A recent pilot study of sexual minority men diagnosed with prostate cancer observed that participants who received radiation therapy were more likely to engage in posttreatment intercourse compared to those who received surgical treatment (Lee et al., 2013).

Two recent studies suggest sexual minority men experience reduced sexual QoL, psychological distress, and depression as prostate cancer survivors compared to heterosexual men and they have difficulty finding social or psychological supportive care services (Ussher Perz, Kellett, et al., 2016; Ussher, Perz, Rose, et al., 2016). Social support affects QoL in all men with prostate cancer (Paterson, Jones, Rattray, & Lauder, 2013). Prior work has focused predominantly on heterosexual men, the vast majority of whom were married at the time of diagnosis and treatment (Blank, 2005). For gay men, both observational and intervention studies addressing the impact of social support may require consideration of support from sources other than a married or partnered relationship, to include friends or the lesbian, gay, bisexual, and transgender (LGBT) community more broadly (Blank, 2005). Additionally, the sources and extent of social support may be limited for sexual minority men who are not open about their sexual orientation.

In a national U.S. study comparing health behaviors among male cancer survivors (25% diagnosed with prostate cancer), gay men were less likely to engage in moderate exercise and reported higher levels of alcohol consumption when compared to heterosexual male survivors (Kamen et al., 2014). Additionally, qualitative research on prostate cancer in gay male survivors identified their frustrations with the heterosexual orientation of survivorship care as well as concerns about homophobia among oncology health care professionals (Filiault, Drummond, &

Smith, 2008). Because recommendations for positive health behaviors may occur at lower rates among gay prostate cancer survivors, future health promotion efforts should be tailored to address these behaviors as well as being culturally relevant to gay men (Fredriksen-Goldsen, Hoy-Ellis, Goldsen, Emlet, & Hooyman, 2014).

For transgender women, removal of the prostate is not typical, and hormone treatment has not been shown to be preventive against prostate cancer. Although androgen deprivation treatment reduces the size of the prostate, potential for development of prostate cancer remains, especially among those starting hormone treatment after 50 years of age (Sattari, 2015). Two recent case studies present an occurrence of metastatic prostate cancer at ages 75 and 78 years in transgender women who had gender confirmation surgery at ages 43 and 45 years, respectively (Ellent & Matrana, 2016; Turo, Jallad, Prescott, & Cross, 2013); however, larger scale studies of transgender women are needed to fully understand the burden and impact of prostate cancer. As with the previous discussion of cervical cancer screening among transgender men, providers must be aware of the gender dissonance and discomfort that transgender women may face during discussions of and screening for prostate cancer.

CANCER AMONG TRANSGENDER MEN AND WOMEN

As with many outcomes discussed throughout this book, published research concerning cancer among transgender women and men is scarce and largely limited to case studies and small sample sizes in observational studies. As such, drawing firm conclusions from the existing body of research is not indicated. There is a significant opportunity for new research to greatly advance our understanding of cancer among transgender populations, especially with an aging transgender population, as well as with greater opportunities to pool data from datasets throughout the world. However, it will be difficult to move beyond case studies without advance planning and a significant investment in innovative research on transgender health.

There are several issues regarding cancer risk among transgender populations. One is the underutilization of health care in general, often related to fears regarding discrimination and stigma (Bradford, Cahill, Grasso, & Makadon, 2012; Bradford, Reisner, Honnold, & Xavier, 2013). Another is the concept of gender identity mismatch or gender dissonance in that, for example, a person with male reproductive organs who identifies as female may forego prostate screening or avoid addressing prostate-related symptoms (Turo et al., 2013). Other important issues for transgender populations include finding, and comfortably working with, gender minority–friendly health care providers who are knowledgeable about physical and mental health issues distinct to transgender patients. This would apply equally to primary care providers, cancer specialists, survivorship clinics, and the institutions in which care is provided.

STRATEGIES FOR IMPROVING ACCESS

Noah is a 21-year-old college student at a Midwestern university. After learning his school offers free health care services at an on-campus clinic, he decides to stop in for a general check-up. He's also heard from other students that the clinic offers free condoms, and hopes to obtain some. When he arrives at the office, he completes a patient questionnaire and shares his reasons for the visit with the nurse. The doctor soon arrives and reviews Noah's concerns, as noted by the patient questionnaire. Noticing that Noah has not answered any questions regarding sexual orientation and sexual practices, Dr. Avery comments, "I noticed that a couple of items were blank on our intake form. Can you share your sexual orientation as well as any details concerning the gender you identify with most strongly?" Noah is encouraged by his open and friendly demeanor and advises Dr. Avery that he is gay. Upon further questioning, Noah also informs Dr. Avery that he is casually dating. Dr. Avery responds, "Before we address the things that you came in to discuss today, I want to cover a few important points with you. I always like to remind my patients that it's important to be tested for HIV. It's also important that we talk about HPV vaccination as well. As you are a young man who is currently dating other men, you face an elevated risk for acquiring HPV. Common strains of HPV can lead to certain cancers that are more prevalent in the LGBTQ population, so I'd like you to seriously consider starting your first dose today." Dr. Avery goes on to educate Noah regarding the importance of protected sex and assures him that the clinic will provide him with a free supply of condoms. Noah agrees to HPV vaccination as well as HIV testing. As he left the clinic, Noah reflected positively on Dr. Avery's deftness in addressing what were potentially sensitive issues and decided he would recommend Dr. Avery and the clinic to his friends.

With GSM health disparities becoming more evident, it is crucial to implement effective strategies to address and eliminate them. Interventions to assist GSM patients with cancer health care access and decision making are needed. An avenue for patients to find GSM-friendly services is through the Healthcare Equality Index (HEI). HEI was created by the Human Rights Campaign Foundation as a way for health care facilities to affirm that they comply with the Joint Commission and Centers for Medicare and Medicaid Services (CMS) requirements for GSM equity, are committed to GSM patient-centered care, and extend nondiscrimination protection to their GSM employees (Snowdon, 2016). Medical institutions, physicians, nurse educators, and practitioners play critical roles in the accessibility and promotion of cancer-related health care by building trust and cultivating partnerships with the LGBT community (Hanssmann, Morrison, Russian, Shiu-Thornton, & Bowen, 2010; Snowdon, 2016). The availability of a provider directory and facilities that promote health care equity will be even more necessary for patients as awareness of unique health care needs among GSM health increases.

For the first time, *Healthy People 2020* has acknowledged health disparities in the GSM population. One goal of GSM health improvement is to "increase the number of population based data systems used to monitor *Healthy People 2020* objectives that include in their core a standardized set of questions that identify lesbian, gay, bisexual and transgender populations" (U.S. Department of Health and Human Services, 2012). The inclusion of GSM status within electronic medical records is essential to provide a foundation for understanding the cancer-related needs of the population (Cahill & Makadon, 2014; Callahan et al., 2014; IOM, 2013).

Largely due to the minimal information available in existing research, there is a lack of evidence-based guidelines with regard to the cancer-related clinical care of GSM populations. Regardless of the type of cancer, clinical teams should focus on eliciting patient preferences, concerns, and needs pertaining to treatment plans, goals of treatment and, when appropriate, end-of-life care (Harding, Epiphaniou, & Chidgey-Clark, 2012). Discussions about plans of care should be inclusive of patients' partners, family of origin (as appropriate), and family of choice, given the important role they play in decision making (Harding et al., 2012). The medical rights of patients, their partners, and their families need to be acknowledged by health care providers. Clinical and cultural competency training with regard to GSM patients is needed so health care providers and their staff can acquire the skills and knowledge needed to treat GSM patients effectively and to reduce disparities affecting this population. The American Medical Association (2016) recently updated its policies on GSM issues and noted that not obtaining sexual orientation and gender identity from patients was akin to a failure to screen or diagnose. This underscores the professional duty of clinicians to create safe environments for disclosure of and attention to this important aspect of a patient's social history.

CONCLUSION

It is known that the LGBT community has increased risks for some cancers, not because of their sexual orientation and/or gender identity, but because cancer-related risk behaviors are more prevalent in this population due to a variety of factors discussed throughout this book. These risk factors include higher rates of obesity, smoking, and alcohol use. The conundrum of these risk behaviors is that they are likely to have developed as a result of perceptions of stigmatization, marginalization, and overt discrimination. Society in general is gradually becoming more accepting of GSM groups, but the negative impact of discrimination related to sexual orientation and gender identity, combined with barriers to health related to intersectionality, remains high. As with the vicious circle of risk behaviors and increased cancer risk, it will take greater acceptance of the LGBT community in the health care setting for disclosure to occur more routinely. Health care providers should be trained to respond to that disclosure in affirming ways that address the needs of their patients.

A welcoming environment conducive to disclosure is a key element in improving the quality of care for GSM patients. As evidenced throughout this chapter, the collection of sexual orientation and gender identity information and an accurate sexual history is necessary for GSM patients to receive proper screening, diagnosis, and treatment for their cancer health care needs. Equally important is ensuring that health care providers and staff are properly educated on the increased prevalence of risk factors as well as the specific needs of the GSM population in regard to cancer care (while at the same time avoiding stereotyping and offensive assumptions regarding their GSM patients).

There is much that is still not known about prevalence, risk, incidence, and mortality of cancer and QoL among survivors within the GSM population. As large databases such as Surveillance, Epidemiology, and End Results (SEER) registries begin to add sexual orientation and gender identity data to their demographic information, knowledge will improve. To address the dearth of information, the National Institutes of Health and the CDC are working to improve available funding for research that focuses on improved understanding of GSM cancer health needs and disparities (Coulter, Kenst, Bowen, & Scout, 2014). The U.S. Department of Health and Human Services included the health and well-being of GSM individuals in its objectives for Fiscal Year 2016 by requiring, among other things, the inclusion of sexual orientation and gender identity questions in CMS enrollment as well as working with the Office of the National Coordinator for Health Information Technology (ONC) to ensure that information is collected in electronic health records (EHRs) for all health care entities participating in EHR Incentive Programs (Assistant Secretary for Health, 2015). While the status of these changes is in question as of the publication of this book due to changes in the political climate, if these efforts are realized, knowledge of cancer care among the GSM population will improve, thereby improving the quality of care.

■ REFERENCES

Agénor, M., Bailey, Z., Krieger, N., Austin, S. B., & Gottlieb, B. R. (2015). Exploring the cervical cancer screening experiences of Black lesbian, bisexual, and queer women: The role of patient-provider communication. *Women & Health, 55*(6), 717–736.

Agénor, M., Krieger, N., Austin, S. B., Haneuse, S., & Gottlieb, B. R. (2014). Sexual orientation disparities in Papanicolaou test use among US women: The role of sexual and reproductive health services. *American Journal of Public Health, 104*(2), e68–e73.

Agénor, M., Peitzmeier, S. M., Bernstein, I. M., McDowell, M., Alizaga, N. M., Reisner, S. L., ... Potter, J. (2016). Perceptions of cervical cancer risk and screening among transmasculine individuals: Patient and provider perspectives. *Culture, Health & Sexuality, 18*(10), 1192–1206. doi:10.1080/13691058.2016.1177203

Agénor, M., Peitzmeier, S. M., Gordon, A. R., Haneuse, S., Potter, J. E., & Austin, S. B. (2015). Sexual orientation identity disparities in awareness and initiation of the human papillomavirus vaccine among U.S. women and girls: A national survey. *Annals of Internal Medicine, 163*(2), 99–106. doi:10.7326/m14-2108

Alexander, S. C., Fortenberry, J. D., Pollak, K. I., Bravender, T., Østbye, T., & Shields, C. G. (2014). Physicians' use of inclusive sexual orientation language during teenage annual visits. *LGBT Health, 1*(4), 283–291. doi:10.1089/lgbt.2014.0035

American Cancer Society. (2015). Breast cancer prevention and early detection. Retrieved from http://www.cancer.org/cancer/breastcancer/moreinformation/breastcancer earlydetection/breast-cancer-early-detection-acs-recs

American Cancer Society. (2016). Cancer facts & figures 2016. Retrieved from http://www .cancer.org/acs/groups/content/@research/documents/document/acspc-047079.pdf

American Medical Association. (2016). H-160.991 Health care needs of the homosexual population. Policies on lesbian, gay, bisexual, transgender & queer (LGBTQ) issues. Retrieved from https://www.ama-assn.org/delivering-care/policies-lesbian-gay-bisexual -transgender-queer-lgbtq-issues

American Psychiatric Association. (2013). *Diagnostic and Statistical Manual of Mental Disorders* (5th ed.). Arlington, VA: American Psychiatric Publishing.

Assistant Secretary for Health. (2015). LGBT health and well-being. Retrieved from http:// www.hhs.gov/programs/topic-sites/lgbt/reports/health-objectives-2015.html

Barbara, A. M., Quandt, S. A., & Anderson, R. T. (2001). Experiences of lesbians in the health care environment. *Women & Health, 34*(1), 45–62.

Bazzi, A. R., Whorms, D. S., King, D. S., & Potter, J. (2015). Adherence to Mammography Screening Guidelines among transgender persons and sexual minority women. *American Journal of Public Health, 105*(11), 2356–2358. doi:10.2105/AJPH.2015.302851

Bernat, D. H., Gerend, M. A., Chevallier, K., Zimmerman, M. A., & Bauermeister, J. A. (2013). Characteristics associated with initiation of the human papillomavirus vaccine among a national sample of male and female young adults. *Journal of Adolescent Health, 53*(5), 630–636. doi:10.1016/j.jadohealth.2013.07.035

Bilimoria, K. Y., Bentrem, D. J., Rock, C. E., Stewart, A. K., Ko, C. Y., & Halverson, A. (2009). Outcomes and prognostic factors for squamous-cell carcinoma of the anal canal: Analysis of patients from the National Cancer Data Base. *Diseases of the Colon and Rectum, 52*(4), 624–631. doi:10.1007/DCR.0b013e31819eb7f0

Blank, T. O. (2005). Gay men and prostate cancer: Invisible diversity. *Journal of Clinical Oncology, 23*(12), 2593–2596. doi:10.1200/JCO.2005.00.968

Boehmer, U., & Bowen, D. J. (2009). Examining factors linked to overweight and obesity in women of different sexual orientations. *Preventive Medicine, 48*(4), 357–361. doi:10.1016/j.ypmed.2009.02.003

Boehmer, U., Bowen, D. J., & Bauer, G. R. (2007). Overweight and obesity in sexual-minority women: Evidence from population-based data. *American Journal of Public Health, 97*(6), 1134–1140. doi:10.2105/AJPH.2006.088419

Boehmer, U., & Case, P. (2004). Physicians don't ask, sometimes patients tell: Disclosure of sexual orientation among women with breast carcinoma. *Cancer, 101*(8), 1882–1889. doi:10.1002/cncr.20563

Boehmer, U., Freund, K. M., & Linde, R. (2005). Support providers of sexual minority women with breast cancer: Who they are and how they impact the breast cancer experience. *Journal of Psychosomatic Research, 59*(5), 307–314. doi:10.1016/j.jpsychores.2005.06.059

Boehmer, U., Glickman, M., Milton, J., & Winter, M. (2012). Health-related quality of life in breast cancer survivors of different sexual orientations. *Quality of Life Research, 21*(2), 225–236. doi:10.1007/s11136-011-9947-y

Boehmer, U., Glickman, M., Winter, M., & Clark, M. A. (2013). Long-term breast cancer survivors' symptoms and morbidity: Differences by sexual orientation? *Journal of Cancer Survivorship, 7*(2), 203–210. doi:10.1007/s11764-012-0260-8

Boehmer, U., Linde, R., & Freund, K. M. (2005). Sexual minority women's coping and psychological adjustment after a diagnosis of breast cancer. *Journal of Women's Health, 14*(3), 214–224. doi:10.1089/jwh.2005.14.214

Boehmer, U., Miao, X., Maxwell, N. I., & Ozonoff, A. (2014). Sexual minority population density and incidence of lung, colorectal and female breast cancer in California. *BMJ Open, 4*(3), e004461. doi:10.1136/bmjopen-2013-004461

Boehmer, U., Miao, X., & Ozonoff, A. (2011). Cancer survivorship and sexual orientation. *Cancer, 117*(16), 3796–3804. doi:10.1002/cncr.25950

Boehmer, U., Ozonoff, A., & Potter, J. (2015). Sexual minority women's health behaviors and outcomes after breast cancer. *LGBT Health, 2*(3), 221–227. doi:10.1089/lgbt.2014.0105

Boehmer, U., Ozonoff, A., Timm, A., Winter, M., & Potter, J. (2014). After breast cancer: Sexual functioning of sexual minority survivors. *Journal of Sex Research, 51*(6), 681–689. doi:10.1080/00224499.2013.772087

Bonvicini, K. A., & Perlin, M. J. (2003). The same but different: Clinician–patient communication with gay and lesbian patients. *Patient Education & Counseling, 51*(2), 115–122. doi:10.1016/S0738-3991(02)00189-1

Bouvier, A. M., Jooste, V., Bonnetain, F., Cottet, V., Bizollon, M. H., Bernard, M. P., & Faivre, J. (2008). Adjuvant treatments do not alter the quality of life in elderly patients with colorectal cancer: A population-based study. *Cancer, 113*(4), 879–886. doi:10.1002/cncr.23629

Bradford, J., Cahill, S., Grasso, C., & Makadon, H. (2012). *How to gather data on sexual orientation and gender identity in clinical settings*. Boston, MA: The Fenway Institute. Retrieved from http://thefenwayinstitute.org/documents/Policy_Brief_HowtoGather..._v3_01.09.12.pdf

Bradford, J., Reisner, S. L., Honnold, J. A., & Xavier, J. (2013). Experiences of transgender-related discrimination and implications for health: Results from the Virginia Transgender Health Initiative Study. *American Journal of Public Health, 103*(10), 1820–1829. doi:10.2105/AJPH.2012.300796

Brown, J. P., & Tracy, J. K. (2008). Lesbians and cancer: An overlooked health disparity. *Cancer Causes & Control, 19*(10), 1009–1020. doi:10.1007/s10552-008-9176-z

Brown, M. L., Potosky, A. L., Thompson, G. B., & Kessler, L. G. (1990). The knowledge and use of screening tests for colorectal and prostate cancer: Data from the 1987 National Health Interview Survey. *Preventive Medicine, 19*(5), 562–574.

Buchmueller, T., & Carpenter, C. S. (2010). Disparities in health insurance coverage, access, and outcomes for individuals in same-sex versus different-sex relationships, 2000–2007. *American Journal of Public Health, 100*(3), 489–495. doi:10.2105/ajph.2009.160804

Burns, J. (2011). Insurers move toward more equitable care for LGBT population. Discrimination persists in many areas, but slow progress is being made. *Managed care (Langhorne, Pa.), 20*(11), 39–42, 49.

Cahill, S., & Makadon, H. (2014). Sexual orientation and gender identity data collection in clinical settings and in electronic health records: A key to ending LGBT health disparities. *LGBT Health, 1*(1), 34–41. doi:10.1089/lgbt.2013.0001

Callahan, E. J., Sitkin, N., Ton, H., Eidson-Ton, W. S., Weckstein, J., & Latimore, D. (2014). Introducing sexual orientation and gender identity into the electronic health record: One academic health center's experience. *Academic Medicine, 90*(2), 154–160. doi:10.1097/acm.0000000000000467

Campos-Lobato, L. F., Alves-Ferreira, P. C., Lavery, I. C., & Kiran, R. P. (2011). Abdominoperineal resection does not decrease quality of life in patients with low rectal cancer. *Clinics, 66*(6), 1035–1040.

Centers for Disease Control and Prevention. (2012). National and state vaccination coverage among adolescents aged 13–17 years—United States, 2011. *Morbidity and Mortality Weekly Report, 61*(34), 671–677.

Chen, R. C., Chang, P., Vetter, R. J., Lukka, H., Stokes, W. A., Sanda, M. G.,... Sandler, H. M. (2014). Recommended patient-reported core set of symptoms to measure in prostate cancer treatment trials. *Journal of the National Cancer Institute, 106*(7). doi:10.1093/jnci/dju132

Clavelle, K., King, D., Bazzi, A. R., Fein-Zachary, V., & Potter, J. (2015). Breast cancer risk in sexual minority women during routine screening at an urban LGBT Health Center. *Women's Health Issues, 25*(4), 341–348. doi:10.1016/j.whi.2015.03.01

Cochran, S. D., & Mays, V. M. (2012). Risk of breast cancer mortality among women cohabiting with same sex partners: Findings from the National Health Interview Survey, 1997–2003. *Journal of Women's Health, 21*(5), 528–533. doi:10.1089/jwh.2011.3134

Coulter, R. W., Kenst, K. S., Bowen, D. J., & Scout. (2014). Research funded by the National Institutes of Health on the health of lesbian, gay, bisexual, and transgender populations. *American Journal of Public Health, 104*(2), e105–e112. doi:10.2105/ajph.2013.301501

Crawford, E. D. (2003). Epidemiology of prostate cancer. *Urology, 62*(6 Suppl. 1), 3–12.

Cuzick, J., Thorat, M. A., Andriole, G., Brawley, O. W., Brown, P. H., Culig, Z.,... Wolk, A. (2014). Prevention and early detection of prostate cancer. *Lancet Oncology, 15*(11), e484–e492. doi:10.1016/S1470-2045(14)70211-6

Das, P., Crane, C. H., Eng, C., & Ajani, J. A. (2008). Prognostic factors for squamous cell cancer of the anal canal. *Gastrointestinal Cancer Research, 2*(1), 10–14.

Davis, K. M., Kelly, S. P., Luta, G., Tomko, C., Miller, A. B., & Taylor, K. L. (2014). The association of long-term treatment-related side effects with cancer-specific and general quality of life among prostate cancer survivors. *Urology, 84*(2), 300–306. doi:10.1016/j.urology.2014.04.036

Dibble, S. L., Roberts, S. A., & Nussey, B. (2004). Comparing breast cancer risk between lesbians and their heterosexual sisters. *Women's Health Issues, 14*(2), 60–68. doi:10.1016/j.whi.2004.03.004

Eliason, M. J., & Dibble, S. L. (2015). Provider-patient issues for the LGBT cancer patient. In U. Boehmer & R. Elk (Eds.), *Cancer and the LGBT community* (pp. 187–202). New York, NY: Springer.

Ellent, E., & Matrana, M. R. (2016). Metastatic prostate cancer 35 years after sex reassignment surgery. *Clinical Genitourinary Cancer, 14*(2), e207–e209.

Fethers, K., Marks, C., Mindel, A., & Estcourt, C. S. (2000). Sexually transmitted infections and risk behaviours in women who have sex with women. *Sexually Transmitted Infections, 76*(5), 345–349.

Filiault, S. M., Drummond, M. J., & Smith, J. A. (2008). Gay men and prostate cancer: Voicing the concerns of a hidden population. *Journal of Men's Health, 5*(4), 327–332. doi:10.1016/j.jomh.2008.08.005

Fredriksen-Goldsen, K. I., Hoy-Ellis, C. P., Goldsen, J., Emlet, C. A., & Hooyman, N. R. (2014). Creating a vision for the future: Key competencies and strategies for culturally competent practice with lesbian, gay, bisexual, and transgender (LGBT) older adults in the health and human services. *Journal of Gerontological Social Work, 57*(2–4), 80–107. doi:10.1080/01634372.2014.890690

Gates, G. J. (2011). *How many people are lesbian, gay, bisexual and transgender?* Los Angeles, CA: Williams Institute. Retrieved from http://williamsinstitute.law.ucla.edu/research/census-lgbt-demographics-studies/how-many-people-are-lesbian-gay-bisexual-and-transgender/

Gilligan, T., Wang, P. S., Levin, R., Kantoff, P. W., & Avorn, J. (2004). Racial differences in screening for prostate cancer in the elderly. *Archives of Internal Medicine, 164*(17), 1858–1864. doi:10.1001/archinte.164.17.1858

Giuliano, A. R., Nyitray, A. G., Kreimer, A. R., Pierce Campbell, C. M., Goodman, M. T., Sudenga, S. L.,... Franceschi, S. (2015). EUROGIN 2014 roadmap: Differences in human papillomavirus infection natural history, transmission and human papillomavirus–related cancer incidence by gender and anatomic site of infection. *International Journal of Cancer, 136*(12), 2752–2760.

Gorgos, L. M., & Marrazzo, J. M. (2011). Sexually transmitted infections among women who have sex with women. *Clinical Infectious Diseases, 53*(Suppl. 3), S84–S91. doi:10.1093/cid/cir697

Grulich, A. E., Poynten, I. M., Machalek, D. A., Jin, F., Templeton, D. J., & Hillman, R. J. (2012). The epidemiology of anal cancer. *Sexual Health, 9*(6), 504–508. doi:10.1071/SH12070

Hanssmann, C., Morrison, D., Russian, E., Shiu-Thornton, S., & Bowen, D. (2010). A community-based program evaluation of community competency trainings. *Journal of the Association of Nurses in AIDS Care, 21*(3), 240–255. doi:10.1016/j.jana.2009.12.007

Harding, R., Epiphaniou, E., & Chidgey-Clark, J. (2012). Needs, experiences, and preferences of sexual minorities for end-of-life care and palliative care: A systematic review. *Journal of Palliative Medicine, 15*(5), 602–611. doi:10.1089/jwh.2007.0447

Hart, S. L., & Bowen, D. J. (2009). Sexual orientation and intentions to obtain breast cancer screening. *Journal of Women's Health, 18*(2), 177–185. doi:10.1089/jwh.2007.0447

Hart, T. L., Coon, D. W., Kowalkowski, M. A., Zhang, K., Hersom, J. I., Goltz, H. H.,... Latini, D. M. (2014). Changes in sexual roles and quality of life for gay men after prostate cancer: Challenges for sexual health providers. *Journal of Sexual Medicine, 11*(9), 2308–2317. doi:10.1111/jsm.12598

Hawkes, S., & Lewis, D. A. (2014). HPV vaccine strategies: Equitable and effective? *Sexually Transmitted Infections, 90*(7), 510–511. doi:10.1136/sextrans-2014-051637

Heslin, K. C., Gore, J. L., King, W. D., & Fox, S. A. (2008). Sexual orientation and testing for prostate and colorectal cancers among men in California. *Medical Care, 46*(12), 1240–1248. doi:10.1097/MLR.0b013e31817d697f

Hicks, C. W., Wick, E. C., Leeds, I. L., Efron, J. E., Gearhart, S. L., Safar, B., & Fang, S. H. (2015). Patient symptomatology in anal dysplasia. *JAMA Surgery, 150*(6), 563–569. doi:10.1001/jamasurg.2015.28

Hutchinson, M. K., Thompson, A. C., & Cederbaum, J. A. (2006). Multisystem factors contributing to disparities in preventive health care among lesbian women. *Journal of Obstetric, Gynecologic, and Neonatal Nursing, 35*(3), 393–402. doi:10.1111/j.1552-6909.2006.00054.x

Institute of Medicine. (2011). *The health of lesbian, gay, bisexual, and transgender people: Building a foundation for better understanding*. Washington, DC: National Academies Press.

Institute of Medicine. (2013). *Collecting sexual orientation and gender identity data in electronic health records: Workshop summary*. Washington, DC: National Academies Press.

Jabson, J. M., Donatelle, R. J., & Bowen, D. J. (2011). Relationship between sexual orientation and quality of life in female breast cancer survivors. *Journal of Women's Health, 20*(12), 1819–1824. doi:10.1089/jwh.2011.2921

Johnson, M. J., Nemeth, L. S., Mueller, M., Eliason, M. J., & Stuart, G. W. (2016). Qualitative study of cervical cancer screening among lesbian and bisexual women and transgender men. *Cancer Nursing, 39*(6), 455–463. doi:10.1097/NCC.0000000000000338

Kamen, C., Palesh, O., Gerry, A. A., Andrykowski, M. A., Heckler, C., Mohile, S.,... Mustian, K. (2014). Disparities in health risk behavior and psychological distress among gay versus heterosexual male cancer survivors. *LGBT Health, 1*(2), 86–92. doi:10.1089/lgbt.2013.0022

Koskan, A. M., LeBlanc, N., & Rosa-Cunha, I. (2016). Exploring the perceptions of anal cancer screening and behaviors among gay and bisexual men infected with HIV. *Cancer Control, 23*(1), 52–58.

Lee, T. K., Breau, R. H., & Eapen, L. (2013). Pilot study on quality of life and sexual function in men-who-have-sex-with-men treated for prostate cancer. *Journal of Sexual Medicine, 10*(8), 2094–2100. doi:10.1111/jsm.12208

Leonard, D., Beddy, D., & Dozois, E. J. (2011). Neoplasms of anal canal and perianal skin. *Clinics in Colon and Rectal Surgery, 24*(1), 54–63. doi:10.1055/s-0031-1272824

Machalek, D. A., Poynten, M., Jin, F., Fairley, C. K., Farnsworth, A., Garland, S. M.,... Grulich, A. E. (2012). Anal human papillomavirus infection and associated neoplastic lesions in men who have sex with men: A systematic review and meta-analysis. *Lancet Oncology, 13*(5), 487–500. doi:10.1016/s1470-2045(12)70080-3

Marrazzo, J. M., & Stine, K. (2004). Reproductive health history of lesbians: Implications for care. *American Journal of Obstetrics and Gynecology, 190*(5), 1298–1304. doi:10.1016/j.ajog.2003.12.001

McNair, R., Power, J., & Carr, S. (2009). Comparing knowledge and perceived risk related to the human papilloma virus among Australian women of diverse sexual orientations. *Australian and New Zealand Journal of Public Health, 33*(1), 87–93. doi:10.1111/j.1753-6405.2009.00345.x

McRee, A. L., Katz, M. L., Paskett, E. D., & Reiter, P. L. (2014). HPV vaccination among lesbian and bisexual women: Findings from a national survey of young adults. *Vaccine, 32*(37), 4736–4742. doi:10.1016/j.vaccine.2014.07.001

Motofei, I. G., Rowland, D. L., Popa, F., Kreienkamp, D., & Paunica, S. (2011). Preliminary study with bicalutamide in heterosexual and homosexual patients with prostate cancer: A possible implication of androgens in male homosexual arousal. *BJU International, 108*(1), 110–115. doi:10.1111/j.1464-410X.2010.09764.x

Nadarzynski, T., Smith, H., Richardson, D., Jones, C. J., & Llewellyn, C. D. (2014). Human papillomavirus and vaccine-related perceptions among men who have sex with men: A systematic review. *Sexually Transmitted Infections, 90*(7), 515–523. doi:10.1136/sextrans-2013-051357

Parent, M. C., DeBlaere, C., & Moradi, B. (2013). Approaches to research on intersectionality: Perspectives on gender, LGBT, and racial/ethnic identities. *Sex Roles, 68*(11–12), 639–645. doi:10.1007/s11199-013-0283-2

Paterson, C., Jones, M., Rattray, J., & Lauder, W. (2013). Exploring the relationship between coping, social support and health-related quality of life for prostate cancer survivors: A review of the literature. *European Journal of Oncology Nursing, 17*(6), 750–759. doi:10.1016/j.ejon.2013.04.002

Petrosky, E., Bocchini, J. A., Jr., Hariri, S., Chesson, H., Curtis, C. R., Saraiya, M., . . . Markowitz, L. E. (2015). Use of 9-valent human papillomavirus (HPV) vaccine: Updated HPV vaccination recommendations of the Advisory Committee on Immunization Practices. *Morbidity and Mortality Weekly Report, 64*(11), 300–304.

Pfaendler, K. S., Wenzel, L., Mechanic, M. B., & Penner, K. R. (2015). Cervical cancer survivorship: Long-term quality of life and social support. *Clinical Therapeutics, 37*(1), 39–48. doi:10.1016/j.clinthera.2014.11.013

Quach, C., Sanoff, H. K., Williams, G. R., Lyons, J. C., & Reeve, B. B. (2015). Impact of colorectal cancer diagnosis and treatment on health-related quality of life among older Americans: A population-based, case-control study. *Cancer, 121*(6), 943–950.

Quinn, G. P., Sanchez, J. A., Sutton, S. K., Vadaparampil, S. T., Nguyen, G. T., Green, B. L., . . . Schabath, M. B. (2015). Cancer and lesbian, gay, bisexual, transgender/transsexual, and queer/questioning (LGBTQ) populations. *Cancer Journal for Clinicians, 65*(5), 384–400. doi:10.3322/caac.21288

Reiter, P. L., & McRee, A. L. (2015). Cervical cancer screening (Pap testing) behaviours and acceptability of human papillomavirus self-testing among lesbian and bisexual women aged 21–26 years in the USA. *Journal of Family Planning and Reproductive Health Care, 41*(4), 259–264. doi:10.1136/jfprhc-2014-101004

Rimer, B. K., Harper, H., & Witte, O. N. (2014). Accelerating HPV vaccine uptake: Urgency for action to prevent cancer. Retrieved from http://deainfo.nci.nih.gov/advisory/pcp/annualReports/HPV/#sthash.v7EV3G0E.NWWAVXAK.dpbs

Rounds, K. E., McGrath, B. B., & Walsh, E. (2013). Perspectives on provider behaviors: A qualitative study of sexual and gender minorities regarding quality of care. *Contemporary Nurse, 44*(1), 99–110. doi:10.5172/conu.2013.44.1.99

Russo, J., Moral, R., Balogh, G. A., Mailo, D., & Russo, I. H. (2005). The protective role of pregnancy in breast cancer. *Breast Cancer Research, 7*(3), 131–142. doi:10.1186/bcr1029

Sattari, M. (2015). Breast cancer in male-to-female transgender patients: A case for caution. *Clinical Breast Cancer, 15*(1), e67–e69. doi:10.1016/j.clbc.2014.08.004

Schiffman, M., Castle, P. E., Jeronimo, J., Rodriguez, A. C., & Wacholder, S. (2007). Human papillomavirus and cervical cancer. *Lancet, 370*(9590), 890–907. doi:10.1016/s0140-6736(07)61416-0

Scott, J. L., & Kayser, K. (2009). A review of couple-based interventions for enhancing women's sexual adjustment and body image after cancer. *Cancer Journal, 15*(1), 48–56. doi:10.1097/PPO.0b013e31819585df

Serup-Hansen, E., Linnemann, D., Skovrider-Ruminski, W., Høgdall, E., Geertsen, P. F., & Havsteen, H. (2014). Human papillomavirus genotyping and p16 expression as prognostic factors for patients with American Joint Committee on Cancer stages I to III carcinoma of the anal canal. *Journal of Clinical Oncology, 32*(17), 1812–1817. doi:10.1200/JCO.2013.52.3464

Sherman, M. D., Kauth, M. R., Shipherd, J. C., & Street, R. L. (2014). Provider beliefs and practices about assessing sexual orientation in two veterans health affairs hospitals. *LGBT Health, 1*(3), 185–191. doi:10.1089/lgbt.2014.0008

Shetty, G., Sanchez, J. A., Lancaster, J. M., Wilson, L. E., Quinn, G. P., & Schabath, M. B. (2016). Oncology healthcare providers' knowledge, attitudes, and practice behaviors regarding LGBT health. *Patient Education and Counseling, 99*(10), 1676–1684. doi:10.1016/j.pec.2016.05.004

Shiels, M. S., Goedert, J. J., Moore, R. D., Platz, E. A., & Engels, E. A. (2010). Reduced risk of prostate cancer in U.S. Men with AIDS. *Cancer Epidemiology, Biomarkers & Prevention, 19*(11), 2910–2915. doi:10.1158/1055-9965.epi-10-0741

Smith, R. A., Manassaram-Baptiste, D., Brooks, D., Doroshenk, M., Fedewa, S., Saslow, D.,… Wender, R. (2015). Cancer screening in the United States, 2015: A review of current American Cancer Society guidelines and current issues in cancer screening. *Cancer Journal for Clinicians, 65*(1), 30–54. doi:10.3322/caac.21261

Snowdon, S. (2016). *Healthcare Equality Index 2016: Promoting equitable and inclusive care for lesbian, gay, bisexual, and transgender patients and their families.* Washington, DC: Human Rights Campaign. Retrieved from http://www.hrc.org/campaigns/healthcare-equality-index

Stevens, P. E. (1992). Lesbian health care research: A review of the literature from 1970 to 1990. *Health Care for Women International, 13*(2), 91–120. doi:10.1080/07399339209515984

Thompson, J. A., Reiter, P. L., McRee, A. L., Moss, J. L., & Brewer, N. T. (2015). Gay and bisexual men's willingness to use a self-collected anal cancer screening test. *Journal of Lower Genital Tract Disease, 19*(4), 354–361. doi:10.1097/LGT.0000000000000118

Turo, R., Jallad, S., Prescott, S., & Cross, W. R. (2013). Metastatic prostate cancer in transsexual diagnosed after three decades of estrogen therapy. *Canadian Urological Association Journal, 7*(7–8), E544–E546. doi:10.5489/cuaj.175

United States Preventive Services Task Force. (2012). *The guide to clinical preventive services: Screening for cervical cancer* (Vol. *AHRQ* Publication No. 11-05156-EF-3). Baltimore, MD: Lippincott Williams & Wilkins.

U.S. Department of Health and Human Services. (2012). *Healthy People 2020 topics & objectives: Lesbian, gay, bisexual, and transgender health.* Retrieved from http://www.healthypeople.gov/2020/topicsobjectives2020/overview.aspx?topicid=25.

Ussher, J. M., Perz, J., Kellett, A., Chambers, S., Latini, D., Davis, I. D.,… Williams, S. (2016). Health-related quality of life, psychological distress, and sexual changes following prostate cancer: A comparison of gay and bisexual men with heterosexual men. *Journal of Sexual Medicine, 13*(3), 425–434. doi:10.1016/j.jsxm.2015.12.026

Ussher, J. M., Perz, J., Rose, D., Dowsett, G. W., Chambers, S., Williams, S.,… Latini, D. (2016). Threat of sexual disqualification: The consequences of erectile dysfunction and other sexual changes for gay and bisexual men with prostate cancer. *Archives of Sexual Behavior,* 1–15.

Wassersug, R. J., Lyons, A., Duncan, D., Dowsett, G. W., & Pitts, M. (2013). Diagnostic and outcome differences between heterosexual and nonheterosexual men treated for prostate cancer. *Urology, 82*(3), 565–571. doi:10.1016/j.urology.2013.04.022

Waterman, L., & Voss, J. (2015). HPV, cervical cancer risks, and barriers to care for lesbian women. *The Nurse Practitioner, 40*(1), 46–53. doi:10.1097/01.NPR.0000457431.20036.5c

Zaritsky, E., & Dibble, S. L. (2010). Risk factors for reproductive and breast cancers among older lesbians. *Journal of Women's Health, 19*(1), 125–131. doi:10.1089/jwh.2008.1094

CHAPTER **6**

Chronic Illnesses and Conditions in Gender and Sexual Minority Individuals

Jane A. McElroy and Maria T. Brown

Current trends in population growth, an aging population, and improved medical care with concomitant increased survival rates foretell increased prevalence of chronic conditions across all populations (Goodman, Posner, Huang, Parekh, & Koh, 2013). A standardized definition of chronic conditions has yet to be established, and as described by Goodman and colleagues (2013), heterogeneity in definitions varies on many characteristics such as requiring medical attention or inability to be cured. Two characteristics are consistent among the various definitions: duration (typically existing for at least a year) and limitation in function, often provided from participants' self-reports (Goodman et al., 2013). As discussed throughout this book, gender and sexual minority (GSM) individuals experience health inequalities, and these may translate into a higher prevalence in selected chronic conditions for this population (Conron, Mimiaga, & Landers, 2010; Fredriksen-Goldsen, Kim, Barkan, Muraco, & Hoy-Ellis, 2013; Ward, Dahlhamer, Galinsky, & Joestl, 2014); however, at present, the state of the literature is somewhat limited.

Two theories have been posited regarding aging, disparity, and chronic condition prevalence. Compression of morbidity theory suggests that as one grows old, the disparity gap narrows since only the hardiest individuals survive (Beckett, 2000; House, Lantz, & Herd, 2005). In essence, mortality drives this narrowing or elimination of health disparities among disadvantaged minority groups in old age. The cumulative disadvantage hypothesis suggests the opposite—a widening of the health disparity gap due to accumulation of burden over time (Dupre, 2007; J. Kim & Durden, 2007; Lauderdale, 2001). The concept of chronic stress experienced by GSM individuals over a lifetime translates into a wearing down of biological coping systems and thereby results in an increased prevalence of chronic conditions (Cohen, Kessler, & Gordon, 1995). Establishing prevalence of chronic conditions over the life course among GSM groups compared to cisgender heterosexual groups can provide support for either or both of these theories, depending on the outcome and results.

Based on an extensive review of the existing literature, the 2011 Institute of Medicine (IOM) report on *The Health of Lesbian, Gay, Bisexual, and Transgender People: Building a Foundation for Better Understanding* recommended population-based collection of data on GSM individuals through the inclusion of sexual orientation and gender identity questions in population-based health surveys (IOM, 2011). Subsequently, an increasing number of national or state surveillance studies (e.g., Behavioral Risk Factor Surveillance Study [BRFSS], state studies, pooled data, California Health Interview Study, Los Angeles County Study, and the National Health Interview Survey [NHIS]) have published data on the prevalence of a selected number of chronic conditions based on self-reported sexual orientation (Blosnich, Farmer, Lee, Silenzio, & Bowen, 2014; Boehmer, Miao, Linkletter, & Clark, 2012, 2014; Conron et al., 2010; Diamant & Wold, 2003; Fredriksen-Goldsen et al., 2013; Garland-Forshee, Fiala, Ngo, & Moseley, 2014; Ward et al., 2014). Although in these population-based studies between 2% and 10% of the respondents self-identify as GSM, these relatively small sample sizes limit the analysis of multiple social identities within the GSM population.

For this chapter, prevalence of four chronic conditions—hypertension/cardiovascular disease (CVD), asthma, diabetes, and self-reported poor health among GSM as compared to cisgender heterosexual populations—is described. However, only one study to date describes prevalence of chronic conditions (i.e., asthma and diabetes) among transgender individuals, using the Massachusetts BRFSS survey (Conron, Scott, Stowell, & Landers, 2012). This state of affairs mirrors early sexual minority research in which little was known about the health of sexual minority individuals. In the mid-20th century, most of the research was on nonheterosexual sexual orientation as a disease (Moleiro & Pinto, 2015). Starting in the 1980s, the focus of research was primarily on HIV/AIDS/sexually transmitted infections, and then when other health conditions were considered, before the beginning of the 21st century, nonprobability samples were primarily available (Fredriksen-Goldsen & Muraco, 2010; Snyder, 2011). Consequently, for research about sexual minority participants, data from probability sampling using population-based samples will be reported later; however, for research about transgender participants, any published data will be reported.

RISK FACTORS FOR CHRONIC DISEASE

To frame our subsequent discussion of individual chronic diseases, it is important to also examine the differences in risk factors for chronic disease that have been examined within GSM populations. Comparison of health-related risk factors between GSM and cisgender heterosexual individuals has been published for decades using large convenience samples with high consistency in findings (IOM, 2011). These findings have been confirmed in more recent surveillance studies. Some risk factors are closely tied to certain chronic conditions. For example, physical inactivity, obesity, tobacco use, and excessive alcohol consumption are well-established major risk factors for CVD, hypertension, diabetes, and poor health (Booth, Roberts, & Laye, 2012; Sturm, 2002). As indicated in the IOM report, GSM populations have the highest rates of tobacco use and excess alcohol consumption (IOM, 2011). Boehmer et al. (2012) compared prevalence by sex of current smoking status, alcohol consumption, and binge drinking among other health behaviors by age cohort (dichotomous <50 and ≥50 years). Both age groups of lesbians and only the younger age group of bisexual women were significantly more likely to smoke and binge drink, compared to heterosexual, cisgender female participants. However, the pattern was less consistent for sexual minority men. Only gay men in the younger age group were significantly more likely to smoke and drink alcohol during the last month, but were not more likely to binge drink compared to heterosexual, cisgender men. In contrast, only bisexual men in the older age group were more likely to smoke (Boehmer et al., 2012). The implication of these findings is that reporting GSM population health statistics as a homogeneous group is problematic, as is extrapolating the effect of risk factors engaged in earlier in adulthood as influential on chronic disease risk later in life (Boehmer, Miao, Linkletter, & Clark, 2014).

With regard to weight status, lesbians and bisexual women are consistently reported to be more likely to be overweight or obese (Boehmer, Bowen, & Bauer, 2007; Eliason et al., 2015; McElroy & Jordan, 2014). In comparing the health effects of three risk factors (i.e., obesity, smoking, or excessive alcohol consumption), Sturm (2002) reported that the obesity effect was significantly more influential than current smoking or excessive drinking on health. Obesity was equivalent to 20 years of aging with associated risk of chronic conditions associated with this older age.

GSM populations may experience lower levels of preventive health behaviors, such as screening and access to care (Diamant et al., 2000). Access to care impacts the interpretability of health statistics due to the potential for undiagnosed conditions—that is, a failure to find a difference in diagnosis rates may not actually reflect a difference in underlying presence of disease. In the U.S. population, 15% of adults have undiagnosed hypertension (Mozaffarian et al., 2015) and 3% have undiagnosed diabetes (Centers for Disease Control and Prevention [CDC], 2014). Two other modifiable risk factors for many chronic diseases—physical activity and healthy dietary choices—also vary by sexual orientation, though these findings are inconsistent (Minnis et al., 2016). Stress may influence biological processes, such as inflammatory processes, resulting in higher allostatic load, thereby influencing CVD risk (McEwen, 1998; McEwen & Stellar, 1993). GSM individuals have higher stress levels compared to cisgender heterosexual individuals (McElroy, Wintemberg, Cronk, & Everett, 2016). Taken together, the higher prevalence of health risk factors, decreased access to health care, and higher stress levels among GSM subgroups may lead to a higher prevalence of chronic conditions (Boehmer et al., 2014). For additional discussion of health risks, see Chapter 3.

In the next section, specific chronic diseases are described, followed by a review of the literature comparing GSM to cisgender heterosexual participants.

■ HYPERTENSION AND CARDIOVASCULAR DISEASE

Hypertension (i.e., high blood pressure [BP]) is the most common primary diagnosis among U.S. adults and a leading cause of CVD (e.g., heart disease and stroke; James et al., 2014). Thus, hypertension is one of the best surrogate measures for CVDs (Desai, Stockbridge, & Temple, 2006; Fleming & Powers, 2012; Lassere, Johnson, Schiff, & Rees, 2012; Micheel & Ball, 2010). Although estimates vary, hypertension currently affects about one in three Americans (Nwankwo, Yoon, Burt, & Gu, 2013; Whelton, 2015). Average BP is not a static number until late in life. Specifically, systolic BP tends to increase until individuals reach their 70s or 80s and then tends to remain constant. In contrast, diastolic BP tends to increase until individuals reach their 50s or 60s and then tends to remain constant or decrease (Whelton, 1994). About 90% of individuals will have high BP during their lifetimes (Vasan et al., 2002). Among those with high BP, approximately one half to two thirds will have uncontrolled high BP (James et al., 2014; Wang & Vasan, 2005).

CVD continues to be the leading cause of death in the United States for both men and women (Mozaffarian et al., 2015). However, the incidence of CVD in women is lower until the sixth decade of life at which time incidence rates are similar between men and women (Kazis, Selim, Rogers, Qian, & Brazier, 2012). Since the late 1990s, CVD mortality rates have continued to decline in the United States; however, approximately one death per minute is attributable to CVD (Mozaffarian et al., 2015; Xu, Murphy, Kochanek, & Bastian, 2016).

Epidemiology in GSM Populations

In a systematic review of lesbian and bisexual women completed in 2016, Simoni, Smith, Oost, Lehavot, and Fredriksen-Goldsen (2016) did not find strong evidence of higher prevalence of hypertension among sexual minority compared to cisgender heterosexual women, even though a higher obesity prevalence among sexual minority women is consistently documented. Simoni and colleagues (2016) speculate that the lack of evidence of hypertension among sexual minority women may be related to relatively young participants in the studies. For sexual minority men, the evidence is mixed, with some studies showing no increased prevalence of hypertension (Dilley, Simmons, Boysun, Pizacani, & Stark, 2010; Fredriksen-Goldsen et al., 2013; Ward, Joestl, Galinsky, & Dahlhamer, 2015) and others showing an increased prevalence (Everett & Mollborn, 2013; Wallace, Cochran, Durazo, & Ford, 2011) compared to cisgender heterosexual men.

With regard to CVD, Fredriksen-Goldsen and colleagues (2013) reported a statistically significant increased risk of being diagnosed with CVD for lesbians and bisexual women aged 50 years and older compared to similarly aged cisgender heterosexual women. This differed from another study that reported both lesbians and gay men younger than 40 years of age, but not groups aged 40 years or older, have significantly greater odds of being diagnosed with CVD compared to cisgender heterosexual individuals of similar age and gender (Boehmer et al., 2014). One study using 1997 Los Angeles County surveillance data did not find elevated CVD risk for sexual minority women when compared to cisgender heterosexual participants (Diamant et al., 2000). In contrast, another study using 1999 Los Angeles County surveillance data found a significant risk of CVD for lesbians and bisexual females compared to cisgender heterosexual women (Diamant & Wold, 2003). Both of these studies enrolled a small number (i.e., 36–69) of GSM participants, which is a likely factor in the instability of the results.

In pooled BRFSS data from 10 states, bisexual men (but not gay men), lesbians, and bisexual women were significantly more likely to be diagnosed with CVD (Blosnich et al., 2014). Other population-based studies report no significant differences in CVD risk for GSM individuals compared to cisgender heterosexual individuals (Blosnich & Silenzio, 2013; Conron et al., 2010, 2012; Garland-Forshee et al., 2014; Wallace et al., 2011). None of these studies were stratified by age. In addition, all but two of the aforementioned null studies (i.e., Blosnich's Veterans study and Wallace's study of participants aged 50–70 years) were made up of participants with a median or mean age of 38 to 44 years, well before the general age at which CVD reaches its peak impact as a leading cause of death. The lack of consistency of findings points to the need for robust epidemiologic studies of CVD among GSM people, as they are likely at an increased risk of reduced life expectancy from CVD events due to the stress of living in high-prejudice communities (i.e., structural stigma; Hatzenbuehler et al., 2014).

Researchers hypothesize that aging, longer duration of hormonal therapy for some transgender individuals, and gender transition later in life may increase the risk for CVD events (Witten & Whittle, 2004). A meta-analysis of CVD outcomes among a combined group of transgender men and women who used hormone therapy found that participants did not report significant CVD events, though fasting serum triglyceride levels were significantly increased (Elamin, Garcia, Murad, Erwin, & Montori, 2010). The authors also indicated that the quality of the studies used in the meta-analysis was very low, and small sample sizes did not allow for stratification by gender (a highly relevant factor). Increased cardiovascular mortality observed in randomized clinical trials of the higher dose of estrogens given to presumably heterosexual, cisgender men who had experienced a myocardial infarction (Stamler, 1977) and increased cardiovascular events in postmenopausal women in the Women's Health Initiative (WHI; lesbians were included in this initiative) using estrogen are suggestive of an association between hormone use and increased risk of CVD (Hulley et al., 1998; Rossouw et al., 2002; Wierckx et al., 2013). However, whether these findings translate to transgender women using estrogen has not been fully tested, although it is suggestive (Gooren, Wierckx, & Giltay, 2014). Similarly, long-term testosterone therapy for transgender men may increase the risk of CVD, although further research is needed (Futterweit, 1998). Finally, use of hormones acquired outside of the health care system with poor adherence or nonstandard dosage may also be associated with CVD (Feldman & Bockting, 2003; M. E. Williams & Freeman, 2007).

■ ASTHMA

Asthma is a condition that causes difficulty in breathing due to swelling and narrowing of airways. Symptoms include wheezing, coughing, shortness of breath, and chest tightness (Mitani, 2013). Asthma can be life threatening, and approximately 10 Americans die each day from asthma (Akinbami et al., 2012). Studies determining asthma prevalence in survey research can be categorized into two groups. One group obtains data on self-reported lifetime diagnosis, which includes childhood asthma, which is "outgrown" by adulthood in more than two thirds of patients (Sears et al., 2003). The other group obtains data on self-reported current asthma, which includes adult onset as well as unresolved childhood asthma (de Nijs, Venekamp, & Bel, 2013). In the United States, approximately 8.8% of adults aged 20 years and older self-report current asthma status, with a higher prevalence among obese females (14.6%) compared to normal-weight females (7.9%; Akinbami & Fryar, 2016).

Epidemiology in GSM Populations

Approximately one third of population-based studies that evaluated asthma prevalence between GSM and cisgender heterosexual populations assessed current asthma status. Compared to cisgender heterosexual participants, lesbians (Dilley et al., 2010), bisexual women (Dilley et al., 2010; Garland-Forshee et al., 2014), and heterosexual men and women with a history of same-sex sexual partners (Cochran & Mays, 2007) have been found to be at increased risk for current asthma diagnosis. In contrast, two studies did not find differences in current asthma prevalence between more general samples of sexual minorities and cisgender heterosexuals (Cochran & Mays, 2007; Ward et al., 2015).

Findings on lifetime asthma prevalence are mixed. Lifetime asthma prevalence has been found to be greater for lesbians (Boehmer et al., 2014; Conron et al., 2010; Heck & Jacobson, 2006) and bisexual women (Boehmer et al., 2014; Conron et al., 2010) when compared to cisgender heterosexual women. However, studies combining lesbians and bisexual women have found both a significantly greater prevalence of asthma in this population (Valanis et al., 2000) and a similar prevalence as cisgender heterosexual women (Fredriksen-Goldsen et al., 2013; Matthews & Lee, 2014). Another study combining all sexual minority subgroups found an increased prevalence for sexual minority veterans compared to cisgender heterosexual veterans (Blosnich & Silenzio, 2013). However, a study that merged 10 states of BRFSS data found that only bisexual men had a significantly greater prevalence of lifetime asthma compared to the cisgender heterosexual population (Blosnich et al., 2014). Finally, other studies have found that sexual minority men have a greater prevalence than cisgender heterosexual men (Fredriksen-Goldsen et al., 2013; Heck & Jacobson, 2006). When considering gender minorities, a study of Massachusetts BRFSS data found (albeit with major methodological concerns) that lifetime asthma prevalence among those who identified as transgender was not significantly different from cisgender participants (Conron et al., 2012). Further, a needs assessment performed by the Massachusetts Department of Public Health found that those who identified as transgender had the lowest prevalence of lifetime asthma compared to cisgender gay/lesbian, bisexual, and heterosexual participants (Landers & Gilsanz, 2009). It is clear that a consensus has not yet been reached in the literature, and additional studies that define the different groups: those who had childhood asthma only, those who have adult onset, and those who had asthma in childhood and continue to have asthma, may help to clarify similarities and differences in asthma prevalence between GSM and cisgender heterosexual populations.

◼ DIABETES

Diabetes mellitus (DM) is a chronic metabolic disorder that demonstrated steadily increasing prevalence each year during 1990 to 2008 followed by a leveling off from 2008 to 2012 (Geiss et al., 2014). Approximately 100 years ago, an initial distinction was made between type 1 and type 2 DM (Swidorski, 2014). Type 1 DM, formerly known as juvenile diabetes, in which the body does not produce insulin, is usually diagnosed in children and young adults. Approximately 5% of those diagnosed with DM have type 1. In contrast, type 2 DM (formally known as "noninsulin-dependent DM" and formerly known as "adult-onset diabetes") is associated with insulin resistance, relative insulin deficiency, and hyperglycemia (Olokoba, Obateru, & Olokoba, 2012). DM is the seventh leading cause of death in the United States and has an estimated 29.1 million cases (of which approximately one-fourth are undiagnosed; CDC, 2014). Men with type 1 DM lose an estimated 11 years of life, and women with type 1 DM lose an estimated 13 years of life because of their condition (Livingstone et al., 2015). For type 2 DM, the number of years lost increases with diagnosis earlier in adulthood. For example, newly diagnosed 40-year-old men and women will lose about 12 years of life. In contrast, about 1.8 years loss will occur for those 65 years or older and having been diagnosed with type 2 DM for less than 10 years (Engelmann et al., 2016). Most surveillance studies that ask participants about chronic illnesses make no distinction between type 1 and type 2 diabetes. Consequently, the subsequent section on diabetes prevalence in the GSM population does not distinguish between the two types of diabetes.

Epidemiology in GSM Populations

Data from studies comparing diabetes prevalence between GSM and cisgender heterosexual populations are inconsistent. Fredriksen-Goldsen et al. (2013) reported a significantly higher adjusted odds of diabetes for bisexual men (19.74%) than for gay men (9.50%; adjusted odds ratio [AOR] = 2.33; P < .01), but not when comparing either group to cisgender heterosexual men or women. Yet, when Wallace et al. (2011) compared diabetes prevalence between sexual minority and cisgender heterosexual samples aged 50 to 70 years, they reported that sexual minority men, but not sexual minority women, had a significantly greater diabetes prevalence. Another study found that only bisexual women had an increased risk of DM (Dilley et al., 2010). Finally, one study divided its population into three age groups (i.e., <40 years, 40–59 years, and ≥60 years) by gender and found that lesbians 60 years or older were twice as likely to be diagnosed with diabetes (AOR:

2.05, 95% confidence interval [CI] 1.13–3.73) compared to cisgender heterosexual women (Boehmer et al., 2014). In contrast, Blosnich and Silenzio (2013) reported a decreased diabetes prevalence among a combined group of sexual minority men and women compared to cisgender heterosexual men and women (AOR: 0.55, 95% CI 0.34–0.89). However, several studies have reported no significant difference in diabetes prevalence between sexual minority individuals and cisgender hetero-sexual individuals (Blosnich et al., 2014; Conron et al., 2010; Garland-Forshee et al., 2014; Ward et al., 2015). Reasons for the inconsistency may be related to age of the participants, number of female participants, obesity prevalence by gender, and/or combining sexual minority men and women into one group.

One area in which diabetes has particular relevance to GSM populations is for individuals receiving treatment for HIV. Metabolic perturbations including DM and insulin resistance have been linked to antiretroviral therapy use in HIV-infected adults, with an older regime of antiretroviral therapy potentially having played a critical role (Nix & Tien, 2014). A Danish HIV cohort study reported that an older cohort of HIV-infected patients showed an increased risk of DM, but this increased risk was not found in a more recent cohort (Rasmussen et al., 2012). They suggested that the highly active antiretroviral therapy (HAART) regimen including indinavir, saquinavir, stavudine, and didanosine, rarely used in the modern era of antiretroviral therapy, may be a causal factor for the increased DM risk only in the older cohort (Nix & Tien, 2014; Rasmussen et al., 2012). A meta-analysis of three studies suggested that coinfection of hepatitis C and HIV increases the risk of DM in comparison to HIV+ (only) controls ($OR_{unadjusted}$ = 1.82, 95% CI 1.27–2.38), though only three studies were used for the analysis (White, Ratziu, & El-Serag, 2008).

A needs assessment performed by the Massachusetts Department of Public Health using a convenience sample reported that those who identified as transgen-der had the lowest prevalence of DM compared to cisgender gay/lesbian, bisex-ual, and heterosexual participants (Landers & Gilsanz, 2009). Wierckx et al. (2013) separately evaluated transgender men and women who were taking hormones compared to age- and gender-matched control individuals. Both transgender men and women had higher prevalence of diabetes compared to cisgender participants, but this prevalence was observed before starting hormone therapy in transgender women. Further, diabetes incidence was higher in transgender men during hor-mone therapy than cisgender control men and women (Wierckx et al., 2013).

◼ SELF-REPORTED HEALTH

The single item asking, "Would you say your health, in general, is excellent, very good, good, fair, or poor" has been shown in numerous studies to be a valid and reliable measure of general health status (Ferraro & Yu, 1995; Frankenberg & Jones, 2004). However, few studies have been conducted to understand exactly what criteria respondents use when quantifying their health, and no studies have evaluated what health means to GSM populations when answering this question. Consequently, the overall findings of GSM individuals reporting poorer health than cisgender heterosexual individuals may be due to a different emphasis on the constructs of health (e.g., including social support, health promotion behaviors, health-related risk factors, comorbidities, physical functioning) or different established beliefs about health (e.g., health optimists or pessimists; Bailis, Segall, & Chipperfield, 2003) between the two groups rather than an indication of a higher number of chronic conditions. With this caveat in mind, we will report on the studies that compared responses to the question about the self-rating of health between GSM and cisgender heterosexuals.

Epidemiology in GSM Populations

The largest differences in self-reported fair/poor health status between sexual minority and cisgender heterosexual samples were found in the youngest age groups: 16–25 years (Branstrom, Hatzenbuehler, & Pachankis, 2016); 18–29 years; and 30–39 years (Thomeer, 2013). Dilley and colleagues' (2010) sample of young participants found that larger proportions of lesbians, bisexual women, and gay men, but not bisexual men, reported poor health compared to cisgender heterosexual participants. In contrast, one study of participants aged 50 to 70 years found that all sexual minority subgroups had higher prevalence of self-reported fair/poor health than cisgender heterosexual participants (Wallace et al., 2011).

Thomeer (2013) also evaluated self-reported health for men and women by separately comparing those reporting recent same-sex and opposite-sex relationships, while adjusting for year of interview, age, race, marital status, educational attainment, and income. Women in recent same-sex relationships were approximately twice as likely to report fair or poor health compared to women in opposite-sex relationships, while men showed no significant difference based on reported relationship (Thomeer, 2013). Similarly, in an adjusted model, female veterans who identified as a sexual minority were more likely to report poor health compared to their cisgender heterosexual counterparts (Blosnich, Foynes, & Shipherd, 2013). Analyses of the 2013 NHIS data also found that lesbians were more likely to report poor health compared to cisgender heterosexual women (Ward et al., 2014).

In a more detailed analysis using pooled data from the 2013 and 2014 NHIS, Hsieh and Ruther (2016) reported sexual minority status by race (White vs. non-White). They found that White and non-White lesbians and bisexual women, White bisexual men, and non-White gay men reported poorer health compared to White, cisgender heterosexual men in a model conditioned on sociodemographic factors. The one known study evaluating transgender health that reported on general health status did not find a difference between transgender participants and sexual minority and cisgender heterosexual participants (Conron et al., 2012). Again, however, these results should be interpreted with caution given the potential ambiguity of the core question of self-reported health within the context of GSM individuals' different lived experience.

■ RACE/ETHNICITY AND CHRONIC DISEASE

The current research on the prevalence of selected chronic conditions suggests there are differences in prevalence between GSM and cisgender heterosexual populations. However, the particulars of this disparity have yet to be adequately explored. Although understanding who among GSM individuals are at increased risk is important, the relatively small sample sizes of GSM individuals in surveillance studies have meant that, to date, stratification on other social identities has been limited. For example, H. J. Kim and Fredriksen-Goldsen (2012) suggested that elevated asthma prevalence in Hispanic lesbians compared to bisexual and heterosexual Hispanic or non-Hispanic White women may be due to the cumulative risk faced by Hispanic lesbians from their sexual as well as ethnic minority status. In contrast to the increased asthma prevalence among Hispanic lesbians, in a convenience sample of African American lesbians attending the Zuna Institute's National Black Lesbian conference, the prevalence of hypertension was comparable to that of the U.S. population (Dibble, Eliason, & Crawford, 2012). This suggested that the triply disadvantaged (i.e., African American, lesbian, and women) did not appear to have a higher cumulative risk for hypertension in this selected group of educated women leaders. These two examples demonstrate the need for adequately powered studies to investigate multiple social identities within the GSM population to thoroughly examine risks and prevalence of chronic condition (this and related topics are discussed in more detail in Chapter 15).

Oversampling of a target population is often required to increase the reliability and precision of estimates in subgroups (Andresen, Diehr, & Luke, 2004). For example, both the National Health and Nutrition Examination Survey (NHANES) and the NHIS currently oversample African American/Black, Hispanic, and Asian populations, as well as persons aged 60 years and older (National Center for Health Statistics, 2015). All of the single-state BRFSS studies mentioned in this chapter required the pooling of data over 3 to 9 years to create an adequate sample size. Even using probability sampling of a population does not necessarily overcome the potential for a lack of representativeness in samples. Most of the studies mentioned in this chapter relied on relatively young groups of respondents, and this is often listed as a limitation in the discussion of their findings. In addition, for lesbian studies, the majority of participants are often White college-educated women. These selection biases create concern about the generalizability of study findings.

■ THE ROLE OF AGE

Another social identity that may be of critical importance in determination of both chronic disease prevalence and modifiable risk factors is age. To date, only two longitudinal studies—the Nurse's Health study (NHS; lesbian: $n = 665$; bisexual: $n = 309$; Case et al., 2004) and the WHI (adult lesbian: $n = 309$; lifetime lesbian: $n = 264$; bisexual: $n = 740$; Valanis et al., 2000)—incidentally enrolled lesbian and bisexual women. For the NHS, enrollment began in 1989 and sexual orientation questions were asked in 1995. In contrast, the WHI asked sexual behavior at baseline in 1997 to classify their 50- to 79-year-old participants. The NHS, which has the capacity to evaluate modifiable risk factors associated with chronic condition prevalence over a 20-year period, has not published on this chapter's selected chronic conditions by sexual orientation to date. However, the WHI has reported significantly increased lifetime asthma prevalence, but similar hypertension prevalence, when comparing sexual minority women and cisgender heterosexual participants in their older sample (Valanis et al., 2000).

One surveillance study considered chronic conditions in younger (<40 years), middle (40–59 years), and older (≥60 years) ages by sexual orientation (Boehmer et al., 2014). Of the four chronic conditions, none of the groups of older gay or bisexual men were at increased risk compared to cisgender heterosexual men. In contrast, the groups of older lesbians were at increased risk for diabetes and asthma. Only the age groups of younger lesbians and bisexual men and women were at increased risk for fair/poor self-rated health (Boehmer et al., 2014). Boehmer and colleagues (2012) also evaluated sexual minorities' risk factors collapsing the ages into a broad age range: less than 50 years and 50 years or older. They found several risk factors elevated in both the younger and older sexual minority women groups, but generally elevated only in the group of younger sexual minority men. These findings suggest that consideration of age may be important in understanding chronic disease prevalence.

OUTNESS AND TIMING OF IDENTITY DEVELOPMENT

Increased chronic condition or mortality risk associated with GSM identity rests on the fixation of a person's identity at the time of the survey itself, regardless of GSM identification at previous or future time points. Stress associated with GSM status as well as degree of "outness" (disclosure of GSM identity to others) may also be a defining agent between GSM and cisgender heterosexual populations; however, the stresses associated with outness can vary dramatically over time for an individual. There is some empirical evidence to support this idea, beyond the theory proposed by Meyer (2003) that sexual minority stress is associated with mental health burden. Cole and colleagues have written a series of papers that provide evidence that both HIV+ and HIV− gay men's physical health is negatively influenced by concealment of their sexual orientation (Cole, Kemeny, Taylor, Visscher, & Fahey, 1996; Cole, Kemeny, Taylor, & Visscher, 1996; Cole, Kemeny, & Taylor, 1997). On the flip side, Juster, Smith, Ouellet, Sindi, and Lupien (2013) reported significantly better health status among sexual minority men, but not among sexual minority women, who are completely "out" compared to their cisgender heterosexual peers. Beyond sexual orientation and gender identity, studies should also assess the broader sociocultural context of the individual to better elucidate potential differences in chronic diseases between GSM and cisgender heterosexual populations.

Intertwined with the important construct of degree of "outness" is the concept of variability in timing of awareness or embracing of one's gender identity and sexual orientation. Diamond (2008) reported that 67% of women who initially identified as lesbian, bisexual, or "something else" modified how they defined their sexual identity at least once during the 10-year follow-up period. One reason for this may be that the reported identity was strongly linked to current relationship status (Mock & Eibach, 2012). For transgender individuals, the age at which they began living full time as their authentic gender ranged from 18 to 44 years, with transgender men transitioning at an earlier age than transgender women (Grant et al., 2011). Virtually no studies, to our knowledge, have deeply considered the timing issue as it relates to chronic disease disparity experienced by GSM population. However, in the WHI, sexual orientation was determined by classifying women as "lifetime lesbians" who only ever had sex with women, "adult lesbians" who had sex with women only after age of 45 years, and "presumably bisexual women" if the participant reported having had sex with both men and women over their adult lifetime. Differences in the prevalence of several chronic conditions were reported for adult and lifetime lesbians. For example, age-standardized prevalence for asthma was 7.6 for heterosexual women, 8.7 for bisexuals, 11.9 for lifetime lesbians, and 7.2 for adult lesbians (Valanis et al., 2000). Clearly, these statistics suggest that the timing of identifying as a sexual minority may obscure the meaning of differences in chronic conditions.

■ THE ROLE OF MENTAL HEALTH

Strong evidence of mental health disparities between GSM and cisgender heterosexual populations has been documented (see Chapter 10 for a detailed description). For example, in a study by Boehmer and colleagues (2014), all gay and lesbian age groups were at increased risk for mental health needs, and all male and female bisexual age groups, except the oldest female bisexual group, were at increased risk of depression. Evidence indicates that individuals in the general population, even with subthreshold mental disorders, also report more chronic conditions, poorer health status, and increased utilization of health services (Coulehan, Schulberg, Block, Janosky, & Arena, 1990; Katon, 2008; Koopmans & Lamers, 2000; Rucci et al., 2003). The link or pattern of causal relationships between the co-occurrence of these conditions has yet to be fully explored. None of the studies described in this chapter, when evaluating the prevalence of chronic conditions among GSM people, adjusted their models or stratified their analyses for subthreshold mental disorders.

■ THE ROLE OF ACCESS

A disparity gap in access to care for GSM individuals is often cited with numerous reasons given. For example, in a study of sexual minority women, Cochran and colleagues (2001) reported that 72% (68.9%–76.7%) of their lesbian and bisexual sample had received a pelvic exam within the past 2 or 3 years. This was substantially lower than estimates for an overall sample of U.S. women at 87.4% (86%–88.7%). The study standardized the overall sample to age, race/ethnicity, educational level, and geographical region of the sexual minority sample (Cochran et al., 2001). Studies addressing this disparity have concluded that the lower utilization of health screening in sexual minority women results from: (a) lack of insurance (Mayer et al., 2008); (b) negative experiences or fear of discrimination at the doctor's office (Tracy, Lydecker, & Ireland, 2010); (c) lower utilization of routine gynecological care (Cochran et al., 2001; Dolan & Davis, 2003); (d) physician ignorance about the need for screening, particularly for lesbians (Dolan & Davis, 2003; Ferris, Batish, Wright, Cushing, & Scott, 1996; Marrazzo, Koutsky, Kiviat, Kuypers, & Stine, 2001); (e) reduced perception of risk for cervical cancer among sexual minority women (Price, Easton, Telljohann, & Wallace, 1996); and (f) lack of health promotion targeting sexual minority women (Phillips-Angeles et al., 2004; Power, McNair, & Carr, 2009; Richardson, 2000). Similarly, a considerably higher percentage of transgender individuals (30%–40%) may not have regular medical care. Those without medical care often use the emergency room for their health care needs (Feldman & Bockting, 2003). It is not unreasonable to extrapolate from these examples that a higher proportion of GSM individuals may be living with undiagnosed chronic conditions, such as hypertension and diabetes (M. E. Williams & Freeman, 2007).

BIOLOGIC CAUSALITY

Research on the underlying mechanism(s) associated with health disparities faced by GSM populations should be pursued so that strategies can be implemented to eliminate these. Three physiological pathways have been suggested (Lick, Durso, & Johnson, 2013). The first is altered functioning of the hypothalamic–pituitary–adrenal axis. This axis has a significant role in controlling reactions to stress as well as regulating the immune system among other body processes. One hypothesized mechanism is heightened cortisol response when self-identity is or could be negatively judged by others (Dickerson & Kemeny, 2004). A second mechanism is autonomic nervous system (ANS) reactivity. ANS reactivity is typically measured by heart rate and BP. Discrimination has been strongly associated with cardiovascular reactivity with the downstream effect on CVD, especially among African Americans (D. R. Williams & Mohammed, 2009). One study evaluated ANS reactivity in a laboratory setting involving gay men who did and did not disclose their sexual orientation to others by having participants talk about difficulties associated with concealing one's sexual orientation (Perez-Benitez, O'Brien, Carels, Gordon, & Chiros, 2007). Overall, the authors argued that sexual orientation concealment is stressful and can be associated with chronic cardiovascular reactivity (Perez-Benitez et al., 2007). The third pathway is alteration of immune functioning. Segerstrom and Miller (2004) evaluated over 300 studies and concluded that chronic stress was associated with numerous measures of immune dysregulation, such as inflammatory engagement and poor antibody responses. One could argue that because many GSM individuals face antigay and/or transphobic stigma, these experiences may affect the immune system. As mentioned previously, Cole and colleagues' (1996) research has demonstrated that sexual orientation concealment among sexual minority men was associated with increased risk of several infectious diseases such as pneumonia, bronchitis, sinusitis, and tuberculosis. These mechanisms are a promising area of research that might provide empirical evidence to help explain the disparity in the selected chronic condition described in this chapter.

CONCLUSION

Demographic trends indicate future increases in the prevalence of chronic conditions across all populations (Goodman et al., 2013). In particular, GSM populations have been identified as experiencing health inequalities that may translate into higher prevalence rates of selected chronic conditions. Although the data explored in this chapter suggest there are differences in prevalence of selected chronic conditions—hypertension, CVD, asthma, diabetes, and poor self-rated health—between GSM and cisgender heterosexual populations, the particular causes of these disparities have yet to be fully explored. There are several issues in existing research on GSM populations that limit both our understanding of the factors influencing chronic condition prevalence in this population and the generalizability of findings generated by research on this question.

Regardless of the underlying reasons for disparities in access to medical care and utilization of recommended health screenings, it is generally understood that lack of access increases the likelihood of GSM individuals living with undiagnosed chronic conditions such as hypertension or diabetes. Strategies for eliminating the health disparities experienced by GSM populations require a better understanding of their underlying mechanism(s). Future health research with GSM populations should explore these mechanisms and improve our understanding of the disparities in chronic conditions in this population. Finally, there is a strong need to capture GSM identity on all national surveillance surveys, which would undoubtedly help to advance the field.

■ REFERENCES

Akinbami, L. J., & Fryar, C. D. (2016). Asthma prevalence by weight status among adults: United States, 2001–2014 (NCHS Data Brief No. 239). Retrieved from http://www.cdc.gov/nchs/data/databriefs/db239.pdf

Akinbami, L. J., Moorman, J. E., Bailey, C., Zahran, H. S., King, M., Johnson, C. A., & Liu, X. (2012). Trends in asthma prevalence, health care use, and mortality in the United States, 2001–2010 (NCHS Data Brief No. 94). Retrieved from http://www.cdc.gov/nchs/products/databriefs/db94.htm

Andresen, E. M., Diehr, P. H., & Luke, D. A. (2004). Public health surveillance of low-frequency populations. *Annual Review of Public Health, 25,* 25–52. doi:10.1146/annurev.publhealth.25.101802.123111

Bailis, D. S., Segall, A., & Chipperfield, J. G. (2003). Two views of self-rated general health status. *Social Science & Medicine, 56*(2), 203–217.

Beckett, M. (2000). Converging health inequalities in later life: An artifact of mortality selection. *Journal of Health & Social Behavior, 41*(1), 106–119.

Blosnich, J. R., Farmer, G. W., Lee, J. G., Silenzio, V. M., & Bowen, D. J. (2014). Health inequalities among sexual minority adults: Evidence from ten U.S. states, 2010. *American Journal of Preventive Medicine, 46*(4), 337–349.

Blosnich, J. R., Foynes, M. M., & Shipherd, J. C. (2013). Health disparities among sexual minority women veterans. *Journal of Women's Health, 22*(7), 631–636. doi:10.1089/jwh.2012.4214

Blosnich, J. R., & Silenzio, V. M. (2013). Physical health indicators among lesbian, gay, and bisexual U.S. veterans. *Annals of Epidemiology, 23*(7), 448–451. doi:10.1016/j.annepidem.2013.04.009

Boehmer, U., Bowen, D. J., & Bauer, G. R. (2007). Overweight and obesity in sexual-minority women: Evidence from population-based data. *American Journal of Public Health, 97*(6), 1134–1140. doi:10.2105/AJPH.2006.088419

Boehmer, U., Miao, X., Linkletter, C., & Clark, M. A. (2012). Adult health behaviors over the life course by sexual orientation. *American Journal of Public Health, 102*(2), 292–300. doi:10.2105/AJPH.2011.300334

Boehmer, U., Miao, X., Linkletter, C., & Clark, M. A. (2014). Health conditions in younger, middle, and older ages: Are there differences by sexual orientation? *LGBT Health, 1*(3), 168–176. doi:10.1089/lgbt.2013.0033

Booth, F. W., Roberts, C. K., & Laye, M. J. (2012). Lack of exercise is a major cause of chronic diseases. *Comprehensive Physiology, 2*(2), 1143–1211. doi:10.1002/cphy.c110025

Branstrom, R., Hatzenbuehler, M. L., & Pachankis, J. E. (2016). Sexual orientation disparities in physical health: Age and gender effects in a population-based study. *Social Psychiatry and Psychiatric Epidemiology, 51*(2), 289–301. doi:10.1007/s00127-015-1116-0

Case, P., Austin, S. B., Hunter, D. J., Manson, J. E., Malspeis, S., Willett, W. C., & Spiegelman, D. (2004). Sexual orientation, health risk factors, and physical functioning in the Nurses' Health Study II. *Journal of Women's Health, 13*(9), 1033–1047.

Centers for Disease Control and Prevention. (2014). *National Diabetes Statistics Report: Estimates of diabetes and its burden in the United States, 2014.* Atlanta, GA: U.S. Department of Health and Human Services. Retrieved from https://www.cdc.gov/diabetes/pubs/statsreport14/national-diabetes-report-web.pdf

Cochran, S. D., & Mays, V. M. (2007). Physical health complaints among lesbians, gay men, and bisexual and homosexually experienced heterosexual individuals: Results from the California Quality of Life Survey. *American Journal of Public Health, 97*(11), 2048–2055.

Cochran, S. D., Mays, V. M., Bowen, D., Gage, S., Bybee, D., Roberts, S. J.,...White, J. (2001). Cancer-related risk indicators and preventive screening behaviors among lesbians and bisexual women. *American Journal of Public Health, 91*(4), 591–597.

Cohen, S., Kessler, R. C., & Gordon, L. U. (1995). Strategies for measuring stress in studies of psychiatric and physical disorders. In S. Cohen, R. C. Kessler, & L. G. Underwood (Eds.), *Measuring stress: A guide for health and social scientists* (pp. 3–28). New York, NY: Oxford University Press.

Cole, S. W., Kemeny, M. E., & Taylor, S. E. (1997). Social identity and physical health: Accelerated HIV progression in rejection-sensitive gay men. *Journal of Personality & Social Psychology, 72*(2), 320–335.

Cole, S. W., Kemeny, M. E., Taylor, S. E., & Visscher, B. R. (1996). Elevated physical health risk among gay men who conceal their homosexual identity. *Health Psychology, 15*(4), 243–251.

Cole, S. W., Kemeny, M. E., Taylor, S. E., Visscher, B. R., & Fahey, J. L. (1996). Accelerated course of human immunodeficiency virus infection in gay men who conceal their homosexual identity. *Psychosomatic Medicine, 58*(3), 219–231.

Conron, K. J., Mimiaga, M. J., & Landers, S. J. (2010). A population-based study of sexual orientation identity and gender differences in adult health. *American Journal of Public Health, 100*(10), 1953–1960. doi:10.2105/AJPH.2009.174169

Conron, K. J., Scott, G., Stowell, G. S., & Landers, S. J. (2012). Transgender health in Massachusetts: Results from a household probability sample of adults. *American Journal of Public Health, 102*(1), 118–122. doi:10.2105/AJPH.2011.300315

Coulehan, J. L., Schulberg, H. C., Block, M. R., Janosky, J. E., & Arena, V. C. (1990). Depressive symptomatology and medical co-morbidity in a primary care clinic. *International Journal of Psychiatry in Medicine, 20*(4), 335–347.

de Nijs, S. B., Venekamp, L. N., & Bel, E. H. (2013). Adult-onset asthma: Is it really different? *European Respiratory Review, 22*(127), 44–52. doi:10.1183/09059180.00007112

Desai, M., Stockbridge, N., & Temple, R. (2006). Blood pressure as an example of a biomarker that functions as a surrogate. *AAPS Journal, 8*(1), E146–E152. doi:10.1208/aapsj080117

Diamant, A. L., & Wold, C. (2003). Sexual orientation and variation in physical and mental health status among women. *Journal of Women's Health, 12*(1), 41–49.

Diamant, A. L., Wold, C., Spritzer, K., Gelberg, L., Diamant, A. L., Wold, C.,...Gelberg, L. (2000). Health behaviors, health status, and access to and use of health care: A population-based study of lesbian, bisexual, and heterosexual women. *Archives of Family Medicine, 9*(10), 1043–1051.

Diamond, L. M. (2008). Female bisexuality from adolescence to adulthood: Results from a 10-year longitudinal study. *Developmental Psychology, 44*(1), 5–14. doi:10.1037/0012-1649.44.1.5

Dibble, S. L., Eliason, M. J., & Crawford, B. (2012). Correlates of well-being among African American lesbians. *Journal of Homosexuality, 59*(6), 820–838. doi:10.1080/00918369.2012.69476

Dickerson, S. S., & Kemeny, M. E. (2004). Acute stressors and cortisol responses: A theoretical integration and synthesis of laboratory research. *Psychological Bulletin, 130*(3), 355–391. doi:10.1037/0033-2909.130.3.355

Dilley, J. A., Simmons, K. W., Boysun, M. J., Pizacani, B. A., & Stark, M. J. (2010). Demonstrating the importance and feasibility of including sexual orientation in public health surveys: Health disparities in the Pacific Northwest. *American Journal of Public Health, 100*(3), 460–467. doi:10.2105/AJPH.2007.130336

Dolan, K. A., & Davis, P. W. (2003). Nuances and shifts in lesbian women's constructions of STI and HIV vulnerability. *Social Science & Medicine, 57*(1), 25–38.

Dupre, M. E. (2007). Educational differences in age-related patterns of disease: Reconsidering the cumulative disadvantage and age-as-leveler hypotheses. *Journal of Health & Social Behavior, 48*(1), 1–15.

Elamin, M. B., Garcia, M. Z., Murad, M. H., Erwin, P. J., & Montori, V. M. (2010). Effect of sex steroid use on cardiovascular risk in transsexual individuals: A systematic review and meta-analyses. *Clinical Endocrinology, 72*(1), 1–10. doi:10.1111/j.1365-2265.2009.03632.x

Eliason, M. J., Ingraham, N., Fogel, S. C., McElroy, J. A., Lorvick, J., Mauery, D. R., & Haynes, S. (2015). A systematic review of the literature on weight in sexual minority women. *Women's Health Issues, 25*(2), 162–175. doi:10.1016/j.whi.2014.12.001

Engelmann, J., Manuwald, U., Rubach, C., Kugler, J., Birkenfeld, A. L., Hanefeld, M., & Rothe, U. (2016). Determinants of mortality in patients with type 2 diabetes: A review. *Reviews in Endocrine & Metabolic Disorders, 17*(1), 129–137. doi:10.1007/s11154-016-9349-0

Everett, B., & Mollborn, S. (2013). Differences in hypertension by sexual orientation among U.S. young adults. *Journal of Community Health, 38*(3), 588–596. doi:10.1007/s10900-013-9655-3

Feldman, J., & Bockting, W. (2003). Transgender health. *Minnesota Medicine, 86*(7), 25–32.

Ferraro, K. F., & Yu, Y. (1995). Body weight and self-ratings of health. *Journal of Health & Social Behavior, 36*(3), 274–284.

Ferris, D. G., Batish, S., Wright, T. C., Cushing, C., & Scott, E. H. (1996). A neglected lesbian health concern: Cervical neoplasia. *Journal of Family Practice, 43*(6), 581–584.

Fleming, T. R., & Powers, J. H. (2012). Biomarkers and surrogate endpoints in clinical trials. *Statistics in Medicine, 31*(25), 2973–2984. doi:10.1002/sim.5403

Frankenberg, E., & Jones, N. R. (2004). Self-rated health and mortality: Does the relationship extend to a low income setting? *Journal of Health & Social Behavior, 45*(4), 441–452.

Fredriksen-Goldsen, K. I., Kim, H. J., Barkan, S. E., Muraco, A., & Hoy-Ellis, C. P. (2013). Health disparities among lesbian, gay, and bisexual older adults: Results from a population-based study. *American Journal of Public Health, 103*(10), 1802–1809. doi:10.2105/AJPH.2012.301110

Fredriksen-Goldsen, K. I., & Muraco, A. (2010). Aging and sexual orientation: A 25-year review of the literature. *Research on Aging, 32*(3), 372–413. doi:10.1177/0164027509360355

Futterweit, W. (1998). Endocrine therapy of transsexualism and potential complications of long-term treatment. *Archives of Sexual Behavior, 27*(2), 209–226.

Garland-Forshee, R. Y., Fiala, S. C., Ngo, D. L., & Moseley, K. (2014). Sexual orientation and sex differences in adult chronic conditions, health risk factors, and protective health practices, Oregon, 2005–2008. *Preventing Chronic Disease, 11*, E136. doi:10.5888/pcd11.140126

Geiss, L. S., Wang, J., Cheng, Y. J., Thompson, T. J., Barker, L., Li, Y.,...Gregg, E. W. (2014). Prevalence and incidence trends for diagnosed diabetes among adults aged 20 to 79 years, United States, 1980–2012. *Journal of the American Medical Association, 312*(12), 1218–1226. doi:10.1001/jama.2014.11494

Goodman, R. A., Posner, S. F., Huang, E. S., Parekh, A. K., & Koh, H. K. (2013). Defining and measuring chronic conditions: Imperatives for research, policy, program, and practice. *Preventing Chronic Disease, 10*, E66. doi:10.5888/pcd10.120239

Gooren, L. J., Wierckx, K., & Giltay, E. J. (2014). Cardiovascular disease in transsexual persons treated with cross-sex hormones: Reversal of the traditional sex difference in cardiovascular disease pattern. *European Journal of Endocrinology, 170*(6), 809–819. doi:10.1530/EJE-14-0011

Grant, J. M., Mottet, L. A., Tanis, J., Harrison, J., Herman, J. L., & Keisling, M. (2011). *Injustice at every turn: A report of the National Transgender Discrimination Survey*. Washington, DC: National Center for Transgender Equality and National Gay and Lesbian Task Force.

Hatzenbuehler, M. L., Bellatorre, A., Lee, Y., Finch, B. K., Muennig, P., & Fiscella, K. (2014). Structural stigma and all-cause mortality in sexual minority populations. *Social Science & Medicine, 103*, 33–41. doi:10.1016/j.socscimed.2013.06.005

Heck, J. E., & Jacobson, J. S. (2006). Asthma diagnosis among individuals in same-sex relationships. *Journal of Asthma, 43*(8), 579–584.

House, J. S., Lantz, P. M., & Herd, P. (2005). Continuity and change in the social stratification of aging and health over the life course: Evidence from a Nationally Representative Longitudinal Study from 1986 to 2001/2002 (Americans' Changing Lives Study). *Journals of Gerontology, Series B: Psychological Sciences and Social Sciences, 60*(Spec. Iss. 2), S15–S26. doi:60/suppl_Special_Issue_2/S15

Hsieh, N., & Ruther, M. (2016). Sexual minority health and health risk factors: Intersection effects of gender, race, and sexual identity. *American Journal of Preventive Medicine, 50*(6), 746–755. doi:10.1016/j.amepre.2015.11.016

Hulley, S., Grady, D., Bush, T., Furberg, C., Herrington, D., Riggs, B., & Vittinghoff, E. (1998). Randomized trial of estrogen plus progestin for secondary prevention of coronary heart disease in postmenopausal women: Heart and Estrogen/progestin Replacement Study (HERS) Research Group. *Journal of the American Medical Association, 280*(7), 605–613.

Institutes of Medicine. (2011). *The health of lesbian, gay, bisexual, and transgender people: Building a foundation for better understanding*. Washington, DC: National Academies Press.

James, P. A., Oparil, S., Carter, B. L., Cushman, W. C., Dennison-Himmelfarb, C., Handler, J.,...Ortiz, E. (2014). 2014 evidence-based guideline for the management of high blood pressure in adults: Report from the panel members appointed to the Eighth Joint National Committee (JNC 8). *Journal of the American Medical Association, 311*(5), 507–520. doi:10.1001/jama.2013.284427

Juster, R. P., Smith, N. G., Ouellet, É., Sindi, S., & Lupien, S. J. (2013). Sexual orientation and disclosure in relation to psychiatric symptoms, diurnal cortisol, and allostatic load. *Psychosomatic Medicine, 75*(2), 103–116. doi:10.1097/PSY.0b013e3182826881

Katon, W. J. (2008). The comorbidity of diabetes mellitus and depression. *American Journal of Medicine, 121*(11 Suppl. 2), S8–S15. doi:10.1016/j.amjmed.2008.09.008

Kazis, L. E., Selim, A. J., Rogers, W., Qian, S. X., & Brazier, J. (2012). Monitoring outcomes for the Medicare Advantage program: Methods and application of the VR-12 for evaluation of plans. *Journal of Ambulatory Care Management, 35*(4), 263–276. doi:10.1097/JAC.0b013e318267468f

Kim, H. J., & Fredriksen-Goldsen, K. I. (2012). Hispanic lesbians and bisexual women at heightened risk for [corrected] health disparities. *American Journal of Public Health, 102*(1), e9–e15. doi:10.2105/AJPH.2011.300378

Kim, J., & Durden, E. (2007). Socioeconomic status and age trajectories of health. *Social Science & Medicine, 65*(12), 2489–2502. doi:10.1016/j.socscimed.2007.07.022

Koopmans, G. T., & Lamers, L. M. (2000). Chronic conditions, psychological distress and the use of psychoactive medications. *Journal of Psychosomatic Research, 48*(2), 115–123.

Landers, S., & Gilsanz, P. (2009). The health of lesbian, gay, bisexual and transgender (LGBT) persons in Massachusetts. Retrieved from http://www.masstpc.org/wp-content/uploads/2012/10/DPH-2009-lgbt-health-report.pdf

Lassere, M. N., Johnson, K. R., Schiff, M., & Rees, D. (2012). Is blood pressure reduction a valid surrogate endpoint for stroke prevention? An analysis incorporating a systematic review of randomised controlled trials, a by-trial weighted errors-in-variables regression, the surrogate threshold effect (STE) and the Biomarker-Surrogacy (BioSurrogate) Evaluation Schema (BSES). *BMC Medical Research Methodology, 12*, 27. doi:10.1186/1471-2288-12-27

Lauderdale, D. S. (2001). Education and survival: Birth cohort, period, and age effects. *Demography, 38*(4), 551–561.

Lick, D. J., Durso, L. E., & Johnson, K. L. (2013). Minority stress and physical health among sexual minorities. *Perspectives on Psychological Science, 8*(5), 521–548.

Livingstone, S. J., Levin, D., Looker, H. C., Lindsay, R. S., Wild, S. H., Joss, N., . . . Colhoun, H. M.; Scottish Diabetes Research Network epidemiology group; Scottish Renal Registry. (2015). Estimated life expectancy in a Scottish cohort with type 1 diabetes, 2008–2010. *Journal of the American Medical Association, 313*(1), 37–44. doi:10.1001/jama.2014.16425

Marrazzo, J. M., Koutsky, L. A., Kiviat, N. B., Kuypers, J. M., & Stine, K. (2001). Papanicolaou test screening and prevalence of genital human papillomavirus among women who have sex with women. *American Journal of Public Health, 91*(6), 947–952.

Matthews, D. D., & Lee, J. G. (2014). A profile of North Carolina lesbian, gay, and bisexual health disparities, 2011. *American Journal of Public Health, 104*(6), e98–e105.

Mayer, K. H., Bradford, J. B., Makadon, H. J., Stall, R., Goldhammer, H., & Landers, S. (2008). Sexual and gender minority health: What we know and what needs to be done. *American Journal of Public Health, 98*(6), 989–995. doi:10.2105/AJPH.2007.127811

McElroy, J. A., & Jordan, J. (2014). Disparate perceptions of weight between sexual minority and heterosexual female college students. *LGBT Health, 1*(2), 122–130. doi:10.1089/lgbt.2013.0021

McElroy, J. A., Wintemberg, J. J., Cronk, N. J., & Everett, K. D. (2016). The association of resilience, perceived stress and predictors of depressive symptoms in sexual and gender minority youths and adults. *Psychology and Sexuality, 7*(2), 116–130. doi:10.1080/19419899.2015.1076504

McEwen, B. S. (1998). Protective and damaging effects of stress mediators. *New England Journal of Medicine, 338*(3), 171–179.

McEwen, B. S., & Stellar, E. (1993). Stress and the individual: Mechanisms leading to disease. *Archives of Internal Medicine, 153*(18), 2093–2101.

Meyer, I. H. (2003). Prejudice, social stress, and mental health in lesbian, gay, and bisexual populations: Conceptual issues and research evidence. *Psychological Bulletin, 129*(5), 674–697.

Micheel, C. M., & Ball, J. R. (Eds.). (2010). *Evaluation of biomarkers and surrogate endpoints in chronic disease* (pp. 1–15). Retrieved from http://books.nap.edu/catalog/12869.html

Minnis, A. M., Catellier, D., Kent, C., Ethier, K. A., Soler, R. E., Heirendt, W., . . . Rogers, T. (2016). Differences in chronic disease behavioral indicators by sexual orientation and sex. *Journal of Public Health Management Practice, 22*(Suppl. 1), S25–S32. doi:10.1097/PHH.0000000000000350

Mitani, A. (2013). Asthma. In M. D. Gellman & J. R. Turner (Eds.), *Encyclopedia of behavioral medicine* (pp. 139–140). Springer reference. New York, NY: Springer.

Mock, S. E., & Eibach, R. P. (2012). Stability and change in sexual orientation identity over a 10-year period in adulthood. *Archives of Sexual Behavior, 41*(3), 641–648. doi:10.1007/s10508-011-9761-1

Moleiro, C., & Pinto, N. (2015). Sexual orientation and gender identity: Review of concepts, controversies and their relation to psychopathology classification systems. *Frontiers in Psychology, 6*, 1511. doi:10.3389/fpsyg.2015.01511

Mozaffarian, D., Benjamin, E. J., Go, A. S., Arnett, D. K., Blaha, M. J., Cushman, M.,...Turner, M. B.; American Heart Association Statistics Committee and Stroke Statistics. (2015). Heart disease and stroke statistics—2015 update: A report from the American Heart Association. *Circulation, 131*(4), e29–e322. doi:10.1161/CIR.0000000000000152

National Center for Health Statistics. (2015). Summary of NCHS surveys and data collection systems. Retrieved from https://www.cdc.gov/nchs/data/factsheets/factsheet_summary.htm

Nix, L. M., & Tien, P. C. (2014). Metabolic syndrome, diabetes, and cardiovascular risk in HIV. *Current HIV/AIDS Reports, 11*(3), 271–278. doi:10.1007/s11904-014-0219-7

Nwankwo, T., Yoon, S. S., Burt, V., & Gu, Q. (2013). Hypertension among adults in the United States: National Health and Nutrition Examination Survey, 2011–2012 (NCHS Data Brief No. 133). Retrieved from http://www.cdc.gov/nchs/data/databriefs/db133.pdf

Olokoba, A. B., Obateru, O. A., & Olokoba, L. B. (2012). Type 2 diabetes mellitus: A review of current trends. *Oman Medical Journal, 27*(4), 269–273. doi:10.5001/omj.2012.68

Perez-Benitez, C. I., O'Brien, W. H., Carels, R. A., Gordon, A. K., & Chiros, C. E. (2007). Cardiovascular correlates of disclosing homosexual orientation. *Stress Health, 23*(3), 141–152.

Phillips-Angeles, E., Wolfe, P., Myers, R., Dawson, P., Marrazzo, J., Soltner, S., & Dzieweczynski, M. (2004). Lesbian health matters: A pap test education campaign nearly thwarted by discrimination. *Health Promotion Practice, 5*(3), 314–325.

Power, J., McNair, R., & Carr, S. (2009). Absent sexual scripts: Lesbian and bisexual women's knowledge, attitudes and action regarding safer sex and sexual health information. *Culture, Health & Sexuality, 11*(1), 67–81. doi:10.1080/13691050802541674

Price, J. H., Easton, A. N., Telljohann, S. K., & Wallace, P. B. (1996). Perceptions of cervical cancer and pap smear screening behavior by women's sexual orientation. *Journal of Community Health, 21*(2), 89–105.

Rasmussen, L. D., Mathiesen, E. R., Kronborg, G., Pedersen, C., Gerstoft, J., & Obel, N. (2012). Risk of diabetes mellitus in persons with and without HIV: A Danish nationwide population-based cohort study. *PlOS ONE, 7*(9), e44575. doi:10.1371/journal.pone.0044575

Richardson, D. (2000). The social construction of immunity: HIV risk perception and prevention among lesbians and bisexual women. *Culture, Health & Sexuality, 2*(1), 33–49.

Rossouw, J. E., Anderson, G. L., Prentice, R. L., LaCroix, A. Z., Kooperberg, C., Stefanick, M. L.,...Ockene, J.; Writing Group for the Women's Health Initiative Investigators. (2002). Risks and benefits of estrogen plus progestin in healthy postmenopausal women: Principal results from the women's health initiative randomized controlled trial. *Journal of the American Medical Association, 288*(3), 321–333.

Rucci, P., Gherardi, S., Tansella, M., Piccinelli, M., Berardi, D., Bisoffi, G.,...Pini, S. (2003). Subthreshold psychiatric disorders in primary care: Prevalence and associated characteristics. *Journal of Affective Disorders, 76*(1–3), 171–181.

Sears, M. R., Greene, J. M., Willan, A. R., Wiecek, E. M., Taylor, D. R., Flannery, E. M.,...Poulton, R. (2003). A longitudinal, population-based, cohort study of childhood asthma followed to adulthood. *New England Journal of Medicine, 349*(15), 1414–1422. doi:10.1056/NEJMoa022363

Segerstrom, S. C., & Miller, G. E. (2004). Psychological stress and the human immune system: A meta-analytic study of 30 years of inquiry. *Psychological Bulletin, 130*(4), 601–630. doi:10.1037/0033-2909.130.4.601

Simoni, J. M., Smith, L., Oost, K. M., Lehavot, K., & Fredriksen-Goldsen, K. (2017). Disparities in physical health conditions among lesbian and bisexual women: A systematic review of population-based studies. *Journal of Homosexuality, 64*(1), 32–44. doi:10.1080/00918369.2016.1174021

Snyder, J. E. (2011). Trend analysis of medical publications about LGBT persons: 1950–2007. *Journal of Homosexuality, 58*(2), 164–188. doi:10.1080/00918369.2011.540171

Stamler, J. (1977). The coronary drug project: Findings with regard to estrogen, dextrothyroxine, clofibrate and niacin. *Advances in Experimental Medicine & Biology, 82,* 52–75.

Sturm, R. (2002). The effects of obesity, smoking, and drinking on medical problems and costs. *Health Affairs, 21*(2), 245–253.

Swidorski, D. (2014). *Diabetes history.* Madeira Beach, FL: Defeat Diabetes Foundation. Retrieved from http://www.defeatdiabetes.org/diabetes-history

Thomeer, M. B. (2013). Sexual minority status and self-rated health: The importance of socioeconomic status, age, and sex. *American Journal of Public Health, 103*(5), 881–888. doi:10.2105/AJPH.2012.301040

Tracy, J. K., Lydecker, A. D., & Ireland, L. (2010). Barriers to cervical cancer screening among lesbians. *Journal of Women's Health, 19*(2), 229–237.

Valanis, B. G., Bowen, D. J., Bassford, T., Whitlock, E., Charney, P., & Carter, R. A. (2000). Sexual orientation and health: Comparisons in the women's health initiative sample. *Archives of Family Medicine, 9*(9), 843–853.

Vasan, R. S., Beiser, A., Seshadri, S., Larson, M. G., Kannel, W. B., D'Agostino, R. B., & Levy, D. (2002). Residual lifetime risk for developing hypertension in middle-aged women and men: The Framingham Heart Study. *Journal of the American Medical Association, 287*(8), 1003–1010.

Wallace, S. P., Cochran, S. D., Durazo, E. M., & Ford, C. L. (2011). *The health of aging lesbian, gay and bisexual adults in California* (Policy Brief No. PB2011-2) Los Angeles: University of California, Los Angeles Center for Health Policy Research.

Wang, T. J., & Vasan, R. S. (2005). Epidemiology of uncontrolled hypertension in the United States. *Circulation, 112*(11), 1651–1662. doi:10.1161/CIRCULATIONAHA.104.490599

Ward, B. W., Dahlhamer, J. M., Galinsky, A. M., & Joestl, S. S. (2014). Sexual orientation and health among U.S. adults: National Health Interview Survey, 2013. *National health statistics reports;* no 77. Hyattsville, MD: National Center for Health Statistics.

Ward, B. W., Joestl, S. S., Galinsky, A. M., & Dahlhamer, J. M. (2015). Selected diagnosed chronic conditions by sexual orientation: A National Study of US Adults, 2013. *Preventing Chronic Disease, 12,* E192. doi:10.5888/pcd12.150292

Whelton, P. K. (1994). Epidemiology of hypertension. *Lancet, 344*(8915), 101–106.

Whelton, P. K. (2015). The elusiveness of population-wide high blood pressure control. *Annual Review of Public Health, 36,* 109–130. doi:10.1146/annurev-publhealth-031914-122949

White, D. L., Ratziu, V., & El-Serag, H. B. (2008). Hepatitis C infection and risk of diabetes: A systematic review and meta-analysis. *Journal of Hepatology, 49*(5), 831–844. doi:10.1016/j.jhep.2008.08.006

Wierckx, K., Elaut, E., Declercq, E., Heylens, G., De Cuypere, G., Taes, Y., . . . T'Sjoen, G. (2013). Prevalence of cardiovascular disease and cancer during cross-sex hormone therapy in a large cohort of trans persons: A case-control study. *European Journal of Endocrinology, 169*(4), 471–478. doi:10.1530/EJE-13-0493

Williams, D. R., & Mohammed, S. A. (2009). Discrimination and racial disparities in health: Evidence and needed research. *Journal of Behavioral Medicine, 32*(1), 20–47. doi:10.1007/s10865-008-9185-0

Williams, M. E., & Freeman, P. A. (2007). Transgender health: Implications for aging and caregiving. *Journal of Gay & Lesbian Social Services, 18*(3–4), 93–108.

Witten, T. M., & Whittle, S. (2004). TransPanthers: The greying of transgender and the law. *Deakin Law Review, 9*(2), 503–522.

Xu, J., Murphy, S. L., Kochanek, K. D., & Bastian, B. A. (2016). Deaths: Final data for 2013. *National Vital Statistics Reports, 64*(2), 1–119.

CHAPTER **7**

Reproductive Health and Parenting in Gender and Sexual Minority Populations

K. Nikki Barefoot, K. Bryant Smalley, and Jacob C. Warren

The sexual/reproductive health and parenting needs and experiences of gender and sexual minority (GSM) individuals are critical components of their overall health and well-being. However, these topics are scarcely represented within GSM health research and are often overlooked or minimized by health care professionals (Institute of Medicine [IOM], 2011). The research that is available highlights that GSM individuals face a multitude of sexual and reproductive health disparities and barriers to care that vary significantly across GSM identities. Therefore, this chapter provides an overview of the unique sexual and reproductive health, family planning, and parenting needs and experiences of cisgender sexual minority women, cisgender sexual minority men, and gender minority individuals separately, in addition to providing recommendations for health care professionals working with these subgroups within the realms of reproductive health and parenting.

■ REPRODUCTIVE HEALTH ISSUES AMONG SEXUAL MINORITY WOMEN

Cisgender sexual minority women face a variety of reproductive health disparities and have unique needs and experiences when it comes to women's health issues and service provision. Most notably, previous research has established that cisgender sexual minority women are at increased risk for the majority of reproductive cancers (e.g., cervical, ovarian, and breast; American College of Obstetricians and Gynecologists [ACOG], 2012; Austin et al., 2012; J. P. Brown & Tracy, 2008; Cochran et al., 2001). This heightened risk is related largely to a combination of greater health risk factors and lower screening rates among sexual minority women, in addition to a multitude of patient-, provider-, and system-level barriers to appropriate and ongoing women's health care (IOM, 2011; Mravcak, 2006). Disparities in reproductive cancer risk factors among sexual minority women include: a higher prevalence of smoking, excessive alcohol use, obesity, nulligravidity (no history of pregnancy), low parity (fewer gestational births), and a lower prevalence of regular physical activity/exercise, breastfeeding, oral contraceptive use, and surgical tubal occlusion (ACOG, 2012; Austin et al., 2012; J. P. Brown & Tracy, 2008; Dibble, Roberts, Robertson, & Paul, 2002; Zaritsky & Dibble, 2010). Sexual minority women have also been found to engage in lower rates of preventive health care including Pap smears, clinical breast exams, and age-appropriate mammograms when compared to their cisgender heterosexual counterparts (Agénor, Krieger, Austin, Haneuse, & Gottlieb, 2014; Bazzi, Whorms, King, & Potter, 2015; Cochran et al., 2001; Diamant, Wold, Spritzer, & Gelberg, 2000; Kerker, Mostashari, & Thorpe, 2006; Tracy, Schluterman, & Greenberg, 2013; Waterman & Voss, 2015). See Chapter 5 for a more in-depth discussion of the reproductive cancer disparities faced by sexual minority women.

Given that the sexual identity, behavior, and practices of cisgender sexual minority women are very diverse, thus too are their sexual and reproductive health needs (Marrazzo & Gorgos, 2012). However, it is often wrongly assumed by patients and providers alike that sexual minority women, especially those who identify as lesbian and/or engage only in same-sex intercourse, have limited reproductive and sexual health risks (e.g., unintended pregnancy, human papillomavirus [HPV], cervical cancer, and HIV/sexually transmitted infections [STIs]) and needs (e.g., contraceptive and family planning services, cervical cancer screenings, and safe-sex education), with the primary rationale being that these health risks and needs are typically associated with opposite-sex intercourse (Bailey, Farquhar, Owen, & Mangtani, 2004; Gorgos & Marrazzo, 2011; Jones & Hoyler, 2006; Marrazzo & Gorgos, 2012; Power, McNair, & Carr, 2009). Despite these misperceptions, there are many unique health needs and risks associated with same-sex intercourse among women, including the fact that HPV and HIV/STIs can be transmitted between female sexual partners (Marrazzo & Gorgos, 2012). Furthermore, the majority of sexual minority women have a history of male sexual partners, including 70% to 80% of those who identify as lesbian (Bailey et al., 2004; Barefoot, Warren, & Smalley, 2017; Gorgos & Marrazzo, 2011; Jones & Hoyler, 2006; Koh, Gómez, Shade, & Rowley, 2005; Marrazzo & Gorgos, 2012). Therefore, it is important for providers working with sexual minority women to take a comprehensive history of patients' sexual identity, behavior, and practices and assess their current reproductive and sexual health needs (e.g., the need for contraceptives, family planning services, appropriate safe-sex education, HIV/STI testing, and cancer screenings) through nonjudgmental and open-ended discourse (ACOG, 2012; Gorgos & Marrazzo,

2011; Mravcak, 2006). See Chapter 13 for further discussion of the sexual health needs and STI disparities faced by sexual minority women.

Similar to their cisgender heterosexual counterparts, sexual minority women may face reproductive health issues related to their menstrual cycle, hormone fluctuations, and other complications with the female reproductive system such as irregular menstruation, menorrhagia, premenstrual syndrome (PMS), premenstrual dysphoric disorder (PMDD), polycystic ovary syndrome (PCOS), uterine fibroids, endometriosis, chronic pelvic pain, and other gynecological conditions. However, it is important for providers to be aware of the unique needs and experiences that sexual minority women may have related to these health concerns and the associated treatments (e.g., oral contraceptives, hormone replacement therapy, hysterectomy), in addition to the sexual orientation disparities that do exist.

Menstrual Cycle, Contraception, and Menopause

Given their lower rates of oral contraceptive use (J. P. Brown & Tracy, 2008; Charlton et al., 2014), which are known to regulate menstrual cycles and bleeding (American Society for Reproductive Medicine, 2011), premenopausal sexual minority women may experience more irregular periods and/or heavier menstrual bleeding. Similar to other cisgender women, sexual minority women may also present with premenstrual symptoms that are consistent with PMS or PMDD. PMS is typically characterized by a pattern of mild to moderate affective (depression, anxiety, irritability, insomnia, and social withdrawal) and somatic (changes in appetite, bloating/weight gain, breast tenderness, headache, abdominal pains, and fatigue) symptoms that occur prior to the start of menstruation (ACOG, 2015), and affects approximately half of reproductive age cisgender women (Direkvand-Moghadam, Sayehmiri, Delpisheh, & Sattar, 2014). What little research is available suggests that sexual minority women experience PMS at rates similar to their cisgender heterosexual counterparts (Moegelin, Nilsson, & Helström, 2010). Approximately 2% to 5% of cisgender women experience a more severe and disabling form of PMS called PMDD (Epperson et al., 2012). According to the *Diagnostic and Statistical Manual of Mental Disorders, 5th edition* (*DSM-5*; American Psychiatric Association, 2013), PMDD is a depressive disorder with onset during ovulation and remission within a few days of menses that is characterized by a persistent pattern of mood disturbances (including mood lability, dysphoria, and anxiety), behavioral and/or physical symptoms (including changes in sleep and eating patterns and somatic symptoms of PMS), and significant functional impairment. Evidence-based treatment options for PMS and/or PMDD include: oral contraceptives containing low doses of estrogen and the progestin drospirenone, serotonergic antidepressant, anxiolytics, gonadotropin-releasing hormone (GnRH) agonists and other ovulation suppressants, calcium supplements, and cognitive behavioral therapy (Rapkin, 2003; Rapkin & Winer, 2008).

Overall, oral contraceptives have many reproductive health uses among cisgender women beyond pregnancy prevention (American Society for Reproductive Medicine, 2011), and some sexual minority women, including those who engage only in same-sex intercourse, may be prescribed these medications to manage the previously mentioned menstrual-related health concerns. Therefore, it is essential for health care professionals to be aware of and assess for this in an affirmative manner (see discussion of language concerns that follows) as part of a thorough medication history and not automatically assume that sexual minority women do not take oral contraceptives or that being prescribed this type of medication is indicative of one's sexual orientation and/or behavior. Furthermore, when oral contraceptives are prescribed to sexual minority women for menstruation management, it is important for health care professionals to provide them with comprehensive education regarding these additional uses of oral contraceptives, in addition to being aware that being prescribed oral contraceptives and/or the reference to these medications as "contraceptives" or "birth control" may conflict with some sexual minority women's sexual and/or gender identity, especially those who present/identify as more masculine (e.g., "butch," "stud," "boi") and cause them discomfort or distress (Chrisler et al., 2016; Hiestand, Horne, & Levitt, 2007). Therefore, health care professionals should be sensitive to these language concerns, and affirming of the individual patient's preferences, when discussing medication history and treatment options with sexual minority women. Other, more neutral ways to refer to these types of medications may include hormone pills/medication, hormone therapy, the actual name of the hormone being supplemented/altered by the medication (e.g., estrogen and/or progesterone), and/or the generic or brand name of the medication. If discomfort with oral contraceptive use persists beyond language concerns, other treatment options, including the previously mentioned nonpharmacologic treatments of PMS/PMDD should be explored with the patient.

As with other cisgender women, sexual minority women typically go through menopause (i.e., the cessation of their menstrual cycle) in their late 40s/early 50s, with the average age of menopause being 51 (Office on Women's Health, 2010). Physical and mental symptoms often associated with menopause include hot flashes, insomnia, night sweats, vaginal and urinary problems (drier vaginal tissues, increases in urinary tract infections, and urinary incontinence), mood changes (including mood swings, tearfulness, and irritability), decreased libido and interest in sex, weight gain, achiness in muscles and joints, forgetfulness, and difficulties with concentration. Moderate to severe symptoms of menopause may be treated with menopausal hormone therapy (MHT), also known as *hormone replacement therapy*, which involves taking estrogen and/or progesterone (Office on Women's Health, 2010). Although there are few studies specifically on menopause among sexual minority women, what little research is available provides valuable insight into their unique needs and experiences related to menopause and MHT. For example, qualitative research suggests that many sexual minority women may feel unprepared for menopause and other age-related changes in their bodies and to their health, including postmenopausal changes in their metabolism and increased difficulties with weight management, while other sexual minority women may have specific concerns related to MHT, including limited knowledge of the treatment indications, benefits, and risks and concerns over sexual side effects (Garbers et al., 2015). Previous research also suggests that discomfort discussing menopause is significantly predictive of delayed or foregone medical care among sexual minority women (White & Dull, 1997). Therefore, it is important for health care providers to facilitate sexual minority women's comfort with discussing menopause and related health concerns through open and affirming communication, in addition to providing them with culturally tailored education on menopause and MHT.

Other Gynecological Conditions

In terms of other gynecological conditions, meta-analysis results suggest that cisgender sexual minority women experience PCOS, endometriosis, and uterine fibroids at rates similar to their heterosexual counterparts; however, bisexual women have higher rates of chronic pelvic pain than heterosexual women (Robinson, Galloway, Bewley, & Meads, 2016). Although sexual minority women are not at increased risk for having PCOS, it is important for health care professionals to be aware that the infertility issues associated with PCOS may exacerbate the barriers to family planning experienced by same-sex female couples (see Family Planning among Same-Sex Female Couples section that follows). This is evident by the finding that approximately 80% of lesbians undergoing fertility treatment have polycystic ovaries, with 38% being diagnosed with PCOS (compared to only 32% and 14% of heterosexual women, respectively; Agrawal et al., 2004).

Hysterectomy is the second most common surgical procedure performed on reproductive-aged cisgender women, with over one third of cigsgender women having had a hysterectomy by the age of 60 years (National Women's Health Network, 2015). Hysterectomy is a common treatment option for a variety of gynecological conditions and concerns (e.g., cervical, ovarian, uterine, or endometrial cancer; endometriosis; uterine fibroids; uterine prolapse; and/or excessive or unusual vaginal bleeding) and can be medically necessary or optional, depending on the type and severity of the problem (Office on Women's Health, 2014). Previous research suggests that sexual minority women have hysterectomies at rates similar to their cisgender heterosexual counterparts (Dibble et al., 2002; IOM, 2011; Valanis et al., 2000). Groff and colleagues (2000) conducted qualitative interviews with sexual minority women regarding their decision-making and attitudes toward hysterectomy and found that sexual minority women may have both positive and negative attitudes toward hysterectomy. Positive aspects of having a hysterectomy identified by sexual minority women include freedom from the burdens of menstrual bleeding and related benefits to their sex lives. Negative aspects identified include: giving up the future option of pregnancy; a feeling of loss related to a physical piece of themselves being taken away; negative changes in mood; and the need for hormone therapy. Many sexual minority women described negative health care experiences related to hysterectomies, including perceptions that physicians were too quick to suggest that they have a hysterectomy. Lastly, sexual minority women expressed a desire to be in charge of their own decisions regarding hysterectomies and felt that education about their diagnoses and treatment options, the experiences and support of others, and second medical options would be important factors in their decision-making process.

Access to Care

As previously noted, sexual minority women face a variety of barriers that significantly diminish their engagement in sexual and reproductive health care and ultimately increase their risks for a variety of health conditions. Most notably, given that contraceptive services are an important entry point into women's health care, sexual minority women may not regularly engage in these types of services and, as a result, are less likely to receive appropriative sexual and reproductive health education and timely health screenings for reproductive cancers and other gynecological-related conditions (Agénor, Krieger, Austin, Haneuse & Gottlieb, 2014). In fact, over half of sexual minority women may not have a regular source of women's health care (i.e., a provider whom they see for gynecologic preventive care; Barefoot et al., 2017). Furthermore, of those who do engage in regular women's health care, many feel that their provider is not knowledgeable about the unique health concerns of sexual minority women, with less than half being asked about their sexual orientation and less than one-fourth being provided appropriate safe-sex education by their provider (Barefoot et al., 2017).

Other sexual minority women may avoid routine health care altogether due to fears of discrimination and/or mistreatment based on past encounters and/ or the reported experiences of others (Barefoot et al., 2017; Hernandez & Fultz, 2006; Hutchinson, Thompson, & Cederbaum, 2006). This may be especially true for sexual minority women who present/identify as more masculine (i.e., those who identify as "butch") who, in comparison to their "femme"-identified counterparts, have been found to experience greater discrimination and maltreatment in medical settings, have greater difficulties finding lesbian, gay, bisexual, and transgender (LGBT)-friendly health care providers, and engage in routine gynecological care less frequently (Hiestand et al., 2007). Other barriers experienced by sexual minority women include: concerns about sexual orientation disclosure and confidentiality; higher uninsured rates/financial barriers; limited understanding of gynecological risks and health needs; not having a regular doctor; and a lack of physician referral for gynecological services (ACOG, 2012; IOM, 2011; Tracy et al., 2013). Lastly, despite the unique sexual and reproductive health needs of sexual minority women, the majority of obstetrician/gynecologists (OB/GYNs) do not receive education on lesbian and bisexual health as part of their medical school or residency training program (Abdessamad, Yudin, Tarasoff, Radford, & Ross, 2013). Therefore, cultural competency training related to the unique health needs of sexual minority women is greatly needed in order to better address and eliminate the sexual and reproductive health disparities faced by this population.

■ REPRODUCTIVE HEALTH ISSUES AMONG SEXUAL MINORITY MEN

Cisgender sexual minority men also have diverse sexual and reproductive health needs and experiences. However, much of the research in this area has focused primarily on HPV-related reproductive cancers, HIV/STIs, and sexual dysfunction, with limited research on sexual minority men's experiences with other nonmalignant conditions of the male reproductive system, including issues with infertility (IOM, 2011). Therefore, what follows is a review of the available literature on these topics and a discussion of other sexual and reproductive health issues that sexual minority men may experience, in addition to the unique patient-, provider-, and system-level barriers to appropriate and ongoing men's health care that they face.

Sexually Transmitted Infections

As discussed more in Chapters 5 and 13, sexual minority men are disproportionately affected by HPV infections and have increased risks for HPV-related diseases, including genital warts and anal and penile cancers (Machalek et al., 2012; Sadlier et al., 2014). Sexual minority men are especially vulnerable to anal cancer, with a risk that is approximately 20 times greater than that of the general population among HIV-negative sexual minority men and 40 times higher among those who are HIV positive (National LGBT Cancer Network, 2009). However, many sexual minority men are unaware of these risks and the associated preventative measures and, as a result, have low rates of HPV vaccination and screenings (D'Souza et al., 2013; Reiter, Brewer, McRee, Gilbert, & Smith, 2010). For example, among a national sample of sexual minority men, overall knowledge of and concern about getting HPV-related disease was very low, with 42% not knowing that HPV can cause health problems for men and only about 30% knowing that HPV can cause anal and penile cancer (Reiter et al., 2010). Among the same sample of men, HPV vaccine acceptability was highest among those who believed that their doctor would recommend it, those who perceived HPV-related diseases as more severe, those who perceived that the vaccine would be effective, and those who anticipated regret if they did not get the vaccine and later contracted HPV. In addition to low knowledge and perceived risk, other common barriers to HPV screenings among sexual minority men include limited access to these services, feelings of embarrassment, and perceived discomfort/pain of the screening (D'Souza et al., 2013; Reed, Reiter, Smith, Pakefsky, & Brewer, 2010). Therefore, it is imperative for health care professionals to openly discuss HPV-related disease prevention with their sexual minority male patients by providing education on both their risks and prevention/detection options while alleviating their concerns through an affirming and nonjudgmental approach.

There are several decades of research on the sexual risks and HIV/STI disparities among sexual minority men discussed in detail in Chapter 13. Of particular relevance to their reproductive health are the findings highlighting that sexual minority men, in comparison to their cisgender heterosexual counterparts, have higher rates of HIV/AIDS, syphilis, chlamydia, and gonorrhea (Abara, Hess, Neblett Fanfair, Bernstein, & Paz-Bailey, 2016; Centers for Disease Control and Prevention [CDC], 2014, 2017), all of which have been shown to increase the risk of infertility among men (Brookings, Goldmeier, & Sadeghi-Nejad, 2013; Kushnir & Lewis, 2011). Also fundamental to their sexual and reproductive health is the fact that many sexual minority men, including those who identify as gay, have a history of both male and female partners. In fact, emerging research suggests that approximately 67% of bisexual-identified men have had opposite-sex intercourse in the past year, with 34% recently having only female sexual partners. For gay-identified men, 5% have had at least one female sexual partner in the past year, while 40% have a lifetime history of opposite-sex intercourse (E. Brown & England, 2016). Therefore, in order to adequately address the reproductive and sexual health needs of sexual minority men, it is essential for health care providers to thoroughly assess their past and current sexual health histories (including previous STI diagnoses; their sexual identity, behavior, and practices; and the gender and number of previous and current sexual partners) in a culturally sensitive and affirmative manner (Knight & Jarrett, 2015; Makadon, Mayer, & Garofalo, 2006). This will allow providers to tailor both the education and treatment recommendations that they provide to the unique needs of the patient.

Sexual Dysfunction

Sexual minority men may also experience a variety of sexual difficulties that can significantly impact their reproductive, sexual, and mental health (Sandfort & de Keizer, 2001), with prevalence estimates of sexual dysfunctions relatively high among this population. Namely, among a large, diverse sample of sexual minority men, 79% reported at least one persistent sexual dysfunction in the past year, with specific rates as follows: erectile difficulties (45%), sexual performance anxiety (44%), not finding sex pleasurable (37%), difficulty in or inability to achieve orgasm (36%), premature ejaculation (34%), and pain during sex (14%; Hirshfield et al., 2010). Furthermore, previous research suggests that sexual minority men may experience erectile dysfunction at rates higher than their cisgender heterosexual counterparts, with concerns over performance failure being strongly predictive of greater difficulties with erection (Bancroft, Carnes, Janssen, Goodrich, & Long, 2005). The heightened cultural pressure and anxiety related to sexual performance experienced by sexual minority men (in comparison to cisgender heterosexual men) may result in greater feelings of distress and embarrassment about erectile difficulties, making it harder for them to admit and discuss with others, including medical providers (Bancroft et al., 2005; Sandfort & de Keizer, 2001). Therefore, it is important for health care professionals to be mindful of this and assess for sexual dysfunction in a sensitive and affirmative manner as part of a comprehensive assessment of the sexual health history and needs of sexual minority men.

Other Reproductive System Issues

As with other cisgender men, sexual minority men can also experience other non-malignant conditions of the male reproductive system, including but not limited to urinary tract infections, prostatitis, penile and perianal yeast infections, benign prostatic hyperplasia (BPH), epididymitis, varicoceles, and Peyronie's disease (PD; discussed in more detail later). However, as previously noted, there is little research that specifically examines sexual minority men's experiences with these conditions. Previous research during the height of the HIV epidemic suggested that penile and/or perianal yeast infections are found in approximately one out of six sexual minority men (David, Walzman, & Rajamanoharan, 1997), with 23% of sexual minority men having a lifetime history of urinary tract infections and 8% having a lifetime history of prostatitis (Breyer, Vittinghoff, Van Den Eeden, Erickson, & Shindel, 2012), indicating that these may be relatively common presenting sexual health concerns among sexual minority men. Recent qualitative interviews with sexual minority men suggest that they have very low awareness and knowledge of most nonmalignant testicular disorders, including epididymitis and varicoceles (Saab, Landers, & Hegarty, 2016). A varicocele is characterized by an abnormal enlargement of the veins in the scrotum and is present in approximately 15% of cisgender men. The swelling of the testicular veins causes them to overheat and can result in infertility (Alsaikhan, Alrabeeah, Delouya, & Zini, 2016). Future research is needed to explore sexual minority men's unique experiences with these conditions in order to better understand and address their sexual and reproductive health needs.

PD is an acquired fibrotic disorder resulting from plaque formation in the penis that typically causes penile deformation and a curved, and sometimes painful, erection. Although the specific prevalence rate among sexual minority men is unknown, recent research estimates that approximately 0.7% to 11.8% of cisgender men have PD (Stuntz, Perlaky, des Vignes, Kyriakides, & Glass, 2016). Farrell, Corder, and Levine (2013) examined the associated psychosocial factors and treatment history of sexual minority men with PD and found that the majority of men indicated that they were self-conscious about their penis (92.9%) and that PD had a negative impact on their emotional functioning (89.0%), with 45% reporting a negative effect on their intimate relationships. Furthermore, 31% reported a decrease in sexual desire and 50% reported a decline in sexual frequency. Of the 27 sexual minority men in the study, 88.9% had received nonsurgical treatment and 29.6% had undergone corrective surgery for PD. Overall, these results suggest that PD can significantly impact the sexual and mental health of sexual minority men. Therefore, it is important for providers to establish trust with their sexual minority male clients in order to appropriately assess for PD and other sexual/reproductive conditions and, when present, related experiences of psychological and relational distress.

Barriers to Care

In addition to the previously mentioned barriers, there are many other obstacles to regular and affirming men's health care that sexual minority men may face. In fact, approximately two thirds of sexual minority men report difficulties accessing regular health care due to financial and/or social barriers, with only about 43% having received primary care services in the past 2 years (McKirnan, Du Bois, Alvy, & Jones, 2013). According to recent estimates, approximately one out of five sexual minority men are uninsured and one out of six have been unable to obtain needed medical care due to cost (Kates, Ranji, Beamesderfer, Salganicoff, & Dawson, 2016). In addition to these financial barriers, mistrust in the health care system and discomfort with discussing one's sexual orientation with medical providers have both been found to be associated with decreased health care access among sexual minority men (McKirnan et al., 2013). Furthermore, when sexual minority men do seek preventive health care services, they often experience these environments as not affirming or knowledgeable of their unique sexual and reproductive health needs and experiences (Knight & Jarrett, 2015). These negative experiences can result in them avoiding subsequent health care and/or not following medical advice, further exacerbating the health disparities that they face (Knight & Jarrett, 2015; Makadon et al., 2006).

■ REPRODUCTIVE HEALTH ISSUES AMONG GENDER MINORITY INDIVIDUALS

As discussed in Chapter 1, "gender minority" is a broad term to describe individuals who experience an incongruity between their gender identity/expression and the binary sex that they were assigned at birth. While identifying as transgender is the best-known of these identities, others include but are not limited to genderqueer, gender fluid, and nonbinary. The standard practice for identifying gender minority patients as part of the intake process and/or health research involves a two-step approach that asks patients to indicate the sex that they were assigned at birth and their current gender identity (Cahill & Makadon, 2014; Tate, Ledbetter, & Youssef, 2013). Gender minority individuals may choose to undergo gender-affirming medical treatment, which can include hormone treatment (i.e., masculinizing or feminizing hormones) and various types of gender confirmation surgery (i.e., masculinizing surgeries: mastectomy, chest contouring, vaginectomy, phalloplasty, scrotoplasty, and/or hysterectomy; and feminizing surgeries: augmentation mammoplasty, penectomy, gonadectomy, and/or vaginoplasty; see Chapter 14 for a more detailed discussion). These procedures are often referred to as "top" and "bottom" surgery (Deutsch, 2016). Overall, gender minority individuals represent a diverse group with regard to both gender identity and transition status and sexual identity, behavior, and practices, and therefore have diverse sexual and reproductive health needs (Unger, 2014). In order to provide appropriate health care to gender minority individuals, it is important for health care providers to be aware of their hormonal status and natal and surgical anatomy (McNamara & Ng, 2016). The discussion necessary to acquire such knowledge requires a constant focus on being affirming of the patient's identity and journey, and an awareness that many gender minority individuals prefer not to discuss their physical and/or biological characteristics. Much of the research on the sexual and reproductive health of gender minority individuals has focused primarily on HIV/STI rates and risk behaviors and pelvic health among transgender persons (Edmiston et al., 2016), with limited research on other sexual and reproductive health concerns, including fertility, and the unique experiences of gender minority individuals who identity outside of the binary.

Gender minority individuals have diverse risks and needs when it comes to reproductive cancer prevention and screening (Unger, 2014). However, the majority of preventive health care providers lack the training, experience, and knowledge needed to adequately address the unique needs of gender minority patients (Edmiston et al., 2016). For example, it is often wrongly assumed by medical providers that transgender men are at low risk for cervical cancer and therefore do not require regular screenings (i.e., Pap tests; Agénor et al., 2016; Potter et al., 2015). However, research suggests that a majority of transgender men do not undergo gender confirmation surgery and/or do not have a total hysterectomy until later in life, if ever. Therefore, most transgender men have a cervix and require routine cancer screenings that follow the exact same guidelines as cisgender women, regardless of their sexual identity, behavior, and practices (Deutsch, 2016; Edmiston et al., 2016; Peitzmeier, Reisner, Harigopal, & Potter, 2014; Potter et al., 2015; Unger, 2014).

Despite these recommendations, transgender men are significantly less likely than cisgender women to engage in regular Pap tests (Peitzmeier, Khullar, Reisner, & Potter, 2014). This is likely due to the previously mentioned provider-level barriers in addition to transgender men's lack of awareness of cervical cancer risks and need for screening; the incongruence between the patient's gender identity and biological sex (and potentially ignoring the existence of one's natal reproductive structures altogether); and/or discomfort and/or distress related to cervical exams (Peitzmeier, Khullar, et al., 2014; Potter et al., 2015). Furthermore, when transgender men do receive cervical cancer screenings, they are more likely to have an inadequate Pap test when compared to cisgender female patients, which may be attributable to testosterone-induced vaginal/cervical atrophy and patient and/or provider discomfort with the procedure (Peitzmeier, Reisner, et al., 2014). When providing preventive health care services to transgender men, it is important for providers to appropriately assess whether transgender male patients have had some or all of their internal pelvic organs removed (Unger, 2014). Furthermore, it is crucial for providers to be aware of the cervical cancer screening guidelines for transgender men, in addition to the previously mentioned challenges that these patients experience with regard to Pap testing in order to provide them with appropriate and affirming preventive care. Specific guidelines and provider recommendations for affirmatively screening transgender male patients for cervical cancer are available and should be followed (e.g., Deutsch, 2016; Potter et al., 2015).

Breast cancer can also occur in gender minority individuals, including both transgender men and transgender women (Deutsch, 2016). However, the majority of gynecologists are unaware of breast cancer screening recommendations for transgender persons (Unger, 2015). According to treatment guidelines, transgender women who are 50 years of age or older and have undergone feminizing hormone therapy for at least 5 to 10 years should be screened for breast cancer via mammography every 2 years, whereas transgender men who have not undergone a bilateral mastectomy or those who have remaining breast tissue following masculinizing chest surgery should follow the same breast cancer screening guidelines as cisgender women (Deutsch, 2016). Despite these recommendations, research suggests that transgender persons, in comparison to their cisgender counterparts, are significantly less likely to adhere to mammography screening guidelines (Bazzi et al., 2015). When considering the appropriate cancer screening services for gender minority individuals, a simple rule for both patients and providers to consider is "if you have it, check it" (Berstein, Potter, & Peitzmeier, 2014; McNamara & Ng, 2016).

Much of the sexual health research among gender minority individuals has focused heavily on HIV/STI-related sexual risks, particularly among transgender women. Therefore, little is known about the reproductive and sexual health needs of gender minority individuals, especially those who identify as genderqueer/nonbinary, beyond HIV/STI risks. In order to provide appropriate health care to gender minority patients, it is important for providers to avoid conflating gender identity and sexual orientation and to recognize that gender minority individuals have diverse sexual identities, behaviors, and practices (McNamara & Ng, 2016). For example, results from the Trans PULSE Project revealed that among transgender men, the gender identity of past-year sexual partners was as follows: 10% other transgender men, 21% cisgender men, 7% transgender women, 44% cisgender women, and 14% genderqueer persons; whereas the gender identity of past-year sexual partners among transgender women was as follows: 4% transgender men, 23% cisgender men, 14% other transgender women, 24% cisgender women, and 3% genderqueer persons (Bauer, Travers, Scanlon, & Coleman, 2012). Therefore, it is important for providers working with gender minority individuals to not assume the sexual orientation or sexual practices of the patient based on their gender identity (i.e., assuming that a transgender man is attracted to women or does not engage in receptive vaginal intercourse) and to take a comprehensive history of the patient's sexual identity, behavior, and practices using nonjudgmental and open-ended questions (McNamara & Ng, 2016). This will allow them to thoroughly assess the patient's current reproductive and sexual health needs and make appropriate recommendations/referrals as needed (including the need for contraceptives, family planning services, appropriate safe-sex education, and HIV/STI screenings).

As discussed more fully in Chapter 14, hormone therapy and/or gender confirmation surgery can significantly impact the fertility of gender minority individuals (Deutsch, 2016). As a result, the informed consent process for either procedure requires that sexual minority patients fully understand the effect hormones/surgery can have on their fertility and future family planning options (Deutsch, 2016; dickey, Ducheny, & Ehrbar, 2016). Fertility preservation options for gender minority individuals prior to hormone therapy and/or sexual reassignment surgery include: pre- or peripubertal–ovarian or testicular tissue cryopreservation; and postpubertal–cryopreservation of oocyte or embryo or sperm banking (Johnson & Finlayson, 2016). Among gender minority individuals who are undergoing hormone therapy, but have otherwise retained their ovaries or testes, ovulation and spermatogenesis may or may not continue. If not, return of fertility may be possible after the discontinuation of hormone therapy (typically within 3–6 months), although permanent loss of fertility is possible and there are other potential physical and psychological ramifications of stopping hormone therapy to attempt fertility. However, given the higher risk for birth defects associated with hormone therapy, either parent should discontinue treatment several months before conception (see Family Planning Among Gender Minority Individuals section; also dickey et al., 2016). Overall, although hormone therapy may reduce the likelihood of an unintended pregnancy, it should not be considered an effective form of contraception alone. Therefore, gender minority individuals who have ovaries/testes and engage in sexual activity that could result in fertilization should be provided with appropriate education on contraceptive options (Deutsch, 2016; dickey et al., 2016).

Gender minority individuals are a vulnerable subgroup of the LGBT community that faces a multitude of patient-, provider-, and system-level barriers to appropriate reproductive and sexual health care (see Chapter 14). Most notably, most health care facilities are not inclusive and welcoming of gender minority individuals, with the majority of medical providers lacking the appropriate training, knowledge, and experience to provide appropriate and affirming reproductive and sexual health services (Edmiston et al., 2016; Unger, 2014). To illustrate, a survey of OB/GYNs from across the United States revealed that 80% had not received training on transgender health as part of their residency program, and 64.7% and 71.0% did not feel comfortable with providing services to transgender women and transgender men, respectively (Unger, 2015). Furthermore, results from the National Transgender Discrimination Survey suggest that 50% of gender minority individuals postpone preventive health care due to financial barriers, and 33% postpone these services due to discrimination by providers (Grant et al., 2011). Yet even when gender minority individuals do engage the health care system, approximately 20% do not follow medical advice (Smalley, Warren, & Barefoot, 2015). Overall, there is a dire need for research that explores the unique sexual and reproductive health needs and experiences of gender minority individuals in order to better serve this population and begin addressing the substantial barriers to care that they face.

GENDER AND SEXUAL MINORITY PARENTING AND FAMILY PLANNING

Parenting and family planning needs and experiences are important health considerations for GSM individuals that can vary significantly across the GSM spectrum (Goldberg & Allen, 2013). Despite the many misconceptions regarding the heteronormativity of family structures in the United States, substantial numbers of GSM individuals are parents (IOM, 2011). In fact, recent national data suggest that approximately 37% of GSM-identified adults are parent to at least one child (Gates, 2013). Furthermore, surveys of GSM individuals reveal that around half of gay men and transgender persons and over one third of lesbians have a desire to become a parent (Riskind & Patterson, 2010; Stotzer, Herman, & Hasenbush, 2014). There are a variety of pathways by which GSM individuals become parents including, but not limited to: (a) having children through a heterosexual relationship/marriage prior to coming out as GSM; (b) having children within a current or previous same- or opposite-sex partnership through sexual intercourse, assisted reproductive technology (ART), foster parenting, or adoption; (c) raising a grandchild, sibling, or other relative or an unrelated child as one's own; (d) coparenting with another GSM nonromantic partner or couple; and/or (e) partnering with someone who already has children by one of the previously mentioned means (Biblarz & Savci, 2010; Gates, 2013; Goldberg & Allen, 2013; Tasker & Patterson, 2008). Following is a discussion of the unique family planning options and needs of GSM couples (i.e., cisgender same-sex couples and couples in which one or both partners identify as a gender minority) who choose to become parents together.

Family Planning Among Cisgender Same-Sex Female Couples

In addition to the previously mentioned pathways to parenthood, many same-sex female couples decide to have children through pregnancy. When cisgender same-sex female couples conceive a child together, third-party sperm donation is required (Greenfeld & Seli, 2016). In addition to deciding on a known or unknown sperm donor, the couple has to determine which partner will be the gestational mother; with multiple pregnancies, this may always be the same partner or, depending on the other partner's desires to experience pregnancy and other psychosocial factors, each partner may eventually carry a child (Bos 2013; Greenfeld & Seli, 2016; Eyler, Pang, & Clark, 2014). Once the couple has decided which partner will be the gestational mother and the known or unknown sperm donor is identified, optional methods of conception include: sexual intercourse with the sperm donor, at-home artificial insemination, intrauterine insemination (IUI), and conventional or reciprocal in vitro fertilization (IVF; Eyler et al., 2014; Greenfeld & Seli, 2016; Puckett, Horne, Levitt, & Reeves, 2011; Yeshua, Lee, Witkin, & Copperman, 2015). Reciprocal IVF, also known as *co-IVF* or *Reception of Oocytes from Partner* (ROPA), is an emerging method of assisted reproduction among cisgender same-sex female couples in which one partner's egg is fertilized by the donor sperm via IVF and the other partner serves as the gestational mother and carries the embryo to term (Eyler et al., 2014; Yeshua et al., 2015). This method allows for the shared experience of biological motherhood, which can have many psychological and emotional benefits to both the couple and child (Yeshua et al., 2015). However, one or both partners in a same-sex female couple may experience fertility difficulties and/or be uncomfortable with bearing a child and, as a result, the couple may decide to use a known or unknown egg donor and/or a traditional or gestational surrogate in order to conceive (Eyler et al., 2014). Lastly, nongestational mothers in same-sex couples, including those who adopt an infant, may ask their physician to assist them with medically inducing lactation so that they are able to breastfeed and strengthen the emotional attachment that they have with their baby (Wahlert & Fiester, 2013).

Family Planning Among Cisgender Same-Sex Male Couples

Many cisgender same-sex male couples adopt and/or coparent with other GSM parents/couples (either as a known sperm donor or with no genetic connection to the child), while other couples may choose to conceive biological children through assisted reproduction (Eyler et al., 2014; Greenfeld & Seli, 2016; Tasker & Patterson, 2008). When cisgender same-sex male couples conceive a child together, egg donation and surrogacy are required (Greenfeld & Seli, 2016). Surrogacy can occur through multiple pathways, including having a traditional surrogate (i.e., the baby is genetically related to the woman carrying it) or having an egg donor and a gestational surrogate (i.e., the baby is genetically related to the egg donor and another woman carries the fertilized embryo to term; Eyler et al., 2014; Greenfeld & Seli, 2016; Lev, 2006; Tasker & Patterson, 2008). In addition to deciding which approach to surrogacy to take and whether or not they want known or unknown egg donors/surrogates, the couple has to determine which partner will provide the sperm for fertilization, or in the case of gestational surrogacy, whether sperm from one or both partners will be used (Greenfeld & Seli, 2016; Lev, 2006). With traditional surrogacy, fertilization can occur through sexual intercourse with the surrogate, at-home artificial insemination, IUI, or IVF (Lev, 2006). With gestational surrogacy, the donated eggs are fertilized by sperm from one or both partners through IVF before transfer of the embryo (or embryos) to the surrogate (Greenfeld & Seli, 2016).

Previous research suggests that approximately 76% of cisgender male couples who utilize gestational surrogacy choose to have both partners fertilize the donated eggs, and when these treatments result in twin pregnancies (i.e., 32% in one study), the infants born are half genetic siblings (Grover, Shmorgun, Moskovtsev, Baratz, & Librach, 2013). Therefore, this approach to surrogacy increases the chances for both partners to experience biological fatherhood together.

Family Planning Among Gender Minority Individuals

As with cisgender men and women, gender minority individuals have diverse sexual identities and behaviors and therefore may partner, and ultimately form a family, with cisgender men, cisgender women, or other gender minority individuals (with either the same or different gender identities as their own; Stotzer et al., 2014). Thus, their family planning options and needs will depend largely on both partners' sexual reproduction organs, transition history (i.e., hormone therapy and/or gender confirmation surgeries), and comfort/openness to traditional and nontraditional means of conception (Deutsch, 2016; dickey et al., 2016). For example, given that the temporary cessation of hormone therapy (i.e., while trying to conceive for transgender women and throughout the entire pregnancy for transgender men) and the use of one's natal reproduction system required for most pathways to biological conception may significantly exacerbate experiences of gender dysphoria and result in depression and anxiety for some gender minority individuals, many may prefer adoption or other nontraditional means of conception to create a family (dickey et al., 2016). However, other gender minority individuals desire a biological connection to their children and choose to have their reproductive cells contribute to the creation of a family (Deutsch, 2016; dickey et al., 2016; Eyler et al., 2014).

If both partners are fertile and have opposite-sex reproductive cells (e.g., a transgender man who is partnered with a cisgender man or a transgender woman), donor egg or sperm may not be required for conception. However, if both partners are fertile and have same-sex reproductive cells (e.g., a transgender man who is partnered with a cisgender woman or two transgender women), donor egg or sperm is needed for conception. Once the partners decide who will be contributing the reproductive cells (i.e., both partners or one partner and a donor), conception options may include: sexual intercourse, at-home insemination, or ART (i.e., IUI or IVF with the potential for a traditional or gestational surrogate; Deutsch, 2016; dickey et al., 2016). Again, the approach that the couple chooses to take will depend largely on the comfort level of each partner (i.e., if a transgender man is not comfortable with being pregnant, the couple may choose to use a surrogate), which is a crucial component of family planning counseling with gender minority individuals (Deutsch, 2016; dickey et al., 2016). However, as noted earlier in the chapter, hormone therapy can significantly impact the health of reproductive cells. Furthermore, if one or both partners have undergone certain gender confirmation surgeries (i.e., a gonadectomy), and did not previously preserve their fertility (i.e., cryopreservation of their egg or sperm cells), the couple's options for conception will be further limited. Therefore, fertility services, donor eggs/sperm, and/or surrogacy may be required regardless of the natal sex of the partners (Deutsch, 2016; dickey et al., 2016; Eyler et al., 2014). Lastly, given that it is possible for lactation to be activated in many gender minority individuals (including both transgender men and transgender women), some gender minority parents may choose to chestfeed their infant for the nutritional benefits and/or to strengthen their parent–child attachment (dickey et al., 2016). Therefore, it is important for providers to recognize that this may be desired and possible for gestational, nongestational, and adoptive gender minority parents, and for them to be willing to assist with medically inducing lactation if it would otherwise be a healthy option for both the parent and the infant (i.e., if a transgender man is comfortable with temporarily ceasing hormone therapy in order to chestfeed).

Systematic Barriers to GSM Family Planning

The legal rights of GSM parents have significantly progressed over the past few years, with the passing of marriage equality nationwide in 2015 technically ensuring that legally married GSM couples have the right to petition for joint and second-parent adoption across all 50 states (Family Equality Council, 2016). However, despite these advances, adoption petitions remain at an individual judge's discretion (and thus subject to discrimination), and GSM couples continue to face other legal barriers to family planning. For example, 55% of GSM individuals live in states where GSM parents cannot petition for second-parent adoption unless they are legally married to their child's other parent. In addition, only 30% live in states that have laws that explicitly support fostering by GSM parents, while several states legally permit state-licensed child welfare agencies to refuse to place children with GSM parents on the basis of their religious beliefs. Moreover, despite GSM couples' legal right to petition for adoption, some states are still not permitting same-sex couples to jointly adopt children from foster care (Family Equality Council, 2016).

In addition to these legal barriers, GSM individuals face other systematic barriers to family planning. Most notably, both adoption and ART (i.e., fertility services and surrogacy) are very expensive processes that many GSM couples simply cannot afford (dickey et al., 2016; Greenfeld & Seli, 2016). Even for those couples that have access to health insurance/coverage, there are only about 14 states that mandate health insurance companies to cover infertility treatments. Furthermore, when they are covered, there are typically strict eligibility criteria for infertility insurance benefits that most GSM couples do not meet (i.e., their infertility condition is not considered to be a "disease" requiring treatment according to their health insurance plan; Eyler et al., 2014). Therefore, most couples end up having to self-pay for adoption and/or fertility services, which, along with legal fees and other costs, can be an insurmountable financial burden (dickey et al., 2016; Eyler et al., 2014; Greenfeld & Seli, 2016). Furthermore, many GSM couples have limited access to LGBT-affirming and competent adoption agencies, reproductive health care providers, and fertility treatment centers, and may face discrimination and mistreatment as they attempt to access family planning services (Berger, Potter, Shutters, & Imborek, 2015; S. Brown, Smalling, Groza, & Ryan, 2009; dickey et al., 2016; Greenfeld & Seli, 2016; IOM, 2011; Light, Obedin-Maliver, Sevelius, & Kerns, 2014). Given these barriers, family planning can be a very stressful and discouraging process that can heighten feelings of minority stress for GSM couples and, if family creation efforts are unsuccessful, result in significant feelings of grief and loss (Greenfeld & Seli, 2016; dickey et al., 2016).

The Health and Well-Being of GSM Parents and Families

Decades of research have established that there are no major differences between children raised by GSM parents and those raised by cisgender heterosexual parents across measures of developmental milestones, cognitive functioning, psychosocial adjustment, mental health, school outcomes, psychosexual development (including sexual orientation/gender identity), peer and romantic relationships, delinquency, and substance use (Crowl, Ahn, & Baker, 2008; Ethics Committee of the American Society of Reproductive Medicine, 2015; IOM, 2011; Stotzer et al., 2014; Tasker & Patterson, 2008), with a plethora of studies highlighting the unique strengths of same-sex and gender minority–led families. For example, parents in same-sex–led families, in comparison to heterosexual parents, report significantly stronger relationships with their children and are less likely to use physical punishment as a form of discipline (Crowl et al., 2008; IOM, 2011). Furthermore, gay fathers have recently been found to report higher levels of subjective well-being when compared to heterosexual fathers (Erez & Shenkman, 2016).

In addition to these strengths, it is important for health care providers to be aware of the unique psychosocial stressors and disparities that GSM families may face as a result of social and systematic discrimination. For example, GSM families may experience: (a) greater barriers to care, including a limited availability of LGBT-affirming pediatricians and other medical and mental health care providers; (b) exposure to negative societal attitudes and beliefs about GSM parenting and families, especially when they interact with traditional institutions within the community (i.e., school, legal, medical, and religious systems); (c) less help and support from the parents' families of origin; (d) limited social support both outside of and within the LGBT community; (e) increased disclosure-related dilemmas and higher levels of anxiety due to fears of legal problems and discrimination; and (f) additional experiences of parenting, relational, and minority stress (Goldberg & Allen, 2013; IOM, 2011; Stotzer et al., 2014; Weber, 2008, 2010).

■ CONCLUSION

Sexual and gender minority individuals have unique reproductive health care needs and experiences, in addition to a variety of disparities, including lower rates of engagement in preventative care and greater fertility-related difficulties. Furthermore, GSM families may experience greater psychosocial stressors due to negative societal attitudes and beliefs. Despite these challenges, research consistently finds that children raised by GSM parents are equally healthy and well-adjusted as those raised by cisgender heterosexual parents. Overall, research suggests that sexual and gender minority individuals face a multitude of patient-, provider-, and system-level barriers to sexual and reproductive health care and family planning services. These include, but are not limited to, a lack of health insurance coverage/financial limitations, the limited available of LGBT-affirming and competent services, and experiences of discrimination and/or mistreatment. It is important for health care professionals to be aware of these barriers and the unique reproductive health care and family planning needs and experiences of sexual and gender minority individuals in order to provide them and their families with appropriate and affirming care. While research in this area is growing, significant gaps in our knowledge of the reproductive health of GSM individuals remain, especially with regard to the needs of sexual minority men and gender minority individuals beyond sexual risks and dysfunction, and the unique reproductive health and family planning experiences of genderqueer/nonbinary individuals. Future research is needed to better understand and address the reproductive health needs of these GSM subgroups.

■ REFERENCES

Abara, W. E., Hess, K. L., Neblett Fanfair, R., Bernstein, K. T., & Paz-Bailey, G. (2016). Syphilis trends among men who have sex with men in the United States and Western Europe: A systematic review of trend studies published between 2004 and 2015. *PLOS ONE, 11*(7), e0159309. doi:10.1371/journal.pone.0159309

Abdessamad, H. M., Yudin, M. H., Tarasoff, L. A., Radford, K. D., & Ross, L. E. (2013). Attitudes and knowledge among obstetrician–gynecologists regarding lesbian patients and their health. *Journal of Women's Health (2002), 22*(1), 85–93. doi:10.1089/jwh.2012.3718

Agénor, M., Krieger, N., Austin, S. B., Haneuse, S., & Gottlieb, B. R. (2014). Sexual orientation disparities in Papanicolaou test use among US women: The role of sexual and reproductive health services. *American Journal of Public Health, 104*(2), e68–e73. doi:10.2105/AJPH.2013.301548

Agénor, M., Peitzmeier, S. M., Bernstein, I. M., McDowell, M., Alizaga, N. M., Reisner, S. L.,... Potter, J. (2016). Perceptions of cervical cancer risk and screening among transmasculine individuals: Patient and provider perspectives. *Culture, Health & Sexuality, 18*(10), 1192–1206. doi:10.1080/13691058.2016.1177203

Agrawal, R., Sharma, S., Bekir, J., Conway, G., Bailey, J., Balen, A. H., & Prelevic, G. (2004). Prevalence of polycystic ovaries and polycystic ovary syndrome in lesbian women compared with heterosexual women. *Fertility and Sterility, 82*(5), 1352–1357.

Alsaikhan, B., Alrabeeah, K., Delouya, G., & Zini, A. (2016). Epidemiology of varicocele. *Asian Journal of Andrology, 18*(2), 179–181. doi:10.4103/1008-682X.172640

American College of Obstetricians and Gynecologists. (2015). Premenstrual syndrome (PMS). Retrieved from http://www.acog.org/Patients/FAQs/Premenstrual-Syndrome-PMS

American College of Obstetricians and Gynecologists, Committee on Health Care for Underserved Women. (2012). Health care for lesbians and bisexual women. Retrieved from https://www.acog.org/-/media/Committee-Opinions/Committee-on-Health-Care-for-Underserved-Women/co525.pdf?dmc=1&ts=20161215T1036423989

American Psychiatric Association. (2013). *Diagnostic and statistical manual of mental disorders* (5th ed.). Arlington, VA: American Psychiatric Publishing.

American Society for Reproductive Medicine. (2011). Noncontraceptive benefits of birth control pills. Retrieved from https://www.asrm.org/FACTSHEET_Noncontraceptive_Benefits_of_Birth_Control_Pills

Austin, S. B., Pazaris, M. J., Rosner, B., Bowen, D. J., Rich-Edwards, J. W., & Spiegelman, D. (2012). Application of the Rosner-Colditz risk prediction model to estimate sexual orientation group disparities in breast cancer risk in a US cohort of premenopausal women. *Cancer Epidemiology and Prevention Biomarkers, 21*(12), 2201–2208. doi:10.1158/1055-9965.EPI-12-0868

Bailey, J. V., Farquhar, C., Owen, C., & Mangtani, P. (2004). Sexually transmitted infections in women who have sex with women. *Sexually Transmitted Infections, 80*(3), 244–246. doi:10.1136/sti.2003.007641

Bancroft, J., Carnes, L., Janssen, E., Goodrich, D., & Long, J. S. (2005). Erectile and ejaculatory problems in gay and heterosexual men. *Archives of Sexual Behavior, 34*(3), 285–297.

Barefoot, K. N., Warren, J. C., & Smalley, K. B. (2017). Women's healthcare: The experiences and behaviors of rural and urban lesbians in the US. *Rural and Remote Health, 17*(1), 3875.

Bauer, G. R., Travers, R., Scanlon, K., & Coleman, T. A. (2012). High heterogeneity of HIV-related sexual risk among transgender people in Ontario, Canada: A province-wide respondent-driven sampling survey. *BMC Public Health, 12*, 292. doi:10.1186/1471-2458-12-292

Bazzi, A. R., Whorms, D. S., King, D. S., & Potter, J. (2015). Adherence to mammography screening guidelines among transgender persons and sexual minority women. *American Journal of Public Health, 105*(11), 2356–2358. doi:10.2105/AJPH.2015.302851

Berger, A. P., Potter, E. M., Shutters, C. M., & Imborek, K. L. (2015). Pregnant transmen and barriers to high quality healthcare. *Proceedings in Obstetrics and Gynecology, 5*(2), 1–12.

Bernstein, I., Potter, J., & Peitzmeier, S. M. (2014) *If you have it, check it: Overcoming barriers to cervical cancer screening with patients on the female-to-male transgender spectrum.* Boston, MA: National LGBT Health Education Center. Retrieved from http://www.lgbthealtheducation.org/wp-content/uploads/Overcoming-Barriers-to-Cervical-Cancer-Screening.pdf

Biblarz, T. J., & Savci, E. (2010). Lesbian, gay, bisexual, and transgender families. *Journal of Marriage and Family, 72*(3), 480–497. doi:10.1111/j.1741-3737.2010.00714.x

Bos, H. (2013). Lesbian-mother families formed through donor insemination. In A. E. Goldberg & K. R. Allen (Eds.), *LGBT-parent families: Possibilities for new research and implications for practice* (pp. 21–37). New York, NY: Springer.

Breyer, B. N., Vittinghoff, E., Van Den Eeden, S. K., Erickson, B. A., & Shindel, A. W. (2012). Impact of sexually transmitted infections, lifetime sexual partner count and recreational drug use on lower urinary tract symptoms in men who have sex with men. *Urology, 79*(1), 188–193. doi:10.1016/j.urology.2011.07.1412

Brookings, C., Goldmeier, D., & Sadeghi-Nejad, H. (2013). Sexually transmitted infections and sexual function in relation to male fertility. *Korean Journal of Urology, 54*(3), 149–156. doi:10.4111/kju.2013.54.3.149

Brown, E., & England, P. (2016). Sexual orientation versus behavior—Different for men and women? *Context: Sexuality and Inequality Research.* Washington, DC: American Sociological Association. Retrieved from https://contexts.org/blog/sexual-orientation-versus-behavior-different-for-men-and-women/

Brown, J. P., & Tracy, J. K. (2008). Lesbians and cancer: An overlooked health disparity. *Cancer Causes & Control, 19*(10), 1009–1020. doi:10.1007/s10552-008-9176-z

Brown, S., Smalling, S., Groza, V., & Ryan, S. (2009). The experiences of gay men and lesbians in becoming and being adoptive parents. *Adoption Quarterly, 12*(3/4), 229–246.

Cahill, S., & Makadon, H. (2014). Sexual orientation and gender identity data collection in clinical settings and in electronic health records: A key to ending LGBT health disparities. *LGBT Health, 1*(1), 34–41. doi:10.1089/lgbt.2013.000

Centers for Disease Control and Prevention. (2017). HIV among gay and bisexual men. Retrieved from https://www.cdc.gov/nchhstp/newsroom/docs/factsheets/cdc-msm-508.pdf

Centers for Disease Control and Prevention. (2014). Sexually transmitted disease surveillance 2014. Retrieved from https://www.cdc.gov/std/stats14/surv-2014-print.pdf

Charlton, B. M., Corliss, H. L., Missmer, S. A., Frazier, A. L., Rosario, M., Kahn, J. A., & Austin, S. B. (2014). Influence of hormonal contraceptive use and health beliefs on sexual orientation disparities in Papanicolaou test use. *American Journal of Public Health, 104*(2), 319–325. doi:10.2105/AJPH.2012.301114

Chrisler, J. C., Gorman, J. A., Manion, J., Murgo, M., Barney, A., Adams-Clark, A., Newton, J. R., & McGrath, M. (2016). Queer periods: Attitudes toward and experiences with menstruation in the masculine of centre and transgender community. *Culture, Health & Sexuality, 18*(11), 1238–1250. doi:10.1080/13691058.2016.1182645

Cochran, S. D., Mays, V. M., Bowen, D., Gage, S., Bybee, D., Roberts, S. J.,... White, J. (2001). Cancer-related risk indicators and preventive screening behaviors among lesbians and bisexual women. *American Journal of Public Health, 91*(4), 591–597.

Crowl, A., Ahn, S., & Baker, J. (2008). A meta-analysis of developmental outcomes for children of same-sex and heterosexual parents. *Journal of GLBT Family Studies, 4*(3), 385–407.

D'Souza, G., Rajan, S. D., Bhatia, R., Cranston, R. D., Plankey, M. W., Silvestre, A.,... Brewer, N. T. (2013). Uptake and predictors of anal cancer screening in men who have sex with men. *American Journal of Public Health, 103*(9), e88–e95. doi:10.2105/AJPH.2013.301237

David, L. M., Walzman, M., & Rajamanoharan, S. (1997). Genital colonisation and infection with candida in heterosexual and homosexual males. *Genitourinary Medicine, 73*(5), 394–396.

Deutsch, M. B. (ed.) (2016). *Guidelines for the primary and gender-affirming care of transgender and gender nonbinary people (2nd ed.).* San Francisco: Center for Excellence in Transgender Health, Department of Family and Community Medicine, University of California, San Francisco. Retrieved from http://transhealth.ucsf.edu/trans?page=guidelines-home

Diamant, A. L., Wold, C., Spritzer, K., & Gelberg, L. (2000). Health behaviors, health status, and access to and use of health care: A population-based study of lesbian, bisexual, and heterosexual women. *Archives of Family Medicine, 9*(10), 1043–1051.

Dibble, S. L., Roberts, S. A., Robertson, P. A., & Paul, S. M. (2002). Risk factors for ovarian cancer: Lesbian and heterosexual women. *Oncology Nursing Forum, 29*(1), E1–E7. doi:10.1188/02.ONF.E1-E7

dickey, L. M., Ducheny, K. M., & Ehrbar, R. D. (2016). Family creation options for transgender and gender nonconforming people. *Psychology of Sexual Orientation and Gender Diversity, 3*(2), 173–179. doi:10.1037/sgd0000178

Direkvand-Moghadam, A., Sayehmiri, K., Delpisheh, A., & Sattar, K. (2014). Epidemiology of premenstrual syndrome (PMS): A systematic review and meta-analysis study. *Journal of Clinical and Diagnostic Research, 8*(2), 106–109. doi:10.7860/JCDR/2014/8024.4021

Edmiston, E. K., Donald, C. A., Sattler, A. R., Peebles, J. K., Ehrenfeld, J. M., & Eckstrand, K. L. (2016). Opportunities and gaps in primary care preventative health services for transgender patients: A systematic review. *Transgender Health, 1*(1), 216–230. doi:10.1089/trgh.2016.0019

Epperson, C. N., Steiner, M., Hartlage, S. A., Eriksson, E., Schmidt, P. J., Jones, I., & Yonkers, K. A. (2012). Premenstrual dysphoric disorder: Evidence for a new category for DSM-5. *The American Journal of Psychiatry, 169*(5), 465–475.

Erez, C., & Shenkman, G. (2016). Gay dads are happier: Subjective well-being among gay and heterosexual fathers. *Journal of GLBT Family Studies.* Advanced online publication, *12*(5), 451–467. doi:10.1080/1550428X.2015.1102668

Ethics Committee of the American Society for Reproductive Medicine. (2015). Access to fertility services by transgender persons: An ethics committee opinion. *Fertility and Sterility, 104*(5), 1111–1115. doi:10.1016/j.fertnstert.2015.08.021

Eyler, A. E., Pang, S. C., & Clark, A. (2014). LGBT-assisted reproduction: Current practice and future possibilities. *LGBT Health, 1*(3), 151–156. doi:10.1089/lgbt.2014.0045

Family Equality Council (2016). Equality maps: Foster and adoption laws. Retrieved from http://www.familyequality.org/get_informed/resources/equality_maps/joint_adoption_laws/

Farrell, M. R., Corder, C. J., & Levine, L. A. (2013). Peyronie's disease among men who have sex with men: Characteristics, treatment, and psychosocial factors. *The Journal of Sexual Medicine, 10*(8), 2077–2083. doi:10.1111/jsm.12202

Garbers, S., McDonnell, C., Fogel, S. C., Eliason, M., Ingraham, N., McElroy, J. A., . . . Haynes, S. G. (2015). Aging, weight, and health among adult lesbian and bisexual women: A meta-synthesis of the multisite "Healthy Weight Initiative" focus groups. *LGBT Health, 2*(2), 176–187. doi:10.1089/lgbt.2014.0082

Gates, G. J. (2013). *LGBT parenting in the United States.* Los Angeles, CA: The Williams Institute. Retrieved from http://williamsinstitute.law.ucla.edu/wp-content/uploads/LGBT-Parenting.pdf

Goldberg, A. E., & Allen, K. R. (Eds.) (2013). *LGBT-parent families: Innovations in research and implications for practice.* New York, NY: Springer.

Gorgos, L. M., & Marrazzo, J. M. (2011). Sexually transmitted infections among women who have sex with women. *Clinical Infectious Diseases, 53*(Suppl 3), S84–S91. doi:10.1093/cid/cir697

Grant, J. M., Mottet, L. A., Tanis, J., Harrison, J., Herman, J. L., & Keisling, M. (2011) Injustice at every turn: A report of the national transgender discrimination survey. Retrieved from http://endtransdiscrimination.org/PDFs/NTDS_Report.pdf

Greenfeld, D. A., & Seli, E. (2016). Same-sex reproduction: Medical treatment options and psychosocial considerations. *Current Opinion in Obstetrics & Gynecology, 28*(3), 202–205. doi:10.1097/GCO.0000000000000266

Groff, J. Y., Mullen, P. D., Byrd, T., Shelton, A. J., Lees, E., & Goode, J. (2000). Decision making, beliefs, and attitudes toward hysterectomy: A focus group study with medically underserved women in Texas. *Journal of Women's Health & Gender-Based Medicine, 9*(2, Suppl 2), 39–50.

Grover, S. A., Shmorgun, Z., Moskovtsev, S. I., Baratz, A., & Librach, C. L. (2013). Assisted reproduction in a cohort of same-sex male couples and single men. *Reproductive Biomedicine Online, 27*(2), 217–221. doi:10.1016/j.rbmo.2013.05.003

Herndandez, M., & Fultz, S. L. (2006). Barriers to health care access. In M. D. Shankle (Ed.), *The handbook of lesbian, gay, bisexual, and transgender public health: A practitioner's guide to service* (pp. 177–200), New York, NY: Routledge.

Hiestand, K. R., Horne, S. G., & Levitt, H. M. (2008). Effects of gender identity on experiences of healthcare for sexual minority women. *Journal of LGBT Health Research, 3*(4), 15–27. doi:10.1080/15574090802263405

Hirshfield, S., Chiasson, M. A., Wagmiller, R. L., Remien, R. H., Humberstone, M., Scheinmann, R., & Grov, C. (2010). Sexual dysfunction in an Internet sample of U.S. men who have sex with men. *The Journal of Sexual Medicine, 7*(9), 3104–3114.

Hutchinson, M. K., Thompson, A. C., & Cederbaum, J. A. (2006). Multisystem factors contributing to disparities in preventive health care among lesbian women. *Journal of Obstetric, Gynecologic, and Neonatal Nursing, 35*(3), 393–402.

Institute of Medicine, Committee on Lesbian, Gay, Bisexual, and Transgender Health Issues and Research Gaps and Opportunities. (2011). *The health of lesbian, gay, bisexual, and transgender people: Building a foundation for better understanding.* Washington, DC: National Academies Press.

Johnson, E. K., & Finlayson, C. (2016). Preservation of fertility potential for gender and sex diverse individuals. *Transgender Health, 1*(1), 41–44. doi:10.1089/trgh.2015.0010

Jones, A. R., & Hoyler, C. L. (2006). HIV/AIDS among women who have sex with women. In F. Fernandez & P. Ruiz (Eds.), *Psychiatric aspects of HIV/AIDS* (pp. 299–307). Philadelphia, PA: Lippincott Williams & Wilkins.

Kates, J., Ranji, U., Beamesderfer, A., Salganicoff, A., & Dawson, L. (2016). *Health and access to care and coverage for lesbian, gay, bisexual, and transgender individuals in the U.S.* (Issue Brief). Menlo Park, CA: The Henry J. Kaiser Family Foundation. Retrieved from http://files.kff.org/attachment/Issue-Brief-Health-and-Access-to-Care-and-Coverage-for-LGBT-Individuals-in-the-US

Kerker, B. D., Mostashari, F., & Thorpe, L. (2006). Health care access and utilization among women who have sex with women: Sexual behavior and identity. *Journal of Urban Health, 83*(5), 970–979. doi:10.1007/s11524-006-9096-8

Knight, D. A., & Jarrett, D. (2015). Preventive health care for men who have sex with men. *American Family Physician, 91*(12), 844–852.

Koh, A. S., Gómez, C. A., Shade, S., & Rowley, E. (2005). Sexual risk factors among self-identified lesbians, bisexual women, and heterosexual women accessing primary care settings. *Sexually Transmitted Diseases, 32*(9), 563–569.

Kushnir, V. A., & Lewis, W. (2011). HIV/AIDS and infertility: Emerging problems in the era of highly active antiretrovirals. *Fertility and Sterility, 96*(3), 546–553. doi:10.1016/j.fertnstert.2011.05.094

Lev, A. I. (2006). Gay dads: Choosing surrogacy. *Lesbian and Gay Psychology Review, 7*(1), 73–77. Retrieved from http://www.choicesconsulting.com/TESTING/assets/pro_writing/Gay_Dads-Choosing_Surrogacy[1].pdf

Light, A. D., Obedin-Maliver, J., Sevelius, J. M., & Kerns, J. L. (2014). Transgender men who experienced pregnancy after female-to-male gender transitioning. *Obstetrics and Gynecology, 124*(6), 1120–1127. doi:10.1097/AOG.0000000000000540

Machalek, D. A., Poynten, M., Jin, F., Fairley, C. K., Farnsworth, A., Garland, S. M., … Grulich, A. E. (2012). Anal human papillomavirus infection and associated neoplastic lesions in men who have sex with men: A systematic review and meta-analysis. *The Lancet Oncology, 13*(5), 487–500. doi:10.1016/s1470-2045(12)70080-3

Makadon, H. J., Mayer, K. H., & Garofalo, R. (2006). Optimizing primary care for men who have sex with men. *Journal of the American Medical Association, 296*(19), 2362–2365.

Marrazzo, J. M., & Gorgos, L. M. (2012). Emerging sexual health issues among women who have sex with women. *Current Infectious Disease Reports, 14*(2), 204–211. doi:10.1007/s11908-012-0244-x

McKirnan, D. J., Du Bois, S. N., Alvy, L. M., & Jones, K. (2013). Health care access and health behaviors among men who have sex with men: The cost of health disparities. *Health Education & Behavior, 40*(1), 32–41. doi:10.1177/1090198111436340

McNamara, M. C., & Ng, H. (2016). Best practices in LGBT care: A guide for primary care physicians. *Cleveland Clinic Journal of Medicine, 83*(7), 531–541. doi:10.3949/ccjm.83a.15148

Moegelin, L., Nilsson, B., & Helström, L. (2010). Reproductive health in lesbian and bisexual women in Sweden. *Acta Obstetricia et Gynecologica Scandinavica, 89*(2), 205–209. doi:10.3109/00016340903490263

Mravcak, S. A. (2006). Primary care for lesbians and bisexual women. *American Family Physician, 74*(2), 279–286.

National LGBT Cancer Network. (2009). Anal cancer, HIV, and gay/bisexual men. Retrieved from http://www.cancer-network.org/cancer_information/gay_men_and_cancer/anal_cancer_hiv_and_gay_men.php#footnotes

National Women's Health Network. (2015). Hysterectomy. Retrieved from https://www.nwhn.org/hysterectomy/

Office on Women's Health, U.S. Department of Health and Human Services. (2010). Menopause and menopause treatments. Retrieved from: https://www.womenshealth.gov/files/assets/docs/fact-sheets/menopause-treatment.pdf

Office on Women's Health, U.S. Department of Health and Human Services. (2014). Hysterectomy. Retrieved from https://www.womenshealth.gov/publications/our-publications/briefs/hysterectomy/hysterectomy.pdf

Peitzmeier, S. M., Khullar, K., Reisner, S. L., & Potter, J. (2014). Pap test use is lower among female-to-male patients than non-transgender women. *American Journal of Preventive Medicine, 47*(6), 808–812. doi:10.1016/j.amepre.2014.07.031

Peitzmeier, S. M., Reisner, S. L., Harigopal, P., & Potter, J. (2014). Female-to-male patients have high prevalence of unsatisfactory Paps compared to non-transgender females: Implications for cervical cancer screening. *Journal of General Internal Medicine, 29*(5), 778–784. doi:10.1007/s11606-013-2753-1

Potter, J., Peitzmeier, S. M., Bernstein, I., Reisner, S. L., Alizaga, N. M., Agénor, M., & Pardee, D. J. (2015). Cervical cancer screening for patients on the female-to-male spectrum: A narrative review and guide for clinicians. *Journal of General Internal Medicine, 30*(12), 1857–1864. doi:10.1007/s11606-015-3462-8

Power, J., McNair, R., & Carr, S. (2009). Absent sexual scripts: Lesbian and bisexual women's knowledge, attitudes and action regarding safer sex and sexual health information. *Culture, Health & Sexuality, 11*(1), 67–81. doi:10.1080/13691050802541674

Puckett, J. A., Horne, S. G., Levitt, H. M., & Reeves, T. (2011). Out in the country: Rural sexual minority mothers. *Journal of Lesbian Studies, 15*(2), 176–186.

Rapkin, A. (2003). A review of treatment of premenstrual syndrome & premenstrual dysphoric disorder. *Psychoneuroendocrinology, 28,* 39–53. doi:10.1016/S0306-4530(03)00096-9

Rapkin, A. J., & Winer, S. A. (2008). The pharmacologic management of premenstrual dysphoric disorder. *Expert Opinion on Pharmacotherapy, 9*(3), 429–445. doi:10.1517/14656566.9.3.429

Reed, A. C., Reiter, P. L., Smith, J. S., Palefsky, J. M., & Brewer, N. T. (2010). Gay and bisexual men's willingness to receive anal Papanicolaou testing. *American Journal of Public Health, 100*(6), 1123–1129. doi:10.2105/AJPH.2009.176446

Reiter, P. L., Brewer, N. T., McRee, A. L., Gilbert, P., & Smith, J. S. (2010). Acceptability of HPV vaccine among a national sample of gay and bisexual men. *Sexually Transmitted Diseases, 37*(3), 197–203. doi:10.1097/OLQ.0b013e3181bf542c

Riskind, R. G., & Patterson, C. J. (2010). Parenting intentions and desires among childless lesbian, gay, and heterosexual individuals. *Journal of Family Psychology, 24*(1), 78–81.

Robinson, K., Galloway, K. Y., Bewley, S., & Meads, C. (2016). Lesbian and bisexual women's gynaecological conditions: A systematic review and exploratory meta–analysis. *BJOG: An International Journal of Obstetrics & Gynaecology, 124*(3), 381–392. doi:10.1111/1471-0528.14414

Saab, M. M., Landers, M., & Hegarty, J. (2016). Exploring awareness and help-seeking intentions for testicular symptoms among heterosexual, gay, and bisexual men in Ireland: A qualitative descriptive study. *International Journal of Nursing Studies, 67,* 41–50. doi:10.1016/j.ijnurstu.2016.11.016

Sadlier, C., Rowley, D., Morley, D., Surah, S., O'Dea, S., Delamere, S.,...Bergin, C. (2014). Prevalence of human papillomavirus in men who have sex with men in the era of an effective vaccine: A call to act. *HIV Medicine, 15*(8), 499–504. doi:10.1111/hiv.12150

Sandfort, T. G., & de Keizer, M. (2001). Sexual problems in gay men: An overview of empirical research. *Annual Review of Sex Research, 12*(1), 93–120.

Smalley, K. B., Warren, J. C., & Barefoot, K. N. (2015). Differences in health risk behaviors across understudied LGBT subgroups. *Health Psychology, 35*(2), 103–114.

Stotzer, R. L., Herman, J. L., & Hasenbush, A. (2014). *Transgender parenting: A review of existing research.* Los Angeles, CA: The Williams Institute. Retrieved from http://williams institute.law.ucla.edu/wp-content/uploads/transgender-parenting-oct-2014.pdf

Stuntz, M., Perlaky, A., des Vignes, F., Kyriakides, T., & Glass, D. (2016). The prevalence of Peyronie's disease in the United States: A population-based study. *PLOS ONE, 11*(2), e0150157. doi:10.1371/journal.pone.0150157

Tasker, F., & Patterson, C. J. (2008). Research on gay and lesbian parenting: Retrospect and prospect. *Journal of GLBT Family Studies, 3*(2–3), 9–34. doi:10.1300/J461v03n02_02

Tate, C. C., Ledbetter, J. N., & Youssef, C. P. (2013). A two-question method for assessing gender categories in the social and medical sciences. *Journal of Sex Research, 50*(8), 767–776. doi:10.1080/00224499.2012.690110

Tracy, J. K., Schluterman, N. H., & Greenberg, D. R. (2013). Understanding cervical cancer screening among lesbians: A national survey. *BMC Public Health, 13,* 442. doi:10.1186/1471-2458-13-442

Unger, C. A. (2014). Care of the transgender patient: The role of the gynecologist. *American Journal of Obstetrics and Gynecology, 210*(1), 16–26. doi:10.1016/j.ajog.2013.05.035

Unger, C. A. (2015). Care of the transgender patient: A survey of gynecologists' current knowledge and practice. *Journal of Women's Health, 24*(2), 114–118. doi:10.1089/jwh.2014.4918

Valanis, B. G., Bowen, D. J., Bassford, T., Whitlock, E., Charney, P., & Carter, R. A. (2000). Sexual orientation and health: Comparisons in the women's health initiative sample. *Archives of Family Medicine, 9*(9), 843–853.

Wahlert, L., & Fiester, A. (2013). Induced lactation for the nongestating mother in a lesbian couple. *The Virtual Mentor, 15*(9), 753–756. doi:10.1001/virtualmentor.2013.15.9.ecas2-1309

Waterman, L., & Voss, J. (2015). HPV, cervical cancer risks, and barriers to care for lesbian women. *The Nurse Practitioner, 40*(1), 46–53. doi:10.1097/01.NPR.0000457431.20036.5

Weber, S. (2008). Parenting, family life, and well-being among sexual minorities: Nursing policy and practice implications. *Issues in Mental Health Nursing, 29*(6), 601–618.

Weber, S. (2010). A stigma identification framework for family nurses working with parents who are lesbian, gay, bisexual, or transgendered and their families. *Journal of Family Nursing, 16*(4), 378–393. doi:10.1177/1074840710384999

White, J. C., & Dull, V. T. (1997). Health risk factors and health-seeking behavior in lesbians. *Journal of Women's Health, 6*(1), 103–112.

Yeshua, A., Lee, J. A., Witkin, G., & Copperman, A. B. (2015). Female couples undergoing IVF with partner eggs (co-IVF): Pathways to parenthood. *LGBT Health, 2*(2), 135–139. doi:10.1089/lgbt.2014.0126

Zaritsky, E., & Dibble, S. L. (2010). Risk factors for reproductive and breast cancers among older lesbians. *Journal of Women's Health (2002), 19*(1), 125–131. doi:10.1089/jwh.2008.1094

CHAPTER **8**

Intimate Partner Violence Among Gender and Sexual Minority Groups

Rita M. Melendez and Jillian Crystal Salazar

Intimate partner violence (IPV) impacts health in several ways. IPV refers to abusive behaviors occurring within the context of a sexual relationship. Abusive behaviors take the form of sexual abuse (forcing individuals to have sex with the perpetrator or others), physical abuse (hitting, kicking, or other forms of physical violence), and/or emotional abuse (controlling behaviors, verbal harassment; Reuter, Newcomb, Whitton, & Mustanski, 2016). IPV is distinct from hate crimes (Herek, 2009) and childhood physical and sexual abuse (Roberts, Austin, Corliss, Vandermorris, & Koenen, 2010), but often coincides with both.

Previous research on IPV focused primarily on cisgender women and their abusive male partners (Cannon & Buttell, 2015). A focus on cisgender women as victims of IPV resulted in a decreased understanding of and services for gender and sexual minority (GSM) individuals. The focus on cisgender women as victims in IPV led to an association with heterosexual relationships, where women are victims and men perpetrators. This historical link between IPV and gender is problematic. When IPV is associated with heterosexual couples it makes invisible the plight of GSM individuals, as well as male victims of female perpetrators (Messinger, 2011).

The consequence of the generalized association of IPV with heterosexual relationships has far-reaching implications. For example, the Violence Against Women

Act (VAWA) of 1998 did not protect GSM survivors of IPV. In 2012, the VAWA was reissued without any protections for GSM individuals, and only in 2013 was inclusive language added (Modi, Palmer, & Armstrong, 2014). Previous to the added provision, GSM survivors could be turned away from IPV shelters due to gender identity or sexual orientation. When policies do not recognize GSM issues relating to IPV, there are very real consequences for individuals including physical and mental health repercussions (Coker, Smith, Bethea, King, & McKeown, 2000).

While there are likely differences between and within each of the groups represented within the umbrella term *GSM*, there seems to be an increased risk of experiencing IPV among GSM individuals. The National Violence Against Women (NVAW) survey finds that 20% of women in opposite-sex couples report physical abuse in their lifetimes, as do 7% of men in opposite-sex couples. By contrast, among those in same-sex couples, 21% of men and 35% of women report physical abuse in their lifetimes (Tjaden & Thoennes, 2000). Those who identified as bisexual from the NVAW survey were the most likely to have experienced IPV (Messinger, 2011). In a separate study, transgender individuals seem to have even higher rates of IPV than their cisgender sexual minority counterparts, with 34% of transgender participants reporting IPV compared to 14% of gay and lesbian individuals (Landers & Gilsanz, 2009). Unfortunately, because experiences with stigma may have occurred in organizations that provide medical and social services, GSM individuals may be less likely to report IPV (Addis, Davies, Greene, MacBride-Stewart, & Shepherd, 2009), complicating both their ability to receive needed support services and our underlying understanding of IPV within the community.

This chapter highlights important issues surrounding IPV among GSM individuals. Each primary lesbian, gay, bisexual and transgender (LGBT) subgroup is addressed separately to demonstrate the specific and important characteristics of each group in relation to IPV. A case study of Juan is provided to demonstrate issues related to IPV among Latino sexual minority men. The chapter ends with best practices of community-based organizations and recommendations to provide services for GSM individuals experiencing IPV.

■ JUAN'S STORY

As part of a research study on Latino immigrants' access to care, we conducted interviews with 127 Latino immigrants who are HIV positive and currently living in the San Francisco Bay Area (Zepeda, Melendez, Samaniego, & Alaniz, 2012). Many participants experienced IPV and shared their stories. "Juan" is a composite of many of the participants and will illustrate some issues with IPV and barriers to care.

Juan emigrated from Mexico to the San Francisco Bay Area to escape ridicule and stigma associated with being gay. Even though his family accepted his sexual orientation, he faced discrimination from people outside of his home that made his life unbearable. For example, when his coworkers found out that Juan is gay, they assumed that he had AIDS. One coworker soaked a cup he had used in bleach before placing it back in the cupboard. Because of these experiences, Juan decided to leave Mexico and arrive in San Francisco where he hoped people would be more open to his sexual orientation.

Juan was lonely without his family. He was also dependent on a network of immigrants from Mexico to tell him about work opportunities. He wanted to escape the stigma he experienced in Mexico, but continued to feel he could not be open about being gay in the United States. His network of immigrant peers was equally insulting to gay men. If they knew Juan was gay, they would not let him know about work opportunities; therefore, Juan kept his gay life separate and secret from his peers.

When Juan started dating another Mexican immigrant, he was happy to have found a boyfriend and they both agreed to keep their relationship a secret. Even though his partner was controlling and told Juan what to do, Juan still liked having a boyfriend and having someone around whom he could be himself. Soon his relationship became violent. Juan felt there was no one to whom to turn for help. His boyfriend threatened to out Juan if he went to talk to someone about their relationship. Since Juan had no family in the United States and his network would not want to help him and would reject him for being gay, he felt trapped. Juan felt he would be better off putting up with violence that occurred once in a while rather than being alone and isolated, or worse, to be outed by his partner.

Juan's Barriers to Care

Juan's inability to seek help for the violence he experiences is a direct result of a number of factors. While researchers have noted the importance of screening for IPV among women (Waalen, Goodwin, Spitz, Petersen, & Saltzman, 2000), there is little research exploring how to screen for IPV among GSM individuals. Since many individuals in same-sex relationships may not publicly identify with a sexual minority group and may not wish to share their same-sex behaviors with their medical providers, it seems that screening in medical establishments may be challenging.

Homophobia and heteronormativity among medical providers lead many GSM individuals to not discuss their same-sex relationships (Freedberg, 2006). Juan does not always identify himself as gay. When asked, he sometimes says "yes" and sometimes "no." His openness about his sexual orientation is dependent on how safe he feels. Since he has had many experiences of stigma related to his sexual orientation, he does not always feel comfortable discussing his same-sex relationships. Importantly, organizations trained to handle GSM health issues and with training around issues of GSM IPV may not reach people like Juan, because they do not have staff who speak Spanish and because they do not actively recruit for Spanish-speaking clients. Additionally, since Juan is not fully "out," he may not feel comfortable entering a medical or service establishment that is LGBT-identified because he may fear people finding out that he is gay (Melendez & Pinto, 2009).

To screen for IPV you also need access to medical care and services. Juan, like many other immigrants (Zepeda et al., 2012), may not have access to health services. Screening by trained professionals will reach only the people who already have the resources to visit a medical provider. For immigrants who are undocumented, access to health care can vary greatly. For immigrants who are documented, they must have private health insurance or wait 5 years before being able to join a health care provider available through the Affordable Care Act (Zepeda et al., 2012). Juan may need to seek free services catering to undocumented immigrants. Because these services are also accessed by Juan's social network of immigrants, he may be uncomfortable discussing his sexuality there.

■ IPV AND GSM HEALTH OUTCOMES

IPV impacts several areas of GSM health. Direct effects to health relate to the physical pain and suffering inflicted in IPV. The indirect effects to health, such as depression, posttraumatic stress disorder (PTSD), substance use, and dissociation (World Health Organization [WHO], 2012), are less visible than bruises and broken bones, but have a long-lasting impact in the lives of survivors of IPV. The indirect effects of IPV combine with stigma and discrimination related to being a member of a gender and/or sexual minority group and can lead to negative, long-lasting effects on health. As Minority Stress Theory postulates, the accumulation of stressors takes an increased toll on the health outcomes of GSM individuals (Meyer, 1995). For example, those who experience IPV in same-sex relationships rate their health status as poorer than those in opposite-sex relationships (Blosnich & Bossarte, 2009).

Depression

Research demonstrates a strong correlation between mental health issues and IPV, especially depression (Buller, Devries, Howard, & Bacchus, 2014) and PTSD (Roberts et al., 2010). GSM survivors of IPV are more likely to experience verbal and emotional abuse as opposed to physical and sexual abuse (Messinger, 2011). The increase in emotional and verbal abuse may make IPV less visible among survivors and may make it more challenging for survivors to seek treatment for their abuse. The combination of these factors often leads GSM individuals who have experienced IPV to need mental health and support services. For example, one study found that GSM individuals are more likely to report symptoms of PTSD corresponding to IPV than cisgender individuals in opposite-sex relationships (Roberts et al., 2010).

Substance Use

Many researchers point to the increased risk of substance use among individuals identifying as a gender and/or sexual minority (Wong, Weiss, Ayala, & Kipke, 2010). Substance use may be an overall risk factor for causing IPV in relationships (Klostermann, Kelley, Milletich, & Mignone, 2011). While some studies show increased substance abuse among GSM survivors of IPV (Buller et al., 2014), others find no association (Reuter et al., 2016). Substance use may also be a means of coping with IPV (Wong et al., 2010).

Sexual Health

Sexual health is another important consideration for IPV among GSM individuals. Studies find a correlation between HIV risk and experiences with IPV (Feldman, Díaz, Ream, & El-Bassel, 2008; Heintz & Melendez, 2006; Ramachandran, Yonas, Silvestre, & Burke, 2010). HIV transmission in relationships where IPV is present can occur directly through forced unprotected sex. However, for many who experience IPV, the route to HIV is indirect. For example, many researchers cite the difficulties that individuals who have experienced IPV face when trying to negotiate safer sex with their partners (Eaton et al., 2008; Feldman et al., 2008; Heintz & Melendez, 2006; Simpson & Helfrich, 2007), such as fear of being physically abused, threatened, or accused of infidelity by partners when discussing sexual issues such as condom use. Another factor limiting the ability of negotiating safer sex is the process of dissociation, whereby survivors of sexual violence feel paralyzed with fear and outside of their bodies when engaging in sexual behaviors, thus limiting their ability to consent to sex and negotiate safer sex (Iverson et al., 2013; Morin, 2014).

■ IPV AMONG LESBIANS

Research shows that the percentage of women who have been abused by a female intimate partner ranges from 11% to 47% (Hassouneh & Glass, 2008; Waldner-Haugrud, Gratch, & Magruder, 1997). Of 79 women in a same-sex relationship, 11% reported experiencing rape or physical assault by a female intimate partner at some point in their lives (Tjaden, Thoennes, & Allison, 1999). The highest prevalence rates of 47% came from a study of 118 lesbians (Waldner-Haugrud et al., 1997). This study expanded the criteria of IPV in lesbian relationships to include threats, pushing, slapping, punching, being struck with an object, and use of a weapon (Waldnder-Haugrud et al., 1997). Further, a review of 11 studies found that lesbian women experienced sexual assault, sexual abuse, or rape at rates ranging from 2% to 45%, with a median rate of 12% (Rothman, Exner, & Baughman, 2011).

Western gender roles for women influence IPV among lesbians. Namely, traditional gender roles expect women to be feminine, nonviolent, and nurturing (Hassouneh & Glass, 2008). Women who do not fit these gender roles are not given the same legitimacy in the context of IPV (Hassouneh & Glass, 2008). Victims are sometimes ignored because it is assumed that women do not hit other women and, if they do, it must not be that serious (Hassouneh & Glass, 2008). Lesbians perceived as feminine are more likely to be treated as legitimate victims, while lesbians perceived as masculine are more likely to be treated as perpetrators (Little & Terrance, 2010). Stereotypes about lesbian relationships also affect experiences of IPV. Lesbian communities are thought by many to be nonviolent because there are no cisgender men (Hassouneh & Glass, 2008). Gender stereotypes about women and lesbians can even lead to victims not being able to recognize when abuse is occurring (Donovan & Hester, 2008).

Risk factors associated with IPV are higher among African American lesbians who are more likely to face obstacles seeking services when compared to White lesbians (Hill, Woodson, Ferguson, & Parks, 2012). Further, lesbians of color who seek intimate relationships with women of the same ethnic background may find a high degree of closeness with their partners that makes it difficult to disentangle from these relationships if their partners are abusive (Kanuha, 2013).

IPV AMONG GAY MEN

Due to historical views that IPV is male perpetrated, many have thought that IPV among gay men would be high; however, research shows that while IPV is higher for GSM individuals, it is not higher for men than for women in same-sex relationships (Messinger, 2011). In a study of 989 gay men, most felt that IPV was common among gay men and seen as both problematic and severe (Finneran & Stephenson, 2013). The study also found that gay men's previous experiences with homophobia resulted in decreased expectations of helpfulness with regard to the police and reporting IPV to them (Finneran & Stephenson, 2013). One study of 403 sexual minority men found that men in romantic relationships with men who are of another ethnicity were more likely to report IPV (Stephenson, Sato, & Finneran, 2013). As in the previous discussion regarding lesbians, it is unclear if this lower reported rate of IPV reflects differences in underlying incidence rates or in likelihood of reporting.

IPV among gay men is linked to several health issues. Studies exploring the correlation of IPV with early childhood physical and sexual abuse find that gay men who reported either were more likely to be both victims and perpetrators of IPV as adults (Welles, Corbin, Rich, Reed, & Raj, 2011). Several studies link IPV with increased HIV risk (Feldman et al., 2008; Heintz & Melendez, 2006; Ramachandran et al., 2010). Other studies have likewise demonstrated increased depression, PTSD, and suicide (as well as suicidal thoughts and attempts) among male survivors of IPV (Randle & Graham, 2011).

For sexual minority men who are members of racial and/or ethnic minority groups, IPV can occur within a racial/ethnic context that is less accepting (Finneran & Stephenson, 2014). The issues related to sexual minority men of color exemplify the challenges of seeking services for issues related to sexual behaviors without the ability to be as open about those behaviors. Given that research finds that men in relationships that are closeted tend to have increased incidence of IPV (Stephenson et al., 2013), there may be a disproportionate burden of IPV among men who experience additional pressures to conceal their sexual orientation from others (e.g., racial/ethnic minority).

IPV AMONG BISEXUAL INDIVIDUALS

Research demonstrates that bisexual individuals have higher rates of IPV when compared to gay and lesbian individuals (Messinger, 2011; West, 2012), and that bisexual women have higher rates of IPV than bisexual men (Walters, Chen, & Breiding, 2013). In one study, rates of IPV for bisexual individuals were associated with opposite-sex relationships rather than same-sex relationships (Goldberg & Meyer, 2013), while in another it was higher in same-sex relationships (Freedner, Freed, Yang, & Austin, 2002).

Despite the high rates of IPV found among bisexual individuals, there still exists a dearth of robust research. Since many studies explore sexual behaviors versus the sexual orientation of individuals, bisexual individuals may remain invisible in many studies. For example, if a bisexual individual is with a same-sex partner, they may be classified as gay or lesbian. When with an opposite sex partner, they may be classified as heterosexual.

Research has shown that partners may feel threatened by their bisexual partner's identity and past relationships with either opposite- or same-sex partners (Spalding & Peplau, 1997). This may lead to increased risk for IPV among bisexual individuals and may also lead to decreased support for bisexual individuals seeking help for IPV. Researchers exploring issues related to bisexual individuals in relationships cite the notion that bisexual individuals are frequently perceived as unfaithful (McLean, 2004), which may also lead to an increased rate of IPV.

IPV AMONG TRANSGENDER INDIVIDUALS

Studies demonstrate that transgender individuals experience high levels of violence throughout their lives (Stotzer, 2009). For example, transgender individuals experience more than twice the national rate of criminal victimization (Herek, 2009). In a national survey of 402 transgender respondents, over half of all individuals reported some experience with violence, with 47% of respondents reporting being assaulted and 14% experiencing rape or attempted rape (Lombardi, Wilchins, Priesing, & Malouf, 2002)). IPV is a particularly important focus area in preventing violence against transgender people, as in 2015, 23% of transgender homicide victims were killed by intimate partners (Human Rights Campaign & Trans People of Color Coalition, 2015).

Considering prior research demonstrating homophobia's role as a major factor in sexual minority experiences of IPV, transphobia is also likely a major risk factor for IPV among transgender individuals (Langenderfer-Magruder, Whitfield, Walls, Kattari, & Ramos, 2016). The lack of employment opportunities as well as discrimination against transgender individuals is directly related to their vulnerability with sexual partners. Many transgender individuals feel isolated and discriminated against, and may stay with their abusive partners because they have no one else who offers them support and comfort (Melendez & Pinto, 2007).

As transgender individuals navigate the care available to them, they face unequal treatment and awareness from providers (Yerke & DeFeo, 2016). Providers are often unprepared to handle issues that arise for transgender individuals due to a lack of appropriate training (Ford, Slavin, Hilton, & Holt, 2013). Transgender IPV survivors may experience discrimination when seeking help, such as mistaking their gender, blaming them for violence, or turning them away because of their gender identity (GLBT Domestic Violence Coalition & Jane Doe Inc., 2005). The intersecting marginalized identities that many transgender individuals hold are also risk factors for discrimination in care settings. Race, ethnicity, class, educational level, citizenship, age, and disability may contribute to care providers' poor treatment of transgender people (Bradford, Reisner, Honnold, & Xavier, 2013; Lombardi, 2009; Seelman, 2015).

Transgender youth are especially vulnerable to IPV (Brown & Herman, 2015). They may fear being outed as transgender by their abusers. If outed, they may feel vulnerable to other types of violence. Some abusive partners instill fear in their transgender partners by telling them that no one will like them if they find out they are transgender (FORGE, 2011). Perpetrators want their partners to feel like they need to stay closeted. Outing as a form of abuse can be especially traumatizing and lead to isolation (Dank, Lachman, Zweig, & Yahner, 2014; Freedner et al., 2002).

"Trans panic" or a very strong emotional reaction to a sexual partner's previously unknown transgender identity that results in violence is a specific form of IPV (Shepherd, 2013). "Trans panic" has been used as a legal defense for perpetrators of violence against transgender individuals. However, as of 2013, it has been rejected as an acceptable legal defense by the American Bar Association (Shepherd, 2013).

■ ADDRESSING IPV AMONG GSM INDIVIDUALS

As awareness of IPV for GSM individuals grows, there are more organizations dedicated to serving their needs. Crucial to the resilience and support of GSM survivors of IPV is the contribution of community-based organizations. They fill necessary gaps for survivors living at the margins, whether it be for temporary housing, crisis support, legal aid, community organizing, or other needs. Unfortunately, there is a clear need for continued education and training regarding IPV within the LGBT community as general crisis center staff have been found to take cases of same-sex IPV less seriously than instances of heterosexual IPV (L. S. Brown & Pantalone, 2011).

On a national level, organizations such as the National Coalition of Anti-Violence Programs focus on GSM survivors of violence. Examples of local organizations that focus on GSM survivors include the Community United Against Violence (CUAV), the San Francisco Gay & Lesbian Center, and the Los Angeles Gay & Lesbian Center. Larger structural injustices such as heterosexism and homophobia drive the mission of many organizations, such as the Texas Council on Family Violence. They adapted the Duluth Gender and Control Wheel created by the Domestic Abuse Intervention Project (1984) for GSM individuals. The adapted model for GSM individuals addresses issues of heterosexism, homophobia, biphobia, and transphobia to illustrate that IPV occurs within larger societal inequalities. The adapted model has been used by many organizations as a teaching tool.

Many organizations provide a 24-hour hotline for GSM survivors to call. Survivors are able to seek emergency crisis counseling and receive short-term counseling. Hotline operators are trained in crisis management, safety planning, and assisting the survivor in locating local resources for ongoing help. Group and peer counseling is often offered to survivors. Group counseling dedicated to GSM survivors provides a safe space for healing and allows participants to see they are not alone. Peer counseling can be mixed with short-term case management to ensure that survivors are able to work with a trained counselor one-on-one to begin the healing process and be connected to other resources they may need such as shelters, immigration services, and legal assistance, among others.

Many organizations also offer assistance navigating law enforcement, medical establishments, and the judicial system for GSM survivors. Organizations such as the New York City Anti-Violence Project and San Francisco Women Against Rape train advocates to accompany survivors to institutions that can be intimidating, confusing, and discriminatory, especially GSM survivors who are further marginalized due to race, ethnicity, and socioeconomic or immigration status.

Policies work hand-in-hand with community-based organizations in addressing the needs of GSM individuals with regard to IPV. There are a few policies already in existence that support GSM survivors of IPV. The reauthorization of the VAWA in 2013 added protections for GSM survivors of IPV and included a provision that prohibited shelters from discriminating against individuals based on sexual orientation or gender identity (Violence Against Women Act, 2013). However, not all states protect GSM survivors—Louisiana, Montana, and South Carolina explicitly deny protection to survivors whose assailant is the same sex as them (American Bar Association Commission on Domestic Violence, 2008). Virginia does not have case law to discriminate against GSM survivors; however, according to an Attorney General opinion, the law does not include GSM survivors (American Bar Association Commission on Domestic Violence, 2008).

A report published in December 2015 indicates that while the annual incidence and economic burden of sexual violence is significantly higher than cancer, cardiovascular disease, diabetes, and HIV/AIDS, preventive funding allocated to these chronic diseases far exceeds that devoted to IPV (Waechter & Ma, 2015). If funding is used as a measure for priority, sexual violence is low on the list of priorities for policy makers. When considering marginalized populations such as GSM individuals, policies addressing IPV are scarce. Some have pushed to consider sexual violence a public health issue rather than just a social justice issue (Modi et al., 2014; Waechter & Ma, 2015). The recategorization as a public health issue is significant because efforts can be focused on prevention rather than on reaction. While the WHO made this distinction over 20 years ago, the issue of sexual violence continues to be underprioritized and underfunded (García-Moreno et al., 2015).

In a victory for anti-sexual violence advocates, the State of California signed into law the "Yes Means Yes" bill in September 2014. SB 967 states that state-funded universities must employ an understanding of consent that is affirmative—partners need a continual "yes" to engage in consensual sex. Affirmative consent differs from a "no means no" understanding of consent. SB 967 applies only in the state of California and only in the context of state-funded universities. Despite this narrow coverage, the impact of this law will make it easier to identify sexual violence as well as to identify consent regardless of previous consent or relationship status. SB 967 can stand as an example for other states and at the federal level.

■ RECOMMENDATIONS

A number of community-based organizations as well as researchers have discussed recommendations or best practices for addressing issues of IPV among GSM individuals (see Table 8.1). The recommendations are still evolving, but often reveal simple, easy-to-implement practices that are available to many providers.

TABLE 8.1: Review of Best Practices to Address IPV in GSM Patients

BEST PRACTICES FOR COMMUNITY-BASED ORGANIZATIONS	
Train staff and volunteers on the prevalence of IPV and stereotypes/assumptions about GSM survivors	Ford et al. (2013)
Make GSM materials available and visible; ensure that entrance, waiting room, and posters/signage make GSM survivors feel welcome	The Northwest Network of Bisexual, Trans, Lesbian & Gay Survivors of Abuse (2001)
Agencies must intentionally establish themselves as serving GSM individuals	Duke and Davidson (2009)
Transgender individuals need services based on their gender identification, including shelter	Hines and Douglas (2011)
Nonidentified LGBT clinics need to be trained for GSM patients who may desire to receive their services	Melendez and Pinto (2009)
Address and reduce minority stressors	Edwards, Sylaska, and Neal (2015)
Solicit feedback to ensure agency is meeting needs of GSM individuals	Helfrich and Simpson (2006)
BEST PRACTICES FOR MEDICAL AND HEALTH CARE PROVIDERS	
Use inclusive language when working with survivors (such as "partner" vs. "wife" or "husband")	Ard and Makadon (2011)
Be knowledgeable of local GSM resources and of health risks associated with IPV	Ard & Makadon (2011)
Screening for IPV should routinely be done with GSM individuals	Langenderfer-Magruder et al. (2016)
Discuss safer sex negotiation in the context of IPV	Heintz and Melendez (2006)
Develop safer sex safety plans in addition to physical safety plans	Heintz and Melendez (2006)
Explicitly state commitment to fight multiple sites of systemic oppression that GSM survivors face such as racism and heterosexism	Singh and McKleroy (2011)
Ensure gender-neutral bathrooms are available	Singh and McKleroy (2011)
BEST PRACTICES FOR LAW ENFORCEMENT	
Provide training on the needs of GSM individuals of all races and backgrounds using inclusive language	Morrison (2003)

(continued)

TABLE 8.1: Review of Best Practices to Address IPV in GSM Patients *(continued)*

Outreach to LGBT communities to increase reporting of IPV	Finneran and Stephenson (2013)
Provide training about biases due to stereotypes around gender and sexual orientation	Hassouneh and Glass (2008)
BEST PRACTICES FOR EDUCATORS	
Create an inclusive environment focusing on ideas and beliefs of healthy relationships rather than a focus on gender and heterosexuality	Donovan and Hester (2008)
Offer IPV prevention and intervention programs for GSM youth	Freedner et al. (2002)
Create peer-led groups to increase awareness of teen dating violence for GSM youth	Dank et al. (2014)
Conduct educational programs that reduce homo-/bi-/transphobia	GLBT Domestic Violence Coalition and Jane Doe Inc. (2005)
BEST PRACTICE FOR POLICY AND LAW MAKERS	
Include protections for undocumented immigrants in the Violence Against Women Act	Modi, Palmer, and Armstrong (2014)
Include all genders and sexual orientations when creating policy	Langenderfer-Magruder et al. (2016)
Understand IPV as a public health issue in need of public funding	Waechter and Ma (2015)

GSM, gender and sexual minority; IPV, Intimate partner violence; LGBT, lesbian, gay, bisexual and transgender.

For example, a simple technique recommended by the authors is to avoid the use of gendered language when discussing issues of IPV. Instead of assuming an individual is with an opposite sex partner, use nongender-specific language—such as "your partner."

Conclusion

A unique consideration for GSM survivors of IPV relates to the provision of LGBT-identified services. While some GSM individuals may be more comfortable seeking services in an LGBT-identified organization, others may feel more comfortable seeking services in an organization that is not specific for GSM individuals (Melendez & Pinto, 2009). Many individuals who may not choose to outwardly identify as GSM may be more comfortable in a location that is a family clinic for example, as they may not want others to infer regarding their sexual orientation or gender identity based upon their presence at the clinic.

The issue of having LGBT-identified providers as well as non-LGBT-identified providers points to the need for diverse approaches and techniques in addressing issues related to IPV. Just as GSM individuals stem from a multitude of communities, approaches to both prevention and supportive services need to be diverse and varied. For this reason, community-based organizations are in a unique location to rapidly and creatively address the issues of their specific community members.

■ REFERENCES

Addis, S., Davies, M., Greene, G., Macbride-Stewart, S., & Shepherd, M. (2009). The health, social care and housing needs of lesbian, gay, bisexual and transgender older people: A review of the literature. *Health & Social Care in the Community, 17*(6), 647–658. doi:10.1111/j.1365-2524.2009.00866.x

American Bar Association Commission on Domestic Violence. (2008). Overview of CPO protections for LGBT victims of domestic violence. Retrieved from http://www .americanbar.org/content/dam/aba/migrated/domviol/pdfs/CPO_Protections_ for_LGBT_Victims_7_08.authcheckdam.pdf

Ard, K. L., & Makadon, H. J. (2011). Addressing intimate partner violence in lesbian, gay, bisexual, and transgender patients. *Journal of General Internal Medicine, 26*(8), 930–933.

Blosnich, J. R., & Bossarte, R. M. (2009). Comparisons of intimate partner violence among partners in same-sex and opposite-sex relationships in the United States. *American Journal of Public Health, 99*(12), 2182–2184. doi:10.2105/AJPH.2008.139535

Bradford, J., Reisner, S. L., Honnold, J. A., & Xavier, J. (2013). Experiences of transgender-related discrimination and implications for health: Results from the Virginia Transgender Health Initiative Study. *American Journal of Public Health, 103*(10), 1820–1829. doi:10.2105/AJPH.2012.300796

Brown, L. S., & Pantalone, D. (2011). Lesbian, gay, bisexual, and transgender issues in trauma psychology: A topic comes out of the closet. *Traumatology, 17*(2), 1–3. doi:10.1177/1534765611417763

Brown, T. N. T., & Herman, J. L. (2015). *Intimate partner violence and sexual abuse among LGBT people: A review of existing research.* Los Angeles, CA: The Williams Institute. Retrieved from http://williamsinstitute.law.ucla.edu/wp-content/uploads/Intimate-Partner -Violence-and-Sexual-Abuse-among-LGBT-People.pdf

Buller, A. M., Devries, K. M., Howard, L. M., & Bacchus, L. J. (2014). Associations between intimate partner violence and health among men who have sex with men: A systematic review and meta-analysis. *PLOS Medicine, 11*(3), e1001609. doi:10.1371/journal. pmed.1001609

Cannon, C., & Buttell, F. (2015). Illusion of Inclusion: The failure of the gender paradigm to account for intimate partner violence in LGBT relationships. *Partner Abuse, 6*(1), 65–77. doi:10.1891/1946-6560.6.1.65

Coker, A. L., Smith, P. H., Bethea, L., King, M. R., & McKeown, R. E. (2000). Physical health consequences of physical and psychological intimate partner violence. *Archives of Family Medicine, 9*(5), 451–457.

Dank, M., Lachman, P., Zweig, J. M., & Yahner, J. (2014). Dating violence experiences of lesbian, gay, bisexual, and transgender youth. *Journal of Youth and Adolescence, 43*(5), 846–857. doi:10.1007/s10964-013-9975-8

Domestic Abuse Intervention Project. (1984). Power and control wheel. Retrieved from http://www.theduluthmodel.org/pdf/PowerandControl.pdf

Donovan, C., & Hester, M. (2008). 'Because she was my first girlfriend, I didn't know any different': Making the case for mainstreaming same-sex sex/relationship education. *Sex Education, 8*(3), 277–287. doi:10.1080/14681810802218155

Duke, A., & Davidson, M. M. (2009). Same-sex intimate partner violence: Lesbian, gay, and bisexual affirmative outreach and advocacy. *Journal of Aggression, Maltreatment & Trauma, 18*(8), 795–816.

Eaton, L., Kaufman, M., Fuhrel, A., Cain, D., Cherry, C., Pope, H., & Kalichman, S. C. (2008). Examining factors co-existing with interpersonal violence in lesbian relationships. *Journal of Family Violence, 23*(8), 697–705. doi:10.1007/s10896-008-9194-3

Edwards, K., Sylaska, K., & Neal, A. M. (2015). Intimate partner violence among sexual minority populations: A critical review of the literature and agenda for future research. *Psychology of Violence, 5*(2), 112–121. doi:10.1037/a0038656

Feldman, M. B., Díaz, R. M., Ream, G. L., & El-Bassel, N. (2008). Intimate partner violence and HIV sexual risk behavior among Latino gay and bisexual men. *Journal of LGBT Health Research, 3*(2), 9–19.

Finneran, C., & Stephenson, R. (2013). Gay and bisexual men's perceptions of police helpfulness in response to male-male intimate partner violence. *Western Journal of Emergency Medicine, 14*(4), 354–362. doi:10.5811/westjem.2013.3.15639

Finneran, C., & Stephenson, R. (2014). Intimate partner violence, minority stress, and sexual risk-taking among U.S. men who have sex with men. *Journal of Homosexuality, 61*(2), 288–306. doi:10.1080/00918369.2013.839911

Ford, C. L., Slavin, T., Hilton, K. L., & Holt, S. L. (2013). Intimate partner violence prevention services and resources in Los Angeles: Issues, needs, and challenges for assisting lesbian, gay, bisexual, and transgender clients. *Health Promotion Practice, 14*(6), 841–849. doi:10.1177/1524839912467645

FORGE. (2011). Transgender domestic violence and sexual assault resource sheet. Retrieved from https://avp.org/wp-content/uploads/2017/04/2011_FORGE_Trans_DV_SA_Resource_Sheet.pdf

Freedberg, P. (2006). Health care barriers and same-sex intimate partner violence: A review of the literature. *Journal of Forensic Nursing, 2*(1), 15–25. doi:10.1111/j.1939-3938.2006.tb00049.x

Freedner, N., Freed, L. H., Yang, Y. W., & Austin, S. B. (2002). Dating violence among gay, lesbian, and bisexual adolescents: Results from a community survey. *The Journal of Adolescent Health, 31*(6), 469–474. doi:10.1016/S1054-139X(02)00407-X

García-Moreno, C., Hegarty, K., d'Oliveira, A. F., Koziol-McLain, J., Colombini, M., & Feder, G. (2015). The health-systems response to violence against women. *The Lancet, 385*(9977), 1567–1579. doi:10.1016/S0140-6736(14)61837-7

GLBT Domestic Violence Coalition, & Jane Doe Inc. (2005). Shelter/housing needs for lesbian, bisexual and transgender (GLBT) victims of domestic violence. Retrieved from http://www.ncdsv.org/images/shelterhousingneedsforglbtvictimsdv.pdf

Goldberg, N. G., & Meyer, I. H. (2013). Sexual orientation disparities in history of intimate partner violence results from the California health interview survey. *Journal of Interpersonal Violence, 28*(5), 1109–1118. doi:10.1177/0886260512459384

Hassouneh, D., & Glass, N. (2008). The influence of gender role stereotyping on women's experiences of female same-sex intimate partner violence. *Violence Against Women, 14*(3), 310–325. doi:10.1177/1077801207313734

Heintz, A. J., & Melendez, R. M. (2006). Intimate partner violence and HIV/STD risk among lesbian, gay, bisexual, and transgender individuals. *Journal of Interpersonal Violence, 21*(2), 193–208. doi:10.1177/0886260505282104

Helfrich, C. A., & Simpson, E. K. (2006). Improving services for lesbian clients: What do domestic violence agencies need to do? *Health Care for Women International, 27*(4), 344–361. doi:10.1080/07399330500511725

Herek, G. M. (2009). Hate crimes and stigma-related experiences among sexual minority adults in the United States: Prevalence estimates from a national probability sample. *Journal of Interpersonal Violence, 24*(1), 54–74. doi:10.1177/0886260508316477

Hill, N. A., Woodson, K. M., Ferguson, A. D., & Parks, C. W. (2012). Intimate partner abuse among African American lesbians: Prevalence, risk factors, theory, and resilience. *Journal of Family Violence, 27*(5), 401–413. doi:10.1007/s10896-012-9439-z

Hines, D. A., & Douglas, E. M. (2011). Symptoms of posttraumatic stress disorder in men who sustain intimate partner violence: A study of helpseeking and community samples. *Psychology of Men & Masculinity, 12*(2), 112.

Human Rights Campaign, & Trans People of Color Coalition. (2015). Addressing anti-transgender violence: Exploring realities, challenges and solutions for policymakers and community advocates. Retrieved from http://hrc-assets.s3-website-us-east-1.amazonaws.com//files/assets/resources/HRC-AntiTransgenderViolence-0519.pdf

Iverson, K. M., Litwack, S. D., Pineles, S. L., Suvak, M. K., Vaughn, R. A., & Resick, P. A. (2013). Predictors of intimate partner violence revictimization: The relative impact of distinct PTSD symptoms, dissociation, and coping strategies. *Journal of Traumatic Stress, 26*(1), 102–110. doi:10.1002/jts.21781

Kanuha, V. K. (2013). "Relationships so loving and so hurtful": The constructed duality of sexual and racial/ethnic intimacy in the context of violence in Asian and Pacific Islander lesbian and queer women's relationships. *Violence Against Women, 19*(9), 1175–1196. doi:10.1177/1077801213501897

Klostermann, K., Kelley, M. L., Milletich, R. J., & Mignone, T. (2011). Alcoholism and partner aggression among gay and lesbian couples. *Aggression and Violent Behavior, 16*(2), 115–119. doi:10.1016/j.avb.2011.01.002

Landers, S. J., & Gilsanz, P. (2009). The health of lesbian, gay, bisexual and transgender (LGBT) persons in Massachusetts: A survey of health issues comparing LGBT persons with their heterosexual and non-transgender counterparts. Retrieved from http://masslib-dspace.longsight.com/handle/2452/112258

Langenderfer-Magruder, L., Whitfield, D. L., Walls, N. E., Kattari, S. K., & Ramos, D. (2016). Experiences of intimate partner violence and subsequent police reporting among lesbian, gay, bisexual, transgender, and queer adults in Colorado: Comparing rates of cisgender and transgender victimization. *Journal of Interpersonal Violence, 31*(5), 855–871. doi:10.1177/0886260514556767

Little, B., & Terrance, C. (2010). Perceptions of domestic violence in lesbian relationships: stereotypes and gender role expectations. *Journal of Homosexuality, 57*(3), 429–440. doi:10.1080/00918360903543170

Lombardi, E. L. (2009). Varieties of transgender/transsexual lives and their relationship with transphobia. *Journal of Homosexuality, 56*(8), 977–992. doi:10.1080/00918360903275393

Lombardi, E. L., Wilchins, R. A., Priesing, D., & Malouf, D. (2002). Gender violence: Transgender experiences with violence and discrimination. *Journal of Homosexuality, 42*(1), 89–101. doi:10.1300/J082v42n01_05

McLean, K. (2004). Negotiating (non) monogamy: Bisexuality and intimate relationships. *Journal of Bisexuality, 4*(1–2), 83–97. doi:10.1300/J159v04n01_07

Melendez, R. M., & Pinto, R. (2007). 'It's really a hard life': Love, gender and HIV risk among male-to-female transgender persons. *Culture, Health & Sexuality, 9*(3), 233–245. doi:10.1080/13691050601065909

Melendez, R. M., & Pinto, R. M. (2009). HIV prevention and primary care for transgender women in a community-based clinic. *The Journal of the Association of Nurses in AIDS Care, 20*(5), 387–397. doi:10.1016/j.jana.2009.06.002

Messinger, A. M. (2011). Invisible victims: Same-sex IPV in the National Violence Against Women Survey. *Journal of Interpersonal Violence, 26*(11), 2228–2243. doi:10.1177/0886260510383023

Meyer, I. H. (1995). Minority stress and mental health in gay men. *Journal of Health and Social Behavior, 36*(1), 38–56.

Modi, M. N., Palmer, S., & Armstrong, A. (2014). The role of Violence Against Women Act in addressing intimate partner violence: A public health issue. *Journal of Women's Health, 23*(3), 253–259. doi:10.1089/jwh.2013.4387

Morin, C. (2014). Re-traumatized: How gendered laws exacerbate the harm for same-sex victims of intimate partner violence. *New England Journal on Criminal & Civil Confinement, 40(2)*, 477–497.

Morrison, A. M. (2003). Queering domestic violence to straighten out criminal law: What might happen when queer theory and practice meet criminal law's conventional responses to domestic violence. *South Carolina Review of Law and Women's Studies, 13*, 81.

The Northwest Network of Bi, Trans, and Gay Survivors of Abuse (2001). Quick Organizational Audit: LGBT Visibility and Inclusion. Retrieved from VAWnet: http://vawnet.org/material/quick-organizational-audit-lgbt-visibility-and-inclusion

Ramachandran, S., Yonas, M. A., Silvestre, A. J., & Burke, J. G. (2010). Intimate partner violence among HIV-positive persons in an urban clinic. *AIDS Care, 22*(12), 1536–1543. doi:10.1080/09540121.2010.482199

Randle, A. A., & Graham, C. A. (2011). A review of the evidence on the effects of intimate partner violence on men. *Psychology of Men & Masculinity, 12*(2), 97–111. doi:10.1037/a0021944

Reuter, T. R., Newcomb, M. E., Whitton, S. W., & Mustanski, B. (2016). Intimate partner violence victimization in LGBT young adults: Demographic differences and associations with health behaviors. *Psychology of Violence,7*(1), 101–109. Advance online publication. doi:10.1037/vio0000031

Roberts, A. L., Austin, S. B., Corliss, H. L., Vandermorris, A. K., & Koenen, K. C. (2010). Pervasive trauma exposure among US sexual orientation minority adults and risk of posttraumatic stress disorder. *American Journal of Public Health, 100*(12), 2433–2441. doi:10.2105/AJPH.2009.168971

Rothman, E. F., Exner, D., & Baughman, A. L. (2011). The prevalence of sexual assault against people who identify as gay, lesbian, or bisexual in the United States: A systematic review. *Trauma, Violence & Abuse, 12*(2), 55–66. doi:10.1177/1524838010390707

Seelman, K. L. (2015). Unequal treatment of transgender individuals in domestic violence and rape crisis programs. *Journal of Social Service Research, 41*(3), 307–325. doi:10.1080/01488376.2014.987943

Shepherd, W. (2013). Resolution 113A. American Bar Association, Criminal Justice Section. Retrieved from http://www.americanbar.org/content/dam/aba/directories/policy/2013_hod_annual_meeting_113A.docx

Simpson, E. K., & Helfrich, C. A. (2007). Lesbian survivors of intimate partner violence: Provider perspectives on barriers to accessing services. *Journal of Gay & Lesbian Social Services, 18*(2), 39–59. doi:10.1300/J041v18n02_03

Singh, A. A., & McKleroy, V. S. (2011). "Just getting out of bed is a revolutionary act": The resilience of transgender people of color who have survived traumatic life events. *Traumatology, 17*(2), 34–44. doi:10.1177/1534765610369261

Spalding, L. R., & Peplau, L. A. (1997). The unfaithful lover: Heterosexuals' perceptions of bisexuals and their relationships. *Psychology of Women Quarterly, 21*(4), 611–625. doi:10.1111/j.1471-6402.1997.tb00134.x

Stephenson, R., Sato, K. N., & Finneran, C. (2013). Dyadic, partner, and social network influences on intimate partner violence among male-male couples. *The Western Journal of Emergency Medicine, 14*(4), 316–323. doi:10.5811/westjem.2013.2.15623

Stotzer, R. L. (2009). Violence against transgender people: A review of United States data. *Aggression and Violent Behavior, 14*(3), 170–179. doi:10.1016/j.avb.2009.01.006

The Northwest Network of Bi, Trans, and Gay Survivors of Abuse. (2001). Quick organizational audit: LGBT visibility and inclusion. Retrieved from VAWnet: http://vawnet.org/material/quick-organizational-audit-lgbt-visibility-and-inclusion

Tjaden, P. G., & Thoennes, N. (2000). *Extent, nature, and consequences of intimate partner violence: Findings from the National Violence Against Women Survey* (NCJ Publication No. 181867). Washington, DC: U.S. Department of Justice, Office of Justice Programs. Retrieved from http://www.ncjrs.gov/App/abstractdb/AbstractDBDetails.aspx?id=181867

Tjaden, P., Thoennes, N., & Allison, C. J. (1999). Comparing violence over the life span in samples of same-sex and opposite-sex cohabitants. *Violence and Victims, 14*(4), 413–415.

Violence Against Women Act, S. 47. (2013). Retrieved from https://www.gpo.gov/fdsys/pkg/BILLS-113s47enr/pdf/BILLS-113s47enr.pdf

Waalen, J., Goodwin, M. M., Spitz, A. M., Petersen, R., & Saltzman, L. E. (2000). Screening for intimate partner violence by health care providers: Barriers and interventions. *American Journal of Preventive Medicine, 19*(4), 230–237. doi:10.1016/S0749-3797(00)00229-4

Waechter, R., & Ma, V. (2015). Sexual violence in America: Public funding and social priority. *American Journal of Public Health, 105*(12), 2430–2437. doi:10.2105/AJPH.2015.302860

Waldner-Haugrud, L. K., Gratch, L. V., & Magruder, B. (1997). Victimization and perpetration rates of violence in gay and lesbian relationships: Gender issues explored. *Violence and Victims, 12*(2), 173–184.

Walters, M. L., Chen J., & Breiding, M. J. (2013). *The National Intimate Partner and Sexual Violence Survey (NISVS): 2010 findings on victimization by sexual orientation.* Atlanta, GA: National Center for Injury Prevention and Control, Centers for Disease Control and Prevention. Retrieved from https://www.ncjrs.gov/App/Publications/abstract.aspx?ID=263171

Welles, S. L., Corbin, T. J., Rich, J. A., Reed, E., & Raj, A. (2011). Intimate partner violence among men having sex with men, women, or both: Early-life sexual and physical abuse as antecedents. *Journal of Community Health, 36*(3), 477–485. doi:10.1007/s10900-010-9331-9

West, C. M. (2012). Partner abuse in ethnic minority and gay, lesbian, bisexual, and transgender populations. *Partner Abuse, 3*(3), 336–357.

Wong, C. F., Weiss, G., Ayala, G., & Kipke, M. D. (2010). Harassment, discrimination, violence, and illicit drug use among young men who have sex with men. *AIDS Education and Prevention, 22*(4), 286–298. doi:10.1521/aeap.2010.22.4.286

World Health Organization. (2012). Understanding and addressing violence against women. Retrieved from http://apps.who.int/iris/bitstream/10665/77432/1/WHO_RHR_12.36_eng.pdf

Yerke, A. F., & DeFeo, J. (2016). Redefining intimate partner violence beyond the binary to include transgender people. *Journal of Family Violence, 31*(8), 975–979. doi:10.1007/s10896-016-9887-y

Zepeda, J., Melendez, R. M., Samaniego, R., & Alaniz, G. (2012, July). Proyecto Acceso: Access to health care for HIV-positive Latino immigrants to the U.S. Paper presented at the International AIDS Conference, Washington DC.

CHAPTER 9

The Needs of Gender and Sexual Minority Persons Living With Disabilities

Franco Dispenza, Tameeka L. Hunter, and Asha Kumar

Disability discourse has undergone drastic changes over the past 30 years, creating substantial tensions that leave scholars in a state of flux when attempting to tackle the very nature of disability (DePoy & Gilson, 2004). Changes in laws, sociopolitical attitudes, health sciences, and language have all contributed to this state of flux, while challenging hegemonic ideals of impairment, ability, functionality, and disability culture. Incidentally, this state of tension has also allowed scholars and members of the greater public to devise advances in technology and health care to better improve the quality of life for persons living with disabilities (Smart & Smart, 2006). There have even been advances to be more inclusive of persons with disabilities in the social environment, despite the fact that persons with disabilities are still socially and economically marginalized (Fassinger, 2008).

As a facet of human diversity, disability is a normative experience (Smart & Smart, 2006). According to the U.S. Census Bureau (2012), approximately 56.7 million Americans reported living with a disability in 2010. The Centers for Disease Control and Prevention (2016) estimated that another 117 million Americans are living with one or more chronic illnesses. Disability and chronic illness conditions include blindness, deafness, developmental and intellectual delays, chronic medical illnesses (e.g., HIV/AIDS and cancer), neurological impairments, traumatic brain and spinal cord injuries, and orthopedic and musculoskeletal impairments, as well as psychiatric illnesses and behavioral-related issues (e.g., substance abuse in recovery; Falvo, 2014).

Since disability is situated within the context of human diversity, many different culturally diverse groups have the capacity to encounter the experience of disability. In particular, sexual minority persons (e.g., lesbian, gay, bisexual, pansexual, and queer) and gender minority persons (e.g., transgender, genderqueer, two spirit, and nonbinary) are two culturally diverse groups that have the capacities to develop disabilities (Fraley, Mona, & Theodore, 2007). Although there are no exact population estimates that account for how many gender and sexual minority (GSM) persons are living with a disability or chronic illness, Lipton (2004) inferred that there could be upwards of 9.3 million.

Of course, over the course of their lifespans, GSM persons could develop one or multiple disabilities—impairing, limiting, and restricting autonomous participation in various aspects of daily living (e.g., employment, education, and community involvement). Despite not having exact estimates as to how many GSM persons are living with disabilities, scholars have noted that disability rates are significantly higher among sexual minority individuals when compared to cisgender heterosexual individuals (Fredriksen-Goldsen, Kim, & Barkan, 2012; Kim & Fredriksen-Goldsen, 2012; Wallace, Cochran, Durazo, & Ford, 2011). Using probabilistic sampling procedures from Washington's Behavioral Risk Factor Surveillance System, Fredriksen-Goldsen et al. (2012) found that the odds of lesbians and bisexual women endorsing a disability were respectively 1.9 and 2.7 times as high as cisgender heterosexual women. The odds of gay and bisexual men endorsing a disability were respectively 1.4 and 2.8 times as high as cisgender heterosexual men. Fredriksen-Goldsen et al. (2012) also found that among those with disabilities, sexual minority individuals were significantly more likely to be younger than their heterosexual counterparts living with disabilities. Sexual minority individuals are also more likely to indicate that their physical health status interferes with their ability to engage in everyday physical activities (Conron, Mimiaga, & Landers, 2010) and that they are more likely to need assistive technology or modifications to adjust to their disability (Fredriksen-Goldsen et al., 2012). Although there are no comparison studies to date that have directly compared gender minority persons with cisgender persons, one international survey conducted with 1,963 transgender persons found that approximately 27% reported living with a disability (Witten, 2014).

GSM persons living with disabilities are a highly marginalized and vulnerable group in the United States (Dispenza, Harper, & Harrigan, 2016). Medical physicians, health care workers, human service providers, and scholars have to be culturally competent when providing services or conducting research with this population. As an overview, this chapter first provides a contextualized view on the lives of GSM persons living with disabilities, which is followed by a discussion of implications for meeting the needs of GSM individuals living with disabilities. Particular emphasis is made with regard to the utility of an affirmative rehabilitation team to help improve the quality of life of GSM persons living with disabilities. Secondly, considerations for universal design (UD) is also made with special attention to its application with GSM individuals living with disabilities.

◼ THE LIVES OF GSM INDIVIDUALS LIVING WITH DISABILITIES

The extent to which individuals experience their disability is contingent on the severity of the disability, the age of onset, culture, environment (physical, social, and political), personal demographics (age, gender, race, and ethnicity), psychological determinants (e.g., personality, temperament, coping, and intelligence), and social and familial support systems (Berens, 2014; DePoy & Gilson, 2004; Falvo, 2014). In conjunction with disability, sexual orientation and gender identity add contextual layers that have the capacity of enriching the human experience, but may also present novel challenges for health care workers, human service providers, and scholars. In particular, health care workers, human service providers, and scholars must particularly attend to identity, disparities in health and health care, and stigma.

Identity

Although sexual orientation and gender identity are not the only identities that play a significant role in the lives of persons with disabilities, they are the two identities that are most often ignored (Glover-Graf, 2012). Other culturally relevant factors could play a significant role, and therefore, when conceptualizing adequate care and even research, providers and scholars may find it beneficial to use an intersectionality framework with GSM persons living with disabilities (Dispenza, Viehl, Sewell, Burke, & Gaudet, 2016). For instance, a White gay man who encountered a catastrophic traumatic brain injury (TBI) might have more access to health resources because he lives in a major metropolitan city, but he may encounter more stigma from the community for having a disability. Alternatively, an African American identified transgender woman living with a psychiatric disability might have less access to mental health–related resources if she were living in a small town, but may have more affirming social support networks. The intersections of sexual orientation and gender identity are unique and highly nuanced, necessitating that practitioners and service providers critically exercise sensitivity when working with GSM individuals living with disabilities.

Sexual orientation, gender identity, and disability also emerge at different points in the life course, and can intersect with one another at any point during one's lifespan development (Dispenza & DeBlaere, 2017). These identities can develop in succession of one another, or emerge all at one time. For instance, an individual could be born with a congenital disability (e.g., autism, cerebral palsy, and spina bifida) and come out as transgender during puberty. Another person could acquire a disability, such as a TBI, and reveal that they are bisexual to others soon after. Identity development becomes an important factor to consider in the context of lifespan development because of its associations with one's sense of self (i.e., values, virtues, ethics, and interests), navigating the social environment, developing pride, and establishing roots with a cultural community (Chaney & Marszalek, 2014; DePoy & Gilson, 2004; Matthews, 2007).

Health Disparities

In conjunction with a primary disability, secondary and tertiary health issues are also common, leading to potential exacerbations of disability symptoms, poor prognosis, or complications to treatment (Falvo, 2014). Although there is hardly any research that addresses health disparities among GSM individuals living with disabilities, GSM individuals are already at risk for developing significantly high rates of physical chronic health conditions (Fredriksen-Goldsen et al., 2014; Witten, 2014; see also Chapter 6). For instance, GSM individuals are more likely than cisgender heterosexual individuals to subjectively report poorer physical health (Lick, Durso, & Johnson, 2013). When compared to heterosexual-identified persons, sexual minority individuals in certain studies also report higher instances of cardiovascular disease (Diamant & Wold, 2003), cancer (Brandenburg, Matthews, Johnson, & Hughes, 2007; Case et al., 2004; Dibble, Roberts, & Nussey, 2004), pulmonary and respiratory conditions (Heck & Jacobson, 2006; Steele, Ross, Dobinson, Veldhulzen, & Tinmouth, 2009), hypertension (Wallace et al., 2011; Wang, Hausermann, Counatsou, Aggleton, & Weiss, 2007), arthritis (Kim & Fredriksen-Goldsen, 2012), and diabetes (Dilley, Simmons, Boysun, Pizacani, & Stark, 2010). Additionally, GSM individuals are at higher risk for developing chronic psychiatric conditions, such as mood and anxiety disorders (Hatzenbuehler, 2009), or posttraumatic stress disorders (Bandermann & Szymanski, 2014; Roberts, Austin, Corliss, Vandermorris, & Koenen, 2010), and have higher rates of overall psychological distress (Riggle, Rostosky, & Horne, 2010; Wallace et al., 2011). Transgender persons are also more likely to report a history of suicidal ideation and suicidal attempts (dickey, Reisner, & Juntunen, 2015).

Relatedly, persons with disabilities have less access to adequate health care, and disparities have been found in relation to both cancer and oral health care screenings (Armour, Swanson, Waldman, & Perlman, 2008; Reichard, Stolze, & Fox, 2011). Scholars have attributed inequity in health care access among persons with disabilities to physical inaccessibility of facilities, communication difficulties, and a lack of competence to work with persons with disabilities by health care professionals (Dovey & Webb, 2000). GSM individuals also have limited access to health care, including limited insurance coverage, prejudice among health care professionals, and reduced practitioner competence to effectively work with GSM individuals (Fredriksen-Goldsen et al., 2014; Lick et al., 2013); therefore, it stands to reason that GSM individuals living with disabilities would be doubly impacted by problems with accessing care.

Stigma in the Lives of GSM Persons Living With Disabilities

GSM individuals living with disabilities are also subject to a variety of discriminatory and oppressive experiences throughout their lifespans (Dispenza et al., 2016). Not only are they subject to be discriminated against because of their GSM identities (covered more in depth in other chapters), but they are also likely to have discriminatory experiences related to age, race or ethnicity, income, education, living arrangements, and relationship status (Fredriksen-Goldsen, Kim, Muraco, & Mincer, 2009). Additionally, caregivers of GSM individuals are likely to experience discrimination (Fredriksen-Goldsen et al., 2009). Although the Americans with Disabilities Act (ADA) protects persons living with a variety of disability conditions from being discriminated against in housing, employment, and public accommodations, there are no uniform legislations that protect persons from being discriminated against because of their sexual orientation or gender identity.

In addition to discrimination, heterosexism, and transphobia, GSM individuals living with disabilities are likely to encounter both *ableism* and *disablism* (Dispenza & DeBlaere, 2017). Ableism constitutes a series of attitudes, practices, and policies that favor persons who are thought of as being fully capable of exercising their physical, cognitive, emotional, and behavioral capacities (Berens, 2014). For instance, a queer man who utilizes a wheelchair for mobility purposes may experience an ableist environment when he discovers that a local community gay bar is not physically accessible for persons who use wheelchairs (i.e., no ramp or elevator to gain access). Disablism, on the other hand, is a series of attitudes and beliefs that regard persons with disabilities as inferior to those not living with disabilities (Miller, Parker, & Gillinson, 2004). Furthermore, disablism includes systemic barriers and discriminatory behaviors that are harmful toward persons with disabilities. For example, a qualified applicant for a job who is blind and a transgender woman may be denied employment for the fact that she is transgender and has a disability.

◼ THE NEEDS OF GSM PERSONS LIVING WITH DISABILITIES

The Affirmative Rehabilitation Team

GSM individuals living with a disability will encounter a variety of specialists, health care professionals, and service providers. Depending on the onset, type, and severity of the disability, persons living with a disability are likely to work with a *rehabilitation team*, a group of providers committed to returning an individual living with a disability to their highest level of quality of life (Behm & Gray, 2012). Rehabilitation team members work collaboratively and synergistically to make decisions that produce optimal outcomes, while working to increase the identified patient's motivation for success (Gage, 1998; Sheehan, Robertson, & Ormond, 2007). Rehabilitation teams are most popularly used in psychiatric, mental health, substance abuse as well as trauma and catastrophic injury–related facilities (e.g., spinal cord, traumatic brain, and amputations). A rehabilitation team most often comprises physicians, nurses, case managers, physical and occupational therapists, psychologists, social workers and counselors, and vocational rehabilitation counselors (Butt & Caplan, 2010). In some instances, there may be other health care and service professionals who constitute the makeup of a rehabilitation team, and the specific roles of each member in the rehabilitation team are likely to change across various health care and human service–related settings. Refer to Table 9.1 for a list of potential rehabilitation team members and a description of their roles.

Service providers and health care professionals may also encounter GSM youth, and need to be aware of *individualized education programming (IEP)*. Authorized by the Individuals with Disabilities Education Act (IDEA), IEP teams specifically work

TABLE 9.1: Rehabilitation Team Members and Their Roles

Physiatrist	A medical physician who specializes in rehabilitation and treats medical conditions affecting the brain, nervous system, bones, and muscles
Occupational Therapist	Help persons living with disabilities develop, recover, or improve skills and activities related to daily living
Speech-Language Pathologist	Diagnose, treat, and rehabilitate deficits and disorders in communication, swallowing, and hearing
Prosthetist/Orthotist	Create medical support devices, including artificial limbs and braces
Child Life Specialist	Work with children and families to better adjust and cope with medical illnesses and disabilities
Rehabilitation Counselor	Professional counselors who address both the vocational and clinical mental health needs of persons with disabilities
Rehabilitation Nurse	Provide holistic and comprehensive treatment and education to persons living with a wide variety of chronic illnesses and disabilities
Physical Therapist	Assess and treat issues related to movement, mobility; help reduce physical pain; help maximize physical functioning; and help to improve overall physical health
Psychologist	Diagnose, test, evaluate, and provide psychological care to a wide variety of mental health issues, including diagnosing and treating psychiatric disabilities and behavioral health-related disabilities
Therapeutic Recreational Specialist	Assess and help persons with disabilities to engage in leisure activities
Social Worker	Help individuals and families with disabilities to improve psychosocial functioning, and connect persons with disabilities to community resources

to assess and devise plans that maximize the full learning and developmental potential of a student with a disability. Often times, IEP teams consist of the child with the disability, parents or guardian of the child, teachers, school psychologists, school social workers, attorneys, and transition counselors or vocational rehabilitation counselors. On rare occasions, health care providers may be asked to consult on IEPs or to take part in the programming. In some instances, health care services may even be written into the formal plan, which would potentially require the school district to pay for those services. Lastly, service and health care providers need to be aware that GSM youth living with disabilities often receive minimal to no sex education in school, and more often, receive no educational information on same-sex relationships or transgender identities (Duke, 2011). For more information regarding GSM youth overall, please refer to Chapter 17.

Clear communication, systematic decision making, appropriate goal setting, organization, and attending to the components that facilitate team processes are the key characteristics to good team functioning (Nijhuis et al., 2007). Optimal team processes consist of fluid leadership committing to a common set of values that assure successful rehabilitation outcomes, maintaining and instilling hope, preventing rivalry between team members, and keeping the person with a disability at the center of the rehabilitation process (Butt & Caplan, 2010).

Operating from both a patient-centered and strengths-based approach also helps contribute to optimal outcomes in the rehabilitation process (Butt & Caplan, 2010), and this implies that a patient's identities, including sexual orientation and gender identity, are central to the rehabilitation process. Because of the need to navigate a variety of institutional systems to access care and services, GSM individuals living with a disability are presented with an increased risk of encountering homophobia, heterosexism, and transphobia (Greene, 2007). This occurs partly because persons living with a disability are often sexually stigmatized and viewed as asexual, reproductively defective, or lacking any capacity to possess a sexual identity (Glover-Graf, 2012). Often, if sexuality is assumed, persons living with disability are thought to be heterosexual. Thus, it is incumbent on members of the rehabilitation team to be affirmative in their scope of practice, and recognize that their patients (or identified student in the context of IEPs) may not be heterosexual or cisgender.

To practice affirmatively with GSM persons means to genuinely believe that all expressions of sexuality and gender are equally valid in society and that practitioners proactively work toward developing the appropriate knowledge, skills, and respectful attitudes to work with GSM persons (Dispenza et al., 2016; Greene, 2007; Matthews, 2007). Furthermore, regardless of how culturally competent they may seem, health care and service providers live in a heterosexist and transphobic society. Practitioners and service providers are all subject to heterosexist and cisgender prejudices and oppression, and therefore, may unconsciously harbor certain beliefs about GSM persons that may unknowingly manifest in practice (Matthews, 2007). Thus, affirmative practices require that health care and service providers working with GSM persons take personal reflective inventory of their own attitudes, beliefs, and biases (Chaney & Marszalek, 2014), and explore how their personal beliefs could facilitate or hinder affirmative rehabilitation care.

Furthermore, affirmative practices include opposing negative sociopolitical messages and not pathologizing same-sex behaviors (e.g., affection and intimacy) or diverse gender expressions (American Psychological Association [APA], 2012, 2015). Affirmative practices also include helping to minimize feelings of stigma, validating the legitimacy of having a sexual or gender minority identity, instilling pride, as well as acknowledging the influence of oppression, stigma, and discrimination that exists in society (Langdridge, 2007). Most importantly, affirmative approaches help facilitate positive identity development among GSM individuals and help promote better psychological adjustment (Matthews, 2007).

Conceptualizing the Affirmative Rehabilitation Team

To place this in context, let us consider DJ, a biracial, cisgender, gay man. DJ served during the Iraq war in 2003 and was discharged from the military after incurring third and fourth degree burns on the left leg during combat. His burns were so severe that it necessitated amputation below the knee. Overall, DJ was intermittently seeking medical care for a period of 3 years for the injuries that he incurred. During that time, DJ worked closely with his rehabilitation team, which consisted of a neurologist, dermatologist, rheumatologist, rehabilitation nurse, psychologist, occupational therapist, prosthetist, social worker, and rehabilitation counselor.

The team members exercised affirmative care in several ways. First, they included DJ's partner, whom he later married, all throughout the rehabilitation planning process. This provided the team an opportunity to motivate and engage DJ's closest social support system as part of his rehabilitation. Secondly, when DJ mentioned that his parents were still having difficulties accepting his gay identity, the psychologist and rehabilitation counselor held joint family therapy sessions with DJ's family in order to process the family's concerns. Not addressing the family's concerns could have exacerbated stress that could have delayed DJ's adjustment and adaptation to his disability.

Thirdly, the rehabilitation team intentionally explored their own heterosexist beliefs and thoughts following an incident that happened in the early rehabilitation planning stages. At the time, one of the physicians requested a second round of HIV testing for DJ. DJ declined the need for the test, as he reported that he and his partner were exclusively monogamous and that they had both been continuously tested as HIV negative. When the physician insisted again that DJ consider the HIV test, DJ left the physician's office and filed a formal complaint against the physician. The physician claimed that DJ was being resistant and noncompliant. Members of the research team objectively explored the complaints made by DJ, and the social worker gently challenged the physician to contemplate the necessity for the testing. After discussing the impact of stigma, history of HIV/AIDS, homophobia, as well as the power dynamics between the physician and DJ, the physician had more context for understanding DJ's motives for not wanting to be tested a second time.

Universal Design

Accessible design, or *accessibility*, is one of the most widely used concepts in the field of disability. To suggest that some aspect of the environment is "accessible" means that physical, social, and technological environments can be easily attained (DePoy & Gilson, 2004). An example would include making a historical building accessible by adding a ramp so persons with mobility-related disabilities or impairments could access the building. However, critics of the accessible design movement indicate that to make structural alteration to accommodate a group of people happens to cater to persons who diverge from the norm. Ultimately, principles of accessible design reinforce segregation and stigma, suggesting that persons with disabilities are in essence a separate population (Iwarsson & Stahl, 2003).

Alternatively, UD operates under the principle that there is never only one population that needs to be considered (Iwarsson & Stahl, 2003). As a practical design strategy, UD insists that all products, environments, services, and social experiences be usable for all persons (Lid, 2014). The conceptual framework of UD reflects the understanding that disability is one of many normative forms of diversity

(Tagayuna, Stodden, Chang, Zeleznik, & Whelley, 2005; Stodden, Whelley, Chang, & Harding, 2001), and that the purpose of UD is to maximize usability to the greatest extent possible, without the need for modifications, alterations, or specialized designs (Higbee, 2003; Lid, 2014). Furthermore, UD is a process that emphasizes changing social attitudes, upholding democratic principles, and striving for equity and global citizenship (Iwarsson & Stahl, 2003).

Both *queer* and *crip* theories (e.g., McRuer, 2006) make it possible to apply principles of UD with GSM persons. According to Myers and Crockett (2013), the application of UD as a framework to conceptualize the lives of GSM persons rests on three assumptions. The first assumption holds that all human bodies and minds are normative, regardless of ability or disability. As such, all sexual orientations and gender identities are normative, including the sexual orientations and gender identities of persons with disabilities. Secondly, physical, social, technological, political, and economic environments are usable by all persons, including persons with diverse sexualities and gender identities. Historically, persons with disabilities, sexual minority persons, and gender minority persons have been excluded from having equal access to employment, education, and health care (Fassinger, 2008). Lastly, intentionally designing physical, social, technological, political, and economic environments to be inclusive benefits all persons, regardless of ability status, sexual orientation, gender identity, or any other diverse identities (Daniels & Geiger, 2010).

Conceptualizing UD With GSM Individuals

UD has been applied to the design of buildings, commercial products, information technology, schools, teaching and learning processes, and even health care settings (Burgstahler & Cory, 2008; Burgstahler & Russo-Gleicher, 2015; Center for Universal Design, 2016). The principles of UD include: (a) equitable use; (b) flexibility in use; (c) simple and intuitive use; (d) perceptible information; (e) tolerance for error; (f) low physical effort; and (g) size and space for approach and use (Center for Universal Design, 2016; Hennessey & Koch, 2007; Winance, 2014).

Myers and Crockett (2013) specifically addressed how each of the UD principles could be applied to GSM persons. Please refer to Table 9.2 to see a list of UD principles and a summary of Myers and Crockett's (2013) application to GSM persons. To place UD in context of GSM individuals living with disabilities, let us consider the case of "Destiny." Destiny is a 27-year-old, African American, gender nonbinary, queer-identified individual. Approximately 12 months ago, Destiny was involved in a motor vehicle accident and lost consciousness at the site of the accident. Destiny was quickly transported to a hospital and began to show the first signs of consciousness after being extubated. At the time, a CT scan indicated a C-spine fracture at C6 and C7. It was determined that Destiny had incomplete quadriplegia. Destiny was then transferred to a rehabilitation center, and underwent physical therapy and occupational therapy 5 days per week. Given the severity of the accident, Destiny was given a dual diagnosis of a TBI in addition to a spinal cord injury (SCI). Approximately 25% to 60% of individuals with acute SCI are reported to have sustained a concomitant brain injury, as manifested by the presence of cognitive deficits, primarily in the areas of new learning and memory

TABLE 9.2: Universal Design Principles

UNIVERSAL DESIGN (UD) CENTER FOR UNIVERSAL DESIGN (2016)	QUEER UD (MYERS & CROCKETT, 2013)
Equitable use: The design is useful and marketable to people with diverse abilities.	Equitable use: Social institutions are equitably available to people with diverse GSM orientations.
Flexibility in use: The design accommodates a wide range of individual preferences and abilities.	Flexibility in use: Social institutions accommodate a wide range of individual, family, and lifestyle preferences.
Simple and intuitive use: Use of the device is easy to understand, regardless of the user's experience, knowledge, language skills, or current concentration level.	Simple and intuitive use: Requirements are easy to understand; no additional requirements based on gender or sexual orientation.
Perceptible information: The design communicates necessary information effectively to the user, regardless of ambient conditions or the user's sensory abilities.	Perceptible information: Information is clearly and accurately transmitted in a way that demonstrates awareness and sensitivity to queer lives.
Tolerance for errors: Design minimizes hazards and the adverse consequences of accidental or unintended actions.	Tolerance for ambiguity: ambiguous, conflicting, and changing GSM orientations are welcomed and seen as normal.
Low physical effect: The design can be used efficiently and comfortably and with a minimum of fatigue.	Freedom from violence: People are free from physical and sexual violence, both in and out of intimate relationships.
Size and space for approach and use: Appropriate size and space is provided for approach, reach, manipulation, and use regardless of user's body size, posture, or mobility.	Privacy: People have the privacy to disclose or not disclose their gender or sexual orientation.

functioning (Falvo, 2014). Since the accident, Destiny now uses a motorized wheelchair for mobility. Destiny has minimal use of upper extremities, and is unable to grip items with either hand. Since the accident, Destiny has not been able to return to work. Destiny subsequently lost employment and Destiny's ex, Sandra, ended their 2-year relationship 3 months after the motor vehicle accident.

The *equitable use principle* indicates that the design of any space, environment, or social experience should be useful and marketable to people with a variety of abilities (Center for Universal Design, 2016; Hennessey & Koch, 2007). Should Destiny go to a physician's office, a height adjustable examination table could benefit Destiny by making it easier to transfer to the examination table from the motorized wheelchair. Besides reducing Destiny's risk of injury, it also reduces the risk of any medical staff encountering an injury. An adjustable exam table would also benefit older adults, shorter individuals, and persons who have strength and endurance issues. Other examples of equitable use include powered doors with sensors that open automatically when an individual's presence is detected,

TABLE 9.3: Recommendations for Universal Design

Mobility and Space	Corridors that are at least 5-feet wide
	Corridors are unobstructed paths of travel
	Adequate clearing space around medical equipment
	Adjustable examination tables and lower sections of reception desk for easier communication with staff
	Adequate and varied seating options, as well as open space for parking mobility aids
Cognitive and Learning	Present information in a logical, straightforward manner, avoiding unnecessary jargon and complexity
	Avoid using metaphors, analogies, sarcasm, etc.
	Essential information presented in a clear, concise manner
	Downloadable information in accessible file formats (e.g., Word, .RTF, and PDFs created with Adobe Pro X or higher) to be read in advance or with text-reading software
Vision and Hearing	Provide accessible websites that can be read using screen-reading software, like JAWS, allows for on-screen text enlargement, and/or the ability to change the level of contrast
	Provide medical sign language interpreter
	Caption all videos on website

Source: Center for Universal Design (2016).

automatic sensors on restroom sinks and towel dispensers, or electronic formats of documents. Please refer to Table 9.3 to see other examples of UD.

In relation to GSM individuals, the space (whether it be a physical building, social institution, or policy, etc.) needs to also be equitably available (Myers & Crockett, 2013). Destiny should not have to encounter barriers, discrimination, or instances of prejudice for being queer identified, nor should Destiny be the victim of bureaucratic policy that would prohibit Destiny from receiving the highest standard of care. For instance, inclusive language on all paperwork can prove helpful and reassuring to a variety of people. One example of how language use can exemplify the equitable use principle is the ability for one to select "significant other," or "partner" on a form, in addition to either "husband" or "wife." This language is inclusive and affirming of all sexual orientations and gender identities, and provides relevant information about an individual's social support. Equitable use ensures that no one person is segregated, targeted, or stigmatized as a result of their identity. Another example is the inclusion of same-sex partners, husbands, and wives as part of the rehabilitation process. Before the U.S. Supreme Court struck bans that prohibited same-sex couples from getting married, Destiny's partner did not have any legal rights to even be in the same hospital room following the accident. Rather, legal documentation would be necessary for her to have any rights to attend to Destiny's needs. All married heterosexual couples would have to do is inform the hospital staff that they were their partner's husband or wife.

Creating systems that support the involvement of partners and significant others in the rehabilitation process is essential in creating supportive, effective care systems.

The *flexibility in use principle* indicates that a design should accommodate a wide range of individuals, including their preferences and abilities (Center for Universal Design, 2016). GSM individuals would easily benefit from this principle should social institutions allow for wide accommodations (Myers & Crockett, 2013). For instance, having a designated wheelchair-accessible, unisex restroom in a physician's office or shopping mall happens to benefit persons with disabilities who use an attendant, a single parent who needs to accompany their child to the restroom, or an older adult who needs to provide some assistance to their spouse. Providing Destiny with the option of a unisex restroom limits any discomfort or potential stigmatization for using a specific gender-assigned restroom. Also, in this particular example with Destiny, UD provides one of the most important aspects to human experience—it provides Destiny dignity and respect.

The *simple and intuitive use principle* is exemplified by a design that makes its use easy to understand, regardless of the user's experience, knowledge, language skills, or current concentration level (Center for Universal Design, 2016). This principle seeks to eliminate complexity, simplify design by being consistent with all user expectations and intuition, arranging information consistent with its importance (e.g., the most important information appears first), and providing effective prompting and feedback during and after a task completion (Burgstahler & Cory, 2008). Given Destiny's cognitive capabilities, using the *Wong-Baker Faces Pain Rating Scale* (Wong-Baker FACES Foundation, 2016) would be an effective way of assessing any pain that may be present. Regardless of any person's education, nationality, or language ability, a person could effectively communicate their current pain level because the emotions represented on the rating scale are universal. With respect to GSM persons, institutional policies in particular should not have to require additional paperwork and intentionally create unnecessary barriers because Destiny identifies as gender nonconforming and queer (Myers & Crockett, 2013). In particular, policies and materials regarding gender, sexuality, and sexual orientation should be easy to understand regardless of Destiny's experience, knowledge, or language capabilities. For example, any print or virtual material regarding sexual health (e.g., HIV and sexually transmitted infections screening, and birth control) should include photographs, illustrations, or video clips while being inclusive of diverse sexualities and gender expressions.

A major element of the *perceptible information principle* is that the design communicates necessary information to the user, regardless of the user's sensory abilities (Center for Universal Design, 2016). Some general guidelines when employing this principle are to use different modes for the presentation of essential information (e.g., pictorial, verbal, and tactile) and provide adequate contrast between essential information and its surroundings (Hennessey & Koch, 2007). It is also important to maximize comprehension of essential information, differentiate elements in ways that can be described (i.e., make it easy to give instructions or directions), and provide compatibility with a variety of techniques or devices used by people with different abilities (Hennessey & Koch, 2007). Providing Destiny with software (e.g., Kurzweil) that reads text on a computer screen may prove beneficial. It also accommodates people with other conditions, such as reading disabilities and visual impairments.

Myers and Crockett (2013) applied this principle slightly differently with GSM persons. In obtaining information efficiently, this principle upholds that accurate and relevant information regarding GSM persons is communicated accurately and prominently. Furthermore, should information regarding sexuality and gender be made available to the wider public, same-sex relationships and diverse gender expressions also should be presented. This upholds the accuracy of GSM diversity.

The *tolerance for error principle* seeks to minimize hazards and the adverse consequences of accidental or unintended actions (Center for Universal Design, 2016). Much like an undo button, it is expected that one will make errors, but those errors can be minimized or corrected. With respect to Destiny, the fluidity of Destiny's gender identity expression should be accepted as normative and not stigmatized as an error or pathology. Myers and Crockett (2013) view it as society's attempt to tolerate ambiguity in one's sexuality and gender expression.

The *low physical effort* principle indicates that design can be used efficiently and comfortably without fatigue. The *size and space for approach and use principle* indicates that appropriate size and space be provided, regardless of one's body, size, posture, or mobility. Myers and Crockett (2013) interpret both of these principles in context of psychological space. GSM persons should be free from physical and psychological violence, including stigma, prejudice, and discrimination. Furthermore, a space needs to be affirming so that someone could have the choice to disclose sexual orientation or gender identity (Myers & Crockett, 2013). Persons working to help maximize Destiny's full rehabilitation potential need to be conscientious of the space with which Destiny interacts on a daily basis. Is it value laden with heteronormativity and gender binaries? Is it hostile toward GSM individuals? These are just some questions to consider when attempting to apply the last two UD principles with GSM persons.

■ CONCLUSION

This chapter sought to provide some context related to the lives of GSM persons living with disabilities. As mentioned previously, there are approximately 56.7 million Americans reportedly living with a disability (U.S. Census Bureau, 2012), and an additional 117 million Americans living with one or more chronic illnesses (Centers for Disease Control and Prevention, 2016). Both disability and chronic illness conditions are significantly higher among GSM persons (Fredriksen-Goldsen et al., 2012; Kim & Fredriksen-Goldsen, 2012; Lick et al., 2012; Wallace et al., 2011), and health care providers should exercise cultural competence and sensitivity when working with GSM persons living with disabilities. First, it is recommended that health care providers consider the advantages of employing affirmative rehabilitation teams. Rehabilitation team members work together with the goal of producing successful outcomes for persons living with disabilities, and they should work toward keeping a person's multiple identities, including sexual orientation and gender identity, centrally focused during the rehabilitation process. Another strategy is to implement UD principles, which seek to reduce the segregation and stigma faced by persons with chronic illnesses and/or disabilities. Our hope is that discussing challenges and strategies will help health care professionals prepare for and improve the quality of health care services provided to GSM populations that experience chronic illness and/or disability.

■ REFERENCES

American Psychological Association. (2012). Guidelines for psychological practice with lesbian, gay, and bisexual clients. *American Psychologist, 67*(1), 10–42.

American Psychological Association. (2015). Guidelines for psychological practice with transgender and gender nonconforming people. *American Psychologist, 70*(9), 832–864.

Armour, B. S., Swanson, M., Waldman, H. B., & Perlman, S. P. (2008). A profile of state-level differences in the oral health of people with and without disabilities, in the U.S., in 2004. *Public Health Reports, 123*(1), 67–75.

Bandermann, K. M., & Szymanski, D. M. (2014). Exploring coping mediators between heterosexist oppression and posttraumatic stress symptoms among lesbian, gay, and bisexual persons. *Psychology of Sexual Orientation and Gender Diversity, 1*(3), 213–224. doi:10.1037/sgd0000044

Behm, J., & Gray, N. (2012). Interdisciplinary rehabilitation team. In K. Mauk (Ed.), *Rehabilitation nursing: A contemporary approach to practice* (pp. 51–62). Sudbury, MA: Jones & Bartlett.

Berens, D. E. (2014). Disability, ableism, and ageism. In D. G. Hays & B. T. Erford (Eds.), *Developing multicultural counseling competence: A systems approach.* (pp. 189–217). Upper Saddle River, NJ: Pearson.

Brandenburg, D. L., Matthews, A. K., Johnson, T. P., & Hughes, T. L. (2007). Breast cancer risk and screening: A comparison of lesbian and heterosexual women. *Women & Health, 45*(4), 109–130.

Burgstahler, S., & Cory, R. C. (2008). Indicators of institutional change. In S. E. Burgstahler & R. C. Cory (Eds.), *Universal design in higher education: From principles to practice* (pp. 247–254). Cambridge, MA: Harvard Education.

Burgstahler, S., & Russo-Gleicher, R. (2015). Applying universal design to address the needs of postsecondary students on the autism spectrum. *Journal of Postsecondary Education & Disability, 28*(2), 199–212.

Butt, L., & Caplan, B. (2010). The rehabilitation team. In R. G. Frank, M. R. Rosenthal, & B. Caplan (Eds.), *Handbook of rehabilitation psychology* (pp. 451–457). Washington, DC: American Psychological Association.

Case, P., Austin, S. B., Hunter, D. J., Manson, J. E., Malspeis, S., Willett, W. C., & Spiegelman, D. (2004). Sexual orientation, health risk factors, and physical functioning in the Nurses' Health Study II. *Journal of Women's Health, 13*(9), 1033–1047. doi:10.1089/jwh.2004.13.1033

Center for Universal Design. (2016, November 16). Retrieved from https://www.ncsu.edu/ncsu/design/cud

Centers for Disease Control and Prevention. (2016). Chronic diseases: The leading causes of death and disability in the United States. Retrieved from http://www.cdc.gov/chronicdisease/overview

Chaney, M. P., & Marszalek, J. (2014). Sexual orientation and heterosexism. In D. G. Hays & B. T. Erford (Eds.), *Developing multicultural counseling competence: A systems approach.* (pp. 127–158). Upper Saddle River, NJ: Pearson.

Conron, K. J., Mimiaga, M. J., & Landers, S. J. (2010). A population-based study of sexual orientation identity and gender differences in adult health. *American Journal of Public Health, 100*(10), 1953–1960. doi:10.2105/AJPH.2009.174169

Daniels, J. R., & Geiger, T. J. (2010, November). *Universal design and LGBTQ (lesbian, gay, transgender, bisexual, and queer) issues: Creating equal access and opportunities for success.* Paper presented at the Annual Meeting of the Association for the Study of Higher Education, Indianapolis, IN.

DePoy, E., & Gilson, S. F. (2004). *Rethinking disability: Principles for professional and social change.* Belmont, CA: Brooks/Cole—Thomson.

Diamant, A. L., & Wold, C. (2003). Sexual orientation and variation in physical and mental health status among women. *Journal of Women's Health, 12*(1), 41–49.

Dibble, S. L., Roberts, S. A., & Nussey, B. (2004). Comparing breast cancer risk between lesbians and their heterosexual sisters. *Women's Health Issues, 14*(2), 60–68.

dickey, l. m., Reisner, S. L., & Juntunen, C. L. (2015). Non-suicidal self-injury in a large online sample of transgender adults. *Professional Psychology: Research and Practice, 46*(1), 3–11. doi:10.1037/a0038803

Dilley, J. A., Simmons, K. W., Boysun, M. J., Pizacani, B. A., & Stark, M. J. (2010). Demonstrating the importance and feasibility of including sexual orientation in public health surveys: Health disparities in the Pacific Northwest. *American Journal of Public Health, 100*(3), 460–467. doi:10.2105/AJPH.2007.130336

Dispenza, F., & DeBlaere C. (2017). Sexual orientation and ability status. In K. L. Nadal (Ed.), *The SAGE encyclopedia of psychology and gender.* Thousand Oaks, CA: Sage.

Dispenza, F., Harper, L. S., & Harrigan, M. A. (2016). Subjective health among LGBT persons living with disabilities: A qualitative content analysis. *Rehabilitation Psychology, 61*(3), 251–259. doi:10.1037/rep0000086

Dispenza, F., Viehl, C., Sewell, M. H., Burke, M. A., & Gaudet, M. M. (2016). A model of affirmative intersectional rehabilitation counseling with sexual minorities. *Rehabilitation Counseling Bulletin, 59*(3), 143–157. doi:10.1177/0034355215579916

Dovey, S., & Webb, O. J. (2000). General practitioners' perception of their role in care for people with intellectual disability. *Journal of Intellectual Disability Research, 44*(Pt 5), 553–561.

Duke, T. S. (2011). Lesbian, gay, bisexual, and transgender youth with disabilities: A meta-synthesis. *Journal of LGBT Youth, 8*(1), 1–52. doi:10.1080/19361653.2011.519181

Falvo, D. (2014). *Medical and psychosocial aspects of chronic illness and disability* (5th ed.). Boston, MA: Jones & Bartlett.

Fassinger, R. E. (2008). Workplace diversity and public policy. *American Psychologist, 63*(4), 252–268. doi:10.1037/0003-066X.63.4.252.

Fraley, S. S., Mona, L. R., & Theodore, P. S. (2007). The sexual lives of lesbian, gay, and bisexual people with disabilities: Psychological perspectives. *Sexuality Research & Social Policy, 4*(1), 15–26.

Fredriksen-Goldsen, K. I., Kim, H. J., & Barkan, S. E. (2012). Disability among lesbian, gay, and bisexual adults: Disparities in prevalence and risk. *American Journal of Public Health, 102*(1), e16–e21. doi:10.2105/AJPH.2011.300379

Fredriksen-Goldsen, K. I., Kim, H. J., Muraco, A., & Mincer, S. (2009). Chronically ill midlife and older lesbians, gay men, and bisexuals and their informal caregivers: The impact of the social context. *Sexuality Research & Social Policy, 6*(4), 52–64.

Fredriksen-Goldsen, K. I., Simoni, J. M., Kim, H. J., Lehavot, K., Walters, K. L., Yang, J.,…Muraco, A. (2014). The health equity promotion model: Reconceptualization of lesbian, gay, and bisexual, and transgender (LGBT) health disparities. *American Journal of Orthopsychiatry, 84*(6), 653–663.

Gage, M. (1998). From independence to interdependence: Creating synergistic healthcare teams. *Journal of Nursing Administration, 28*(4), 17–26.

Glover-Graf, N. M. (2012). Sexuality and disability. In I. Marini, N. M. Glover-Graf, M. J. Millington (Eds.), *Psychosocial aspects of disability: Insider perspectives and counseling strategies* (pp. 195–233). New York, NY: Springer Publishing.

Greene, B. (2007). Delivering ethical psychological services to lesbian, gay, and bisexual clients. In K. J. Bieschke, R. M. Perez, & K. A. DeBord, (Eds.), *Handbook of counseling and psychotherapy with lesbian, gay, bisexual, and transgender clients* (pp. 181–200). Washington, DC: American Psychological Association.

Hatzenbuehler, M. L. (2009). How does sexual minority stigma "get under the skin?" A psychological mediation framework. *Psychological Bulletin, 135*, 707–730. doi:10.1037/a0016441

Heck, J. E., & Jacobson, J. S. (2006). Asthma diagnosis among individuals in same-sex relationships. *Journal of Asthma, 43*(8), 579–584.

Hennessey, M., & Koch, L. (2007). Universal design for instruction in rehabilitation counselor education. *Rehabilitation Education, 21*(3), 187–194.

Higbee, J. (2003). *Curriculum transformation and disability: Implementing universal design in higher education.* Minneapolis: University of Minnesota, Center for Research on Developmental Education and Urban Literacy.

Iwarsson, S., & Ståhl, A. (2003). Accessibility, usability and universal design–positioning and definition of concepts describing person–environment relationships. *Disability and Rehabilitation, 25*(2), 57–66.

Kim, H. J., & Fredriksen-Goldsen, K. I. (2012). Hispanic lesbians and bisexual women at heightened risk for [corrected] health disparities. *American Journal of Public Health, 102*(1), e9–e15. doi:10.2105/AJPH.2011.300378

Langdridge, D. (2007). Gay affirmative therapy: A theoretical framework and defense. *Journal of Gay & Lesbian Psychotherapy, 11*(1–2), 27–43.

Lick, D. J., Durso, L. E., & Johnson, K. L. (2013). Minority stress and physical health among sexual minorities. *Perspectives on Psychological Science, 8*(5), 521–548. doi:10.1177/1745691613497965

Lid, I. M. (2014). Universal Design and disability: An interdisciplinary perspective. *Disability and Rehabilitation, 36*(16), 1344–1349. doi:10.3109/09638288.2014.931472

Lipton, B. (2004). Gay men living with non-HIV chronic illnesses. *Journal of Gay & Lesbian Social Services, 17*(2), 1–23. doi:10.1300/J041v17n02_01

Matthews, C. R. (2007). Affirmative lesbian, gay, and bisexual counseling with all clients. In K. J. Bieschke, R. M. Perez, & K. DeBord (Eds.), *Handbook of counseling and psychotherapy with lesbian, gay, bisexual, and transgender clients* (pp. 201–220). Washington, DC: American Psychological Association.

McRuer, R. (2006). *Crip theory: Cultural signs of queerness and disability.* New York: New York University Press.

Miller, P., Parker, S., & Gillinson, S. (2004). *Disablism: How to tackle the last prejudice.* London, England: Demos.

Myers, M., & Crockett, J. (2013). Manifesto for queer universal design. *Journal of Queer Studies in Finland, 6*(1–2), 58–64.

Nijhuis, B. J., Reinder-Messelink, H. A., de Blecourt, A. C., Olijive, W. G., Groothoof, J. W., Nakken, H., & Postema, K. (2007). A review of salient elements defining team collaboration in pediatric rehabilitation. *Clinical Rehabilitation, 21*(3), 195–211.

Reichard, A., Stolzle, H., & Fox, M. H. (2011). Health disparities among adults with physical disabilities or cognitive limitations compared to individuals with no disabilities in the United States. *Disability and Health Journal, 4*(2), 59–67. doi:10.1016/j.dhjo.2010.05.003

Riggle, E. D. B., Rostosky, S. S., & Horne, S. G. (2010). Does it matter where you live? Nondiscrimination laws and the experiences of LGB residents. *Sexuality Research & Social Policy, 7*, 168–172. doi:10.1007/s131780100016z.

Roberts, A. L., Austin, S. B., Corliss, H. L., Vandermorris, A. K., & Koenen, K. C. (2010). Pervasive trauma exposure among US sexual orientation minority adults and risk of posttraumatic stress disorder. *American Journal of Public Health, 100*(12), 2433–2441.

Sheehan, D., Robertson, L., & Ormond, T. (2007). Comparison of language used and patterns of communication in interprofessional and multidisciplinary teams. *Journal of Interprofessional Care, 21*(1), 17–30.

Smart, J. F. & Smart, D. W. (2006). Models of disability: Implications for the counseling profession. *Journal of Counseling and Development, 84*, 29–40. doi:10.1002/j.1556-6678.2006 .tb00377.x

Steele, L. S., Ross, L. E., Dobinson, C., Veldhuizen, S., & Tinmouth, J. M. (2009). Women's sexual orientation and health: Results from a Canadian population-based survey. *Women & Health, 49*(5), 353–367. doi:10.1080/03630240903238685

Stodden, R., Whelley, T., Chang, C., & Harding, T. (2001). Current status of educational support provisions to students with disabilities in postsecondary education. *Journal of Vocational Rehabilitation, 16*(3), 189–198.

Tagayuna, A., Stodden, R. A., Chang, C., Zeleznik, M. E., & Whelley, T. A. (2005). A two-year comparison of support provision for persons with disabilities in postsecondary education. *Journal of Vocational Rehabilitation, 22*(1), 13–21.

U.S. Census Bureau (2012, July). Nearly 1 in 5 people have a disability in the U.S. Census Bureau reports. Retrieved from https://www.census.gov/newsroom/releases/ archives/miscellaneous/cb12-134.html

Wallace, S. P., Cochran, S. D., Durazo, E. M., & Ford, C. L. (2011). *The health of aging lesbian, gay, and bisexual adults in California.* Los Angeles: University of California, Los Angeles Center for Health Policy Research.

Wang, J., Hausermann, M., Counatsou, P., Aggleton, P., & Weiss, M. G. (2007). Health status, behavior, and care utilization in the Geneva Gay Men's Health Study. *Preventive Medicine, 44*(1), 70–75.

Winance, M. (2014). Universal design and the challenge of diversity: Reflections on the principles of UD, based on empirical research of people's mobility. *Disability & Rehabilitation, 36*(16), 1334–1343. doi:10.3109/09638288.2014.936564

Witten, T. M. (2014). End of life, chronic illness, and trans-identities. *Journal of Social Work in End-of-Life & Palliative Care, 10*, 34–58. doi:10.1080/15524256.2013.877864

Wong-Baker FACES Foundation (2016). Wong-Baker FACES® pain rating scale. Retrieved with permission from http://www.WongBakerFACES.org

CHAPTER **10**

The Mental Health of Gender and Sexual Minority Groups in Context

Tracy J. Cohn, Stephen P. Casazza, and Elizabeth M. Cottrell

Exploring an individual's mental health without understanding the cultural and environmental context in which an individual exists is an impossible endeavor. In an effort to address mental health for gender and sexual minority (GSM) populations, the scope of this chapter is threefold. First, context is provided to understand the lived experiences of GSM individuals in the United States beginning with discussion of societal acceptance of GSM populations, followed by prevalence rates of mental health at large, the history of diagnosing mental illness in GSM populations, and finally by exploring minority stress theory as a foundation for understanding higher rates of certain disorders. Second, summaries of prevalence rates are provided for specific mental disorders and symptoms among those in the lesbian, gay, bisexual, and transgender (LGBT) community, as well as disparities in prevalence between those in the LGBT community and the general population. Third, treatment interventions and programs specifically tailored toward the unique needs of GSM populations are addressed with attention placed on positive psychology, an important psychological theory and framework for understanding individual strengths.

SOCIETAL ACCEPTANCE OF GSM INDIVIDUALS

Although one may perceive that acceptance of sexual minority individuals by the general public moves at a glacial pace, findings from Gallup Polls suggest rather rapid shifts. In 1984, when queried as to whether respondents felt homosexuality was "acceptable" as a lifestyle, 34% of the residents in the United States said "yes." In 2008, the same question garnered an approval rating of 57% (Gallup Politics, 2012). When asked if people were born gay, 51% of respondents reported the affirmative in 2015 versus only 13% in 1977 (Gallup Politics, n.d.). Before the ruling by the U.S. Supreme Court in 2015 that legalized same-sex marriage in the United States, approval rating on the issue was 58%, and remained steady following the ruling from the Court (Gallup Politics, n.d.). Although ratings suggest that GSM individuals have more "approval" as a group, Schmidt, Miles, and Welsh (2011) have argued that discrimination remains widely prevalent and that "discrimination based on sexual orientation remains a socially sanctioned form of prejudice and includes traditional heterosexism devaluing the gay and lesbian equality movement, aversion to lesbians and gay men, among other overt and covert hostilities" (p. 296). Although gay and lesbian individuals are increasingly accepted in the United States, findings have suggested a different experience for gender minority people. Although data vary, especially given the more recent emergence of gender minority people in the media in the United States, researchers have found that gender minority individuals face substantial risk of discrimination in employment, housing, health care, and relationships (Bryant & Schilt 2008; Grant et al., 2011). Moreover, gender minority individuals are more likely to experience violence due to gender expression and transphobia (Grant et al., 2011). Additionally, Norton and Herek (2013) concluded that attitudes toward gender minority individuals are overwhelmingly more negative than attitudes toward sexual minority individuals. Recognizing that the environment in which GSM individuals live is ripe for discrimination and prejudice helps one understand the multifaceted stressors experienced by GSM individuals.

THE HISTORY OF "DIAGNOSIS"

A second contextual component of mental health is the instrument used to render a diagnosis. The *Diagnostic and Statistical Manual of Mental Disorders, 5th Edition* (*DSM-5*; American Psychiatric Association, 2013), is the standard taxonomy in the United States used to provide a mental health diagnosis. Although one might assume that a taxonomy of mental disorders would be value-neutral (i.e., free from bias), there is a long and complicated history between the *DSM* and minority populations. The act of engaging in, and the desire for, same-sex sexual contact (i.e., *homosexuality*), was a diagnosable mental disorder until 1973, at which time the diagnosis was modified and renamed "sexual orientation disturbance" (SOD), intended as a diagnosis for those individuals who experience clinical distress due to their sexual orientation, without acknowledging that the distress was largely normative and adaptive to the stressors faced by sexual minority individuals. In the 1987 *DSM-III*, SOD was removed and replaced by ego-dystonic homosexuality (EDH), continuing to pathologize people who experienced distress due to same-sex attraction (Krajeski, 1996). In the most recent version of the *DSM* (5th edition), homosexuality is no longer considered a diagnosable mental disorder. Along similar lines, gender minority individuals have experienced an evolution of diagnosis, beginning with "gender identity disorder," and currently, individuals who experience distress related to their gender identity generally meet the diagnostic criteria of "gender dysphoria." The continued use of a formal mental health diagnosis associated with gender identity remains controversial, however (see Chapter 14 for a more in-depth discussion). A number of other writers have written about the use of the *DSM* to control and regulate populations (see Caplan, 1995).

PREVALENCE RATES AT LARGE

Although much of this chapter examines prevalence rates for GSM populations, it is important to consider those findings within the general population. The most recent data from the National Comorbidity Survey Replication (NCS-R; Kessler, Chiu, Demler, & Walters, 2005), based on a random national sample of 9,000 adults, concluded that mental illness has been experienced by 26.2% to 32.4% of individuals in the last 12 months (exclusive of individuals who were homeless, individuals in institutions, and individuals who were non-native-speakers of English). As evidenced in this chapter, certain disorders are diagnosed at higher rates in GSM samples, and, when available, comparison between GSM populations and cisgender heterosexual populations are provided. In general, Meyer (2013) found that rates of mental disorders were higher for GSM individuals in comparison to cisgender heterosexual populations. It is essential, though, that the reader is cognizant that although the rates of many disorders are higher for GSM populations, it is not identification as a gender and/or sexual minority that increases risk. Rather, what is proposed is that the hostile and tense environment in which GSM individuals exist, termed *minority stress*, results in mental health disparities (Meyer, 2013).

MINORITY STRESS AND CONCEALMENT

Bruce, Harper, and Bauermeister (2015) suggested that increased rates of depression and other mental health concerns among those in the LBGT community may be explained by stigma and discrimination that results from living in heterosexist societies. Bullying, verbal abuse, violence, and other forms of victimization that result from sexual orientation status have been linked to a variety of negative mental health outcomes, including depression and suicide attempts (Baams, Grossman, Russell, 2015; Bruce et al., 2015; Hightow-Weidman et al., 2011). The concept that the stress and strain associated with being identified as a sexual minority results in health disparities is termed the *minority stress model* or *minority stress theory*. (Bruce et al., 2015) that seeks to shift the understanding of health disparities within GSM groups from the identity itself to the societal pressures associated with the identity.

Concealment of sexual orientation has also been associated with distress. Concealment of sexual minority status may be a method of reducing or avoiding stigma, discrimination, and victimization, and therefore, may reduce mental health outcomes associated with being open with one's sexual orientation. However, concealment of sexual minority status has also been associated with increased symptoms of mental illness (Cohen, Blasey, Taylor, Weiss, & Newman, 2016). Concealment status can be further complicated by gender. For instance, Pachankis, Cochran, and Mays (2015) suggested that although males who were open with their sexual minority identity showed increased rates of depression compared to cisgender heterosexual individuals, females who were open about their sexual minority status showed lower levels of depression.

Minority stress has also been considered in the context of psychological distress among gender minority individuals. Transgender individuals may experience misclassification of their gender identity, or misgendering, as well as internalized anti-transgender attitudes, experiences of prejudice and discrimination, or fear of anti-transgender stigma (McLemore, 2016; Tebbe & Moradi, 2016). McLemore (2016) found that approximately 65% of gender minority individuals report being misgendered by others "sometimes," "often," or "always" with these misgendering experiences contributing significantly to feelings of stigmatization. In turn, perceived stigmatization and frequency of misgendering was positively associated with psychological distress. Furthermore, minority stressors including prejudice and discrimination, internalized anti-transgender attitudes, and fear of anti-transgender stigma have been associated with negative mental health outcomes such as depression and suicide risk (Tebbe & Moradi, 2016).

Having provided context for understanding differential rates of diagnosis, specific information based on mental health concerns is now provided.

■ DEPRESSION

In the general population, the 12-month prevalence rate for a diagnosis of major depressive disorder is 7% (American Psychiatric Association, 2013), with higher rates of individuals experiencing depressive symptoms that may not meet the criteria for major depressive disorder. However, research has consistently shown higher rates of depressive symptoms among samples of sexual minority individuals when compared to the rates of the general population and/or their heterosexual counterparts (Cohen et al., 2016; Ngamake, Walch, & Raveepatarakul, 2016; Roi, Kretschmer, Dijkstra, Veenstra, & Oldehinkel, 2016). There may be differences in gender identity when considering increased risk for major depressive disorder. For example, S. D. Cochran, Mays, and Sullivan (2003) previously found that those who identified as male and gay or bisexual were three times more likely to meet criteria for major depressive disorder than those males who identified as heterosexual. However, there were no differences found between rates of depression for those who identified as female and lesbian/gay or heterosexual in the same study (S. D. Cochran et al., 2003). However, more recently, Cohen and colleagues (2016) found significantly higher rates of clinical level symptoms of depression in both gay men and lesbians when compared to their heterosexual counterparts.

There also exist disparities in rates of depressive symptomatology for those who identify as a gender minority; namely, research has found that those who identify as a gender minority have higher levels of depressive symptoms and are nearly twice as likely to meet clinical cutoffs for depression than their cis-gender counterparts (i.e., 52% for gender minority individuals, 27% for cisgender females, and 25% for cisgender males; Reisner, Katz-Wise, Gordon, Corliss, & Austin, 2016).

ANXIETY

Anxiety can take many different forms such as specific phobias, panic and panic attacks, generalized anxiety, or anxiety caused by social situations. Similar to the increased rates of depression found in GSM individuals, minority stress can lead to increased levels of anxiety symptoms. For instance, Ngamake and colleagues (2016) suggested that perceived discrimination explained increased levels of anxiety and stress among sexual minority individuals.

In the general population, prevalence rate estimates for specific anxiety disorders range from 2% to 7% depending on the disorder (American Psychiatric Association, 2013), with higher rates of individuals experiencing some symptoms of anxiety, but not necessarily enough to meet diagnostic criteria for an anxiety disorder. Findings on prevalence rates among GSM individuals vary, but have consistently been found to be higher than rates of cisgender heterosexual comparison groups (Cohen et al., 2016; Ngamake et al., 2016). When considering anxiety disorders as a whole, findings have suggested that GSM individuals have 1.5 times the risk for developing an anxiety disorder compared to cisgender heterosexual individuals (Hartman, 2013). However, increased rates of anxiety found among GSM individuals vary by specific disorder (Cohen et al., 2016).

One factor that has been increasingly studied in relation to the rates of anxiety and other mental health concerns among sexual minority individuals is internalized homophobia/transphobia (i.e., when a GSM individual internalizes external negative messages regarding sexual orientation and/or gender identity; Lock, 1998). For instance, Walch, Ngamake, Bovornusvakool, and Walker (2016) studied the relationship between discrimination, internalized homophobia, and mental health in sexual minority individuals. They found that negative mental health outcomes in sexual minority individuals resulting from perceived discrimination were explained only through an indirect path through internalized homophobia (Walch et al., 2016). This finding suggests that discrimination alone may not adequately explain why GSM individuals report higher rates of anxiety, but it may be the internalized homophobia resulting from discrimination that leads to the higher rates of mental health symptomatology experienced by GSM individuals. However, this was found to be true only when individuals concealed their sexual orientation status. Sexual minority participants in this investigation reported direct negative mental health outcomes, including anxiety, as a result of perceived discrimination when they were "widely" open about their sexual orientation (Walch et al., 2016). This highlights the important role that concealment or openness about sexual orientation may play in sexual minority individuals' mental health; however, one must always consider the implications of physical safety regarding openness, particularly in more conservative climates (e.g., rural areas—see Chapter 18).

Those who identify as a sexual minority and as female who concealed their sexual orientation to others reported increased levels of social phobia (Cohen et al., 2016). These findings support Pachankis, Cochran, and Mays (2015) findings that sexual minority women who were open about their sexual orientation were less likely to experience depressive symptoms. However, no differences were found in levels of anxiety among sexual minority men between those who reported concealment or those who were open about their sexual minority status. It is important to note that investigations examining sexual orientation concealment vary in their findings (McGarrity & Huebner, 2013; Pachankis, 2007; Schrimshaw, Siegel, Downing, & Parsons, 2013). It has been suggested that concealment is a technique that may allow GSM individuals to escape discrimination, stigma, and harassment/assault (Walch, et al., 2016). On the other hand, inability to be open about one's sexual orientation may lead to negative views of one's self (i.e., internalized homophobia/transphobia) and therefore may contribute to negative mental health outcomes (Walch et al., 2016). It is clear that concealment of sexual or gender minority identity is a complicated construct and one that warrants adequate attention when considering mental health of GSM groups.

Research has also supported differences in the prevalence rates of anxiety disorders between gender minority and cisgender groups, absent of sexual orientation. For example, Reisner and colleagues (2016) found that anxiety symptoms were rated higher in gender minority individuals compared to cisgender individuals. Additionally, they found prevalence rates meeting clinical cut offs for anxiety disorders to be higher for gender minority individuals (38%) than cisgender females (30%) and cisgender males (14%; Reisner et al., 2016).

■ TRAUMA

Experiencing traumatic events such as interpersonal violence, combat exposure, natural disasters, witnessing the death of another, or near death experiences can lead to lasting negative mental health outcomes. Negative mental health outcomes as a result of a traumatic experience have been found to occur at higher rates among sexual minority individuals. For instance, on a measure of symptoms associated with posttraumatic stress disorder (PTSD), sexual minority men and women scored significantly higher than heterosexual individuals (Cohen et al., 2016). Additionally, research suggests that sexual minority individuals, as well as heterosexual individuals who have had same-sex partners, are nearly twice as likely to meet criteria for PTSD in their lifetimes when compared to exclusively heterosexual individuals (Roberts, Austin, Corliss, Vandermorris, & Koenen, 2010). Furthermore, Roberts and colleagues (2010) found the sexual orientation disparities in rates of PTSD to be almost completely accounted for by the increased rates of interpersonal violence and childhood abuse or neglect experienced by sexual minority individuals. Gender minority individuals have also been found to report higher prevalence rates of PTSD. For example, Shipherd, Maguen, Skidmore, and Abramovitz (2011) found that not only did gender minority individuals in their study report higher exposure to multiple traumatic events throughout their lives when compared to cisgender individuals, but also that nearly 18% of their gender minority sample met criteria for PTSD (compared to only 5%–10% of the general population).

Additionally, it has been documented that sexual minority individuals are at increased risk for experiencing exposure to traumatic events and victimization, which may not lead to a full diagnosis of PTSD, including childhood maltreatment, bullying, and physical and sexual assault (Balsam & Hughes, 2013). Victimization experienced by sexual minority individuals has been linked to the development of depression, anxiety, suicidality, disordered eating, and substance use as well as higher risk-taking behaviors in gay and bisexual men (Balsam, & Hughes, 2013). GSM individuals may experience victimization due to their minority group status more so than any other minority group, with previous research suggesting that 60% to 70% of GSM individuals have experienced at least one bias-related victimization experience (Grant et al., 2011; Rose & Mechanic, 2002).

Furthermore, not all symptoms related to trauma are the direct result of one specific traumatic experience or even overt heterosexism and intentionally hurtful behaviors of others, especially in marginalized populations such as the LGBT community. Microaggressions—the communications of prejudice and discrimination expressed through seemingly meaningless and unharmful tactics (Shelton, & Delgado-Romero, 2011)—have recently been explored as an additional source to overt heterosexism in contributing to traumatic stress in minority populations. Chronic stress that results from minority status and microaggressions experienced as a result of GSM status have been found to be not only related to PTSD but also increased suicide rates, depression, anxiety-related disorders, as well as a host of other negative mental health outcomes (Sue, 2010).

■ EATING DISORDERS

The most frequently documented forms of disordered eating include anorexia nervosa and bulimia nervosa; however, other eating disorders include pica, rumination disorder, avoidant/restrictive food intake disorder, and binge-eating disorder. Prevalence rates for eating disorders in the general population are generally lower than many other classes of disorders and range from 0.4% to 1.5%. However, there are significant differences in rates by gender and there is little known about the prevalence of certain eating disorders (American Psychiatric Association, 2013).

Research has consistently suggested that GSM individuals report higher prevalence of disordered eating and diagnosable eating disorders. For example, within a sample of over 100,000 college students, Matthews-Ewald, Zullig, and Ward (2014) found that sexual minority men reported clinical eating disorders as well as disordered eating at higher rates than cisgender heterosexual men. Additionally, although not necessarily considered disordered eating, the researchers found that all sexual minority men and women were significantly more likely to report dieting to lose weight when compared to cisgender heterosexual peers.

Similarly, Diemer, Grant, Munn-Chernoff, Patterson, and Duncan (2015) found that transgender individuals reported higher rates of self-reported eating disorders in the past year, and past month vomiting or laxative use, than cisgender heterosexual individuals. Additionally, the researchers found that cisgender sexual minority men and women had significantly higher self-reported levels of eating disorders than cisgender heterosexual individuals; however, sexual minority individuals reported lower rates of disordered eating than did transgender individuals. These findings suggest that although GSM populations as a group experience higher levels of disordered eating than the general population, there are important differences in disordered eating within GSM populations as well.

SUICIDE

Although covered in more detail elsewhere in this publication (Chapter 11), suicidality among GSM individuals warrants mention in the current chapter as suicidality, although not a diagnosable condition, has been associated with many mental health conditions. Sexual minority status has been suggested to be associated with increased risk for suicidal ideation, attempts, and completion. Meta-analytic research has suggested that those who identify as lesbian, gay, or bisexual are twice as likely as their heterosexual counterparts to attempt suicide in their lifetimes (King et al., 2008). Furthermore, recent research suggests that approximately 41% of gender minority individuals have had at least one lifetime suicide attempt (compared to only 1.6% of the general population; Grant et al., 2011), and that lack of a supportive environment increases the risk for suicide attempts by up to 20% (Hatzenbuehler, 2011). Although not a specific diagnostic category, suicidality is clearly an important mental health concern, especially among GSM individuals.

SUBSTANCE ABUSE

Substance abuse, although covered in more detail elsewhere in this text (Chapter 12), also warrants mentioning. Findings have consistently suggested higher rates of alcohol and substance use among GSM individuals (Hughes, Johnson, Steffen, Wilsnack, & Everett, 2014; Ngamake et al., 2016; Pesola, Shelton, & van den Bree, 2014). Several rationales for these findings have been suggested and investigated. For example, Hughes and colleagues (2014) found that victimization accounted for some, but not all, risk of hazardous drinking. Researchers suggested that stigma and discrimination due to gender and/or sexual minority status played an important role in alcohol use. Additionally, Johnson et al. (2013) suggested that sexual minority women who experienced anxiety were more likely to drink in hazardous ways. It could be that GSM individuals report higher rates of substance use than heterosexual individuals due to the increased discrimination and stigma that they experience related to their gender and/or sexual minority status (Pesola et al., 2014).

HIV-ASSOCIATED DEMENTIA

According to the Centers for Disease Control and Prevention (CDC, 2015), approximately 57% of individuals in the United States who are living with a diagnosis of HIV are sexual minority men. Although HIV is not an illness specific to GSM individuals and is covered in detail in Chapter 13, it is worth mentioning in this chapter due to the high rates of individuals diagnosed with HIV who go on to experience mild neurocognitive disorder (NCD) due to HIV (American Psychiatric Association, 2013).

HIV has the potential to result in either major or mild NCD as well as signs and symptoms of neurocognitive impairment that may not meet the diagnostic threshold for NCD. Subclinical symptoms of neurocognitive disturbance impact approximately one-third to over one-half of individuals with HIV (American Psychiatric Association, 2013). According to the American Psychiatric Association (2013), approximately 25% of HIV positive individuals will meet criteria for mild or major NCD, contrasted with only 5% of the general population. Symptoms of advanced NCD due to HIV infection may include prominent neuromotor features such as severe incoordination, ataxia, and motor slowing. Additionally, individuals may display aggressive or inappropriate affect, loss of emotional control, or apathy (American Psychiatric Association, 2013).

■ GENDER DYSPHORIA

Although typically discussed in the context of gender minority individuals, gender dysphoria can occur in heterosexual as well as sexual minority individuals. Updated to a more descriptive terminology from the prior "gender identity disorder" in the *DSM-IV*, gender dysphoria focuses on the dysphoria as the clinical problem, not the identity of the individual, and refers to the distress that may accompany the incongruence between one's experienced or expressed gender and one's assigned gender (American Psychiatric Association, 2013). Gender dysphoria may occur at different rates, and may be categorized by different diagnostic criteria during differing developmental periods.

In their review of the literature to date on gender dysphoria, Dhejne, Van Vlerken, Heylens, and Arcelus (2016) found that transgender individuals reported higher levels of depression and anxiety disorders than cisgender individuals but reported no differences in more severe and persistent mental illnesses such as schizophrenia or bipolar disorder. Although not all those who experience gender dysphoria opt to undergo medical interventions, the researchers suggested that in post-gender-confirming medical intervention, reports of those who had experienced gender dysphoria showed rates of psychiatric diagnoses that were no higher than cisgender comparison groups. Additional information regarding mental health in transgender men and women beyond gender dysphoria is found in Chapter 14.

■ CULTURALLY COMPETENT CARE

The American Psychological Association (2012, 2015) outlined guidelines for psychological practice with GSM clients. These guidelines encourage culturally competent and affirmative practice with GSM clients that are applicable not only to mental health professionals, but also to anyone interacting with GSM clients. The Association's practice guidelines encourage psychologists to utilize interventions that increase clients' sense of safety, reduce stress, resolve residual trauma, and empower clients to combat stigma and discrimination (American Psychological Association, 2012). Affirmative practice necessitates that clinicians understand common terminology, are aware of how their own views affect the care their clients receive, and understand how stigma and discrimination affect the mental health and well-being of GSM clients (American Psychological Association, 2015). For a more comprehensive discussion of recommendations for working with GSM clients, please refer to Chapter 22.

■ OUTCOMES

Research suggests that gay and lesbian adults utilize mental health services at higher rates than heterosexual men and women (Bell & Weinberg, 1978; Morgan, 1992; S. D. Cochran et al., 2003; Grella, Greenwell, Mays, & Cochran, 2009). S. D. Cochran et al. (2003) estimated that 7% of midlife-adults receiving mental health care in the United States identify as lesbian, gay, or bisexual although LGB individuals make up approximately 3% of the population. A study of transgender individuals seeking physical health services found that 53% reported a need for counseling services (Goldberg, Matte, MacMillan, & Hudspith, 2003). A Canadian study found that although transgender individuals were less likely than cisgender sexual minority or heterosexual respondents to see a physician for mental health needs, transgender respondents were slightly more likely to see a counselor or therapist than the sexual minority and heterosexual respondents (Simeonov, Steele, Anderson, & Ross, 2015). Gender minority individuals have also been found to have a higher level of perceived need for psychological services than their cisgender sexual minority counterparts (Warren, Smalley, & Barefoot, 2016).

Researchers have found overall positive treatment outcomes when gender minority clients receive affirmative health care (Byne et al., 2012; Davis & Meier, 2014; Kuhn et al., 2009). Murad and colleagues (2010) conducted a meta-analysis of studies on hormone therapy treatment of gender minority clients. They found that 80% of participants who received affirmative medical care reported an improvement in gender dysphoria, 78% showed improvement in psychological symptoms, and 80% reported improvement in quality of life (Murad et al., 2010).

Additionally, research on substance abuse treatment outcomes for GSM individuals found higher rates of abstinence after completion of the program among those who were in substance abuse treatment programs specialized for GSM persons compared to participants who were not in a specialized treatment program or setting (Senreich, 2010).

■ EXPERIENCES IN TREATMENT

Extensive research has documented the high rates of mental health concerns among GSM individuals, as noted earlier, as well as higher rates of utilization of mental health services by this population (Bell & Weinberg, 1978; Morgan, 1992; S. D. Cochran et al., 2003; Grella et al., 2009). However, few studies have examined GSM individuals' experiences with mental health services. Although minority stress theory helps explain higher levels of mental health concerns in general, studies of mental health and substance abuse treatment providers have reflected a general level of negative or ambivalent attitude toward GSM clients and lack of knowledge about GSM-specific issues (Eliason, 2000). Thus, GSM individuals who are in need of culturally sensitive services may encounter negative environments or incompetent providers.

Avery, Hellman, and Sudderth (2001) examined GSM clients' experiences with mental health care and found that 17.6% of GSM clients reported dissatisfaction with their mental health services compared to 8% of cisgender heterosexual clients. However, a Canadian study found that GSM clients reported high levels of satisfaction with their primary mental health provider, as 81.5% of sexual minority and 87.8% of transgender-identified clients reported being "satisfied" or "very satisfied" with their mental health care (Simeonov et al., 2015). Despite reporting satisfaction with their mental health care, 50% of transgender and 27.7% of sexual minority participants in this study reported discontinuing mental health services due to negative experiences in therapy related to gender identity or sexual orientation. Additionally, Lombardi (2007) found that transgender individuals in substance-use treatment programs reported more transphobic experiences from staff than other patients. Negative experience with mental health care providers can lead to avoidance of further services, potentially causing more severe consequences (Xavier et al., 2013).

Simeonov and colleagues (2015) pointed out that, as many GSM participants reported past negative experiences yet endorsed high levels of satisfaction with their current provider, it was possible that GSM individuals were eventually locating culturally competent, affirmative mental health providers through personal recommendations and social networks. Previous research has also indicated that gay men and lesbians frequently screened mental health providers for affirmative attitudes before scheduling services (Liddle, 1997) and that sexual minority individuals would avoid clinicians who held heterocentric views (Burckell & Goldfried, 2006). The discrepancies among GSM clients' experiences and satisfaction with mental health care highlight the need for additional research.

■ MENTAL HEALTH PROGRAMS

Due to the increased prevalence rates of mental health symptomatology and the unique stressors experienced by GSM individuals, a need exists for specialized programs in mental health that incorporate consideration for such issues. Although GSM individuals encounter similar mental health problems to cisgender heterosexual peers, as noted earlier, research has demonstrated that GSM individuals experience higher rates of many mental health disorders than the general public. One such concern is substance use.

Previous research suggests that GSM clients prefer organizations that incorporate GSM-specific issues (Driscoll, 1982) and that GSM clients in substance abuse treatment have better outcomes when groups and programs integrate GSM-specific issues (Hicks, 2000; Senreich, 2010). Although one can hypothesize that these results are generalizable to other mental health issues, most of the specialized GSM programs are within the realm of substance use (Hicks, 2000; Neisen,

1997). Hicks (2000) describes a specialized substance abuse treatment program for GSM individuals with a dual diagnosis, where staff are specially trained on GSM issues such as discrimination and policy advocacy. The program comprises a multi-disciplinary affirmative staff, which provides educational courses to providers in the community, in addition to the services offered to patients.

However, when B. N. Cochran, Peavy and Robohm (2007) surveyed substance use treatment programs offering specialized services for GSM clients, they found that 70% of the programs that claimed to offer specialized services were providing the same treatment approach to GSM clients as the services marketed to the general public. Although some specialized programs exist, there is a lack of research on the effectiveness of these programs and their availability.

■ TREATMENT CONSIDERATIONS

GSM individuals seek assistance from mental health providers in addressing sexual orientation– and/or gender identity–related concerns as well as other mental health concerns. Many GSM clients seek out mental health services for reasons other than their sexual orientation or gender identity, and thus, it is important for providers to understand that the mental health problems experienced by GSM clients may or may not be related to their sexual orientation and gender identity (see Chapter 22 for more details). Additionally, mental health providers should not assume that an individual's gender and/or sexual minority status means that mental health services are required.

Career and employment issues are common concerns for transgender individuals, as those who are not out at work often have concern about their transgender identity being discovered (Berg, Mimiaga, & Safren, 2008; Israel & Tarver, 1997). They may have concerns about the disclosure process, possible repercussions, or negative responses from coworkers. Due to these concerns, transgender clients may seek out counseling for support on coming out to work, or help navigating gender identity concerns at work. Other career-related concerns include general vocational concerns, employment discrimination, on the job transitions, hostile work environments, and overall high rates of unemployment among gender minority individuals (Korell & Lorah, 2007).

■ COGNITIVE-BEHAVIORAL THERAPY

Although not a specific treatment intervention, one psychological theory for addressing concerns of GSM individuals is cognitive behavioral therapy (CBT), which focuses on altering clients' thoughts and perceptions of events as a way to change behaviors and emotions (Beck, 1993). CBT can be adapted to incorporate aspects of minority stress theory discussed previously in this chapter. For example, empirical research as well as case studies have indicated that affirmative CBT is effective for treating depression among GSM individuals (Martell, Safren, & Prince, 2004; Zapor & Stuart, 2016). Additional studies are needed, but early research suggests that adapting CBT interventions to address the causes of depression hypothesized by the minority stress model are effective at reducing symptoms for GSM individuals (Craig, Austin, & Alessi, 2013; Ross, Doctor, Dimito, Kuehl, & Armstrong, 2008).

Pachankis (2014) adapted evidence-based interventions, primarily cognitive behavioral therapy, to address minority stress in gay and bisexual men. A preliminary study examined the effectiveness of affirmative cognitive behavioral therapy (CBT) for gay and bisexual men (Pachankis, Hatzenbuehler, Rendina, Safren, & Parsons, 2015). The authors utilized a transdiagnostic cognitive behavioral approach, which was adapted to address the minority stress experienced by gay and bisexual men. The study showed initial support for the approach, which addresses the minority stress origin of co-occurring health problems, including anxiety, depression, and alcohol use (Pachankis, Hatzenbuehler, et al., 2015).

An adaptation of CBT for use with transgender individuals was also offered by Austin and Craig (2015). The transgender affirmative model includes psychoeducation, enhancing social support, and changing maladaptive thoughts (Austin & Craig, 2015). Additionally, Rutter and Camarena (2015) provided a multicultural and gay affirmative approach to counseling African American and Latino sexual minority men. The authors integrated existing multicultural theories and approaches with gay affirmative strategies. They also provided suggestions for therapy, including cognitive interventions and psychoeducation (Rutter & Camarena, 2015).

■ POSITIVE PSYCHOLOGY

Positive psychology focuses on individuals' strengths, and encourages alternative perspectives that depathologize human experiences (Seligman & Csikszentmihalyi, 2000). Although researchers have focused on psychosocial vulnerabilities of GSM individuals, including depression, substance abuse, and suicide, protective factors for GSM individuals such as family acceptance and connectedness (Eisenberg & Resnick, 2006; Ryan, Russell, Huebner, Diaz, & Sanchez, 2010) have also been studied, particularly with young adults. Recent research has focused on resilience, or the ability to adapt to and overcome adversity or stressors. Positive psychology research has provided a deeper understanding of the personal characteristics and social factors that help people be resilient under stressful circumstances (Hart & Sasso, 2011; Luthar & Cicchetti, 2000). Researchers have used the positive psychology framework to examine strengths among GSM individuals (Vaughan & Rodriguez, 2014). Kwon (2013) proposed a theoretical framework for resilience among sexual minority individuals. Kwon argued that social support, emotional openness, and hope and optimism lower reactivity to prejudice, ultimately leading to psychological health and well-being. Although research on resilience in transgender individuals is scarce, Singh, Hays, and Watson (2011) identified common themes of resilience in transgender individuals. These themes included social activism, cultivating hope for the future, serving as a role model, and connection with a supportive community. Resilience in GSM individuals can also include LGBT community support, which can partially compensate for parental rejection (Shilo, Antebi, & Mor, 2015).

Meta-analyses on the effectiveness of positive psychology interventions, including activities to encourage positive feelings, behaviors, and thoughts, have reflected an increase in psychological well-being and decrease in depressive symptoms (Sin & Lyubomirsky, 2009). Findings suggest that interventions focused on strengths are effective at not only promoting wellness but also reducing negative mental health outcomes. Additional research supports the utilization of a strength-based approach in working with GSM individuals (Lytle, Vaughan, Rodriguez, & Shmerler, 2014; Vaughan & Rodriguez, 2014) and in the treatment of mental health disorders (Fava et al., 2005; Galvez, Thommi, & Ghaemi, 2011; Resnick & Rosenheck, 2006).

■ CONCLUSION

The focus of this chapter was on understanding the mental health needs, risks, and interventions associated with GSM individuals. Although a number of findings have suggested an increased risk of mental illness, understanding sexual minority individuals in context, that is, within the frame of minority stress theory, helps illuminate the impact of discrimination, stigma, and hostile environments in which GSM individuals live. Although rates of suicide, substance use, and psychological distress are alarming, it is imperative that readers be aware that tailored interventions which are strength-based and that work to foster resilience and recovery, are available for GSM individuals.

■ REFERENCES

American Psychiatric Association. (2013). *Diagnostic and statistical manual of mental disorders* (5th ed.). Arlington, VA: American Psychiatric Publishing.

American Psychological Association. (2012). Guidelines for psychological practice with lesbian, gay, and bisexual clients. *American Psychologist, 67*(1), 10–42. doi:10.1037/a0024659

American Psychological Association. (2015). Guidelines for psychological practice with transgender and gender nonconforming people. *American Psychologist, 70*(9), 832–864. doi:10.1037/a0039906

Austin, A., & Craig, S. L. (2015). Transgender affirmative cognitive behavioral therapy: Clinical considerations and applications. *Professional Psychology: Research and Practice, 46*(1), 21–29. doi:10.1037/a0038642

Avery, A. M., Hellman, R. E., & Sudderth, L. K. (2001). Satisfaction with mental health services among sexual minorities with major mental illness. *American Journal of Public Health, 91*(6), 990–991. doi:10.2105/aJph.91.6.990

Baams, L., Grossman, A. H., & Russell, S. T. (2015). Minority stress and mechanisms of risk for depression and suicidal ideation among lesbian, gay, and bisexual youth. *Developmental Psychology, 51*(5), 688–696. doi:10.1037/a0038994

Balsam, K., & Hughes, T. (2013). Sexual orientation, victimization, and hate crimes. In C. J. Patterson & A. R. D'Augelli (Eds.), *Handbook of psychology and sexual orientation* (pp. 267–280). New York, NY: Oxford University Press.

Beck, A. T. (1993). Cognitive therapy: Past, present, and future. *Journal of Consulting and Clinical Psychology, 61*(2), 194–198.

Bell, A. P. & Weinberg, M. S. (1978). *Homosexualities: A study of diversity among men and women.* New York, NY: Simon & Schuster.

Berg, M. B., Mimiaga, M. J., & Safren, S. A. (2008). Mental health concerns of gay and bisexual men seeking mental health services. *Journal of Homosexuality, 54*(3), 293–306. doi:10.1080/00918360801982215

Bruce, D., Harper, G. W., & Bauermeister, J. A. (2015). Minority stress, positive identity development, and depressive symptoms: Implications for resilience among sexual minority male youth. *Psychology of Sexual Orientation and Gender Diversity, 2*(3), 287–296. doi:10.1037/sqd0000128

Bryant, K., & Schilt, K. (2008). Transgender people in the U.S. military: Summary and analysis of the 2008 transgender American Veterans Association survey. Retrieved from http://www.palmcenter.org/node/1137

Burckell, L. A., & Goldfried, M. R. (2006). Therapist qualities preferred by sexual-minority individuals. *Psychotherapy, 43*(1), 32–49.

Byne, W., Bradley, S. J., Coleman, E., Eyler, A. E., Green, R., Menvielle, E. J., . . . Tompkins, D. A. (2012). Report of the American Psychiatric Association Task Force on treatment of gender identity disorder. *Archives of Sexual Behavior, 41*(4), 759–796. doi:10.1007/s10508-012-9975-x

Caplan, P. J. (1995). *They say you're crazy: How the world's most powerful psychiatrists decide who's normal.* Reading, MA: Addison-Wesley/Longman.

Centers for Disease Control and Prevention. (2015). HIV among gay and bisexual men. Retrieved from http://www.cdc.gov/hiv/group/msm

Cochran, B. N., Peavy, K. M., & Robohm, J. S. (2007). Do specialized services exist for LGBT individuals seeking treatment for substance misuse? A study of available treatment programs. *Substance Use & Misuse, 42*(1), 161–176.

Cochran, S. D., Mays, V. M., & Sullivan, J. G. (2003). Prevalence of mental disorders, psychological distress, and mental health services use among lesbian, gay, and bisexual adults in the United States. *Journal of Consulting and Clinical Psychology, 71*(1), 53–61.

Cohen, J. M., Blasey, C., Taylor, C. B., Weiss, B. J., & Newman, M. G. (2016). Anxiety and related disorders and concealment in sexual minority young adults. *Behavioral Therapy, 46*, 91–101. doi:10.1016/j.beth.2015.09.006

Craig, S., Austin, A., & Alessi, E. (2013). Gay affirmative cognitive behavioral therapy for sexual minority youth: A clinical adaptation. *Clinical Social Work Journal, 41*(3), 258–266. doi:10.1007/s10615-012-0427-9

Davis, S. A., & Meier, S. C. (2014). Effects of testosterone treatment and chest reconstruction surgery on mental health and sexuality in female-to-male transgender people. *International Journal of Sexual Health, 26*(2), 113–128. doi:10.1080/19317611.2013.833152

Dhejne, C., Van Vlerken, R., Heylens, G., & Arcelus, J. (2016). Mental health and gender dysphoria: A review of the literature. *International Review of Psychiatry, 28*(1), 44–57. doi:10.3109/09540261.2015.1115753

Diemer, E. W., Grant, J. D., Munn-Chernoff, M. A., Patterson, D. A., & Duncan, A. E. (2015). Gender identity, sexual orientation, and eating-related pathology in a national sample of college students. *Journal of Adolescent Health, 57*(2), 144–149. doi:10.1016/j.jadohealth.2015.03.003

Driscoll, R. (1982). A gay-identified alcohol treatment program: A follow-up study. *Journal of Homosexuality, 7*(4), 71–80.

Eisenberg, M. E., & Resnick, M. D. (2006). Suicidality among gay, lesbian and bisexual youth: The role of protective factors. *Journal of Adolescent Health, 39*(5), 662–668. doi:10.1016/j.jadohealth.2006.04.024

Eliason, M. J. (2000). Substance abuse counsellor's attitudes regarding lesbian, gay, bisexual, and transgendered clients. *Journal of Substance Abuse, 12*(4), 311–328.

Fava, G. A., Ruini, C., Rafanelli, C., Finos, L., Salmaso, L., Mangelli, L., & Sirigatti, S. (2005). Well-being therapy of generalized anxiety disorder. *Psychotherapy and Psychosomatics, 74*(1), 26–30.

Gallup Politics. (n.d.). Gay and lesbian rights. Retrieved from http://www.gallup.com/poll/1651/gay-lesbian-rights.aspx

Gallup Politics. (2012). U.S. acceptance of gay/lesbian relations is the new normal. Retrieved from http://www.gallup.com/poll/154634/Acceptance-Gay-Lesbian-Relations-New-Normal.aspx

Galvez, J. F., Thommi, S., & Ghaemi, S. N. (2011). Positive aspects of mental illness: A review in bipolar disorder. *Journal of Affective Disorders, 128*(3), 185–190. doi:10.1016/j.jad.2010.03.017

Goldberg, J., Matte, N., MacMillan, M., & Hudspith, M. (2003). Community survey: Transition/crossdressing services in BC: Final report. Retrieved from http://www.spectrumwny.org/info/bcsurvey.pdf

Grant, J. M., Mottet, L. A., Tanis, J., Harrison, J., Herman, J. L., & Keisling, M. (2011). Injustice at every turn: A report of the national transgender discrimination survey. Retrieved from http://endtransdiscrimination.org/PDFs/NTDS_Report.pdf

Grella, C. E., Greenwell, L., Mays, V. M., & Cochran, S. D. (2009). Influence of gender, sexual orientation, and need on treatment utilization for substance use and mental disorders: Findings from the California Quality of Life Survey. *BMC Psychiatry, 9,* 52. doi:10.1186/1471-244X-9-52

Hart, K. E. & Sasso, T. (2011). Mapping the contours of contemporary positive psychology. *Canadian Psychology, 52*(2), 82–92. doi:10.1037/a0023118

Hartman, C. (2013). Are lesbian, gay, bisexual, and transgender patients at higher risk for mental health disorders? *Evidence-Based Practice, 16*(3), 7.

Hatzenbuehler, M. L. (2011). The social environment and suicide attempts in lesbian, gay, and bisexual youth. *Pediatrics, 127*(5), 896–903. doi:10.1542/peds.2010-3020

Hicks, D. (2000). The importance of specialized treatment programs for lesbian and gay patients. *Journal of Gay and Lesbian Psychotherapy, 3*(3–4), 81–94.

Hightow-Weidman, L. B., Phillips, H., II, Jones, K. C., Outlaw, A. Y., Fields, S. D., Smith, J. C. (2011). Racial and sexual identity-related maltreatment among minority YMSM: Prevalence, perceptions, and the association with emotional distress. *AIDS Patient Care and STDs, 25,* S39–S45. doi:10.1089/apc.2011.9877

Hughes, T. L., Johnson, T. P., Steffen, A. D., Wilsnack, S. C., & Everett, B. (2014). Lifetime victimization, hazardous drinking, and depression among heterosexual and sexual minority women. *LGBT Health, 1*(3), 192–203. doi:10.1089/lgbt.2014.0014

Israel, G. E., & Tarver, D. E., II. (Eds.) (1997). *Transgender care: Recommended guidelines, practical information, and personal accounts.* Philadelphia, PA: Temple University Press.

Johnson, T. P., Hughes, T. L., Cho, Y. I., Wilsnack, S. C., Aranda, F., & Szalacha, L. A. (2013). Hazardous drinking, depression, and anxiety among sexual-minority women: Self-medication or impaired functioning? *Journal of Studies on Alcohol and Drugs, 74*(4), 565–575.

Kessler, R. C., Chiu, W. T., Demler, O., Merikangas, K. R., & Walters, E. E. (2005). Prevalence, severity, and comorbidity of 12-month DSM-IV disorders in the National Comorbidity Survey Replication. *Archives of General Psychiatry, 62*(6), 617–627. doi:10.1001/archpsyc.62.6.617

King, M., Semlyen, J., Tai, S. S., Killaspy, H., Osborn, D., Popelyuk, D., & Nazareth, I. (2008). A systematic review of mental disorder, suicide, and deliberate self harm in lesbian, gay and bisexual people. *BMC Psychiatry, 8,* 70. doi:10.1186/1471-244X-8-70

Korell, S. C., & Lorah, P. (2007). An overview of affirmative psychotherapy and counseling with transgender clients. In K. J. Bieschke, R. M. Perez, K. A. DeBord, K. J. Bieschke, R. M. Perez, & K. A. DeBord (Eds.), *Handbook of counseling and psychotherapy with lesbian, gay, bisexual, and transgender clients* (2nd ed., pp. 271–288). Washington, DC: American Psychological Association. doi:10.1037/11482-011

Krajeski, J. (1996). Homosexuality and the mental health professions: A contemporary history. In R. P. Cabaj & T. S. Stein (Eds.), *Textbook of homosexuality and mental health* (pp. 17–31). Arlington, VA: American Psychiatric Association.

Kuhn, A., Bodmer, C., Stadlmayr, W., Kuhn, P., Mueller, M. D., & Birkhäuser, M. (2009). Quality of life 15 years after sex reassignment surgery for transsexualism. *Fertility and Sterility, 92*(5), 1685–1689.e3. doi:10.1016/j.fertnstert2008.08.126.

Kwon, P. (2013). Resilience in lesbian, gay, and bisexual individuals. *Personality and Social Psychology Review, 17*(4), 371–383. doi:10.1177/1088868313490248

Liddle, B. J. (1997). Gay and lesbian clients' selection of therapists and utilization of therapy. *Psychotherapy: Theory, Research, Practice, Training, 34*(1), 11–18.

Lock, J. (1998). Treatment of homophobia in a gay male adolescent. *American Journal of Psychotherapy, 52*(2), 202–214.

Lombardi, E. (2007). Substance use treatment experiences of transgender/transsexual men and women. *Journal of LGBT Health Research, 3*(2), 37–47.

Luthar, S. S., & Suchman, N. E. (2000). Relational Psychotherapy Mothers' Group: A developmentally informed intervention for at-risk mothers. *Development and Psychopathology, 12*(2), 235–253.

Lytle, M. C., Vaughan, M. D., Rodriguez, E. M., & Shmerler, D. L. (2014). Working with LGBT individuals: Incorporating positive psychology into training and practice. *Psychology of Sexual Orientation and Gender Diversity, 1*(4), 335–347. doi:10.1037/sgd0000064

Martell, C. R., Safren, S. A., & Prince, S. E. (2004). *Cognitive-behavioral therapies with lesbian, gay, and bisexual clients.* New York, NY: Guilford Press.

Matthews-Ewald, M. R., Zullig, K. H., & Ward, R. M. (2014). Sexual orientation and disordered eating behaviors among self-identified male and female college students. *Eating Behaviors, 15*(3), 441–444. doi:10.1016/j.eatbeh.2014.05.002

McGarrity, L., & Huebner, D. (2013). Is being out about sexual orientation uniformly healthy? The moderating role of socioeconomic status in a prospective study of gay and bisexual men. *Annals of Behavioral Medicine, 47*(1), 28–38. doi:10.1007/s12160-013-9575-6

McLemore, K. A. (in press). A minority stress perspective on transgender individuals' experience with misgendering. *Stigma and Health.* Advanced online publication. doi:10.1037/sah0000070

Meyer, I. H. (2013). Prejudice, social stress, and mental health in lesbian, gay, and bisexual populations: Conceptual issues and research evidence. *Psychology of Sexual Orientation and Gender Diversity, 1,* 3–26. doi:10.1037/2329-0382.1.S.3

Morgan, K. S. (1992). Caucasian lesbians' use of psychotherapy: A matter of attitude? *Psychology of Women Quarterly, 16*(1), 127–130. doi:10.1111/j.1471-6402.1992.tb00244.x

Murad, M. H., Elamin, M. B., Garcia, M. Z., Mullan, R. J., Murad, A., Erwin, P. J., & Montori, V. M. (2010). Hormonal therapy and sex reassignment: A systemic review and meta-analysis of quality of life and psychosocial outcomes. *Clinical Endocrinology, 72*(2), 214–231. doi:10.1111/j.1365-2265.2009.03625.x

Neisen, J. H. (1997). An inpatient psychoeducational group model for gay men and lesbians with alcohol and drug abuse problems. In L. D. McVinney (Ed.), *Chemical dependency treatment: Innovative group approach* (pp. 37–51). New York, NY: Haworth Press.

Ngamake, S. T., Walch, S. E., & Raveepatarakul, J. (2016). Discrimination and sexual minority mental health: Mediation and moderation effects of coping. *Psychology of Sexual Orientation and Gender Diversity, 3*(2), 213–226. doi:10.1037/sgd0000163

Norton, A. T., & Herek, G. M. (2013). Heterosexuals' attitudes toward transgender people: Findings from a national probability sample of U.S. adults. *Sex Roles, 68*(11), 738–753. doi:10.1007/s11199-011-0110-6

Pachankis, J. E. (2007). The psychological implications of concealing a stigma: A cognitive-affective-behavioral model. *Psychological Bulletin, 133*(2), 328–345. doi:10.1037/0033-2909.133.2.328

Pachankis, J. E. (2014). Uncovering clinical principles and techniques to address minority stress, mental health, and related health risks among gay and bisexual men. *Clinical Psychology, 21*(4), 313–330.

Pachankis, J. E., Cochran, S. D., & Mays, V. M. (2015). The mental health of sexual minority adults in and out of the closet: A population-based study. *Journal of Consulting and Clinical Psychology, 83*(5), 890–901. doi:10.1037/ccp0000047

Pachankis, J. E., Hatzenbuehler, M. L., Rendina, H. J., Safren, S. A., & Parsons, J. T. (2015). LGB-affirmative cognitive-behavioral therapy for young adult gay and bisexual men: A randomized controlled trial of a transdiagnostic minority stress approach. *Journal of Consulting & Clinical Psychology, 83*(5), 875–889. doi:10.1037/ccp0000037

Pesola, R., Shelton, K. H., & van den Bree, M. B. M. (2014). Sexual orientation and alcohol problem use among UK adolescents: An indirect link through depressed mood. *Addiction, 109*(7), 1072–1080. doi:10.1111/add.12528

Reisner, S. L., Katz-Wise, S. L., Gordon, A. R., Corliss, H. L., & Austin, S. B. (2016). Social epidemiology of depression and anxiety by gender identity. *Journal of Adolescent Health, 59*(2), 203–208. doi:10.1016/j.jadohealth.2016.04.006

Resnick, S. G., & Rosenheck, R. A. (2006). Recovery and positive psychology: Parallel themes and potential synergies. *Psychiatric Services, 57*(1), 120–122.

Roberts, A. L., Austin, S. B., Corliss, H. L., Vandermorris, A. K., & Koenen, K. C. (2010). Pervasive trauma exposure among US sexual orientation minority adults and risk of posttraumatic stress disorder. *American Journal of Public Health, 100*(12), 2433–2441. doi:10.2105/AJPH.2009.168971

Roi, C. L., Kretschmer, T., Dijkstra, J. K., Veenstra, R., & Oldehinkel, A. J. (2016). Disparities in depressive symptoms between heterosexual and lesbian, gay, and bisexual youth in a Dutch cohort: The TRAILS Study. *Journal of Youth and Adolescence, 45*(3), 440–456. doi:10.1007/s10964-015-0403-0

Rose, S. M., & Mechanic, M. B. (2002) Pscyhological distress, crime features, and help-seeking behaviors related to homophobic bias incidents. *American Behavioral Scientist, 46*, 14–26.

Ross, L. E., Doctor, F., Dimito, A., Kuehl, D., & Armstrong, M. S. (2008). Can talking about oppression reduce depression? Modified CBT group treatment for LGBT people with depression. *Journal of Gay & Lesbian Social Services, 19*(1), 1–15. doi:10.1300/J041v19n01_01

Rutter, P. A., & Camarena, J. (2015). Decolonizing sex: A multicultural and gay affirmative approach to counseling with African American and Latino men who have sex with men. *Journal of LGBT Issues in Counseling, 9*(1), 57-68. doi:10.1080/15538605.2014.997330

Ryan, C., Russell, S. T., Huebner, D., Diaz, R., & Sanchez, J. (2010). Family acceptance in adolescence and the health of LGBT young adults. *Journal of Child and Adolescent Psychiatric Nursing, 23*(4), 205–213. doi:10.1111/j.1744-6171.2010.00246.x

Schmidt, C. K., Miles, J. R., & Welsh, A. C. (2011). Perceived discrimination and social support: The influences on career development and college adjustment of LGBT college students. *Journal of Career Development, 38*(4), 293–309. doi:10.1177/0894845310372615

Schrimshaw, E. W., Siegel, K., Downing, M. J., & Parsons, J. T. (2013). Disclosure and concealment of sexual orientation and the mental health of non-gay-identified, behaviorally bisexual men. *Journal of Consulting and Clinical Psychology, 81*(1), 141–153.

Seligman, M., & Csikszentmihalyi, M. (2000). Positive psychology: An introduction. *American Psychologist, 55*(1), 5–14.

Senreich, E. (2010). Are specialized LGBT program components helpful for gay and bisexual men in substance abuse treatment? *Substance Use & Misuse, 45*(7–8), 1077–1096.

Shelton, K., & Delgado-Romero, E. A. (2011). Sexual orientation microaggressions: The experience of lesbian, gay, bisexual, and queer clients in psychotherapy. *Journal of Counseling Psychology, 58*(2), 210–221.

Shilo, G., Antebi, N., & Mor, Z. (2015). Individual and community resilience factors among lesbian, gay, bisexual, queer and questioning youth and adults in Israel. *American Journal of Community Psychology, 55*(1–2), 215–227. doi:10.1007/s10464-014-9693-8

Shipherd, J. C., Maguen, S., Skidmore, W. C., & Abramovitz, S. M. (2011). Potentially traumatic events in a transgender sample: Frequency and associated symptoms. *Traumatology, 17*(2), 56–67. doi:10.1177/1534765610395614

Simeonov, D., Steele, L. S., Anderson, S., & Ross, L. E. (2015). Perceived satisfaction with mental health services in the lesbian, gay, bisexual, transgender, and transsexual communities in Ontario, Canada: An internet-based survey. *Canadian Journal of Community Mental Health, 34*(1), 31–44 doi:10.7870/cjcmh-2014-037

Sin, N. L., & Lyubomirsky, S. (2009). Enhancing well-being and alleviating depressive symptoms with positive psychology interventions: A practice-friendly meta-analysis. *Journal of Clinical Psychology, 65*(5), 467–487. doi:10.1002/jclp.20593

Singh, A. A., Hays, D. G., & Watson, L. S. (2011). Strength in the face of adversity: Resilience strategies of transgender individuals. *Journal of Counseling & Development, 89*(1), 20–27. doi:10.1002/j.1556-6678.2011.tb00057.x

Sue, D. W. (2010). *Microaggressions and marginality: Manifestations, dynamics, and impact.* Hoboken, NJ: Wiley.

Tebbe, E. A., & Moradi, B. (2016). Suicide risk in trans populations: An application of minority stress theory. *Journal of Counseling Psychology, 63*(5), 520–533. doi:10.1037/cou0000152

Vaughan, M. D., & Rodriguez, E. M. (2014). LGBT strengths: Incorporating positive psychology into theory, research, training, and practice. *Psychology of Sexual Orientation and Gender Diversity, 1*(4), 325–334. doi:10.1037/sgd0000053

Walch, S. E., Ngamake, S. T., Bovornusvakool, W., & Walker, S. V. (2016). Discrimination, internalized homophobia, and concealment in sexual minority physical and mental health. *Psychology of Sexual Orientation and Gender Diversity, 3*(1), 37–48. doi:10.1037/sgd0000146

Warren, J. C., Smalley, K. B., & Barefoot, K. N. (2016). Psychological well-being among transgender and genderqueer individuals. *International Journal of Transgenderism, 17*(3–4), 114–123. doi:10.1080/15532739.2016.1216344

Xavier, J., Bradford, J., Hendricks, M., Safford, L., McKee, R., Martin, E., & Honnold, J. A. (2013). Transgender health care access in Virginia: A qualitative study. *International Journal of Transgenderism, 14*(1), 3–17. doi:10.1080/15532739.2013.689513

Zapor, H., & Stuart, G. L. (2016). Affirmative cognitive behavioral therapy for a male with depression following sexual orientation discrimination. *Clinical Case Studies, 15*(2), 143–156. doi:10.1177/1534650115604928

▪ FURTHER READINGS

To learn more about mental health, recovery, and resilience, the authors recommend the following resources:

Chung, Y. B., Szymanski, D. M., & Markle, E. (2012). Sexual orientation and sexual identity: Theory, research, and practice. In N. A. Fouad, J. A. Carter, & L. M. Subich (Eds.), *APA handbook of counseling psychology, vol. 1: Theories, research, and methods* (pp. 423–451). doi:10.1037/13754-016

Ferguson, A. D. (2016). Cultural issues in counseling lesbians, gays, and bisexuals. In I. Marini & M. A. Stebnicki (Eds.), *The professional counselor's desk reference* (2nd ed., pp. 159–162). New York, NY: Springer Publishing.

Hancock, K. A. (2013). Psychotherapy with lesbian, gay, and bisexual clients. In G. P. Koocher, J. C. Norcross, & B. A. Greene (Eds.), *Psychologists' desk reference* (3rd ed., pp. 234–237). doi:10.1093/med:psych/9780199845491.003.0047

Smith, L. C. (2015). Queering multicultural competence in counseling. In R. D. Goodman & P. C. Gorski (Eds.), *International and cultural psychology: Decolonizing "multicultural" counseling through social justice* (pp. 23–39). doi:10.1007/978-1-4939-1283-4_3

CHAPTER **11**

Suicide and Self-Injury in Gender and Sexual Minority Populations

Kimberly H. McManama O'Brien, Richard T. Liu, Jennifer M. Putney, Taylor A. Burke, and Laika D. Aguinaldo

In addition to being the most fatal manifestation of mental suffering, suicide often has a profound and lasting negative impact on the family and friends of the suicide decedent (Brent et al., 1992; Clark & Goldney, 2000). Among the groups that have been consistently found to be at heightened risk for engaging in suicidal behavior and death by suicide are gender and sexual minority (GSM) populations (Haas et al., 2011; Hawton, Saunders, & O'Connor, 2012; Turecki & Brent, 2016). GSM youth, in particular, have recently been identified as a priority for the development of effective research-based suicide prevention strategies to reduce rates of suicide and suicidal behavior (National Action Alliance for Suicide Prevention, 2014). In this chapter, we provide a review of the current literature on self-injurious thoughts and behaviors in GSM individuals. We begin with an overview of conceptually distinct forms of these phenomena, their prevalence rates in the general population, and findings on risk for these outcomes in GSM individuals. Drawing on the GSM literature, we then present a theoretical framework for understanding elevated risk for these phenomena in GSM populations. Guided by this conceptual framework, we then summarize the findings on risk and protective factors that may be of particular relevance in accounting for the higher prevalence of self-harm in these communities. Finally, we conclude with a discussion of considerations for prevention and intervention efforts to reduce the risk for GSM self-harm.

■ SELF-INJURIOUS THOUGHTS AND BEHAVIORS: DEFINITIONS AND PREVALENCE

Suicide, defined as the purposeful act of ending one's own life (Klonsky, May, & Saffer, 2016), is a major cause of death worldwide. Indeed, it ranks as the 15th leading cause of death according to recent estimates, accounting for approximately 1.5% of all mortality (World Health Organization, 2014). This issue is particularly a concern with the young. In the United States, for example, suicide is the 11th leading cause of death in children of ages 5 to 11 years, and has recently risen to being the second leading cause of death across the ages of 10 to 34 years (Centers for Disease Control and Prevention [CDC], 2015). Furthermore, while mortality rates for other leading causes of death, including cancer, heart disease, and stroke, have experienced appreciable declines in recent decades (Mokdad, Marks, Stroup, & Gerberding, 2004), suicide remains a persistent public health concern, with one recent national study reporting a 24% *increase* in suicides over the last 15 years (CDC, 2016) and another study projecting a 50% increase in the global suicide rates between 2002 and 2030 (Mathers & Loncar, 2006).

Arriving at accurate estimates of suicide in GSM individuals relative to the general population is especially challenging, as sexual orientation and gender identity are not typically included in death certificates. Compounding this problem, psychological autopsy studies (i.e., studies conducted with family and friends of suicide decedents) may be biased toward underreporting of GSM status insofar as some informants were unaware or nonaccepting of the decedent's sexual orientation and/or gender identity (Haas et al., 2011; Renaud, Chagnon, Turecki, & Marquette, 2005). Consequently, estimates of risk have often been achieved indirectly. For example, in one population-based study where same-sex registered domestic partnerships functioned as a proxy for same-sex orientation, cisgender men in these partnerships were eight times more likely to die by suicide than were heterosexually married counterparts and almost twice as likely as never-married individuals (Mathy, Cochran, Olsen, & Mays, 2011). In addition to such studies, higher risk for suicide has been often assumed based on the more well-characterized finding of higher prevalence of suicide attempts, commonly defined as the intentional infliction of self-harm with at least some intent to end one's life (Silverman, Berman, Sanddal, O'Carroll, & Joiner, 2007), in GSM populations (Haas & Lane, 2015). This assumption is informed in large part by the finding that a history of suicide attempts is associated with a substantially elevated risk for eventual death by suicide (Bridge, Goldstein, & Brent, 2006; Christiansen & Jensen, 2007). A degree of caution should be taken, however, in forming such inferences, as higher rates of suicide attempts do not always correspond with higher rates of suicides. One well-established example of this is gender differences in both phenomena; although women are more likely to attempt suicide, men are more likely to die from it, largely attributed to a consequence of their tendency to adopt more lethal methods (Conner, 2004; Nock et al., 2013). Until data on sexual orientation and gender identity are systematically and accurately collected as part of death records, it will be impractical (if not impossible) to produce reliable estimates of the prevalence of suicide in GSM populations (Haas & Lane, 2015).

In addition to suicide, nonfatal manifestations of suicidality—suicidal ideation and suicide attempts—are clinically important phenomena. The lifetime prevalence rate for suicidal ideation (defined as the desire to die or to kill oneself) is approximately 9.2% worldwide, and although the mildest form of suicidality, it is clinically significant in part because most individuals who transition from ideation to suicide attempts do so within a year of onset of ideation (Nock et al., 2008). Suicidal ideation may therefore serve as an early warning sign of risk for suicidal behavior. In a meta-analysis of suicidality, sexual minority individuals have two times the risk of experiencing suicidal ideation within their lifetimes relative to cisgender individuals who identify as heterosexual (King et al., 2008). Studies of transgender individuals indicate a greater risk for suicidal ideation relative to cisgender counterparts, with lifetime estimates for the former group ranging from 32% to 58.1% (Marshall, Claes, Bouman, Witcomb, & Arcelus, 2016; Reisner, White, Bradford, & Mimiaga, 2014). It should be noted, however, that these studies generally featured small numbers of transgender respondents, leading to relatively unstable estimates, and the percentage of cisgender respondents who endorsed a lifetime history of suicidal ideation was sometimes also higher than in the general population (e.g., 20.6%; Reisner et al., 2014), perhaps reflecting the naturally elevated levels of psychopathology in the sample source.

The lifetime prevalence rate of suicide attempts in the general population is 2.7% (Nock et al., 2008). In a recent meta-analysis of studies directly comparing sexual minority adults to cisgender heterosexual counterparts, the lifetime prevalence rate was significantly higher among sexual minority individuals (11%) than cisgender heterosexual individuals (4%; Hottes, Bogaert, Rhodes, Brennan, & Gesink, 2016). In studies of transgender individuals, the lifetime prevalence of suicide attempts ranged from 18% to 45% (Haas, Rodgers, & Herman, 2014; Marshall et al., 2016). Despite the wide range in prevalence rates, these studies consistently reported substantially higher rates than are found in the general population.

A related clinical phenomenon that has received increasing recognition over the last decade is nonsuicidal self-injury (NSSI), defined as the direct and deliberate destruction of one's own bodily tissue in the absence of any suicidal intent (Nock, 2010). NSSI has traditionally been perceived as a less severe form of self-harm, falling on the lower end of the same continuum as suicidal behavior, and has consequently been the focus of substantially less empirical and clinical attention. In recent years, however, NSSI has come to be considered a clinically important concern in its own right. Moreover, the *Diagnostic and Statistical Manual of Mental Disorders, fifth edition (DSM-5)* introduced NSSI disorder as a clinical syndrome warranting further consideration (American Psychiatric Association, 2013). There is recent evidence that NSSI is an even stronger predictor of future suicidal behavior than is a history of suicidal behavior (Asarnow et al., 2011; Ribeiro et al., 2016; Wilkinson, Kelvin, Roberts, Dubicka, & Goodyer, 2011). Furthermore, although suicidal behavior and NSSI do share some similarities, and these phenomena often co-occur, important differences also exist, particularly with regard to their neurobiology, response to treatment, and long-term trajectory (Brent, 2011; Mars et al., 2014; Muehlenkamp, 2005; Muehlenkamp & Gutierrez, 2007; Wichstrøm, 2009). Lifetime prevalence estimates for NSSI vary considerably, in large part due to differences in method of assessment, but in one recent meta-analysis, lifetime prevalence estimates were found to be 17.2% among adolescents and 5.5% among adults (Swannell, Martin, Page, Hasking, & St John, 2014), with recent epidemiologic research indicating a 5.9% lifetime prevalence in adults (Klonsky, 2011).

Although few studies to date have directly compared sexual minorities to heterosexual counterparts in terms of prevalence of NSSI, there appears to be emerging evidence of greater risk associated with sexual minority status, with a recent meta-analysis finding the odds of this behavior in sexual minorities being three times that of heterosexual individuals (Batejan, Jarvi, & Swenson, 2015). In this study, the risk for NSSI was especially elevated in sexual minority adolescents, with odds of this behavior being nearly six times that of cisgender heterosexual counterparts. Studies of NSSI prevalence among gender minority populations are even rarer, and epidemiologic estimates are currently unavailable. There is emerging evidence, however, that transgender individuals may be at greater risk for NSSI relative to their cisgender counterparts. Although lifetime rates of NSSI varied widely across three studies in this area with adult samples, ranging from 19% to 41.9% (Claes et al., 2015; Davey, Arcelus, Meyer, & Bouman, 2015; dickey, Reisner, & Juntunen, 2015), these figures are uniformly and considerably higher than those observed in the general population. In studies with transgender adolescents, the percentage of youth with a history of NSSI ranged from 24% to 39% (Marshall et al., 2016). In addition to sample size limitations being common in the small number of existing studies in this area, prevalence estimates are likely influenced by the number of NSSI methods assessed and the nature of the sample (e.g., sample source and stage of transition). For these reasons, more reliable estimates of NSSI prevalence in these populations await future investigation.

■ CONCEPTUAL FRAMEWORK

In their landmark lesbian, gay, bisexual, and transgender (LGBT) health report, the Institute of Medicine ([IOM]; 2011) asserts that the social ecology perspective, minority stress model, intersectionality perspective, and life course perspective provide a conceptual blueprint for research related to GSM health. Taken together, these models lend a comprehensive framework for inquiry into the risk and protective factors for suicide and NSSI among GSM individuals. By using these conceptual frameworks as a model for examining risk and protective factors, we have the potential to design more impactful prevention and intervention efforts with this population.

The social ecology perspective, in particular, provides a broad framework with which to conceptualize the mental health of GSM groups. It asserts that people and their ecological environments reciprocally shape each other, such that individuals can be best understood in the context of their family, peer, community, cultural, and political contexts (Bronfenbrenner, 1979; McLeroy, Bibeau, Stecklet, & Glanz, 1988). Further, the theory suggests that individual-level psychological distress and suicidality may represent destructive attempts to cope with stigma, rejection, discrimination, systematically inequitable opportunity structures, and lack of legal protections based on sexual orientation, gender identity, race, and ethnicity. Hong, Espalage, and Kral (2011) applied the social ecology perspective to a review of available literature on suicide risk among sexual minority youth and delineated the relevant spheres of influence at multiple levels. Parental and peer rejection based on sexual orientation and gender expression, for example, appeared to predict suicide attempts and depression (Ryan, Huebner, Diaz, & Sanchez, 2009). At the community level, perceived discrimination and associated alienation can contribute to higher rates of suicidal behavior (Halpert, 2002). The social ecology perspective suggests multiple possibilities for interventions at the individual, family, peer, school, work, community, and political levels. Where environments are more responsive and affirming, individuals are more likely to thrive. The limitation of the social ecology perspective, however, is that it falls short of offering more specific information about which risk and protective factors are more or less predictive and which interventions hold promise. Accordingly, the minority stress model is consistent with the social ecology perspective, and yet addresses this limitation by offering more specificity.

The minority stress model offers another empirically supported conceptual framework to understand suicide-related thoughts and behaviors among GSM populations. Brooks (1981) asserts that minority stress results from "culturally sanctioned, categorically ascribed inferior status, social prejudice and discrimination" (p. 107). This model assumes that minority stress is unique, chronic, and specific to GSM identities. It is perpetuated by stable social structures that maintain systems of inequity (Meyer, 2003, 2007). Minority stress is created by distal conditions, such as discriminating social policies, and related proximal reactions, such as internalized homophobia/transphobia, concealment of identity, and expectations of rejection. The increased risk for suicide-related thoughts and behaviors may be due, in part, to the complex processes of minority stress that involve internalized stigma related to repeated, chronic exposure to hostile social environments (Meyer, 2003). Recent inquiries have partially supported this model as a mechanism to understand the disproportionately high rate of suicide-related behavior among sexual minority populations (Baams, Grossman, & Russell, 2015; Michaels, Parent, & Torrey, 2016). The minority stress model offers a promising yet understudied framework to explain the risk and protective factors for suicide among gender minority individuals as well (Tebbe & Moradi, 2016). This framework suggests that possible interventions include familial support, welcoming school and work environments, inclusive social policies, and affirming mental health treatment.

In combination with the social ecology perspective and the minority stress model, the intersectional perspective offers a useful way to conceptualize the complex risk and protective factors for suicidality among GSM populations. Disparities in suicidal behavior need to be considered in the context of individuals' multiple identities, including race, ethnicity, gender, sexual orientation, and socioeconomic status, and how they intersect with systems of inequality, such as racism, sexism, heterosexism, and transphobia. Instead of being independent and unidimensional, this paradigm asserts that identity categories are interdependent and that they shape each other. This perspective recognizes that identities are constructed within a social context of systemically unequal distribution of resources and opportunities. The intersectional perspective has preliminary empirical support as a model to understand the relationship between suicidality, forms of discrimination, and multiple social identities (Bostwick et al., 2014; Perez-Brumer, Hatzenbueler, Oldenburg, & Bockting, 2015). More research is needed to more fully understand how race, sexual orientation, ethnicity, gender identity and expression, geographic location, and socioeconomic status intersect in nuanced ways to shape risk and protective factors for suicide and NSSI.

Finally, the life course perspective (Elder, 1998) offers a complementary developmental framework with which to understand the mental health of GSM individuals over the life span. This perspective recognizes that interdependence with other people and interaction with systems (e.g., work, school, and neighborhood) are critical contexts for mental health outcomes. It also suggests that an individual's experiences are shaped, in part, by a particular historical context, such that each age cohort may experience events differently. In sum, the social ecology perspective, minority stress model, intersectionality perspective, and life course perspective emphasize that individuals have multiple identities and are embedded in complex social environments that together may confer risk for suicide and NSSI. To more fully understand suicide and NSSI among GSM individuals, research and related interventions must take into account the interaction between multiple individual- and structural-level factors.

■ RISK AND PROTECTIVE FACTORS FOR SUICIDE AMONG GSM INDIVIDUALS

Despite the evidence that GSM individuals are at higher risk for suicide relative to their heterosexual and/or cisgender counterparts, research on specific risk and protective factors for suicide is lacking for this population. However, the studies that do examine suicide risk among GSM individuals have identified some notable familial and social factors that confer or protect against suicide risk.

The majority of empirical research on risk factors for suicide among GSM groups has focused specifically on the sexual minority population. The most commonly cited risk factors among sexual minority individuals include depression, substance use, early sexual initiation, feeling unsafe at school, inadequate social support, and factors related to sexual minority status such as homophobic victimization and stress (IOM, 2011). Notably, factors related to parental acceptance, family rejection (Ryan et al., 2009), and trauma during childhood (Flynn, Johnson, Bolton, & Mojtabai, 2016) have been shown to also confer risk for suicide. For example, D'Augelli et al. (2005) found that greater parental psychological abuse during childhood and increased parental efforts to discourage childhood gender-atypical behavior increased risk for suicidal behavior among sexual minority youth. In the same study, early openness about sexual orientation and being considered gender atypical in childhood by parents were associated with a higher likelihood of having a suicide attempt that participants reported was directly related to being a sexual minority (D'Augelli et al., 2005).

Although studies on suicide risk among GSM individuals have focused primarily on sexual minority populations, it is important to note that gender minority individuals are at particularly high risk for suicide and are just beginning to garner attention in suicide research. Risk factors for suicide attempts that have been found in studies of gender minority individuals include disclosure of gender identity, family rejection, verbal and physical harassment or bullying at school, sexual assault, treatment refusal by health care providers, and homelessness (Haas et al., 2014). For transgender adults, having a diagnosis of depression, history of substance abuse treatment, experience with gender-based discrimination, and being under the age of 25 have been associated with a higher risk for suicide (Clements-Nolle, Marx, & Katz, 2006). In one study of transgender youth, experiences of past parental abuse (verbal and physical) and lower body esteem were associated with a history of suicide attempt (Grossman & D'Augelli, 2007).

Protective factors are especially relevant to examine when determining targets for prevention and intervention with GSM groups at risk for suicide. Just as negative family, social, and school experiences serve as risk factors for suicide among GSM individuals, evidence suggests that positive supports related to these factors can have a particularly salient buffering effect. For instance, family connectedness, adult caring (Eisenberg & Resnick, 2006), and overall parental and family support (Bauer, Scheim, Pyne, Travers, & Hammond, 2015; Mustanski & Liu, 2013) have been found to protect against the occurrence of suicide attempts among sexual minority youth. More specifically, this support is characterized by family acceptance of sexual and gender identity and supportive reactions by family (Ryan, Russell, Huebner, Diaz, & Sanchez, 2010). The elements of school and social supports which may buffer against suicide risk include school safety (Eisenberg & Resnick, 2006), social support from peers, family support for gender, strong support from leaders (Bauer et al., 2015), and having supportive adults inside and outside the family (Veale, Saewyc, Frohard-Dourlent, Dobson, & Clark, 2015). Among transgender individuals, in particular, access to medical intervention, lower levels of transphobic experiences, and possessing personal identification and documentation that reflected the individual's gender identity were associated with decreased risk for suicidal ideation and attempts in one study (Bauer et al., 2015). In addition, having parental support for gender identity or expression has also been associated with a lower likelihood of suicide attempts among transgender youth (Travers et al., 2012).

When these findings are taken together, the risk for suicide among GSM individuals may be particularly high for those who experience familial or social abuse and rejection due to their sexual and/or gender identities. Conversely, strong familial and social support and acceptance may buffer against suicide risk among GSM individuals.

■ RISK AND PROTECTIVE FACTORS FOR NSSI AMONG GSM INDIVIDUALS

Although literature suggests that GSM individuals are significantly more likely to engage in NSSI as compared to their cisgender heterosexual counterparts, there is a dearth of research examining risk factors for this behavior in the GSM population. However, the small body of extant literature highlights important GSM subgroup, demographic, and psychosocial risk factors.

Among subgroups of sexual orientation, those who identify as bisexual are at the highest risk for engaging in NSSI. Whitlock et al. (2011) found that bisexual undergraduates were 3.8 times as likely to have a history of NSSI compared to cisgender heterosexuals. In comparison, individuals who characterized themselves as "mostly straight," "mostly gay/lesbian," and "gay/lesbian" were 2.6, 2.3, and 1.7 times as likely to have a history of NSSI compared to cisgender heterosexuals, respectively (Whitlock et al., 2011). A recent meta-analysis as well as other individual studies examining the relationship between sexual orientation and NSSI supports this same pattern, finding that bisexual individuals are at higher risk for engaging in NSSI compared to cisgender heterosexual, gay/lesbian, and questioning/other individuals (Batejan et al., 2015; Benau, Jenkins, & Conner, 2017; Silva, Chu, Monahan, & Joiner, 2015; Tsypes, Lane, Paul, & Whitlock, 2016). Transgender individuals have also evidenced a particularly heightened risk for engagement in NSSI as compared to cisgender individuals (House, Van Horn, Coppeans, & Stepleman, 2011; Liu & Mustanski; 2012; Marshall et al., 2016; Walls, Laser, Nickels, & Wisneski, 2010).

Among GSM individuals, female gender and younger age may pose greater risk for engaging in NSSI. Indeed, among several studies of GSM adolescents and young adults, females evidenced significantly greater risk for NSSI as compared to males (House et al., 2011; Liu & Mustanski; 2012; Walls et al., 2010; Whitlock et al., 2011), a finding consistent with NSSI gender patterns found in general populations (Bresin & Schoenleber, 2015). Also consistent with demographic patterns of NSSI in general populations, a recent meta-analysis found that sexual minority youth are at greater risk than sexual minority adults for engaging in NSSI (Batejan et al., 2015). Future research is needed to determine whether race or ethnicity may also differentially affect NSSI risk among GSM individuals.

The body of research examining psychosocial risk factors for NSSI among GSM individuals has not only replicated some of the consistently implicated risk factors for NSSI among general samples, but has also identified GSM-specific risk factors that may help to account for why NSSI rates are particularly elevated in this population. In line with findings evidenced in general populations, history of attempted suicide (Liu & Mustanski, 2012), having friends with a history of attempted suicide (Walls et al., 2010), sensation seeking (Liu & Mustanski, 2012), interpersonal trauma (House et al., 2011), depression (Walls et al., 2010), and physical abuse (Nickels, 2013) each pose risk for engaging in NSSI among GSM individuals.

Beyond demonstrating consistency in risk factors between GSM populations and general populations, however, recent literature has elucidated GSM-specific risk factors for NSSI. This body of research has demonstrated preliminary support for the minority stress model as a framework to understand specific risk factors for NSSI among GSM individuals. In a 2-year longitudinal study of GSM youth, GSM-specific victimization prospectively predicted the occurrence of NSSI (Liu & Mustanski, 2012). Victimization due to gender/sexual minority status was associated with a 2.5-fold increase in risk of engaging in NSSI, acting as the most potent predictor of NSSI in this sample behind suicide attempt history (Liu & Mustanski, 2012). In another sample, youth reporting harassment at school because of their sexual orientation or gender identity were 2.3 times as likely to report engaging in self-cutting behavior (Walls et al., 2010). Additionally, cross-sectional studies have demonstrated a consistent risk relationship between discrimination based on gender/sexual minority status and NSSI among adolescent and young adult GSM samples (Almeida, Johnson, Corliss, Molnar, & Azrael, 2009; House et al., 2011). In a more recent study, Muehlenkamp, Hilt, Ehlinger, and McMillan (2015) attempted to examine the mechanisms through which GSM-specific minority stress leads to increased NSSI. Their results suggested that perceived burdensomeness resulting from the experience of minority stress may, in part, account for this relationship.

Evidence suggests that degree of "outness" may serve as both a risk and a protective factor among GSM individuals (D'Augelli, 2006; Wright & Perry, 2006) and likely plays a role in the extent of minority stress experienced by GSM individuals. In two separate youth samples collected from the same source, greater outness predicted greater likelihood of engaging in NSSI (Nickels, 2013; Walls et al., 2010). These results are inconclusive, given that they reflect only one recruitment source and thus future research is needed to determine if this relationship is generalizable to other GSM samples. Nevertheless, it will be important for future research to elucidate under what conditions (e.g., societal, familial, psychological) degree of outness may be protective against risk for NSSI versus potentially detrimental. For example, it is possible that for some individuals, greater outness may increase minority stress so severely that the benefits of outness (e.g., increased connection to the LGBT community and social support, increased openness and intimacy, decreased efforts to conceal one's identity) may not be realized. Prospective studies are necessary to better elucidate other aspects of minority stress beyond victimization, discrimination, and outness (e.g., expectations of rejection, internalized stigma) that may account for the relationship between GSM status and NSSI risk, as well as to adequately examine the underlying mechanisms through which minority stress may lead to NSSI.

Although a growing body of literature has suggested that specific GSM subgroups (e.g., individuals who identify as bisexual and/or transgender) exhibit particularly heightened levels of risk for NSSI, scarce research has examined subgroups separately to determine if psychosocial risk factors for NSSI differ based on subgroup membership. One exception to this is a study that found that, whereas among gay/lesbian individuals, physical assault, intimate partner violence, and sexual assault were associated with NSSI, among bisexual individuals these risk factors as well as family problems and discrimination also predicted NSSI (Blosnich & Bossarte, 2012). The finding that discrimination was a risk factor among the bisexual group but not the gay/lesbian group lends support to the notion that bisexual individuals may face more discrimination than gay/lesbian individuals (Mulick & Wright, 2011) and that this in turn may explain their higher rates of NSSI. Indeed, theory suggests that bisexual individuals may be faced with a "double closet," such that they may feel pressured to conceal their identity from both heterosexual peers and from other sexual minority individuals (Zinik, 2000). That bisexual individuals face unique discrimination and may additionally suffer from an absence of a distinct community (Dobinson, MacDonnell, Hampson, Clipsham, & Chow, 2005) necessitates greater research to be conducted to better understand how the specific experiences of bisexuals may explain their particularly elevated risk for NSSI compared to other sexual minority groups. Other health factors impacted by this dual discrimination are discussed in Chapter 16.

Similarly, as research suggests that transgender individuals are at particularly elevated risk for NSSI among GSM individuals, more research is needed to understand the unique risk factors faced by this subgroup which may contribute to greater NSSI. Only two studies to our knowledge have examined risk factors for NSSI among a solely transgender population. One study found that compared to transgender adults without a history of NSSI, transgender adults with a history of NSSI were more likely to identify as male, were younger, and evidenced greater psychopathology, lower body satisfaction, lower self-esteem, and lower social support (Davey et al., 2015). In a study examining transgender youth, those assigned female at birth, those with greater general psychopathology, lower self-esteem, greater interpersonal problems, and who experienced more transphobia were significantly more likely to engage in NSSI (Arcelus, Claes, Witcomb, Marshall, & Bouman, 2016).

Very few studies have examined protective factors for NSSI among GSM individuals. However, extant research suggests that social support may be particularly beneficial in this population. One study found that youth who indicated they knew a safe adult with whom they could talk about their sexuality and gender identity were significantly less likely to report a history of NSSI (Walls et al., 2010). Reisner et al. (2014) found that family support was particularly protective against NSSI among sexual minority populations.

Overall, the current literature suggests that GSM individuals not only share risk factors for NSSI with the general population, but additionally face risk factors specific to their sexual and/or gender minority status (e.g., discrimination and victimization). Evidence and theory (e.g., the minority stress model) support the notion that these additional sexual and/or gender minority-specific risk factors may account for the pronounced augmented risk for NSSI observed in GSM populations. Fortunately, similar to findings elucidating protective factors for suicide-related outcomes among GSM individuals, social support, specifically from family, appears to buffer against the risk for engaging in NSSI.

To prevent suicide and NSSI among GSM populations, strategic implementation of targeted programs and protocols in schools, communities, and health care systems is necessary. Prevention strategies currently used with GSM individuals include gatekeeper training, talk and text lines that provide confidential support, and counseling by mental health providers, but unfortunately little is known about the efficacy of these strategies (Russell, 2003). An additional method of mitigating suicidal behaviors and NSSI includes early identification using brief and validated screening instruments, followed by a thorough assessment of both risk and protective factors (Horowitz, Ballard, & Pao, 2009). Moreover, population-based screening studies should include sexual orientation and gender identity questions in accordance with the best practices for identifying GSM populations (Haas et al., 2014) to allow for more accurate prevalence rates.

There is a dearth of research on the development and testing of interventions specifically adapted for the treatment of GSM individuals (Almeida et al., 2009; see also Chapter 21), especially those that aim to reduce suicide and NSSI risk (Mustanski & Liu, 2013). To date, there are two interventions, both group based, that were designed for and tested with GSM populations (Reisner et al., 2011; Ross, Doctor, Dimito, Kuehl, & Armstrong, 2008). Unfortunately, neither of these interventions focused specifically on suicide and/or NSSI risk; instead, they targeted the reduction of depressive symptoms and both physical and mental health outcomes. The first study tested a cognitive behavioral therapy–based group intervention with GSM individuals with depressed mood, and found the intervention to be effective in reducing depressive symptoms and increasing self-esteem from baseline to follow-up (Ross et al., 2008). The intervention group consisted of 14 weekly 2-hour sessions, and included a booster session that took place 2 months after the final intervention session. The treatment protocol followed the first nine chapters of *Mind Over Mood* (Greenberger & Padesky, 1995) and included interventions that targeted antioppression principles related to coming out and internalized homophobia (Ross et al., 2008).

The second study tested a manualized group intervention named "40 & Forward" which targeted the reduction of HIV sexual risk for gay and bisexual men with comorbid mental health concerns via a peer-led group modality consisting of six consecutive weekly 2-hour sessions (Reisner et al., 2011). Given that reducing social isolation and increasing social opportunities was a target for treatment, each meeting consisted of a social dinner group and a didactic discussion. All participants received individualized, facilitated referrals and peer health navigators to guide them in accessing needed health care services. From pre- to post-assessments, participants demonstrated significant reductions in symptoms of depression, social anxiety, loneliness, and fear of negative evaluation (Reisner et al., 2011).

Attachment-Based Family Therapy (ABFT; G. S. Diamond, Reis, Diamond, Siqueland, & Isaacs, 2002) is one intervention with an emerging evidence base for use with sexual minority youth, which has the potential to decrease risk for suicide and NSSI. ABFT was originally designed for adolescents experiencing family trauma or attachment ruptures and specifically targets the management of affective disturbance among youth (G. S. Diamond et al., 2002). The course of AFBT is 16 weeks and uses family-based emotion-focused techniques to alleviate suicide-related thoughts and behaviors by improving the parent–child relationship. In an open trial of ABFT modified for sexual minority youth ($N = 10$), participants demonstrated a reduction in suicidal ideation from baseline to posttreatment (G. M. Diamond et al., 2012), suggesting its promise as a targeted treatment for sexual minority youth who present with suicide-related thoughts and behaviors.

Despite the lack of research on prevention and intervention with GSM individuals at risk for suicide and NSSI (Mustanski & Liu, 2013), emerging findings suggest that interventions that focus on family support and acceptance, as well as peer, school, and social supports, may be effective. These findings are reinforced by the framework of the minority stress model, which suggests that possible interventions should include familial support, welcoming school and work environments, inclusive social policies, and affirming mental health treatment (Tebbe & Moradi, 2016). Importantly, social support is a malleable factor, and thus should be targeted in interventions and prevention programs with GSM individuals in order to buffer against the impact of minority stress on this population.

Transgender individuals who are supported in their gender identity have demonstrated developmentally normative levels of depression and only minimal elevations in anxiety (Olson, Durwood, DeMeules, & McLaughlin, 2016), allowing us to surmise that this may translate to findings related to suicide and NSSI. Gender-affirming therapeutic techniques that focus on psychoeducation, modifying problematic thinking styles, and enhancing social support are recommended (Austin & Craig, 2015). Specifically, techniques that help to modify cognitive cycles related to transgender oppressive contexts, which generate hopelessness and contribute to suicide-related thoughts and behaviors, should be used (Austin & Craig, 2015). In addition to modifying maladaptive thoughts and behaviors, identifying specific factors that encourage resilience within this population will be critical for designing effective interventions and prevention programs. Peer, school, and social support may be a catalyst for the development and/or maintenance of this resilience. Future research on the development and testing of interventions and prevention programs specifically tailored for GSM groups will help to elucidate the mechanisms by which we can reduce the risk for suicide and NSSI among this vulnerable population.

■ CONCLUSION

GSM individuals are at elevated risk for self-injurious thoughts and behaviors relative to cisgender and heterosexual individuals. Social ecology, minority stress, intersectional, and life course perspectives help to elucidate the reasons the LGBT community is at greater risk for suicide and self-harm. Although risk and protective factors vary across gender identities and sexual orientations, familial and/or social abuse and rejection appear to be particularly strong risk factors for GSM individuals, while familial and social support and acceptance seem to buffer against self-injurious thoughts and behaviors. Consistent with underlying theoretical perspectives and empirical evidence on risk and protective factors, research shows that interventions and prevention programs that focus on family support and acceptance, as well as peer, school, and social supports, may be most effective. Future research on interventions tailored to the diverse needs of GSM individuals is needed in order to make advances in the prevention of suicide and self-harm.

REFERENCES

Almeida, J., Johnson, R. M., Corliss, H. L., Molnar, B. E., & Azrael, D. (2009). Emotional distress among LGBT youth: The influence of perceived discrimination based on sexual orientation. *Journal of Youth and Adolescence, 38*(7), 1001–1014. doi:10.1007/s10964-009-9397-9

American Psychiatric Association. (2013). *Diagnostic and statistical manual of mental disorders (5th ed.)*. Arlington, VA: American Psychiatric Publishing.

Arcelus, J., Claes, L., Witcomb, G. L., Marshall, E., & Bouman, W. P. (2016). Risk factors for non-suicidal self-injury among trans youth. *The Journal of Sexual Medicine, 13*(3), 402–412. doi:10.1016/j.jsxm.2016.01.003

Asarnow, J. R., Porta, G., Spirito, A., Emslie, G., Clarke, G., Wagner, K. D.,...Brent, D. A. (2011). Suicide attempts and nonsuicidal self-injury in the treatment of resistant depression in adolescents: Findings from the TORDIA study. *Journal of the American Academy of Child and Adolescent Psychiatry, 50*, 772–781. doi:10.1016/j.jaac.2011.04.003

Austin, A., & Craig, S. L. (2015). Transgender affirmative cognitive behavioral therapy: Clinical considerations and applications. *Professional Psychology: Research and Practice, 46*(1), 21–29. doi:10.1037/a0038642

Baams, L., Grossman, A. H., & Russell, S. T. (2015). Minority stress and mechanisms of risk for depression and suicidal ideation among lesbian, gay, and bisexual youth. *Developmental Psychology, 51*(5), 688–696. doi:10.1037/a0038994

Batejan, K. L., Jarvi, S. M., & Swenson, L. P. (2015). Sexual orientation and non-suicidal self-injury: A meta-analytic review. *Archives of Suicide Research, 19*, 131–150. doi:10.1080/13811118.2014.957450

Bauer, G. R., Scheim, A. I., Pyne, J., Travers, R., & Hammond, R. (2015). Intervenable factors associated with suicide risk in transgender persons: A respondent-driven sampling study in Ontario, Canada. *BMC Public Health, 15*, 525. doi:10.1186/s12889-015-1867-2

Benau, E. M., Jenkins, A. L., & Conner, B. T. (2017). Perceived parental monitoring and sexual orientation moderate lifetime acts of non-suicidal self-injury. *Archives of Suicide Research, 21*(2), 322–340. Advanced online publication. doi:10.1080/13811118.2016.1182092

Blosnich, J., & Bossarte, R. (2012). Drivers of disparity: Differences in socially based risk factors of self-injurious and suicidal behaviors among sexual minority college students. *Journal of American College Health, 60*(2), 141–149. doi:10.1080/07448481.2011.623332

Bostwick, W. B., Meyer, I., Aranda, F., Russell, S., Hughes, T., Birkett, M., & Mustanski, B. (2014). Mental health and suicidality among racially/ethnically diverse sexual minority youths. *American Journal of Public Health, 104*(6), 1129–1136. doi:10.2105/AJPH.2013.301749

Brent, D. (2011). Nonsuicidal self-injury as a predictor of suicidal behavior in depressed adolescents. *The American Journal of Psychiatry, 168*, 452–454. doi:10.1176/appi.ajp.2011.11020215

Brent, D. A., Perper, J., Moritz, G., Allman, C., Friend, A., Schweers, J.,...Harrington, K. (1992). Psychiatric effects of exposure to suicide among the friends and acquaintances of adolescent suicide victims. *Journal of the American Academy of Child and Adolescent Psychiatry, 31*(4), 629–639. doi:10.1097/00004583-199207000-00009

Bresin, K., & Schoenleber, M. (2015). Gender differences in the prevalence of nonsuicidal self-injury: A meta-analysis. *Clinical Psychology Review, 38*, 55–64. doi:10.1016/j.cpr.2015.02.009

Bridge, J. A., Goldstein, T. R., & Brent, D. A. (2006). Adolescent suicide and suicidal behavior. *Journal of Child Psychology and Psychiatry, 47*, 372–394. doi:10.1111/j.1469-7610.2006.01615.x

Bronfenbrenner, U. (1979). *The ecology of human development: Experiments by nature and design.* Cambridge, MA: Harvard University Press.

Brooks, V. R. (1981). *Minority stress in lesbian women*. Lexington, MA: Lexington Books, D. C. Health.

Centers for Disease Control and Prevention. (2015). *Web-based Injury Statistics Query and Reporting System (WISQARS)*. Atlanta, GA: Author.

Centers for Disease Control and Prevention. (2016). Increase in suicide in the United States, 1999–2014. Retrieved from http://www.cdc.gov/nchs/products/databriefs/db241 .htm

Christiansen, E., & Jensen, B. F. (2007). Risk of repetition of suicide attempt, suicide or all deaths after an episode of attempted suicide: A register-based survival analysis. *Australian and New Zealand Journal of Psychiatry, 41*, 257–265. doi:10.1080/00048670601172749

Claes, L., Bouman, W. P., Witcomb, G., Thurston, M., Fernandez-Aranda, F., & Arcelus, J. (2015). Non-suicidal self-injury in trans people: Associations with psychological symptoms, victimization, interpersonal functioning, and perceived social support. *Journal of Sexual Medicine, 12*, 168–179. doi:10.1111/jsm.12711

Clark, S. E., & Goldney, R. D. (2000). The impact of suicide on relatives and friends. In K. Hawton & K. van Heeringen (Eds.), *The international handbook of suicide and attempted suicide* (pp. 467–484). West Sussex, England: John Wiley & Sons. doi:10.1002/9780470698976.ch26

Clements-Nolle, K., Marx, R., & Katz, M. (2006). Attempted suicide among transgender persons: The influence of gender-based discrimination and victimization. *Journal of Homosexuality, 51*(3), 53–69.

Conner, K. R. (2004). A call for research on planned vs. unplanned suicidal behavior. *Suicide & Life-threatening Behavior, 34*, 89–98. doi:10.1521/suli.34.2.89.32780

D'Augelli, A. R. (2006). Developmental and contextual factors and mental health among lesbian, gay, and bisexual youths. In A. E. Omoto & H. M. Kurtzman (Eds.), *Sexual orientation and mental health: Examining identity and development in lesbian, gay, and bisexual people* (pp. 37–53). Washington, DC: American Psychological Association.

D'Augelli, A. R., Grossman, A. H., Salter, N. P., Vasey, J. J., Starks, M. T., & Sinclair, K. O. (2005). Predicting the suicide attempts of lesbian, gay, and bisexual youth. *Suicide & Life-threatening Behavior, 35*(6), 646–660.

Davey, A., Arcelus, J., Meyer, C., & Bouman, W. P. (2015). Self-injury among trans individuals and matched controls: Prevalence and associated factors. *Health & Social Care in the Community, 24*(4), 485–494. doi:10.1111/hsc.12239

Diamond, G. M., Diamond, G. S., Levy, S., Closs, C., Ladipo, T., & Siqueland, L. (2012). Attachment-based family therapy for suicidal lesbian, gay, and bisexual adolescents: A treatment development study and open trial with preliminary findings. *Psychotherapy, 49*(1), 62–71. doi:10.1037/a0026247

Diamond, G. S., Reis, B. F., Diamond, G. M., Siqueland, L., & Isaacs, L. (2002). Attachment-based family therapy for depressed adolescents: A treatment development study. *Journal of the American Academy of Child & Adolescent Psychiatry, 41*(10), 1190–1196. doi:10.1097/00004583-200210000-00008

dickey, l. m., Reisner, S. L., & Juntunen, C. L. (2015). Non-suicidal self-injury in a large online sample of transgender adults. *Professional Psychology: Research and Practice, 46*, 3–11. doi:10.1037/a0038803

Dobinson, C., MacDonnell, J., Hampson, E., Clipsham, J., & Chow, K. (2005). Improving the access and quality of public health services for bisexuals. *Journal of Bisexuality, 5*(1), 39–77. doi:10.1300/j159v05n01_05

Eisenberg, M. E., & Resnick, M. D. (2006). Suicidality among gay, lesbian and bisexual youth: The role of protective factors. *The Journal of Adolescent Health, 39*(5), 662–668.

Elder, G. H. (1998). The life course as developmental theory. *Child Development, 69*(1), 1–12.

Flynn, A. B., Johnson, R. M., Bolton, S. L., & Mojtabai, R. (2016). Victimization of lesbian, gay, and bisexual people in childhood: Associations with attempted suicide. *Suicide & Life-threatening Behavior, 46*(4), 457–470. doi:10.1111/sltb.12228

Greenberger, D., & Padesky, C. A. (1995). *Mind over mood* (1st ed.). New York, NY: Guilford Publications.

Grossman, A. H., & D'Augelli, A. R. (2007). Transgender youth and life-threatening behaviors. *Suicide & Life-threatening Behavior, 37*(5), 527–537.

Haas, A. P., Eliason, M., Mays, V. M., Mathy, R. M., Cochran, S. D., D'Augelli, A. R.,…Clayton, P. J. (2011). Suicide and suicide risk in lesbian, gay, bisexual, and transgender populations: Review and recommendations. *Journal of Homosexuality, 58*(1), 10–51. doi:10.1080/00918369.2011.534038

Haas, A. P., & Lane, A. (2015). Collecting sexual orientation and gender identity data in suicide and other violent deaths: A step towards identifying and addressing LGBT mortality disparities. *LGBT Health, 2*, 84–87. doi:10.1089/lgbt.2014.0083

Haas, A. P., Rodgers, P. L., & Herman, J. L. (2014). Suicide attempts among transgender and gender non-conforming adults: Findings of the national transgender discrimination survey. Retrieved from http://williamsinstitute.law.ucla.edu/wp-content/uploads/AFSP-Williams-Suicide-Report-Final.pdf

Halpert, S. C. (2002). Suicidal behavior among gay male youth. *Journal of Gay & Lesbian Psychotherapy, 6*(3), 53–79.

Hawton, K., Saunders, K. E., & O'Connor, R. C. (2012). Self-harm and suicide in adolescents. *Lancet, 379*, 2373–2382. doi:10.1016/S0140-6736(12)60322-5

Hong, J. S., Espelage, D. L., & Kral, M. J. (2011). Understanding suicide among sexual minority youth in America: An ecological systems analysis. *Journal of Adolescence, 5*(34), 885–894. doi:10.1016/j.adolescence.2011.01.002

Horowitz, L. M., Ballard, E. D., & Pao, M. (2009). Suicide screening in schools, primary care and emergency departments. *Current Opinion in Pediatrics, 21*(5), 620–627. doi:10.1097/MOP.0b013e3283307a89

Hottes, T. S., Bogaert, L., Rhodes, A. E., Brennan, D. J., & Gesink, D. (2016). Lifetime prevalence of suicide attempts among sexual minority adults by study sampling strategies: A systematic review and meta-analysis. *American Journal of Public Health, 106*(5), e1–e12. doi:10.2105/AJPH.2016.303088

House, A. S., Van Horn, E., Coppeans, C., & Stepleman, L. M. (2011). Interpersonal trauma and discriminatory events as predictors of suicidal and nonsuicidal self-injury in gay, lesbian, bisexual, and transgender persons. *Traumatology, 17*(2), 75–85. doi:10.1177/1534765610395621

Institute of Medicine. (2011). *The health of lesbian, gay, bisexual, and transgender people: Building a foundation for better understanding.* Washington, DC: National Academies Press.

King, M., Semlyen, J., Tai, S. S., Killaspy, H., Osborn, D., Popelyuk, D., & Nazareth, I. (2008). A systematic review of mental disorder, suicide, and deliberate self harm in lesbian, gay and bisexual people. *BMC Psychiatry, 8*, 70. doi:10.1186/1471-244X-8-70

Klonsky, E. D. (2011). Non-suicidal self-injury in United States adults: Prevalence, sociodemographics, topography and functions. *Psychological Medicine, 41*, 1981–1986. doi:10.1017/S0033291710002497

Klonsky, E. D., May, A. M., & Saffer, B. Y. (2016). Suicide, suicide attempts, and suicidal ideation. *Annual Review of Clinical Psychology, 12*, 307–330. doi:10.1146/annurev-clinpsy-021815-093204

Liu, R. T., & Mustanski, B. (2012). Suicidal ideation and self-harm in lesbian, gay, bisexual, and transgender youth. *American Journal of Preventive Medicine, 42*(3), 221–228. doi:10.1016/j.amepre.2011.10.023

Mars, B., Heron, J., Crane, C., Hawton, K., Lewis, G., Macleod, J.,…Gunnell, D. (2014). Clinical and social outcomes of adolescent self harm: Population based birth cohort study. *BMJ, 349*, g5954. doi:10.1136/bmj.g5954

Marshall, E., Claes, L., Bouman, W. P., Witcomb, G. L., & Arcelus, J. (2016). Non-suicidal self-injury and suicidality in trans people: A systematic review of the literature. *International Review of Psychiatry, 28*, 58–69. doi:10.3109/09540261.2015.1073143

Mathers, C. D., & Loncar, D. (2006). Projections of global mortality and burden of disease from 2002 to 2030. *PLOS Medicine, 3*, e442. doi:10.1371/journal.pmed.0030442

Mathy, R. M., Cochran, S. D., Olsen, J., & Mays, V. M. (2011). The association between relationship markers of sexual orientation and suicide: Denmark, 1990–2001. *Social Psychiatry and Psychiatric Epidemiology, 46*, 111–117. doi:10.1007/s00127-009-0177-3

McLeroy, K. R., Bibeau, D., Steckler, A., & Glanz, K. (1988). An ecological perspective on health promotion programs. *Health Education Quarterly, 15*(4), 351–377.

Meyer, I. H. (2003). Prejudice, social stress, and mental health in lesbian, gay, and bisexual populations: Conceptual issues and research evidence. *Psychological Bulletin, 129*, 674–697.

Meyer, I. H. (2007). Prejudice and discrimination as social stressors. In I. H. Meyer & M. E. Northridge (Eds.), *The health of sexual minorities: Public health perspectives on lesbian, gay, bisexual, and transgender populations* (pp. 242–267). New York, NY: Springer.

Michaels, M. S., Parent, M. C., & Torrey, C. L. (2016). A minority stress model for suicidal ideation in gay men. *Suicide and Life-threatening Behavior, 46*(1), 23–34. doi:10.1111/sltb.12169

Mokdad, A. H., Marks, J. S., Stroup, D. F., & Gerberding, J. L. (2004). Actual causes of death in the United States, 2000. *The Journal of the American Medical Association, 291*, 1238–1245. doi:10.1001/jama.291.10.1238

Muehlenkamp, J. J. (2005). Self-injurious behavior as a separate clinical syndrome. *The American Journal of Orthopsychiatry, 75*(2), 324–333. doi:10.1037/0002-9432.75.2.324

Muehlenkamp, J. J., & Gutierrez, P. M. (2007). Risk for suicide attempts among adolescents who engage in non-suicidal self-injury. *Archives of Suicide Research, 11*, 69–82. doi:10.1080/13811110600992902

Muehlenkamp, J. J., Hilt, L. M., Ehlinger, P. P., & McMillan, T. (2015). Nonsuicidal self-injury in sexual minority college students: A test of theoretical integration. *Child and Adolescent Psychiatry and Mental Health, 9*(1), 1–8. doi:10.1186/s13034-015-0050-y

Mulick, P. S., & Wright, L. W. (2011). The biphobia scale a decade later: Reflections and additions. *Journal of Bisexuality, 11*, 453–457. doi:10.1080/15299716.2011.620486

Mustanski, B., & Liu, R. T. (2013). A longitudinal study of predictors of suicide attempts among lesbian, gay, bisexual, and transgender youth. *Archives of Sexual Behavior, 42*(3), 437–448. doi:10.1007/s10508-012-0013-9

National Action Alliance for Suicide Prevention. (2014). *A prioritized research agenda for suicide prevention: An action plan to save lives.* Rockville, MD: National Institute of Mental Health and the Research Prioritization Task Force.

Nickels, S. J. (2013). The role of the social environment in non-suicidal self-injury among LGBTQ youth: A mixed methods study (Doctoral dissertation). Retrieved from http://digitalcommons.du.edu/etd/992

Nock, M. K. (2010). Self-injury. *Annual Review of Clinical Psychology, 6*, 339–363. doi:10.1146/annurev.clinpsy.121208.131258

Nock, M. K., Borges, G., Bromet, E. J., Alonso, J., Angermeyer, M., Beautrais, A., . . . Williams, D. (2008). Cross-national prevalence and risk factors for suicidal ideation, plans and attempts. *The British Journal of Psychiatry, 192*, 98–105. doi:10.1192/bjp.bp.107.040113

Nock, M. K., Green, J. G., Hwang, I., McLaughlin, K. A., Sampson, N. A., Zaslavsky, A. M., & Kessler, R. C. (2013). Prevalence, correlates, and treatment of lifetime suicidal behavior among adolescents: Results from the National Comorbidity Survey Replication - Adolescent Supplement (NCS-A). *JAMA Psychiatry, 70*, 300–310. doi:10.1001/2013.jamapsychiatry.55

Olson, K. R., Durwood, L., DeMeules, M., & McLaughlin, K. A. (2016). Mental health of transgender children who are supported in their identities. *Pediatrics, 137*(3), e20153223. doi:10.1542/peds.2015-3223

Perez-Brumer, A., Hatzenbuehler, M. L., Oldenburg, C. E., & Bockting, W. (2015). Individual- and structural-level risk factors for suicide attempts among transgender adults. *Behavioral Medicine, 41*(3), 164–171. doi:10.1080/08964289.2015.1028322

Reisner, S. L., O'Cleirigh, C., Hendriksen, E. S., McLain, J., Ebin, J., Lew, K.,…Mimiaga, M. J. (2011). "40 & forward": Preliminary evaluation of a group intervention to improve mental health outcomes and address HIV sexual risk behaviors among older gay and bisexual men. *Journal of Gay & Lesbian Social Services, 23*(4), 523–545. doi:10.1080/10538720.2011.611113

Reisner, S. L., White, J. M., Bradford, J. B., & Mimiaga, M. J. (2014). Transgender health disparities: Comparing full cohort and nested matched-pair study designs in a community health center. *LGBT Health, 1*, 177–184. doi:10.1089/lgbt.2014.0009

Renaud, J., Chagnon, F., Turecki, G., & Marquette, C. (2005). Completed suicides in a youth centres population. *Canadian Journal of Psychiatry, 50*(11), 690–694.

Ribeiro, J. D., Franklin, J. C., Fox, K. R., Bentley, K. H., Kleiman, E. M., Chang, B. P., & Nock, M. K. (2016). Self-injurious thoughts and behaviors as risk factors for future suicide ideation, attempts, and death: A meta-analysis of longitudinal studies. *Psychological Medicine, 46*, 225–236. doi:10.1017/S0033291715001804

Ross, L. E., Doctor, F., Dimito, A., Kuehl, D., & Armstrong, M. S. (2008). Can talking about oppression reduce depression? Modified CBT group treatment for LGBT people with depression. *Journal of Gay & Lesbian Social Services, 19*(1), 1–15.

Russell, S., (2003). Sexual minority youth and suicide risk. *American Behavioral Scientist, 46*(9), 1241–1257. doi:10.1177/0002764202250667

Ryan, C., Huebner, D., Diaz, R. M., & Sanchez, J. (2009). Family rejection as a predictor of negative health outcomes in White and Latino lesbian, gay, and bisexual young adults. *Pediatrics, 123*(1), 346–352. doi:10.1542/peds.2007-3524

Ryan, C., Russell, S. T., Huebner, D., Diaz, R., & Sanchez, J. (2010). Family acceptance in adolescence and the health of LGBT young adults. *Journal of Child and Adolescent Psychiatric Nursing, 23*(4), 205–213. doi:10.1111/j.1744-6171.2010.00246.x

Silva, C., Chu, C., Monahan, K. R., & Joiner, T. E. (2015). Suicide risk among sexual minority college students: A mediated moderation model of sex and perceived burdensomeness. *Psychology of Sexual Orientation and Gender Diversity, 2*(1), 22–33. doi:10.1037/sgd0000086

Silverman, M. M., Berman, A. L., Sanddal, N. D., O'Carroll, P. W., & Joiner, T. E. (2007). Rebuilding the tower of Babel: A revised nomenclature for the study of suicide and suicidal behaviors. Part II: Suicide-related ideations, communications, and behaviors. *Suicide and Life-threatening Behavior, 37*, 264–277. doi:10.1521/suli.2007.37.3.264

Swannell, S. V., Martin, G. E., Page, A., Hasking, P., & St John, N. J. (2014). Prevalence of nonsuicidal self-injury in nonclinical samples: Systematic review, meta-analysis and meta-regression. *Suicide & Life-threatening Behavior, 44*, 273–303. doi:10.1111/sltb.12070

Tebbe, E. A., & Moradi, B. (2016). Suicide risk in trans populations: An application of minority stress theory. *Journal of Counseling Psychology, 63*(5), 520–533. doi:10.1037/cou0000152

Travers, R., Bauer, G., Pyne, J., Bradley, K., Gale, L., & Papadimitriou, M. (2012). Impacts of strong parental support for trans youth: A report prepared for Children's Aid Society of Toronto and Delisle Youth Services. Retrieved from http://transpulseproject.ca/wp-content/uploads/2012/10/Impacts-of-Strong-Parental-Support-for-Trans-Youth-vFINAL.pdf

Tsypes, A., Lane, R., Paul, E., & Whitlock, J. (2016). Non-suicidal self-injury and suicidal thoughts and behaviors in heterosexual and sexual minority young adults. *Comprehensive Psychiatry, 65*, 32–43. doi:10.1016/j.comppsych.2015.09.012

Turecki, G., & Brent, D. A. (2016). Suicide and suicidal behaviour. *Lancet, 387*, 1227–1239. doi:10.1016/S0140-6736(15)00234-2

Veale, J., Saewyc, E., Frohard-Dourlent, H., Dobson, S., & Clark, B. (2015). Being safe, being me: Results of the Canadian Trans Youth Health Research Survey. Retrieved from http://www.saravyc.ubc.ca/2015/05/05/being-safe-being-me-results-of-the-canadian-trans-youth-health-survey

Walls, N. E., Laser, J., Nickels, S. J., & Wisneski, H. (2010). Correlates of cutting behavior among sexual minority youths and young adults. *Social Work Research, 34*(4), 213–226.

Whitlock, J., Muehlenkamp, J., Purington, A., Eckenrode, J., Barreira, P., Baral Abrams, G., & Chin, C. (2011). Non-suicidal self-injury in a college population: General trends and sex differences. *Journal of American College Health, 59*(8), 691–698. doi:10.1080/07448481.2010.529626

Wichstrøm, L. (2009). Predictors of non-suicidal self-injury versus attempted suicide: Similar or different? *Archives of Suicide Research, 13*, 105–122. doi:10.1080/13811110902834992

Wilkinson, P., Kelvin, R., Roberts, C., Dubicka, B., & Goodyer, I. (2011). Clinical and psychosocial predictors of suicide attempts and nonsuicidal self-injury in the Adolescent Depression Antidepressants and Psychotherapy Trial (ADAPT). *American Journal of Psychiatry, 168*, 495–501. doi:10.1176/appi.ajp.2010.10050718

Wright, E. R., & Perry, B. L. (2006). Sexual identity distress, social support, and the health of gay, lesbian, and bisexual youth. *Journal of Homosexuality, 51*, 81–110. doi:10.1300/j082v51n01_05

World Health Organization. (2014). *Preventing suicide: A global imperative.* Geneva, Switzerland: Author. Retrieved from http://apps.who.int/iris/bitstream/10665/131056/1/9789241564779_eng.pdf?ua=1&ua=1

Zinik, G. (2000). Identity conflict or adaptive flexibility? Bisexuality reconsidered. In P. C. Rust (Ed.), *Bisexuality in the United States: A social science reader* (pp. 55–60). New York, NY: Columbia University Press.

CHAPTER **12**

Substance Use Among Gender and Sexual Minority Youth and Adults

Genevieve Weber and Ashby Dodge

To fully understand the context of substance use among gender and sexual minority (GSM) populations, it is first important to understand the social, cultural, and psychological environment in which GSM individuals seek health and happiness. Considered an at-risk group, GSM people from youth throughout adulthood are exposed to various forms of discrimination and victimization that place them at an increased risk for various outcomes discussed throughout this book, including suicide, dropping out of school, verbal and physical abuse by family or peers, lower social support, homelessness, HIV/AIDS, hopelessness, physical problems, psychological distress (e.g., anxiety and depression), and the topic of the current chapter: substance use (Frost, Levahot, & Meyer, 2015; Grossman, 1997; Meyer, 1995, 2003a, 2003b, 2015; Mustanki & Liu, 2013; Woodford, Kulick, Sinco, & Hong, 2014).

As a result of being gender and/or sexual minorities in a marginalizing society that promotes heterosexuality and the gender binary, GSM individuals experience chronic physical and emotional stress, a phenomenon that Meyer (1995, 2003a, 2003b) refers to as "minority stress." Heterosexism, homophobia, and cisgenderism are cultural ideologies that oppress GSM people. Heterosexism denies, ignores, denigrates, stigmatizes, and ultimately oppresses nonheterosexual forms of emotional/affectional expression, sexual behavior, and peer communities (Herek, 2004), and supports an underlying erroneous and harmful assumption that all individuals are heterosexual. Homophobia has been defined in a number of ways from the irrational fear of, aversion to, or discrimination against GSM behavior or persons (Davies, 1996) to individual hostility toward GSM people (Herek, 2015). Similarly, cisgenderism refers to the nonacceptance and disparagement of individuals' gender identities that do not align with assigned sex at birth as well as resulting behavior, expression, and peer community (Lennon & Mistler, 2014). These constructs are found on individual and societal levels, endorsed through the perpetuation of negative myths and stereotypes about people who are a gender and/or sexual minority, and lead to both subtle and blatant forms of discrimination (Woodford, Kulick, & Atteberry, 2015). It is important to note that bisexual people may experience additional minority stress complicated by marginality from both heterosexual and lesbian/gay communities (see Chapter 16).

Owing to cultural ideologies that perpetuate sexual/gender identity stigma, many GSM individuals hide their sexual/gender identity from others, and feel shame and other negative feelings toward themselves. The phenomenon of internalizing anti-gay attitudes and feeling resistance to accept and express one's sexual minority identity is referred to as "internalized homophobia" (Cabaj, Gorman, Pellicio, Ghindia, & Neisen, 2012). Similarly, the internalizing of cultural prejudices in a society that discriminates against transgender people, condones violence against them, and denies them basic civil rights is referred to as "internalized transphobia" (Keuroghlian, Reisner, White, & Weiss, 2015; Leslie, Perina, & Maqueda, 2012). The negative effects of heterosexism, homophobia, cisgenderism, and internalized homophobia/transphobia for GSM individuals might include the following (Cabaj et al., 2012):

- Self-blame for victimization
- Poor self-concept as a result of negative messages about GSM identities
- Anger directed inward leading to unhealthy behaviors such as substance use
- Feelings of inadequacy, hopelessness, and despair that negatively impact quality of life
- Self-victimization that acts as a barrier to psychological health and development

■ SUBSTANCE USE AS A MEANS OF COPING

As one of several marginalized communities in our society, GSM people often report feelings of isolation, fear, depression, distrust, and anger. Such negative experiences and perceptions place GSM individuals at a higher risk of using substances as a means of coping (Cabaj, 2014). According to the Center for Substance Abuse Treatment ([CSAT], 2012), gay men and lesbians have greater substance use disorders than their cisgender heterosexual counterparts. Furthermore, when compared to the cisgender heterosexual population, GSM individuals are more likely to use substances, have higher rates of moderate to severe substance use, and are more likely to continue substance use into later life (CSAT, 2012).

It is important to recognize that these potential behavioral outcomes result from prejudice and discrimination in society and are *not* a direct consequence of one's sexual orientation and/or gender identity. The process of forming a GSM identity can be a stressful and challenging process as it involves adopting a nontraditional sexual/gender identity, restructuring one's self-concept, and changing one's relationship with society (Reynolds & Hanjorgiris, 2000). GSM individuals may use substances to deal with such stress and the emotional pain associated with internalized homophobia/transphobia (Cabaj, 2014; Cabaj et al., 2012; Keuroghlian et al., 2015). Although substance use provides comfort at times, GSM individuals may experience continued and increased use and possible substance use disorders.

There is a growing body of research that addresses substance use by lesbians and gay men; less research exists on the substance use patterns specifically for bisexual and transgender individuals (who are typically collapsed into a broader GSM umbrella for analysis purposes). Studies on alcohol use have dominated the professional literature, with increasing attention to club drug and methamphetamine use by gay men since the early 1990s. Most studies and clinicians working with GSM people estimate an incidence of substance use of all types to be about 30%, with ranges of 28% to 35%, compared with 10% to 12% in the general population (Cabaj, 2014). There is a body of older research that showed consistent discrepant rates of substance use between the LGBT and the cisgender heterosexual community. For example, McKirnan and Peterson (1989) reported that alcohol problems for lesbians and gay men were greater than those for their cisgender heterosexual counterparts (23% and 8%, 23% and 16%, respectively). Furthermore, in this study, higher numbers of sexual minority individuals used cannabis (56%) and cocaine (23%) than the general population (20% and 9%, respectively). In the Trilogy Project (Skinner & Otis, 1996), higher rates of marijuana, inhalant, and alcohol use were documented for lesbians and gay men when compared to data from the National Household Survey on Drug Abuse (NHSDA). In particular, 87% of lesbians reported alcohol use compared to 64% of heterosexual women from the NHSDA study, and 84% of gay men used alcohol compared to 72% of the NHSDA heterosexual male participants. Sorenson and Roberts (1997) found similar results with 24% of their lesbian participants reporting that they drank two or more drinks per day. In addition, 15% of lesbians identified as alcoholics and 29% indicated that they had attended Alcoholics Anonymous meetings. In a related study, Amadio and Chung (2004) found that 24% of lesbians and bisexual women, and 25% of gay and bisexual men had at least a strong possibility of alcohol abuse (now referred to as "alcohol use disorder" in the *DSM-5*; American Psychiatric Association, 2013). In addition, 15% of lesbians and bisexual women and 11% of gay and bisexual men in the same study met Amadio and Chung's (2004) criteria for drug abuse. Research by Conron, Mimiaga, and Landers (2010) found differential rates of drinking, smoking, and drug use among heterosexual and sexual minority individuals. In particular, sexual minority individuals were more likely to report 30-day drug use and current and former smoking than heterosexual people; bisexual people were more likely than their hetersexual counterparts to report 30-day illicit drug use; and, bisexual women more often reported binge drinking and illict drug use than heterosexual women.

Although the findings of these studies demonstrate concerning levels of substance use in the sexual minority community, many of them have methodological limitations such as poor or absent control groups, non-representative samples, limited generalizability, and inconsistent sexual orientation terminology (Cabaj, 2014). Capturing precise incidence and prevalence rates of substance use in the LGBT community has been difficult due to a lack of reliable information on the size of the GSM population (CSAT, 2012) and other methodological concerns (see Chapter 1). Two of the most popular substance use national surveys—the National Household Survey on Drug Abuse and the Monitoring the Future Study—have not historically included sexual orientation or gender identity as demographic variables in the questionnaires; therefore, the findings from these surveys have not emphasized differences for the LGBT community (S. King, personal communication, July 11, 2016). Further, many empirical studies also either exclude or blend bisexual and/or transgender individuals into their studies; therefore, data specifically related to bisexual and transgender individuals is lacking.

There is increasing research on health and risk issues for transgender people. In the few studies that have been conducted specifically examining substance use in gender minority groups, transgender men and women have a significantly elevated prevalence of alcohol and illicit drug use compared with the general cisgender population (Keuroghlian et al., 2015), with rates as high as 60% (Cabaj, 2014). Transgender women experiencing high levels of enacted stigma (i.e., psychological or physical gender abuse) are three to four times as likely to use alcohol, marijuana, or cocaine and eight times as likely to use drugs overall (Nuttbrock et al., 2014). Substance use among transgender adults is associated with demographic, gender-related, mental health, and societal risk factors that correlate to substance use such as depression and suicidality, limited access to health care, sexual situations where HIV infection may be transmitted, and violence and victimization (Keuroghlian et al., 2015). The first major study on victimization against transgender people in the United States found that 60% of transgender people have experienced some form of harassment and/or violence throughout their lives, and 37% have experienced some form of economic discrimination (Lombardi, Wilchins, Priesing, & Malouf, 2002). Transgender individuals are twice as likely to be unemployed as their cisgender counterparts owing to stigma and discrimination in the workplace (Keuroghlian et al., 2015). Transgender individuals who are unable to "pass" (i.e., to be socially affirmed as the gender with which they identify) may be particularly vulnerable to discrimination and victimization (Keuroghlian et al., 2015). Transgender people also have had negative experiences with medical and mental health services (including finding competent and transgender-sensitive health care providers and getting insurance coverage) based on institutional bias (Leslie et al., 2012). As such, transgender people can be distrustful of health care professionals and treatment recommendations (Leslie et al., 2012). The psychological stress of health care access disparities experienced by transgender individuals might exacerbate already compromised mental health, including substance use as a coping strategy (Keuroghlian et al., 2015), and the lack of available affirming care may prevent gender minority individuals from seeking and/or receiving needed substance use care.

Both the *Healthy People 2010 Companion Document for Lesbian, Gay, Bisexual, and Transgender (LGBT) Health* and the more recent Institute of Medicine's 2011 report on the health of GSM groups noted the concern of substance use among the LGBT community. In these reports, GSM individuals perceived themselves to be at an increased risk for substance use disorders, have an increased need for treatment, and face barriers to substance use treatment (Gay and Lesbian Medical Association, 2001; Institute of Medicine, 2011). Although alcohol and various types of drugs are used, certain drugs appear to be used more often by members of the LGBT community. For example, Cabaj & Smith (2012) discussed that gay men were significantly more likely to have used marijuana, stimulants, sedatives, cocaine, and party drugs when compared with men in the cisgender, heterosexual population. The use of methamphetamines is an epidemic for gay men in some parts of the United States, with rates as high as 25% to 29% (10 times higher than the general population; Balsam, Molina, & Lehavot, 2013; Cabaj & Smith, 2012). Lesbians, on the other hand, exhibit greater diversity in their substance use with no single clear pattern of use behavior within the group (Finnegan, 2012). However, there are stark differences between sexual minority women and heterosexual women with regard to alcohol use: Sexual minority women use alcohol more frequently, consume higher quantities, and report more alcohol-related problems (Balsam et al., 2013).

GSM youth are also at higher risk for substance use than cisgender heterosexual youth (Goldbach & Holleran Steiker, 2011). In a study by Kecojevic et al. (2012), GSM youth not only started misusing prescription drugs at earlier ages than their cisgender heterosexual counterparts, but their GSM identity was also correlated with earlier use of opioids and tranquilizers. There is limited information on substance use rates for GSM youth as well as for assessment, prevention, and treatment services. What the professional literature does emphasize is that although GSM youth and cisgender heterosexual youth face similar developmental tasks, GSM youth face additional challenges in learning how to live in a society with a stigmatized identity (Ryan & Hunter, 2012). Furthermore, Ryan and Hunter (2012) underscore the stress associated with prejudice and discrimination based on one's sexual/gender identity that puts GSM youth at an increased risk for not only substance use, but also psychological distress, homelessness (e.g., teens either run away or are thrown out of their family homes), unprotected sexual activity, and suicide.

One of the most central experiences for GSM people is the process of coming out, which is a lifelong process of developing and disclosing an identity as a GSM person and moving toward self-acceptance (Balsam et al., 2013; Cass, 1979). A series of milestones including awareness of same-gender attractions/transgender identity, negative feelings toward both GSM people as well as heterosexual people, self-identification as a gender and/or sexual minority, disclosure of gender and/or sexual identity to others, engaging in same-gender sexual exploration or transgender expression exploration, and entering into same-gender relationships or transitioning in public daily life are part of the coming out process and GSM identity development (Balsam et al., 2013).

Coming to terms with one's sexual/gender identity can be a challenging time, particularly for youth (Ryan & Hunter, 2012). The reasons that people move through the coming out process, or fail to move, are very complex, understudied, and beyond the scope of this chapter. There is, however, an elevated risk of substance use among GSM adolescents, which is a consequence of the psychosocial stressors associated with coming out as GSM, including gender nonconformity, victimization, lack of support, family problems, suicide attempts by acquaintances, homelessness, substance use, and psychiatric disorders (Suicide Prevention Resource Center, 2008). GSM youth may be at particular risk of using substances to numb feelings associated with negative experiences with the coming out process (Beemyn & Rankin, 2011; Ryan & Hunter, 2012).

■ RISK FACTORS

Reasons for the prevalence of substance use and other mental health disparities among GSM individuals remain underinvestigated (Flentje, Bacca, & Cochran, 2015; Kecojevic et al., 2012). There are numerous factors that place GSM individuals at higher risk of substance use disorders. Cabaj (2014) contextualized current thinking within three categories of contributing factors: biological, social, and psychological. A genetic or biological link that explains higher substance use among GSM people is unlikely. Social and psychological factors, however, are far more likely to contribute to substance use in this community. CSAT (2012) outlined such factors, as supported by Cabaj (2014) and Balsam et al. (2013), to include:

- *Prejudice, discrimination, and victimization*: Societies or cultures in transition have higher rates of substance use; this applies to GSM people who face societal stress from factors such as general mistreatment and anti-gay and/or transphobic violence (physical and sexual abuse); struggles over legally recognized relationships/marriage and related policies and privileges; and job protection. The effects can result in feelings of isolation, fear, depression, anxiety, and anger.
- *Cultural issues*: GSM individuals from an ethnic or racial minority background may face additional challenges coping with their sexual orientation and/or gender identity due to cultural traditions, values, and norms.
- *Legal issues*: Disclosure of one's sexual orientation and/or gender identity can lead to employment problems, denial of housing, and loss of custody of one's children.
- *Accessibility*: Due to homophobia/transphobia and discrimination, some GSM individuals may find it difficult or uncomfortable to access treatment services.
- *Families of origin*: The family of origin's response to one's disclosure of a gender and/or sexual minority identity can have devastating effects on an individual. Unresolved issues with the family of origin can act as emotional triggers to both initial use of substances and relapses.
- *Health issues*: GSM individuals may face a variety of additional health problems such as co-occurring mental health disorders, suicidality, PTSD, HIV/AIDS, sexually transmitted infections, hepatitis, and other injuries that increase the risk of substance use as a means of self-medicating.
- *Gay bars*: Discrimination has often led GSM people to create their own "social fabric" (Cabaj, 2014, p. 710) including neighborhoods that feel safer, more welcoming, and more comfortable in which to live. Common social

outlets that are available to GSM people include bars or organized parties/clubs where alcohol and drugs often play a prominent role. There is a recent increase in alcohol- and drug-free alternatives such as coffeehouses, bookstores, and substance-free clubs, yet they are still limited.

COMING OUT AND INTERNALIZED HOMOPHOBIA/TRANSPHOBIA

Many GSM people have internalized homophobia/transphobia as a result of living in a society that both blatantly and subtly denies nontraditional forms of sexual/gender identities. Based on sexual/gender minority stress theories, substance use disorders among GSM people are increasingly viewed as consequences of this internalized and enacted homophobia/transphobia (Keuroghlian et al., 2015; Weber, 2008). Substance use disconnects GSM people from feelings of shame and anxiety that might result from internalized homophobia/transphobia, while fostering feelings of acceptance, social comfort, and decreased inhibition to reveal feelings and behaviors long suppressed or denied (Cabaj, 2014; Ryan & Hunter, 2012; Weber, 2008).

The coming out experience for GSM people might be delayed or difficult to process owing to how one copes with internalized homophobia. Depending on how supportive the individual's environment may be, a GSM individual may believe that coming out will lead only to loneliness, rejection, sadness, and isolation when, in fact, coming out may be cathartic, rewarding, exciting, and fulfilling (Weber, 2008; Weber, Rose, & Rubinstein, 2011). Substance use might begin in adolescence when GSM individuals become more aware of their differences based on sexual/gender identity; alcohol and drugs might provide comfort to these GSM adolescents as they begin to explore their identities or might numb the discomfort of conflicts of coming out (e.g., family rejection; lack of safety in surroundings; Ryan & Hunter, 2012). Substance use might also allow for the release of suppressed feelings and behaviors, and as such, many first sexual experiences involve some degree of alcohol or drug use (Cabaj, 2014). Cabaj (2014) further posits that this powerful behavioral relationship—that is, the pleasure and release of substance use and the pleasure and release of sexual activity—is a challenge to change or disconnect later in life. The very nature of substance use can exacerbate the feelings and behaviors correlated with internalized homophobia such as depression, self-loathing, anxiety, self-denial, isolation, suicidality, guilt, anger, and hopelessness (Cabaj, 2014). Thus, treatment for substance use can be complicated because the substance use has interrupted the coming out process, and accepting one's sexual/gender identity may be crucial in successfully treating substance use disorders.

INCLUSIVE AND EFFECTIVE TREATMENT

Although GSM individuals are seeking substance use treatment at higher rates than their cisgender heterosexual counterparts (Flentje, Livingston, Roley, & Sorenson, 2015), many of their treatment needs are not being met (Senreich, 2010).

There are special treatment concerns for GSM people including recovery from substance use and the consequences of homophobia/transphobia, and usually require self-acceptance as a gender and/or sexual minority (Cabaj, 2014). In fact, it is currently unclear whether substance use treatment programs and providers are sufficiently aware and knowledgeable of the specific mental and physical health needs of GSM clients (Flentje, et al., 2015). An unsafe treatment environment including GSM individuals being the targets of homophobic/transphobic comments from their peers and helping professionals who lack the awareness, education, and training to treat GSM people is a major concern as it impacts the provision of appropriate services. Without feelings of safety in the treatment environment, GSM people might not explore critical components of their substance use. It is important for a counselor to identify that internalized homophobia/transphobia is the result of living in an anti-LGBT culture, and to encourage the use of counseling and self-help groups (e.g., Alcoholics Anonymous) as a means of expressing and externalizing negative feelings toward self (particularly if such groups are either GSM-specific or delivered by a trained, culturally competent facilitator). Further, discussing experiences with prejudice, discrimination, and victimization is crucial in treatment. Focusing on social support is also important as GSM people might have limited sources of support who relate to them as a GSM person; therefore, giving up fellow substance-using peers and avoiding LGBT social outlets might be particularly difficult (Cabaj, 2014).

Assessment and Treatment Planning

Assessment of GSM people who present for behavioral health services should consistently screen for symptoms of substance use disorders in an affirming, nonjudgmental manner. More in-depth assessment as well as subsequent treatment plans should address the following elements (adapted from Cabaj, 2014):

- Age and adjustment to that age in the life cycle (including any developmental milestones)
- The degree and impact of internalized homophobia
- The stage in the coming out process and the experience of coming out
- Strength of support network (particularly a sober one)
- Current relationship status and history of past relationships
- Relationships with family of origin as well as family of creation
- Degree of comfort with sexual/gender identity, and expression of sexual feelings and gender-affirming behaviors
- Vocational/educational/socioeconomic status
- Current and past health factors

Issues related to sexual/gender identity should be discussed in individual, partner, family, and group counseling, when appropriate. Affirmative counseling groups specific to GSM people are useful in that they create a safe environment where clients can freely discuss their experiences as GSM individuals, and how these experiences have affected their substance abuse behaviors. Although the issues discussed in such groups may have little or nothing to do with sexual/gender identity, the groups still provide a sense of acceptance and support that may provide corrective experiences for GSM clients. Gender-specific groups where lesbians/bisexual women, gay/bisexual males, transgender men, and transgender women can share counseling concerns relevant to their gender and sexual identity that may otherwise not occur in gender-mixed groups may also be helpful.

Gender Minority-Specific Treatment

Substance use treatment for a gender minority client is similar to that for other individuals because it focuses primarily on stopping the substance use that interferes with the well-being of the client. The way that it differs in this community is the need for the treatment to address the clients' feelings about their gender identity and the potential impact transphobia has had on their lives and on their recovery. The client may be harboring the effects of society's negative attitudes which often result in painful and uncomfortable feelings that the client may want to self-medicate (Leslie et al., 2012). Leslie et al. (2012) further underscore that clinicians should have a solid and reliable referral network including helping professionals who are culturally sensitive, and who have a good understanding of the gender minority population and its needs so they can provide effective services.

Using preferred language is critical to an effective helping relationship with a gender minority client. It is important to call the client by their preferred name and always use the pronoun that the client has specified. Counselors should ask a self-identified gender minority client by what name they prefer to be called. Using gender-neutral language until the client says otherwise is a great way to avoid making assumptions. This sensitive use of language can be an important sign of respect and acknowledgment, and help to create a connective and healing environment. Gender minority clients may have additional concerns with which they are dealing, such as lack of family and social supports, isolation, poor self-esteem, and people close to them struggling with transphobia (Leslie et al., 2012). At times, these concerns create intense challenges especially when these individuals are attempting to change their substance use patterns and coping mechanisms that may have worked for them in the past. It is important that counselors avoid the common pitfall of focusing on gender issues as the assumed root cause of the substance use and focus instead on the broader context of the person.

To ensure that the substance use treatment is inclusive and supportive of the needs of transgender clients, some changes may need to be made. For example, programs that use observers when administering urine toxicology testing need to consider the client's comfort and ask which gender observer is preferred. Both inpatient and outpatient treatment facilities should designate a non-gender–specific toilet (and shower when appropriate) to meet the needs of gender minority clients. Intake forms are great opportunities to convey cultural sensitivity and inclusivity by using gender-neutral language and assessing all domains of sexual and gender identity (Levounis, Drescher, & Barber, 2012). Documentation of sexual/gender identity should encourage truthful disclosure by providing many different options from which to choose, and an "other" section where an individual can provide information that might not be listed.

Hormone therapy is also often overlooked or misunderstood by helping professionals (Leslie et al., 2012). Many gender minority clients may be on hormone therapies when entering treatment and should never be asked to discontinue hormone treatment. Hormone treatment is a standard and accepted medical intervention and clients should be encouraged to maintain regular, legally prescribed hormonal treatment under medical supervision without interruption. Helping professionals should be aware that some hormones can impact mood, and some injectable hormones could act as a relapse trigger for those clients in early recovery (Leslie et al., 2012).

Most major metropolitan communities offer a range of substance use treatment centers that provide services for GSM clients. Recovery.org is a great resource for finding appropriate support groups and treatment centers for the LGBT community. The mission at Recovery.org is to connect people and their families with information and resources to help them recover from substance use and behavioral disorders. After accessing the website, readers are prompted to enter the zip code of the location for which they would like to find treatment centers. Once treatment centers are identified, the reader is able to determine the appropriateness for GSM clients (e.g., "exceptionally LGBT friendly" might be listed under "Center Details"). Through its resources and conferences, the National Association of Lesbian and Gay Addictions Professionals (NALGAP) offers addiction professionals, individuals in recovery, and interested others information about training, networking, advocacy, and support related to prevention and treatment of alcoholism, substance use, and other addictions in LGBT communities. The Center for Substance Abuse Treatment (CSAT) of the Substance Abuse and Mental Health Services Administration (SAMHSA) is another important resource to consider when embarking upon substance use treatment work and seeking out best practices. Counselors should be familiar with community resources, and make this information visible and accessible to all clients within the treatment centers.

■ CONCLUSION

GSM individuals experience minority stress as a result of living in a society that has been historically exclusive of people who identify outside of traditional sexual and gender identities. They also use substances at disproportionately higher rates when compared to their heterosexual counterparts. The relationship between minority stress and substance use has been demonstrated in professional literature. As such, professionals who work in settings where GSM individuals might seek substance use treatment services need to be culturally competent and aware of the unique issues that GSM people experience. Substance use treatment providers, counselors, therapists, administrators, and facility directors who are aware, knowledgeable, and skilled to work with GSM individuals will help them receive effective, ethical, and informed care. GSM individuals who use substances are likely experiencing stress related to their stigmatized identities, and as such, treatment should focus on general issues impacting all clients in substance use treatment as well as specific issues related to GSM identities. The most important thing to remember when treating any client, especially clients who belong to marginalized communities, is not to make assumptions. Building rapport and creating a safe environment where GSM individuals can express their genuine selves will set the stage for healthy exploration of substance use concerns. Providing inclusive and culturally sensitive care will help GSM clients with substance use concerns engage in the treatment they need and deserve. With these care provisions in place, outcomes will improve and providers will reach a previously underserved population (CSAT, 2012).

CASE STUDY

You are a clinician at a residential substance use treatment facility and have just completed an intake interview with a new client, Dotty. Soon after Dotty began wearing gender-affirming clothing at the age of 6 or 7, she was caught by her mother and physically disciplined by her father. She became cautious with wearing feminine clothing thereafter and lived with fear that she would be caught by her parents (which she was, and as a result experienced additional painful psychological and physical punishment). After these experiences, Dotty learned to hide her desires to live her life openly as a woman and conformed to her environmental expectations to express and behave like a man. She "passed" as a man for more than a decade until she started seeking out venues where she could wear gender-affirming clothing without the fear of getting caught. Her alcohol and drug use increased around this time, as it allowed her to more easily express her true gender identity and engage in intimate relationships. Her use of alcohol and cocaine increased dramatically in her early 20s; she was using it at private parties and clubs and then would continue for days in her own apartment. She reveals to you that she has been in substance use outpatient treatment before and described a very bad experience. For example, the staff at Dotty's previous treatment center refused to address her as a woman and referred to her by her assigned male birth name. Further, other clients sexually and verbally harassed her based on gender identity and gender expression. She felt very unsafe during her first treatment experience and has carried over some of those fears and overall discomfort to your counseling relationship. At her intake interview in a substance use residential treatment center, Dotty disclosed that her experiences with her parents growing up made it difficult to accept herself, and she was using drugs "to go numb." Dotty disclosed she has felt depressed for years and she knows that her substance use behaviors are a form of slow suicide. Dotty has begun hormone therapy and is preparing for gender confirmation surgery. She is also in a relationship with a cisgender man who accepts her transgender identity yet gave her an ultimatum to seek treatment for her substance use or he would end the relationship. Dotty is also in job jeopardy as her use has impacted her ability to manage a retail clothing shop.

QUESTIONS FOR REFLECTION

1. **How would you protect Dotty and ensure that her negative experiences in her first treatment episode do not reoccur? Keep in mind that this is a residential treatment center where Dotty will be staying for a minimum of 28 days.**

Key Points to Consider

- Accept her into your program and house her as you would other women in your program
- Dorm-type rooms are acceptable; single private room is also acceptable if available
- Designate appropriate time when she can use group showers; if individual showers are available for women, this would be preferable
- Insist that all staff refer to her and treat her as a woman
- Assist in finding outside supportive resources for transgender individuals such as a transgender inclusive self-help group or transgender community center
- Address any client issues as you normally would, through individual counseling
- Engage in staff and client education about transgender individuals, as needed

2. **Social support is very important as an individual enters into and maintains recovery from substance use. Based on the vignette, how would you, as Dotty's counselor, help her utilize and strengthen her support network?**

Key Points to Consider

- Discuss any family involvement with Dotty to determine appropriateness for family therapy (based on abuse, family might or might not participate in family education); invite partner for couples counseling
- Consider additional supports such as friends (e.g., work with Dotty to identify these individuals)
- Help connect Dotty to adjunct supports such as AA/NA—be sure to research and identify a home group where GSM individuals, especially transgender people, attend and are embraced
- Identify a transgender sponsor/main support/mentor who can support Dotty in her early recovery
- Recommend immediately, based on Dotty's mental health history, a psychiatric evaluation with a culturally sensitive psychiatrist who is skilled in working with gender minority clients
- Include individual counseling with a sensitive and skilled clinician; consider group counseling that provides a safe space for Dotty where hostility and cisgenderism are not permitted
- Focus treatment goals on relapse prevention (triggers to use and development of coping strategies); mental health (especially depression); family relationships (history of physical and emotional abuse); social support; vocational and educational strengths (and current job jeopardy due to use); and her transition (particularly internalized transphobia) as it relates to her substance use (remember to not overemphasize gender identity when it is not relevant)

Best practices for counselors working with Dotty (adapted from Leslie et al., 2012):

Do …

- Use proper pronouns and names based on Dotty's self-identity and preference.
- Receive clinical supervision if you have issues or feelings about working with Dotty.

- Require training on transgender competence for all staff.
- Allow Dotty to continue the use of hormones as they are prescribed. If Dotty is using "street" hormones, get immediate medical care.
- Allow Dotty to use bathrooms and showers based on her gender self-identity.
- Require that all clients and staff maintain a safe environment for all transgender clients.
- Post a nondiscrimination policy in the waiting room that explicitly includes sexual orientation and gender identity.

Don't ...

- Call Dotty "he" or "him"; rather, refer to Dotty's preferred pronoun.
- Project your transphobia onto Dotty or share transphobic comments with other staff or clients.
- Make Dotty choose between hormones and treatment/recovery.
- Expect that Dotty educate the staff.
- Make assumptions about Dotty's sexual orientation based on her gender identity and/or the gender of her current partner.
- Make Dotty who is living as female use male facilities.
- Allow staff or clients to make transphobic comments or put Dotty and transgender clients at risk for physical or sexual abuse or harassment.

▉ REFERENCES

Amadio, D. M., & Chung, B. Y. (2004). Internalized homophobia and substance use among lesbian, gay, and bisexual persons. *Journal of Gay and Lesbian Social Services, 17*(1), 83–101. doi:10.1300/J041v17n01_06

American Psychiatric Association. (2013). *Diagnostic and statistical manual of mental disorders* (5th ed.). Arlington, VA: American Psychiatric Publishing.

Balsam, K. F., Molina, Y., & Lehavot, K. (2013). Alcohol and drug use in lesbian, gay, bisexual, and transgender (LGBT) youth and young adults. In P. M. Miller (Ed.), *Principles of addiction* (pp. 563–573). San Diego, CA: Elsevier. doi:10.1016/B978-0-12-398336-7.00058-9

Beemyn, G., & Rankin, S. (2011). *The lives of transgender people.* New York, NY: Columbia University Press.

Cabaj, R. P. (2014). Substance use issues among gay, lesbian, bisexual, and transgender people. In M. Galanter, H. D. Kleber, & K. T. Brady (Eds.), *Textbook of substance abuse treatment* (pp. 707–721). Washington, DC: American Psychiatric Association.

Cabaj, R. P., Gorman, M., Pellicio, W. J., Ghindia, D. J. & Neisen, J. H. (2012). An overview for providers treating LGBT clients. In *A Provider's Introduction to Substance Abuse Treatment for Lesbian, Gay, Bisexual, and Transgender Individuals* (pp. 1–14). HHS Publication No. (SMA) 12-4104. Rockville, MD: U.S. Department of Health and Human Services.

Cabaj, R. P. & Smith, M. (2012). Overview of treatment approaches, modalities, and issues of accessibility in the continuum of care. In *A provider's introduction to substance abuse treatment for lesbian, gay, bisexual, and transgender individuals* (pp. 49–60). HHS Publication No. (SMA) 12-4104. Rockville, MD: U.S. Department of Health and Human Services.

Cass, V. C. (1979). Homosexual identity formation: A theoretical model. *Journal of Homosexuality, 4*(3), 219–235.

Center for Substance Abuse Treatment. (2012). *A provider's introduction to substance abuse treatment for lesbian, gay, bisexual, and transgender individuals.* HHS Publication No. (SMA) 12-4104. Rockville, MD: U.S. Department of Health and Human Services.

Conron, K. J., Mimiaga, M. J., & Landers, S. J. (2010). A population-based study of sexual orientation identity and gender differences in adult health. *American Journal of Public Health, 100*(10), 1953–1960. doi:10.2105/AJPH.2009.174169

Davies, D. (1996). Homophobia and heterosexism. In D. Davies & C. Neal (Eds.), *Pink therapy: A guide for counselors and therapists working with lesbian, gay, and bisexual clients* (pp. 41–65). Buckingham, UK: Open University Press.

Finnegan, D. G. (2012). Clinical issues with lesbians. In *A provider's introduction to substance abuse treatment for lesbian, gay, bisexual, and transgender individuals* (pp. 75–79). HHS Pub. No. (SMA) 12-4104. Rockville, MD: U.S. Department of Health and Human Services.

Flentje, A., Bacca, C. L., & Cochran, B. N. (2015). Missing data in substance abuse research? Researcher's reporting practices of sexual orientation and gender identity. *Drug and Alcohol Dependence, 147*, 280–284. doi:10.1016/j.drugalcdep.2014.11.012

Flentje, A., Livingston, N. A., Roley, J. & Sorenson, J. L. (2015). Mental and physical health needs of lesbian, gay, and bisexual clients in substance abuse treatment. *Journal of Substance Abuse Treatment, 58*, 78–83. doi:10.1016/j.jsat.2015.06.022

Frost, D. M., Lehavot, K., & Meyer, I. H. (2015). Minority stress and physical health among sexual minority individuals. *Journal of Behavioral Medicine, 38*(1), 1–8. doi:10.1007/s10865-013-9523-8

Gay and Lesbian Medical Association (2001). *Healthy People 2010: Companion document for lesbian, gay, bisexual, transgender (LGBT) health.* San Francisco, CA: Author.

Goldbach, J. T., & Holleran Steiker, L. K. (2011). An examination of cultural adaptations performed by LGBT-identified youths to a culturally grounded, evidenced-based substance abuse intervention. *Journal of Gay & Lesbian Social Services, 23*(2), 188–203. doi:10.1080/10538720.2011.560135

Grossman, A. H. (1997). Growing up with a "spoiled identity": Lesbian, gay and bisexual youth at risk. *Journal of Gay and Lesbian Social Services, 6*(3), 45–60. doi:10.1300/J041v06n03_03

Herek, G. M. (2004). Beyond "homophobia": Thinking about sexual stigma and prejudice in the twenty-first century. *Sexuality Research and Social Policy, 1*(2), 6–24. doi:10.1525/srsp.2004.1.2.6

Herek, G. M. (2015). Beyond "homophobia": Thinking more clearly about stigma, prejudice, and sexual orientation. *American Journal of Orthopsychiatry, 85*, S29–S37. doi:10.1037/ort0000092

Institute of Medicine. (2011). *The health of lesbian, gay, bisexual, and transgender people: Building a foundation for better understanding.* Washington, DC: National Academies Press.

Kecojevic, A., Wong, C. F., Schrager, S. M., Silva, K., Jackson Bloom, J., Iverson, E., & Lankenau, S. E. (2012). Initiation into prescription drug misuse: Differences between lesbian, gay, bisexual, transgender (LGBT) and heterosexual high-risk young adults in Los Angeles and New York. *Addictive Behaviors, 37*(11), 1289–1293. doi:10.1016/j.addbeh.2012.06.006

Keuroghlian, A. S., Reisner, S. L., White, J. M., & Weiss, R. D. (2015). Substance use and treatment of substance use disorders in a community sample of transgender adults. *Drug and Alcohol Dependence, 152*, 139–146. doi:10.1016/j.drugalcdep.2015.04.008

Lennon, E. & Mistler, B. J. (2014). Cisgenderism. *Transgender Studies Quarterly, 1*(1–2), 63–64. doi:10.1215/23289252-2399623

Leslie, D. R., Perina, B. A., & Maqueda, M. C. (2012). Clinical issues with transgender individuals. In *A provider's introduction to substance abuse treatment for lesbian, gay, bisexual, and transgender individuals* (pp. 93–100). HHS Pub. No. (SMA) 12-4104. Rockville, MD: U.S. Department of Health and Human Services.

Levounis P., Drescher, J., & Barber, M. D. (2012). *The LGBT casebook.* Washington, DC: American Psychiatric Publishing.

Lombardi, E. L., Wilchins, R. A., Priesing, D. & Malouf, D. (2002). Gender violence: Transgender experiences with violence and discrimination. *Journal of Homosexuality, 42*(1), 89–101.

McKirnan, D. J., & Peterson, P. L. (1989). Alcohol use and drug use among homosexual men and women: Epidemiology and population characteristics. *Addictive Behaviors, 14*(5), 545–553.

Meyer, I. H. (1995). Minority stress and mental health in gay men. *Journal of Health and Social Behavior, 36*(1), 38–56.

Meyer, I. H. (2003a). Prejudice, social stress, and mental health in lesbian, gay, and bisexual populations: Conceptual issues and research evidence. *Psychological Bulletin, 129*(5), 674–697.

Meyer, I. H. (2003b). Prejudice as stress: Conceptual and measurement problems. *American Journal of Public Health, 93*(2), 262–265.

Meyer, I. H. (2015). Resilience in the study of minority stress and health of sexual and gender minorities. *Psychology of Sexual Orientation and Gender Diversity, 2*(3), 209–213. doi:10.1037/sgd0000132

Mustanski, B. & Liu, R. T. (2013). A longitudinal study of predictors of suicide attempts among lesbian, gay, bisexual and transgender youth. *Archives in Sexual Behavior, 42*(3), 437–448. doi:10.1007/s10508-012-0013-9

Nuttbrock, L., Bockting, W., Rosenblum, A., Hwahng, S., Mason, M., Macri, M., & Becker, J. (2014). Gender abuse, depressive symptoms, and substance use among transgender women: A 3-year prospective study. *American Journal of Public Health, 104*(11), 2199–2206. doi:10.2105/AJPH.2014.302106

Reynolds, A. L., & Hanjorgiris, W. F. (2000). Coming out: Lesbian, gay, and bisexual identity development. In R. M. Perez, K. A., DeBord, & K. J. Bieschke (Eds.), *Handbook of counseling and psychotherapy with lesbian, gay, and bisexual clients* (pp. 35–55). Washington, DC: American Psychological Association.

Ryan, C., & Hunter, J. (2012). Clinical issues with youth. In *A provider's introduction to substance abuse treatment for lesbian, gay, bisexual, and transgender individuals* (pp. 101–115). HHS Pub. No. (SMA) 12-4104. Rockville, MD: U.S. Department of Health and Human Services.

Senreich, E. (2010). Are specialized LGBT program components helpful for gay and bisexual men in substance abuse treatment? *Substance Use & Misuse, 45*(7–8), 1077–1096. doi:10.3109/10826080903483855

Skinner, W. F., & Otis, M. D. (1996). Drug and alcohol use among lesbian and gay people in a southern U.S. sample: Epidemiological, comparative, and methodological findings from the Trilogy Project. *Journal of Homosexuality, 30*(3), 59–92.

Sorenson, L., & Roberts, S. J. (1997). Lesbian uses of and satisfaction with mental health services: Results from the Boston Lesbian Health Project. *Journal of Homosexuality, 33*(1), 35–49.

Suicide Prevention Resource Center. (2008). *Suicide risk and prevention for lesbian, gay, bisexual, and transgender youth.* Newton, MA: Education Development Center.

Weber, G. (2008). Using to numb the pain: Substance use and abuse among lesbian, gay, and bisexual individuals. *Journal of Mental Health Counseling, 30,* 31–48. doi:10.17744/mehc.30.1.2585916185422570

Weber, G., Rose, S., & Rubinstein, R. (2011). The impact of internalized homophobia on outness for lesbian, gay, and bisexual individuals. *The Professional Counselor: Research and Practice, 1*(3), 163–175.

Woodford, M.R., Kulick, A., & Atteberry, B. (2015). Protective factors, campus climate, and health outcomes among sexual minority college students. *Journal of Diversity in Higher Education, 8*(2), 73–87. doi:10.1037/a0038552

Woodford, M. R., Kulick, A., Sinco, B. R., & Hong, J. S. (2014). Contemporary heterosexism on campus and psychological distress among LGBQ students: The mediating role of self-acceptance. *American Journal of Orthopsychiatry, 84*(5), 519–529. doi:10.1037/ort0000015

CHAPTER **13**

HIV and Other Sexually Transmitted Infections Within the Gender and Sexual Minority Community

Keith J. Horvath, Nicholas Yared, Sara Lammert,
Alan Lifson, and Shalini Kulasingam

AIDS emerged in Los Angeles in 1981 after five gay men in Los Angeles were hospitalized for a rare form of pneumonia, called *pneumocystis carinii* (Centers for Disease Control and Prevention [CDC], 1981). By the time the first *Morbidity and Mortality Weekly Report* (MMWR) was published, three of the five men had died and other rare conditions (e.g., Kaposi's sarcoma) were emerging among gay men in large U.S. cities. Rates of sexually transmitted infections (STIs), such as syphilis and gonorrhea, in the gay community were known to be high during the 1970s and early 1980s (Weller, as cited in de Vries, 2014). However, no one had seen this constellation of symptoms before in men as young as those who were hospitalized. By August 1981, 108 cases of AIDS had emerged, including 43 deaths (Koop, 2011). In the years to follow, foundational epidemiologic, medical, and biologic studies proved that AIDS was the result of the human immunodeficiency virus, or HIV.

In the 35 years since these initial reports, persons in the lesbian, gay, bisexual, and transgender (LGBT) community continue to be disproportionately affected by HIV/AIDS and other STIs in many regions of the world (UNAIDS, 2016). An

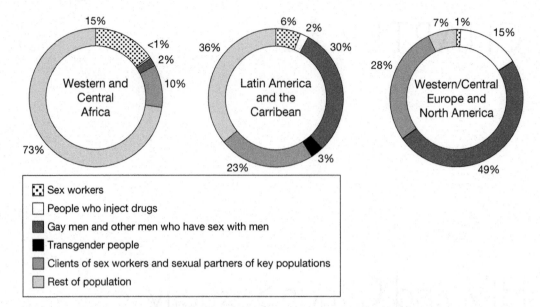

FIGURE 13.1: Distribution of new HIV infections among populations, by selected regions, 2014.
Source: UNAIDS special analysis (2016; selected regions reproduced with permission).

estimated 36.7 million persons are living with HIV worldwide (World Health Organization, 2015), with regional variation in the proportion of estimated new infections that are attributed to sexual minority men (UNAIDS, 2016). As shown in Figure 13.1, while only 2% of new HIV infections in 2014 were attributed to sexual minority men in Western and Central Africa, 30% of infections in Latin America and the Caribbean and 49% of infections in Western/Central Europe and North America were among sexual minority men (UNAIDS, 2016). The number of new infections globally has declined by 35% since 2000, complemented by increasing access to antiretroviral therapy (ART; Friedland, 2016). However, a resurgent epidemic has occurred among sexual minority men in North America and Western Europe. Surveillance data documenting the prevalence and incidence of HIV among sexual minority men in countries with a generalized HIV epidemic are lacking (Baral, Grosso, Holland, & Papworth, 2014), making it difficult to understand the impact of HIV within LGBT communities and, ultimately, to reach prevention and treatment goals (Beyrer et al., 2016).

The purpose of this chapter is to provide an overview of the HIV and STI epidemic among gender and sexual minority (GSM) populations. The remainder of the chapter is devoted primarily to reviewing risk factors associated with HIV acquisition and STI infection, followed by a discussion of recent interventions to address HIV and STI disparities in LGBT communities. Risk factors for HIV and STIs are organized by individual, partner, network, community, and structural levels. It should be acknowledged that while we have attempted to separate risk factors at different levels for clarity, many risk factors (e.g., race/ethnicity) operate at multiple levels (e.g., individual and network level). Finally, a review of recent interventions is organized by biomedical, behavioral, and societal interventions.

It should be noted that a number of decisions had to be made as to what should be emphasized in this chapter. First, HIV infection is prioritized in what follows. HIV has the most severe consequences compared to other STIs and there has yet to be a successful vaccine or cure. In comparison, while hepatitis C infection may lead to liver cirrhosis and ultimately liver failure, this typically occurs over many decades, and new treatments are available with very high demonstrated cure rates. Moreover, many of the risk factors associated with HIV transmission apply to other STIs. Second, this chapter focuses on the epidemic of HIV in LGBT communities in the United States. Although HIV and STIs are prevalent in global communities that are often overburdened and poorly resourced, the highest burden of HIV among GSM populations is found in North America and Western Europe (UNAIDS, 2016). Therefore, given the intended audience for this book and the focus on LGBT communities, we have chosen to focus primarily on the U.S. epidemic. Third, given the massive amount of research and policy literature that has accumulated since the beginning of the HIV epidemic, GSM groups most vulnerable to HIV and other STIs are highlighted. As such, the HIV and STI epidemics in sexual minority men and transgender women are a particular focus of this chapter, with some ancillary discussion of HIV and STIs in other GSM groups. Fourth, to be consistent with terminology throughout the rest of this book, the term *sexual minority men* is used; however, the vast majority of literature regarding HIV and other STIs uses the term *men who have sex with men*, or *MSM*, to be inclusive of individuals who engage in same-sex sexual activity but do not identify as a member of a sexual minority group. For the purposes of this chapter, we include all cisgender men who have sex with men in the umbrella term of *sexual minority men*. Similarly, we include all cisgender women who have sex with women in the umbrella term of *sexual minority women*. We also acknowledge that transgender men and women can have any of a number of sexual orientations; however, much HIV prevention research focused on transgender women does not assess (or report) sexual orientation of its transgender participants. We have elected to use the term *transgender women who have sex with men* or *transgender men who have sex with men* only when the sexual orientation of transgender participants was adequately assessed in the study described; otherwise, we use the term *transgender men* or *transgender women* as appropriate (but acknowledge that this is a limitation of the current literature). Further, we fully affirm the gender identity of all transgender individuals and distinguish, for instance, between sexual minority men and transgender men who have sex with men, only so that it is clear when gender minority status was a part of the study being discussed. Finally, recent advances in HIV and STI research, prevention, and treatment are emphasized over older discoveries. That said, it is critical to acknowledge the previous groundbreaking contributions made by researchers, community agencies, activists, and policy makers. Indeed, it is only through the dedication and efforts of countless persons to address HIV and STIs within LGBT communities that we have radically altered the prevention and treatment landscape, and improved the lives of those infected and affected.

■ OVERVIEW OF THE U.S. HIV EPIDEMIC

At the end of 2013, it was estimated that just under 1 million (950,811) adults and adolescents were living with diagnosed HIV in the United States and six dependent areas, among which 69% are attributed to male-to-male sexual contact (and an additional 7% from male-to-male sexual contact and injection drug use (CDC, 2015). Male-to-male sexual contact is the only transmission category that has seen an increase in HIV diagnoses from 2010 to 2014, increasing 9% during that time (CDC, 2016a). In comparison, HIV diagnoses fell 20% among the heterosexual population, 26% among injection drug users, and 23% among those who report male-to-male sexual contact *and* injection drug use. Although the District of Columbia has the highest prevalence of HIV infection (at 2,696 cases per 100,000), states and territories with the highest infection include New York (784/100,000), the U.S. Virgin Islands (706/100,000), Maryland (641/100,000), Puerto Rico (610/100,000), Florida (606/100,000), Georgia (513/100,000), New Jersey (506/100,000), and Louisiana (502/100,000; CDC, 2016b). Increasingly, the U.S. epidemic has shifted to southern states, which include higher percentages of ethnically and racially diverse persons. The estimated proportion of new HIV diagnoses that were among White sexual minority men decreased from 33% to 30% of all diagnoses in sexual minority men from 2010 to 2014. In comparison, the proportion rose among Hispanic/Latino sexual minority men in the same time period from 24% to 27%, with proportions among Black/African American sexual minority men remaining stable at 38% (CDC, 2016a). If current trends continue, it is estimated that one in two Black sexual minority men and one in four Hispanic/Latino sexual minority men in the United States will be diagnosed with HIV in their lifetimes, compared to 1 in 11 White sexual minority men (Hess, Hu, Lansky, Mermin, & Hall, 2016). For this reason, efforts to address HIV disparities among ethnically and racially diverse sexual minority men—especially those living in the South—have intensified in recent years.

High rates of HIV infection among transgender persons arise from a complex interplay of gender, sexuality, biological vulnerabilities, and social and structural determinants (Reisner et al., 2016). A meta-analysis to estimate the prevalence of HIV infection and risk behaviors of transgender persons within 29 studies showed higher HIV incidence among transgender women (27.7%) than among transgender men (11.8%; Herbst et al., 2008). Alarmingly, 56% of African American transgender women in these studies were found to test positive for HIV. A more recent study examined the electronic health records of young (12–29 years) transgender patients attending a community health center for at least 1 year to determine the proportion of patients who had a laboratory-confirmed positive HIV or STI test (Reisner et al., 2015). Among the 145 patients, 4.8% were HIV-positive and less than 3% had been diagnosed with the following STIs: 2.8% herpes simplex virus, 2.8% syphilis, 2.1% chlamydia, 2.1% gonorrhea, 2.8% hepatitis C, and 1.4% human papillomavirus (HPV; Reisner et al., 2015). Concerns about the vulnerabilities facing transgender persons and the need to address their specific needs (separate from those of sexual minority men) have led to increased interest in transgender-specific research and programs. However, these efforts will require novel approaches and considerations. As Reisner et al. (2016, p. 431) summarized, "within transgender communities, immediate survival needs may supersede perceived health risks and undermine traditional research approaches—research may seem to have little meaning and relevance to people's lives."

RISK FACTORS FOR HIV AND SEXUALLY TRANSMITTED INFECTION TRANSMISSION

Risk factors pertaining to the acquisition of HIV and STIs vary among different subgroups of the U.S. population. A significant body of research has been dedicated to understanding the unique risk factors resulting in the relatively high prevalence of HIV infection in sexual minority men and transgender women. Differential risk for HIV acquisition and transmission among sexual minority men and transgender women is apparent at multiple levels of analysis that encompass individual risk behaviors, partner-level risks, community-level risks, and structural societal features.

Demographic Risks

Race and Ethnicity

The annual incidence of HIV in the United States declined for most groups between 2005 and 2014. However, for African American sexual minority men aged 13 to 24 years, there was an 87% increase in diagnoses (CDC, 2016a). While the early HIV epidemic in the United States involved mostly White sexual minority men, African American and Latino/Hispanic sexual minority men (especially those who are younger) are now at the greatest risk. High risk for HIV infection among African American sexual minority men (Hess et al., 2016) exists despite studies that show that this group has fewer sex partners than White sexual minority men (Crepaz et al., 2009). A study that pooled data from three longitudinal studies of sexual minority men (i.e., HIV Network for Prevention Trials Vaccine Preparedness Study, EXPLORE behavioral efficacy trial, and VAX004 vaccine efficacy trial) found that greater numbers of sexual partners, use of recreational drugs such as methamphetamine, and having had an STI in the past were associated with a greater per contact risk of acquiring HIV (Scott et al., 2014). However, for African American participants, there was a greater per contact risk for condomless anal sex compared to other racial groups despite having the lowest mean number of contacts. In comparison, Latino participants were shown to have an elevated per contact risk for insertive condomless anal intercourse compared with White participants. A meta-analysis of HIV risk behaviors for African American and Caucasian sexual minority men showed that the former were less likely to disclose their gay identity, more likely to have other STIs, and were less likely, if HIV-positive, to be on ART (Millett, Flores, Peterson, & Bakeman, 2007). These, and other factors described later (e.g., see Network-level Risk Factors), may serve to counteract the benefits derived from safer-sex practices among African American sexual minority men.

Age

Age, and the corresponding life transitions that accompany it, are associated with risk for HIV and other STIs (C. F. Wong, Schrager, Chou, Weiss, & Kipke, 2013).

A study of youth (aged 16–20 years) showed that those who were more "disconnected" (defined as neither working nor in school) were more likely to be HIV-positive than those who were more connected (Gayles, Kuhns, Kwon, Mustanski, & Garofalo, 2016). Further subgroup analysis by racial group showed that African American participants were more likely to have a disconnected status and that they were the only group showing an association between disconnection and HIV-positive status, even when controlling for substance use. Similarly, variables correlated to emerging adulthood, such as work status, school enrollment, and residential status, have been shown to variably impact engaging in HIV risk–related behaviors in young sexual minority men; this suggests that the instability and transitional status of this life stage may account for some of the increased risk and rates of HIV infection seen in younger cohorts (C. F. Wong et al., 2013).

Gender

Transgender women face a high burden of HIV disease compared to the general population, with U.S. prevalence estimates as high as 28% (Herbst et al., 2008). Despite the relatively few studies that have examined HIV-related risk behaviors among transgender women and the difficulty addressing unique risks for transgender participants (because studies often group them with cisgender sexual minority participants), recent data have emerged to better characterize risk factors specific to transgender women. A study using both ethnography and longitudinal quantitative data showed that transgender women of color who solely partnered with and/or were attracted to cisgender men had increased risk for HIV acquisition, which in part was due to a greater prevalence of HIV in male partners (Hwahng & Nuttbrock, 2014). Issues related to substance use and mental health also uniquely influence the risk of HIV and STIs in transgender communities. Higher rates of drug use have been found in communities of transgender women of color, serving as a predictor for condomless anal sex (Nemoto, Operario, Keatley, Han, & Soma, 2004). Moreover, mental health problems—sometimes co-occurring with drug use—are frequently seen in transgender communities, with one study demonstrating suicidal ideation in up to 54% of individuals surveyed (Herbst et al., 2008).

Partner- and Network-Level Risks

Decisions between sexual partners that involve which sexual activities to engage in and whether barrier protection is used clearly impact the transmissibility of HIV and STIs. Sexual minority men generally have higher numbers of sexual partners than men who exclusively engage in opposite-sex sexual activity, increasing the probability of HIV and STI transmission among this group (de Vries, 2014). Furthermore, sexual minority men are more likely to engage in receptive and penetrative anal sex, which poses a higher risk for transmission compared to other forms of intercourse (e.g., vaginal intercourse or oral sex) as a result of the ease with which pathogen transmission can occur along the rectal mucosa (Bradford, 2012).

In addition to disparities related to demographic factors, risk of HIV and STI acquisition is also mediated by the characteristics of partnerships and sexual networks found among sexual minority men and transgender women. The number of sexual partners within a network is influenced by shared participant characteristics, including injection drug use, serosorting, and age (Smith, Grierson, Wain, Pitts, & Pattison, 2004). Sexual networks can be determined by demographic factors themselves or form as a result of common interests or patterns of sexual behavior. A good illustration of the former case is a study performed in 2011 that looked at phylogenetic clustering of partnerships among HIV-positive, treatment-naive sexual minority men in the Jackson metropolitan area of Mississippi (Oster et al., 2011). The study found a high degree of homogeneity and demographic insularity of HIV transmission among African American participants, suggesting increased risk of transmission among African American sexual minority men in the United States as a result of having a greater likelihood that someone in their sexual network is HIV-positive compared to other racial groups. As such, while African American sexual minority men engage in less condomless anal sex than their White or Hispanic counterparts, HIV infection rates are higher among African American sexual minority men whose networks are defined by assortative sexual mixing that includes high proportions of persons who are living with HIV.

Subcultures have developed within LGBT communities around shared sexual practices that can have an impact on perceptions of sexual risk and engagement in behaviors that modify the risk of disease transmission. For example, survey data comparing self-identified "leathermen" with sexual minority men not affiliated with the leather community found that the former were 61% more likely to be HIV-positive and reported lower rates of condom use (Moskowitz, Seal, Rintamaki, & Rieger, 2011). Higher rates of condomless anal intercourse with serodiscordant partners have also been found among sexual minority men in the context of group sexual encounters involving more than two individuals (Grov, Rendina, Ventuneac, & Parsons, 2013).

Community-Level Risks

Risk Venues

Historically, in the United States and globally, GSM individuals have had a need to define and create protected spaces in which meeting other similar individuals was permissible, given the level of discrimination targeted against them (Subhrajit, 2014). Included among the various types of spaces that have emerged are physical venues used by some groups for engaging in sexual activity, or sex-on-premises venues. While not necessarily inherent to the structure or purpose of all such venues, and not frequented by a majority of sexual minority men, high-risk behaviors may occur on these premises given their often covert nature and the potential for patrons to engage in sex with multiple partners simultaneously or in quick succession (Melendez-Torres, Nye, & Bonell, 2016). A systematic review of within-subject comparisons of location of sex and sexual risk found a positive association between attendance at sex-on-premises venues (e.g., bathhouses and sex clubs) and engagement in condomless anal intercourse (Melendez-Torres et al., 2016). Moreover, lower rates of HIV status disclosure have also been noted among men attending bathhouses (Grov et al., 2013).

In addition to physical venues, virtual venues have emerged more recently as portals through which GSM individuals can meet potential partners (Melendez-Torres et al., 2016) and connect to engage in sexual activities (Horvath, Bowen, & Williams, 2006). While many of these sites offer a potential way for sexual minorities to meet others with common interests, some sites specifically promote themselves with content encouraging sexual practices that can increase risk of disease transmission (Klein, 2009). Comparisons of sex among individuals using websites to meet partners compared to attendance at physical venues have also revealed how structural differences in such locations result in differences in engagement in risky behavior. For example, the aforementioned study demonstrating lower rates of HIV status disclosure among men attending bathhouses was performed with a comparison to two other types of venues for meeting partners—those who used Craigslist.org, a popular online classified ads site, or those who went to gay bars or clubs. Among the three groups of participants, men seeking sexual partners using the online site were the least likely among the groups to use condoms, whereas men frequenting gay bars or clubs reported the highest amount of alcohol use (Grov et al., 2013).

Homelessness and Health Care Access

Unstable housing presents a significant impediment for individuals seeking services for HIV and STI prevention and treatment since the need to search for a stable location of residence may take precedence over matters related to practicing and maintaining healthy behaviors. Estimates of the risk of homelessness for people living with HIV/AIDS in the United States suggest that as many as 50% of these individuals are at risk of becoming homeless (National Alliance to End Homelessness, 2006). Such instability makes it more difficult for HIV-positive individuals to remain linked to care for their HIV and to maintain viral suppression, thus increasing the possibility of transmitting HIV to their sexual partners (Kidder, Wolitski, Pals, & Campsmith, 2008). The impact of homelessness is particularly acute for young sexual minority men, who may be forced to seek means to survive through engagement in commercial sex work (Bird, LaSala, Hidalgo, Kuhns, & Garofalo, 2016).

Structural-Level Risks

Sexual minority communities exist within a greater social milieu whose structures (e.g., laws, policies, and cultural attitudes) shape patterns of sexual behavior and decision making. These structures impact the risk of exposure to and infection with HIV and other sexually transmitted diseases (STDs). For example, 33 states currently have HIV criminal laws (e.g., making unprotected sex a criminal act) despite a growing body of literature that demonstrates that such laws have little to no public health benefit (Horvath, Meyer, & Rosser, 2016; Lehman et al., 2014). It has been argued that the existence of such laws may undermine empirically supported HIV prevention strategies by implicitly reinforcing a disclosure-based prevention strategy among high-risk groups (Galletly & Pinkerton, 2006).

Prominent among the factors that determine structural risk is the role of stigma experienced by sexual minority men and transgender women who have sex with men (Meyer, 2003; White Hughto, Reisner, & Pachankis, 2015). Low access to information about preventive services has marginalized these groups, contributing to higher rates of HIV both in the United States and globally (Altman et al., 2012). As attitudes toward LGBT communities in the United States have been in flux for the past few decades, differences in levels and types of stigma have emerged across age cohorts. For example, a study of substance-using HIV-negative and unknown status sexual minority men in New York City showed that older men with high anxiety and younger men who identified less with the gay community were both at increased risk for HIV (Lelutiu-Weinberger et al., 2013). Among younger sexual minority men, negative attitudes about persons living with HIV have been connected to increased avoidance of HIV-related educational and health services, contributing to HIV vulnerability (Jeffries et al., 2015). Experienced and anticipated stigma may also be heightened by having HIV, especially for GSMs (CDC, 2016c; Smit et al., 2012). Although attitudes have become more positive toward GSM populations in the United States (Gallup, 2015), there is little evidence that attitudes toward persons with HIV have likewise made gains. Negative attitudes toward people with HIV may suppress HIV status disclosure within sexual partnerships. Indeed, HIV-positive sexual minority men have been found to be less likely to disclose their positive status with their sexual partners compared to HIV-positive heterosexual individuals, contributing to increased risk of HIV transmission among sexual minority men (Przybyla et al., 2013).

Transgender persons also experience high degrees of stigma (White Hughto et al., 2015). A cross-sectional survey of transgender women in San Francisco, CA, revealed that high levels of stigma experienced by this group were independently associated with engaging in condomless anal sex and illicit drug use (Operario, Yang, Reisner, Iwamoto, & Nemoto, 2014). Thus, despite positive changes in the legal climate for GSM groups within the United States that will hopefully contribute to decreasing levels of stigma, the persistence of heterosexism and cisgenderism continues to place sexual minority men and transgender women at a disproportionately high risk for HIV and STI acquisition.

■ SYNDEMIC THEORY

Syndemic theory was developed to better understand how risk factors at the different levels described earlier may interact to impact risk for HIV and STIs. Syndemic theory tries to account for the synergistic effects of behavioral and psychosocial health problems that have converged to result in the higher risk for HIV and STIs seen in young sexual minority men. Illicit substance use, mental health disorders, victimization, and abuse have been identified as convergent factors contributing to higher rates of HIV in this group (Mustanski, Garofalo, Herrick, & Donenberg, 2007). Analysis of survey data of sexual minority men obtained from the Multicenter AIDS Cohort Study showed life-course predictor variables encompassing having suffered abuse or victimization, degree of internalized homophobia and masculinity attainment, social connectedness, and overall life satisfaction as impacting risk factors related to HIV acquisition (Herrick et al., 2013). Additionally, there are data showing that the experience of childhood sexual abuse can impact multiple factors related to HIV and STI acquisition, with sexual minority men reporting childhood sexual abuse more likely to have casual sexual partners and engage in drug use (Lloyd & Operario, 2012).

■ OTHER SEXUALLY TRANSMITTED INFECTIONS IN SEXUAL MINORITY MEN

Looking beyond HIV, sexual minority men are at risk for a number of bacterial STIs, including syphilis, chlamydia, and gonorrhea (Mayer, 2011; Workowski & Bolan, 2015). Factors associated with this increase are varied, and in different studies have included use of recreational drugs such as methamphetamine, use of erectile dysfunction drugs, multiple partners, and seeking partners on the Internet (Klausner, Kent, Wong, McCright, & Katz, 2005; Mayer, 2011; W. Wong, Chaw, Kent, & Klausner, 2005). Although serosorting (sex with partners of the same HIV status) has been adopted by some men as an HIV risk reduction practice (Khosropour et al., 2016), condomless anal intercourse still confers a risk of other STIs.

During 2005 to 2013, the number of primary and secondary syphilis cases reported annually in the United States nearly doubled, with 91% of cases in 2013 among men (Patton, Su, Nelson, & Weinstock, 2014); in those locations where sex partner information was collected, 84% of male cases in 2012 were among sexual minority men. Although cases have occurred in all demographic populations, primary/secondary syphilis rates have been greatest among African Americans, those aged 20 to 29, and those residing in the South and West (Patton, Su, et al., 2014). Syphilis and other genital ulcer diseases are well recognized risk factors for acquiring HIV. Coinfection of HIV and syphilis also increases the risk of neurosyphilis and its complications (Taylor et al., 2008).

Besides increasing awareness about syphilis and encouraging safer sexual practices (including condom use and decreasing the number of partners), annual serologic screening for syphilis is recommended for all sexually active sexual minority men (Workowski & Bolan, 2015); for those with multiple or anonymous partners, more frequent screening (every 3–6 months) is recommended (Patton, Su, et al., 2014). Implementation of these guidelines, however, requires cultural competence and sensitivity among health care workers to prevent the perception among sexual minority patients that they are being stereotyped as promiscuous (for other provider recommendations, see Chapter 22). Although partner notification of sexual minority men has been challenging (especially if there are anonymous partners or mistrust of health departments; Hogben et al., 2005), innovative approaches, including use of social media, have been used (Hunter et al., 2014).

Chlamydia and gonorrhea are both recognized as important STIs in sexual minority men, and many of the same STI risk factors apply. In addition to urogential sites, chlamydia or gonorrhea infection may occur in the oropharynx or rectum. In one analysis of sexual minority men attending 42 STD clinics throughout the United States, 11% tested positive for urogenital gonorrhea, 8% for pharyngeal gonorrhea, 10% for rectal gonorrhea, 8% for urogenital chlamydia, 3% for pharyngeal chlamydia, and 14% for rectal chlamydia (Patton, Kidd, et al., 2014). Studies have reported that STIs in sites such as the rectum may be asymptomatic, and missed if only urethral screening is performed (Kent et al., 2005; Patton, Kidd, et al., 2014). Rectal gonorrhea and chlamydia, especially when recurrent, have been associated with an increased risk of HIV seroconversion in sexual minority men (Bernstein, Marcus, Nieri, Philip, & Klausner, 2010). Screening in extragenital sites with the appropriate lab test is especially important for men who report histories of receptive anal or oral intercourse with multiple recent partners without a barrier.

Among the many viral STIs that sexual minority men may acquire, hepatitis A and B as well as HPV are well recognized, stressing the importance of vaccination (Fairley & Read, 2012). Sexual transmission of hepatitis C virus (HCV) has also been reported, especially among sexual minority men who have HIV coinfection (van de Laar, Matthews, Prins, & Danta, 2010), and screening of HIV-positive sexual minority men for HCV is recommended (especially with current highly effective treatments available for HCV). Other viral infections of importance in sexual minority men include various herpes virus infections. For example, in the National Health and Nutrition Examination surveys in 2001 to 2006, 18% of self-reported sexual minority men had antibodies against herpes virus type 2 (Xu, Sternberg, & Markowitz, 2010a), which also increases the risk of HIV (Freeman et al., 2006).

■ SEXUALLY TRANSMITTED INFECTIONS AMONG SEXUAL MINORITY WOMEN AND TRANSGENDER MEN

Although less well researched than STIs among sexual minority men and transgender women, there is a growing body of literature regarding STIs among sexual minority women in particular, and to a smaller extent, among transgender men. Sexual minority women, especially those who identify as a lesbian and/or engage only in same-sex intercourse, are often assumed to be at low risk for HIV and other STIs (Jones & Hoyler, 2006; Power, McNair, & Carr, 2009). This is largely due to a combination of two major misperceptions regarding the sexual health of sexual minority women. Namely, it is often presumed that (a) lesbian-identified women engage only in same-sex intercourse and (b) that HIV/STIs are transmitted primarily through sexual contact with a male partner, thus diminishing the perceived risks of sexual minority women (Women's Institute, 2009). However, in contrast to these misperceptions, the majority of lesbian-identified women have had at least one male sexual partner (with rates ranging from 70%–80%; Bailey, Farquhar, Owen, & Mangtani, 2004; Barefoot, Warren, & Smalley, 2017; Koh, Gómez, Shade, & Rowley, 2005) and HIV/STIs can in fact be transmitted between female sexual partners (S. K. Chan et al., 2014; Office of Women's Health, U.S. Department of Health and Human Services, 2009). Furthermore, when compared to exclusively heterosexual women, sexual minority women have been found to have a higher prevalence of risky sexual behaviors, including unprotected sexual activity with both male and female partners and a history of multiple sexual partners and/or forced sexual intercourse (Jones & Hoyler, 2006; Mojola & Everett, 2012; Singh, Fine, & Marrazzo, 2011). Despite these added vulnerabilities, many sexual minority women do not perceive themselves to be at risk for contracting HIV/STIs and therefore do not engage in regular screenings, further exacerbating their risks (Kerr, Ding, & Thompson, 2013; Power et al., 2009).

STIs that can easily be transmitted through female-to-female sexual contact include bacterial vaginosis, chlamydia, genital herpes, HPV, and trichomoniasis, whereas (although possible) female-to-female sexual transmission of HIV, gonor-rhea, syphilis, and hepatitis are much more rare (Office of Women's Health, U.S. Department of Health and Human Services, 2009). In addition to sexual contact with female partners, sexual minority women can also contract HIV/STIs through heterosexual intercourse—a history of which, as previously noted, is common even among lesbians—and sharing injection drug needles (Women's Institute, 2009). Approximately 17% of sexual minority women report a lifetime history of at least one STI (Diamant, Schuster, McGuigan, & Lever, 1999; Reisner, Mimiaga, et al., 2010).

Several STIs have been found to be more common among sexual minority women than those who are exclusively heterosexual; these include: bacterial vagi-nosis (i.e., vaginal infections; Fethers, Marks, Mindel, & Estcourt, 2000; Office of Women's Health, U.S. Department of Health and Human Services, 2009), HPV (Reiter & McRee, 2017), and herpes simplex virus type 2 infection (HSV-2; Xu, Sternberg, & Markowitz, 2010b). According to recent data from the National Health and Nutrition Examination Survey, the prevalence rate of HPV infection among sexual minority women ranges from 34.0% (those with no previous male sexual contact) to 55.9% (Reiter & McRee, 2017), while the prevalence rate of HSV-2 among sexual minority women ranges from 8.2% (those who identify as lesbian) to 45.6% (Xu et al., 2010b). The prevalence rate of chlamydia among young sexual minority women also appears to be relatively high, with 7.1% of sexual minor-ity participants testing positive for chlamydia among a clinical sample of women aged 15 to 24 years (Singh et al., 2011).

Due to the scarcity of HIV/STI-related data among transgender men, less is known about the HIV/STI risks of this population (Reisner & Murchison, 2016). Although the sexual identity and behavior of transgender men are very diverse, previous research suggests that the majority of transgender men identify their sex-ual orientation as nonheterosexual (i.e., gay, bisexual, and queer) and many have sex with cisgender men (Clements-Nolle, Marx, Guzman, & Katz, 2001; Kenagy & Hsieh, 2005; Reisner & Murchison, 2016; Reisner, White, Mayer, & Mimiaga, 2014; Rowniak & Chesla, 2013). Transgender men may be particularly vulnerable to HIV and other STIs due to a variety of risky sexual behaviors. For example, when com-pared to transgender women, transgender men have been found to be less likely to have used protection during their last sexual encounter (i.e., 29.0% vs. 59.0%) and more likely to have recently engaged in one or more high-risk sexual activities (80.7% vs. 54.9%; Kenagy & Hsieh, 2005).

Given that many transgender men identify as gay or bisexual and have male sexual partners, most of the research available on the HIV/STI risks of transgender men focuses specifically on those who have sex with men (Reisner & Murchison, 2016). Across two studies of transgender men who have sex with cisgender men, a large percentage of participants reported high-risk sexual behavior such as: recent unprotected sex with a cisgender male whose HIV status was unknown (43.8%); recent use of the Internet to meet sexual partners and engage in sexual activities with anonymous cisgender male partners (62.5%); foregone regular gynecologi-cal care and/or HIV/STD testing (25.0–31.1%; Reisner, Perkovich, & Mimiago, 2010); and inconsistent condom use during receptive vaginal and anal intercourse

(Sevelius, 2009). Prevalence rates of self-reported lifetime history of one or more STIs among samples of transgender men who have sex with men range from 37.5% to 46.7% (Reisner, Perkovich, et al., 2010; Sevelius, 2009), with specific prevalence rates as follows: HIV infection—0% to 3% (Feldman, Romine, & Bockting, 2014; Reisner & Murchison, 2016; Sevelius, 2009); gonorrhea—6.7%; trichomoniasis—6.7% to 12.5%; bacterial vaginosis—6.3% to 8.9%; chlamydia—11.1%; herpes—11.1% to 18.8%; and HPV—24.4% (Reisner et al., 2010; Sevelius, 2009).

■ INTERVENTIONS TO ADDRESS HIV AND STIs

Numerous interventions have been implemented to decrease the incidence of primary HIV infections in sexual minority men as well as improve viral outcomes and reduce risk HIV transmission among sexual minority men. In what follows, we discuss recent interventions and indicate how these interventions can improve GSM health, primarily among sexual minority men and transgender women (the literature regarding prevention of STIs among sexual minority women and transgender men is very scarce). Interventions for sexual minority men and transgender women include biomedical interventions, behavioral interventions, and societal-level interventions.

Cascade of Care/Continuum of Care

HIV interventions for GSM individuals can intervene on multiple levels of the continuum of care, as well as intervene on preventing acquisition of HIV infection. Among those individuals living with HIV, they must first know their status (diagnosis), be linked to care, continue to remain in care, be prescribed and correctly take ART, and be virally suppressed (Mugavero, Amico, Horn, & Thompson, 2013). Research from the CDC (2012) indicates that among sexual minority men, only 79% are diagnosed, 63% are linked to care, 36% are retained in care, 33% are prescribed ART, and 27% are virally suppressed (CDC, 2012). The majority of new infections of HIV in sexual minority men are due to individuals living with HIV who have not been diagnosed or were diagnosed, but not retained in medical care (Skarbinski et al., 2015).

Biomedical Interventions

Treatment as Prevention

Since its introduction for treatment of HIV in 1996, ART has dramatically improved the life expectancy of individuals living with HIV (World Health Organization, 2013). Use of ART has also been shown to reduce viral loads in HIV-infected persons, subsequently reducing the risk of HIV transmission to an uninfected individual (Cohen et al., 2011). The HIV Prevention Trials Network 052 study (although in a heterosexual couple population) showed that early initiation of ART therapy reduced HIV transmission risk by 96% compared to delayed initiation of ART (Cohen et al., 2011). Following this trial, the WHO guidelines changed to indicate that HIV-positive people should be on ART regardless of their CD4 count (World Health Organization, 2016). Among sexual minority men, an observational study followed discordant same-sex male couples who had condomless anal sex for risk of HIV infection when the positive partner was on suppressive ART therapy for approximately 1.3 years per couple (Rodger et al., 2016). Although there were three new HIV infections among the couples, there were no documented cases of transmission between partners, suggesting that transmission occurred outside of the primary relationships (Rodger et al., 2016). Following an additional 5 years of follow-up, there were 78 new HIV infections among 1,763 index participants (Cohen et al., 2016). However, it was determined that new infections occurred only when HIV was not fully suppressed for the index participant (i.e., HIV-positive partner). Early initiation of ART also led to a 93% lower risk of linked HIV infection (i.e., infection from study participant) compared to delayed ART (Cohen et al., 2016). These results suggest that viral suppression among HIV-infected individuals means that they are no longer infectious to seronegative individuals.

Additional studies have shown the effect of an increase in ART treatment coverage in a population on the incidence of new infection in the community. In San Francisco between 2004 and 2008, a reduction in the community viral load and mean individual load was significantly associated with a decrease in new HIV diagnoses (Das et al., 2010). During this time period, there had been an increase in rates of HIV testing as well as expansion of ART coverage (Das et al., 2010).

Preexposure Chemoprophylaxis

In addition to ART regimens being used by HIV-infected individuals, new methods in utilizing ART for HIV prevention are promising, especially preexposure chemoprophylaxis (PrEP). High-risk individuals for acquisition of HIV infection, including unmarried/unpartnered sexual minority men and transgender women, intravenous drug users (IVDUs), and high-risk heterosexual individuals, are prime candidates for PrEP. In a randomized controlled trial, use of once-daily Truvada, compared to a placebo, reduced acquisition of new HIV infection by 44% in a population of seronegative sexual minority men and transgender women who have sex with men (Grant et al., 2010). However, the effectiveness of PrEP is dependent on drug concentrations in the bloodstream, which correlates with an individual's adherence to PrEP (Grant et al., 2014). Among individuals who were randomized to PrEP, HIV incidence differed dramatically by drug concentrations, as shown by the following standardized incidence rates:

- No drug detected: 4.7 infections/100 person-years
- Fewer than 2 tablets/week: 2.3 infections/100 person-years
- 2 to 3 tablets/week: 0.6 infections/100 person-years
- 4 or more tablets/week: 0.0 infections/100 person-years (Grant et al., 2014).

While promising to reduce incidence of HIV, daily adherence to PrEP is crucial to ensure adequate concentrations of treatment in the bloodstream to protect against HIV infection. However, adherence to PrEP medication has been shown to be suboptimal among sexual minority men (Buchbinder & Liu, 2014; P. A. Chan et al., 2016; Liu, Glidden, et al., 2014), as well as in transgender women (Deutsch et al., 2015). In a study of seronegative sexual minority men on PrEP, only 45% self-reported their adherence as excellent, and only 36% reported having perfect adherence over the past 30 days (Liu, Hessoll, et al., 2014). However, these adherence rates vary by subgroup. For example, an observational study among sexual minority men and transgender women in San Francisco, Miami, and Washington DC found that although approximately 80% to 85.6% of participants had adequate protection levels of PrEP (equivalent to 4 tablets/week), African Americans were less likely to have adequate protection levels (at only 56.8%; Liu et al., 2016).

Models run by the CDC indicate that if only 40% of eligible sexual minority men were on PrEP, there would be a 33% reduction in cases over the next 10 years (Jenness et al., 2016). In an evaluation of sexual minority men in San Francisco, approximately 64.1% of sexual minority men were eligible for PrEP, yet only 14.5% of those eligible sexual minority men were using PrEP in 2014 and only 9.2% of sexual minority men overall were prescribed PrEP (Snowden, Chen, McFarland, & Raymond, 2017). However, rates of referrals and initiations of PrEP among the Kaiser Permanente Medical Center in San Francisco have increased since 2012, with no new cases of HIV infection among those individuals (Volk et al., 2015). Similarly, results from the 2014 National HIV Behavioral Surveillance found that although more than 50% of sexual minority men indicated they would take PrEP, only 4% reported being prescribed and using PrEP (Hoots, Finlayson, Nerlander, & Paz-Bailey, 2016).

Tenofovir Gel Study (Women)

The Centre for the AIDS Programme of Research in South Africa (CAPRISA) trial evaluated the effect of a 1% tenofovir vaginal gel in sexually active HIV-negative cisgender women in Africa (Abdool Karim et al., 2010). The 1% tenofovir vaginal gel is inserted before and after sexual intercourse. The tenofovir gel was found to reduce HIV incidence by 39% overall, and reduced incidence in cisgender women who were considered highly adherent to the gel by 54% (Abdool Karim et al., 2010). Even among cisgender women with low gel adherence (<50%), HIV incidence was reduced by 28% (Abdool Karim et al., 2010). Increased concentration of tenofovir in the cervicovaginal fluid is associated with higher protection against new HIV incidence (Kashuba et al., 2015). Studies investigating the use of tenofovir for anal intercourse among sexual minority men and transgender women are still pending, but could prove highly impactful.

Behavioral Interventions

HIV Testing

One of the largest disconnects in the HIV continuum of care is between those who know their status and those who do not; nearly 21% of sexual minority men do not know their status (CDC, 2012). Individuals with unknown status are at increased risk of transmission to other individuals. It is estimated that nearly 91.5% of all new HIV infections in the United States are due to individuals not knowing their HIV diagnosis status or knowing their status and not being retained in care (Skarbinski et al., 2015). One of the CDC's emphases for HIV control is on improving the diagnosis of new HIV infections in the United States (Branson et al., 2006). Focusing resources in nonmedical settings and utilizing technology to improve HIV testing rates in communities at high risk have shown promising results (Bowles et al., 2008; Burns, Keating, & Free, 2016).

Numerous testing interventions in medical settings have been implemented outside of typical primary care settings, including emergency departments (Haukoos et al., 2011; Rothman, Ketlogetswe, Dolan, Wyer, & Kelen, 2003) and dental clinics (Blackstock, King, Mason, Lee, & Mannheimer, 2010). However, they require a coordinated link to HIV primary care settings. Interventions at nonclinical sites more commonly visited by sexual minority men and transgender women, including parks, homeless shelters, and bars, have also shown promising results in improving rates of HIV testing (Bowles et al., 2008).

Many current studies aim at utilizing technology, in particular cellular phones and the Internet, to improve HIV testing rates among sexual minority men (Burns et al., 2016). Platforms such as social media, dating websites, and Internet chat rooms offer a unique opportunity to share information about HIV and locations of HIV testing sites and STD health clinics. Introduction of sexual health information and referral testing sites by social networking sites and gay dating applications has shown that individuals are agreeable to receiving sexual health information via a mobile app (Sun, Stowers, Miller, Bachmann, & Rhodes, 2015), are able to be referred to local HIV and STD sites following chatting via online dating sites (Sun et al., 2015), and demonstrate improved self-reported HIV testing rates (Rhodes et al., 2011). An additional study in London showed that by offering free HIV testing kits to sexual minority men on a gay social networking website sent through the mail, approximately 33% of individuals who requested free HIV testing kits returned them, of which 1.4% of the samples were confirmed as new HIV infections (Elliot, Rossi, McCormack, & McOwan, 2016). However, other studies have found that introducing sexual health information and HIV testing site information or referrals did not lead to increases in HIV testing. For example, a study of an Internet-based social marketing campaign aimed at improving HIV testing rates of MSM in the United Kingdom was not associated with an increase in HIV testing (Hickson et al., 2015).

Sexually Transmitted Infection Testing

Infection with an STI increases the risk for HIV among sexual minority men and a new STI diagnosis has been shown to be associated with a new HIV diagnosis (Katz, Dombrowski, Bell, Kerani, & Golden, 2016; Kelley et al., 2015; Pathela et al., 2017). By offering rescreening 3 months after a diagnosis of a bacterial STI, new incident cases of HIV and bacterial STIs are diagnosed (Harte, Mercey, Jarman, & Benn, 2011). Therefore, improving retesting rates among individuals who have been previously diagnosed with an STI may improve diagnosis of HIV.

Interventions to Improve Antiretroviral Therapy Adherence (Treatment as Prevention and PrEP)

ART has been shown to improve health outcomes and reduce risk of sexual transmission of HIV to partners in sexual minority men as well as prevent HIV acquisition in seronegative individuals (Cohen et al., 2016; Cohen et al., 2011). Adherence to HIV therapies is crucial, yet many sexual minority men and transgender women report low adherence to ART (Liu, Hessol, et al., 2014). Improving adherence to ART medications among individuals will increase the number of individuals virally suppressed and reduce risk of virologic failure, and has subsequently been shown to reduce community viral load and decrease number of new infections (Das et al., 2010).

Recent interventions have focused on utilizing technology, including mobile devices, computers, and social media, to improve adherence to ART and PrEP medications (Young, Swendeman, Holloway, Reback, & Kao, 2015). Recent uses have included daily text message reminders to individuals (Lewis et al., 2013), introduction of ART adherence apps (LeGrand et al., 2016), and online web-based support interventions (Horvath, Oakes, et al., 2013).

Utilization of technology may have strong implications in subpopulations of sexual minority men who are less likely to be engaged in HIV care, including HIV-positive stimulant-using sexual minority men (Horvath, Carrico, et al., 2013). "Thrive with Me" is an online peer-to-peer social support adherence intervention for sexual minority men (Horvath, Carrico, et al., 2013). Although there were no differences in overall adherence for men in the intervention compared to control arm, there was a difference in measures of adherence found among stimulant drug users compared to nonstimulant drug users. Technology-based targeted adherence interventions among individuals at high risk for nonadherence may improve viral outcomes.

Community-Level Interventions

Condom Distribution in Communities

Condoms have been shown to be protective in preventing HIV transmission in sexual minority men. However, studies have shown that 54% of sexual minority men have had condomless anal intercourse over the 12 months (Finlayson et al., 2011). While the findings of such studies are difficult to interpret due to the frequent failure to control for relationship status, it is likely that there is still significant occurrence of condomless sex among sexual minority men not in committed relationships. One frequently reported barrier for consistent use of condoms is cost (Ubrihien, Davies, & Driscoll, 2016).

Many local public health departments, community clinics, and other HIV-related organizations have initiated free condom distribution programs. In an online survey of sexual minority men recruited from social networking sites, nearly 60% had received free condoms in the past year (Khosropour & Sullivan, 2013), with nearly 75% of those individuals using the condoms. While no particular racial or ethnic group was more likely to acquire free condoms, non-Hispanic Black sexual minority men were more likely to use the free condoms (Khosropour & Sullivan, 2013), while individuals with more than three sexual partners in the past 12 months were more likely to acquire the free condoms as well as use them (Khosropour & Sullivan, 2013).

The New York City Department of Health and Mental Hygiene (DOHMH) started the Free Condom Initiative to distribute free condoms to individuals seen at health agencies and social outlets including gay bars. Among patrons to gay bars, only 31% of individuals indicated that they noticed that condoms were available. Among those who noticed the condoms were available, 74% acquired them, while

77% of those who acquired them used them (Renaud et al., 2009). Additionally, other initiatives have been implemented in local community businesses by AIDS organizations to distribute condoms and additional information about HIV (e.g., Rovniak et al., 2010), with the majority of consumers supporting the initiatives (Phillips-Guzman et al., 2011).

These interventions and studies indicate that if free condoms are available to sexual minority men, many will take them and a large proportion of those who acquire the condoms will use them. Large-scale condom distributions that target and are visible to sexual minority men are therefore both necessary and strongly needed.

Condom Distribution Among Incarcerated Sexual Minority Men

One study found that over half of incarcerated sexual minority men and transgender women reported anal sex and two thirds reported oral sex during their incarceration, yet the vast majority of jails and prisons do not provide condoms to the inmates (Harawa, Sweat, George, & Sylla, 2010). A study of a weekly condom distribution program in a Los Angeles Country jail found a 25% reduction in HIV transmissions (Leibowitz, Harawa, Sylla, Hallstrom, & Kerndt, 2013). Inmates were allowed to receive one condom a week. Although 65% of individuals who reported anal sex reported using the provided condoms, 75% of inmates also indicated they had also had condomless anal sex (Harawa et al., 2010). This indicates that more than half of inmates will use a provided condom and suggests that interventions that distribute more condoms may be necessary, particularly in jails and prisons.

Xpress Clinics

Express testing services ("Xpress" clinics) have been introduced in coordination with sexual health clinics (Knight et al., 2013). In this model, asymptomatic patients are eligible to attend either Xpress clinics (including a 15-minute consultation with a nurse, who collected throat and genital swabs, computer-assisted interview questions, and self-collection of genital swabs) or a regular clinic visit. The Xpress clinics reduced patient cost and median wait time for patients, and increased the number of patients seen at the clinic (Knight et al., 2013). A cross-sectional analysis of participating patients indicated that sexual minority men would have gone to the sexual health clinic for screening regardless of whether the Xpress clinic was an option, but would utilize Xpress clinics for future screenings (Martin et al., 2013). Patient satisfaction was high and many indicated they would refer their friends to the Xpress clinic (Martin et al., 2013). Introduction of Xpress clinics to sexual health clinics with high sexual minority male and transgender female patient populations could improve diagnosis rates of HIV and other STIs, and with a coordinated link to care, improve linkage to care in this patient population.

Societal-Level Interventions

Policies and Laws

In 2013, the U.S. Supreme Court Decision *United States v. Windsor* repealed the Defense of Marriage Act, giving same-sex couples full federal marriage rights, and the subsequent ruling in *Obergefell v. Hodges* (2015) legalized same-sex marriage nationwide. Previous research had shown that gay marriage bans increased the rates of HIV infections by four cases per 100,000 people (Francis & Mialon, 2010). The authors hypothesize that increased tolerance may decrease the frequency of high-risk sexual behavior, decreasing the risk of HIV infection (Francis & Mialon, 2010). Following the legalization of same-sex marriages in Massachusetts, health care use, including the frequency of medical and mental health care visits, and mental health care costs decreased compared to before state-level legalization (Hatzenbuehler et al., 2012). Legalization of same-sex marriage may also reduce HIV stigma, which may improve outcomes in those living with HIV. A cross-sectional study of persons living with HIV/AIDS in Los Angeles found that individuals with high levels of internalized HIV stigma were more likely to report poor access to medical care, HIV care, and ART adherence (Sayles, Wong, Kinsler, Martins, & Cunningham, 2009). Although it is too soon to determine the national effect the passage of full marriage rights will have for same-sex couples, particularly incidence of HIV infection among sexual minority men and transgender women, improved access to health care and decreased stigma are to be expected over time (Buffie, 2011).

CDC and Public Health Campaigns

Numerous campaigns have been enacted by the CDC to reduce stigma among the general population as well as target particular populations, including sexual minority men, at highest risk for HIV infection. Targeted interventions for sexual minority men include "Reasons" and "Testing Makes Us Stronger" aimed to improve HIV testing among Latino and African American sexual minority men, respectively, and "Start Talking. Stop HIV," aimed at encouraging sexual minority men to engage in conversations about safe sex including testing, status, condoms, and medications. However, the effect of these public health campaigns on the national rate of HIV infections and additional HIV outcome measures has not been evaluated. However, one campaign, the National HIV Testing Day, has found that over the course of 1 week, an additional 15,000 more HIV tests were given and 100 new HIV infections were diagnosed compared to other weeks in the year and were able to reach populations at highest risk for HIV, including sexual minority men and transgender women (Lecher et al., 2016; Van Handel & Mulatu, 2014).

■ CONCLUSION

HIV and other STIs emerge from similar risk factors and have a profound physical, mental, and cultural impact on the LGBT community. Although a complete review of the literature in this area is far too vast to fully summarize, there are key lessons to be learned from this review and other recent reports describing successes and challenges of addressing these epidemics among the LGBT community (Beyrer et al., 2016). First, risk for HIV and other STIs is multilayered and the intersection of multiple risk factors serves to compound transmission risk. For example, although Black sexual minority men consistently report lower rates of condomless anal intercourse, network, community, and structural risk factors combine to maintain high levels of transmission. Therefore, providing a comprehensive package of prevention programs that addresses risk at all levels will be critical to decrease HIV incidence broadly (Beyrer et al., 2016). Second, increasing the availability and accessibility of biomedical interventions—in particular PrEP—for high-risk groups must be prioritized. These programs, however, must be further supported by behavioral supports to help persons to maintain consistent and sustained adherence to PrEP. Relatedly, universal access to treatment is needed, especially in light of new data supporting the effectiveness of treatment as prevention approaches (Cohen et al., 2016). Finally, in order to assess eligibility for PrEP or treatment, testing in high-risk communities is crucial. Innovations in how to reach HIV testing and how to encourage repeat testing are needed, especially in light of evidence that regular HIV testing is not common among a substantial number of sexual minority men (Mitchell & Horvath, 2013). These efforts will require substantial investments from governmental and nongovernmental agencies to reduce the burden of HIV and STIs among GSM populations. However, we have seen substantial progress over the past 35 years of the HIV epidemic, and there are increased calls for efforts to end the HIV/AIDS epidemic (Sidibe, 2016). While there is still work to do, the path forward is increasingly clear.

■ REFERENCES

Abdool Karim, Q., Abdool Karim, S. S., Frohlich, J. A., Grobler, A. C., Baxter, C., Mansoor, L. E.,...Taylor, D. (2010). Effectiveness and safety of tenofovir gel, an antiretroviral microbicide, for the prevention of HIV infection in women. *Science, 329*(5996), 1168–1174. doi:10.1126/science.1193748

Altman, D., Aggleton, P., Williams, M., Kong, T., Reddy, V., Harrad, D.,...Parker, R. (2012). Men who have sex with men: Stigma and discrimination. *Lancet, 380*(9839), 439–445. doi:10.1016/s0140-6736(12)60920-9

Bailey, J. V., Farquhar, C., Owen, C., & Mangtani, P. (2004). Sexually transmitted infections in women who have sex with women. *Sexually Transmitted Infections, 80*(3), 244–246. doi:10.1136/sti.2003.007641

Baral, S. D., Grosso, A., Holland, C., & Papworth, E. (2014). The epidemiology of HIV among men who have sex with men in countries with generalized HIV epidemics. *Current Opinions in HIV and AIDS, 9*(2), 156–167. doi:10.1097/coh.0000000000000037

Barefoot, K. N., Warren, J. C., & Smalley, K. B. (2017). Women's health care: The experiences and behaviors of rural and urban lesbians in the USA. *Rural and Remote Health, 17*(1), 3875.

Bernstein, K. T., Marcus, J. L., Nieri, G., Philip, S. S., & Klausner, J. D. (2010). Rectal gonorrhea and chlamydia reinfection is associated with increased risk of HIV seroconversion. *Journal of Acquired Immune Deficiency Syndromes, 53*(4), 537–543. doi:10.1097/QAI.0b013e3181c3ef29

Beyrer, C., Baral, S. D., Collins, C., Richardson, E. T., Sullivan, P. S., Sanchez, J.,...Mayer, K. H. (2016). The global response to HIV in men who have sex with men. *Lancet, 388*(10040), 198–206. doi:10.1016/S0140-6736(16)30781-4

Bird, J. D., LaSala, M. C., Hidalgo, M. A., Kuhns, L. M., & Garofalo, R. (2016). "I had to go to the streets to get love": Pathways from parental rejection to HIV risk among young gay and bisexual men. *Journal of Homosexuality.* Advanced online publication. doi:10.1080/00918369.2016.1179039

Blackstock, O. J., King, J. R., Mason, R. D., Lee, C. C., & Mannheimer, S. B. (2010). Evaluation of a rapid HIV testing initiative in an urban, hospital-based dental clinic. *AIDS Patient Care and STDs, 24*(12), 781–785. doi:10.1089/apc.2010.0159

Bowles, K. E., Clark, H. A., Tai, E., Sullivan, P. S., Song, B., Tsang, J.,...Heffelfinger, J. D. (2008). Implementing rapid HIV testing in outreach and community settings: Results from an advancing HIV prevention demonstration project conducted in seven U.S. cities. *Public Health Reports, 123*(Suppl. 3), 78–85.

Bradford, D. (2012). Bisexuality and sexual orientation. In S. Gupta, & B. Kumar (Eds.), *Sexually transmitted infections* (pp. 1174–1178). Haryana, India: Elsevier.

Branson, B. M., Handsfield, H. H., Lampe, M. A., Janssen, R. S., Taylor, A. W., Lyss, S. B., & Clark, J. E. (2006). Revised recommendations for HIV testing of adults, adolescents, and pregnant women in health-care settings. *MMWR Recommendations and Reports, 55*(14), 1–17.

Buchbinder, S. P., & Liu, A. Y. (2014). CROI 2014: New tools to track the epidemic and prevent HIV infections. *Topics in Antiviral Medicine, 22*(2), 579–593.

Buffie, W. C. (2011). Public health implications of same-sex marriage. *American Journal of Public Health, 101*(6), 986–990. doi:10.2105/ajph.2010.300112

Burns, K., Keating, P., & Free, C. (2016). A systematic review of randomised control trials of sexual health interventions delivered by mobile technologies. *BMC Public Health, 16*(1), 778. doi:10.1186/s12889-016-3408-z

Centers for Disease Control and Prevention. (1981). Pneumocystis pneumonia: Los Angeles. *Morbidity and Mortality Weekly Report, 30*(21), 250–252.

Centers for Disease Control and Prevention. (2012). HIV in the United States: The stages of care. Retrieved from https://www.cdc.gov/hiv/pdf/research_mmp_stagesofcare.pdf

Centers for Disease Control and Prevention. (2015). HIV surveillance report, 2014 (Vol. 26). Retrieved from http://www.cdc.gov/hiv/library/reports/surveillance

Centers for Disease Control and Prevention. (2016a). HIV surveillance: Men who have sex with men (MSM). Retrieved from http://www.cdc.gov/hiv/pdf/library/slidesets/cdc-hiv-surveillance-slides-msm.pdf

Centers for Disease Control and Prevention. (2016b). HIV surveillance: Epidemiology of HIV infection (through 2014). Retrieved from http://www.cdc.gov/hiv/pdf/library/slidesets/cdc-hiv-surveillance-genepi.pdf

Centers for Disease Control and Prevention. (2016c). HIV among transgender people. Retrieved from http://www.cdc.gov/hiv/group/gender/transgender

Chan, P. A., Mena, L., Patel, R., Oldenburg, C. E., Beauchamps, L., Perez-Brumer, A. G.,...Nunn, A. (2016). Retention in care outcomes for HIV pre-exposure prophylaxis implementation programmes among men who have sex with men in three US cities. *Journal of the International AIDS Society, 19*(1), 20903. doi:10.7448/ias.19.1.20903

Chan, S. K., Thornton, L. R., Chronister, K. J., Meyer, J., Wolverton, M., Johnson, C. K.,...Sullivan, V. (2014). Likely female-to-female sexual transmission of HIV: Texas, 2012. *Morbidity and Mortality Weekly Report, 63*(10), 209–212.

Clements-Nolle, K., Marx, R., Guzman, R., & Katz, M. (2001). HIV prevalence, risk behaviors, health care use, and mental health status of transgender persons: Implications for public health intervention. *American Journal of Public Health, 91*(6), 915–921.

Cohen, M. S., Chen, Y. Q., McCauley, M., Gamble, T., Hosseinipour, M. C., Kumarasamy, N.,...Fleming, T. R. (2011). Prevention of HIV-1 infection with early antiretroviral therapy. *New England Journal of Medicine, 365*(6), 493–505. doi:10.1056/NEJMoa1105243

Cohen, M. S., Chen, Y. Q., McCauley, M., Gamble, T., Hosseinipour, M. C., Kumarasamy, N.,...Fleming, T. R. (2016). Antiretroviral therapy for the prevention of HIV-1 transmission. *New England Journal of Medicine, 375*(9), 830–839.

Crepaz, N., Marks, G., Liau, A., Mullins, M. M., Aupont, L. W., Marshall, K. J.,...Wolitski, R. J. (2009). Prevalence of unprotected anal intercourse among HIV-diagnosed MSM in the United States: A meta-analysis. *AIDS, 23*(13), 1617–1629. doi:10.1097/QAD.0b013e32832effae

Das, M., Chu, P. L., Santos, G. M., Scheer, S., Vittinghoff, E., McFarland, W., & Colfax, G. N. (2010). Decreases in community viral load are accompanied by reductions in new HIV infections in San Francisco. *PLOS ONE, 5*(6), e11068. doi:10.1371/journal.pone.0011068

de Vries, H. J. (2014). Sexually transmitted infections in men who have sex with men. *Clinics in Dermatology, 32*(2), 181–188. doi:10.1016/j.clindermatol.2013.08.001

Deutsch, M. B., Glidden, D. V., Sevelius, J., Keatley, J., McMahan, V., Guanira, J.,...Grant, R. M. (2015). HIV pre-exposure prophylaxis in transgender women: A subgroup analysis of the iPrEx trial. *Lancet HIV, 2*(12), e512–e519. doi:10.1016/s2352-3018(15)00206-4

Diamant, A. L., Schuster, M. A., McGuigan, K., & Lever, J. (1999). Lesbians' sexual history with men: Implications for taking a sexual history. *Archives of Internal Medicine, 159*(22), 2730–2736.

Elliot, E., Rossi, M., McCormack, S., & McOwan, A. (2016). Identifying undiagnosed HIV in men who have sex with men (MSM) by offering HIV home sampling via online gay social media: A service evaluation. *Sexually Transmitted Infections, 92*(6), 470–473. doi:10.1136/sextrans-2015-052090

Fairley, C. K., & Read, T. R. (2012). Vaccination against sexually transmitted infections. *Current Opinion in Infectious Diseases, 25*(1), 66–72.

Feldman, J., Romine, R. S., & Bockting, W. O. (2014). HIV risk behaviors in the U.S. transgender population: Prevalence and predictors in a large internet sample. *Journal of Homosexuality, 61*(11), 1558–1588. doi:10.1080/00918369.2014.944048

Fethers, K., Marks, C., Mindel, A., & Estcourt, C. S. (2000). Sexually transmitted infections and risk behaviours in women who have sex with women. *Sexually Transmitted Infections, 76*(5), 345–349. doi:10.1136/sti.76.5.345

Finlayson, T. J., Le, B., Smith, A., Bowles, K., Cribbin, M., Miles, I.,...Dinenno, E. (2011). HIV risk, prevention, and testing behaviors among men who have sex with men: National HIV Behavioral Surveillance System, 21 U.S. cities, United States, 2008. *MMWR Surveillance Summaries, 60*(14), 1–34.

Francis, A. M., & Mialon, H. M. (2010). Tolerance and HIV. *Journal of Health Economics, 29*(2), 250–267. doi:10.1016/j.jhealeco.2009.11.016

Freeman, E. E., Weiss, H. A., Glynn, J. R., Cross, P. L., Whitworth, J. A., & Hayes, R. J. (2006). Herpes simplex virus 2 infection increases HIV acquisition in men and women: Systematic review and meta-analysis of longitudinal studies. *AIDS, 20*(1), 73–83.

Friedland, G. (2016). Marking time in the global HIV/AIDS pandemic. *Journal of American Medical Association, 316*(2), 145–146. doi:10.1001/jama.2016.9006

Galletly, C. L., & Pinkerton, S. D. (2006). Conflicting messages: How criminal HIV disclosure laws undermine public health efforts to control the spread of HIV. *AIDS and Behavior, 10*(5), 451–461.

Gallup. (2015). Gay and lesbian rights 2015. Retrieved from http://www.gallup.com/poll/1651/gay-lesbian-rights.aspx

Gayles, T. A., Kuhns, L. M., Kwon, S., Mustanski, B., & Garofalo, R. (2016). Socioeconomic disconnection as a risk factor for increased HIV infection in young men who have sex with men. *LGBT Health, 3*(3), 219–224. doi:10.1089/lgbt.2015.0102

Grant, R. M., Anderson, P. L., McMahan, V., Liu, A., Amico, K. R., Mehrotra, M.,...Glidden, D. V. (2014). Uptake of pre-exposure prophylaxis, sexual practices, and HIV incidence in men and transgender women who have sex with men: A cohort study. *Lancet Infectious Diseases, 14*(9), 820–829. doi:10.1016/s1473-3099(14)70847-3

Grant, R. M., Lama, J. R., Anderson, P. L., McMahan, V., Liu, A. Y., Vargas, L.,...Glidden, D. V. (2010). Preexposure chemoprophylaxis for HIV prevention in men who have sex with men. *New England Journal of Medicine, 363*(27), 2587–2599. doi:10.1056/NEJMoa1011205

Grov, C., Rendina, H. J., Ventuneac, A., & Parsons, J. T. (2013). HIV risk in group sexual encounters: An event-level analysis from a national online survey of MSM in the U.S. *Journal of Sexual Medicine, 10*(9), 2285–2294. doi:10.1111/jsm.12227

Harawa, N. T., Sweat, J., George, S., & Sylla, M. (2010). Sex and condom use in a large jail unit for men who have sex with men (MSM) and male-to-female transgenders. *Journal of Health Care for the Poor and Underserved, 21*(3), 1071–1087. doi:10.1353/hpu.0.0349

Harte, D., Mercey, D., Jarman, J., & Benn, P. (2011). Is the recall of men who have sex with men (MSM) diagnosed as having bacterial sexually transmitted infections (STIs) for re-screening a feasible and effective strategy? *Sexually Transmitted Infections, 87*(7), 577–582. doi:10.1136/sextrans-2011-050144

Hatzenbuehler, M. L., O'Cleirigh, C., Grasso, C., Mayer, K., Safren, S., & Bradford, J. (2012). Effect of same-sex marriage laws on health care use and expenditures in sexual minority men: A quasi-natural experiment. *American Journal of Public Health, 102*(2), 285–291. doi:10.2105/ajph.2011.300382

Haukoos, J. S., White, D. A., Lyons, M. S., Hopkins, E., Calderon, Y., Kalish, B., & Rothman, R. E. (2011). Operational methods of HIV testing in emergency departments: A systematic review. *Annals of Emergency Medicine, 58*(1), S96–S103. doi:10.1016/j.annemergmed.2011.03.017

Herbst, J. H., Jacobs, E. D., Finlayson, T. J., McKleroy, V. S., Neumann, M. S., & Crepaz, N. (2008). Estimating HIV prevalence and risk behaviors of transgender persons in the United States: A systematic review. *AIDS and Behavior, 12*(1), 1–17. doi:10.1007/s10461-007-9299-3

Herrick, A. L., Lim, S. H., Plankey, M. W., Chmiel, J. S., Guadamuz, T. E., Guadamuz, T. T.,...Stall, R. (2013). Adversity and syndemic production among men participating in the multicenter AIDS cohort study: A life-course approach. *American Journal of Public Health, 103*(1), 79–85. doi:10.2105/ajph.2012.300810

Hess, K., Hu, X., Lansky, A., Mermin, J., & Hall, H. I. (2016, February). Estimating the lifetime risk of a diagnosis of HIV infection in the United States (Abstract 52). Paper presented at the Conference on Retroviruses and Opportunistic Infections (CROI), Boston, MA.

Hickson, F., Tomlin, K., Hargreaves, J., Bonell, C., Reid, D., & Weatherburn, P. (2015). Internet-based cohort study of HIV testing over 1 year among men who have sex with men living in England and exposed to a social marketing intervention promoting testing. *Sexually Transmitted Infections, 91*(1), 24–30. doi:10.1136/sextrans-2014-051598

Hogben, M., Paffel, J., Broussard, D., Wolf, W., Kenney, K., Rubin, S., George, D., & Samoff, E. (2005). Syphilis partner notification with men who have sex with men: A review and commentary. *Sexually Transmitted Diseases, 32*(10), S43–S47. doi:10.1097/01.olq.0000180565.54023.bf

Hoots, B. E., Finlayson, T., Nerlander, L., & Paz-Bailey, G. (2016). Willingness to take, use of, and indications for pre-exposure prophylaxis among men who have sex with Men—20 US Cities, 2014. *Clinical Infectious Diseases, 63*(5), 672–677. doi:10.1093/cid/ciw367

Horvath, K. J., Bowen, A. M., & Williams, M. L. (2006). Virtual and physical venues as contexts for HIV risk among rural men who have sex with men. *Health Psychology, 25*(2), 237–242.

Horvath, K. J., Carrico, A. W., Simoni, J., Boyer, E. W., Amico, K. R., & Petroll, A. E. (2013). Engagement in HIV medical care and technology use among stimulant-using and non-stimulant-using men who have sex with men. *AIDS Research and Treatment, 2013*, 121352. doi:10.1155/2013/121352

Horvath, K. J., Meyer, C., & Rosser, B. R. (2016). Men who have sex with men who believe that their state has a HIV criminal law report higher condomless anal sex than those who are unsure of the law in their state. *AIDS and Behavior, 21*(1), 51–58. doi:10.1007/s10461-016-1286-0

Horvath, K. J., Oakes, J. M., Rosser, B. R., Danilenko, G., Vezina, H., Amico, K. R.,...Simoni, J. (2013). Feasibility, acceptability and preliminary efficacy of an online peer-to-peer social support ART adherence intervention. *AIDS and Behavior, 17*(6), 2031–2044. doi:10.1007/s10461-013-0469-1

Hunter, P., Oyervides, O., Grande, K. M., Prater, D., Vann, V., Reitl, I., & Biedrzycki, P. A. (2014). Facebook-augmented partner notification in a cluster of syphilis cases in Milwaukee. *Public Health Reports, 129* (Suppl. 1), 43–49.

Hwahng, S. J., & Nuttbrock, L. (2014). Adolescent gender-related abuse, androphilia, and HIV risk among transfeminine people of color in New York City. *Journal of Homosexuality, 61*(5), 691–713. doi:10.1080/00918369.2014.870439

Jeffries, W. L., Townsend, E. S., Gelaude, D. J., Torrone, E. A., Gasiorowicz, M., & Bertolli, J. (2015). HIV stigma experienced by young men who have sex with men (MSM) living with HIV infection. *AIDS Education and Prevention, 27*(1), 58–71. doi:10.1521/aeap.2015.27.1.58

Jenness, S. M., Goodreau, S. M., Rosenberg, E., Beylerian, E. N., Hoover, K. W., Smith, D. K., & Sullivan, P. (2016). Impact of the Centers for Disease Control's HIV preexposure prophylaxis guidelines for men who have sex with men in the United States. *Journal of Infectious Diseases, 214*(12), 1800–1807.

Jones, A. R., & Hoyler, C. L. (2006). HIV/AIDS among women who have sex with women. In F. Fernandez and P. Ruiz (Eds.), *Psychiatric Aspects of HIV/AIDS* (pp. 299–307). Philadelphia, PA: Lippincott Williams & Wilkins Publishers.

Kashuba, A. D., Gengiah, T. N., Werner, L., Yang, K. H., White, N. R., Karim, Q. A., & Abdool Karim, S. S. (2015). Genital tenofovir concentrations correlate with protection against HIV infection in the CAPRISA 004 trial: Importance of adherence for microbicide effectiveness. *Journal of Acquired Immune Deficiency Syndromes, 69*(3), 264–269. doi:10.1097/qai.0000000000000607

Katz, D. A., Dombrowski, J. C., Bell, T. R., Kerani, R. P., & Golden, M. R. (2016). HIV incidence among men who have sex with men after diagnosis with sexually transmitted infections. *Sexually Transmitted Diseases, 43*(4), 249–254. doi:10.1097/olq.0000000000000423

Kelley, C. F., Vaughan, A. S., Luisi, N., Sanchez, T. H., Salazar, L. F., Frew, P. M., … Rosenberg, E. S. (2015). The effect of high rates of bacterial sexually transmitted infections on HIV incidence in a cohort of Black and White men who have sex with men in Atlanta, Georgia. *AIDS Research and Human Retroviruses, 31*(6), 587–592. doi:10.1089/aid.2015.0013

Kenagy, G. P., & Hsieh, C. M. (2005). The risk less known: Female-to-male transgender persons' vulnerability to HIV infection. *AIDS Care, 17*(2), 195–207. doi:10.1080/19540120512331325680

Kent, C. K., Chaw, J. K., Wong, W., Liska, S., Gibson, S., Hubbard, G., & Klausner, J. D. (2005). Prevalence of rectal, urethral, and pharyngeal chlamydia and gonorrhea detected in 2 clinical settings among men who have sex with men: San Francisco, California, 2005. *Clinical Infectious Diseases, 41*(1), 67–74. doi:10.1086/430704

Kerr, D. L., Ding, K., & Thompson, A. J. (2013). A comparison of lesbian, bisexual, and heterosexual female college undergraduate students on selected reproductive health screenings and sexual behaviors. *Women's Health Issues, 23*(6), e347–e355. doi:10.1016/j.whi.2013.09.003

Khosropour, C. M., Dombrowski, J. C., Swanson, F., Kerani, R. P., Katz, D. A., Barbee, L. A., … Golden, M. R. (2016). Trends in serosorting and the association with HIV/STI risk over time among men who have sex with men. *Journal of Acquired Immune Deficiency Syndromes, 72*(2), 189–197. doi:10.1097/qai.0000000000000947

Khosropour, C. M., & Sullivan, P. S. (2013). Receipt and use of free condoms among US men who have sex with men. *Public Health Reports, 128*(5), 385–392.

Kidder, D. P., Wolitski, R. J., Pals, S. L., & Campsmith, M. L. (2008). Housing status and HIV risk behaviors among homeless and housed persons with HIV. *Journal of Acquired Immune Deficiency Syndromes, 49*(4), 451–455.

Klausner, J. D., Kent, C. K., Wong, W., McCright, J., & Katz, M. H. (2005). The public health response to epidemic syphilis: San Francisco, 1999–2004. *Sexually Transmitted Diseases, 32*(10), S11–S18. doi:10.1097/01.olq.0000180456.15861.92

Klein, H. (2009). Differences in HIV risk practices sought by self-identified gay and bisexual men who use internet websites to identify potential sexual partners. *Journal of Bisexuality, 9*(2), 125–140. doi:10.1080/15299710902881533

Knight, V., Ryder, N., Guy, R., Lu, H., Wand, H., & McNulty, A. (2013). New Xpress sexually transmissible infection screening clinic improves patient journey and clinic capacity at a large sexual health clinic. *Sexually Transmitted Diseases, 40*(1), 75–80. doi:10.1097/OLQ.0b013e3182793700

Koh, A. S., Gómez, C. A., Shade, S., & Rowley, E. (2005). Sexual risk factors among self-identified lesbians, bisexual women, and heterosexual women accessing primary care settings. *Sexually Transmitted Diseases, 32*(9), 563–569.

Koop, C. E. (2011). The early days of AIDS, as I remember them. *Annals of the Forum for Collaborative HIV Research, 13*(2), 5–10.

Lecher, S. L., Hollis, N., Lehmann, C., Hoover, K. W., Jones, A., & Belcher, L. (2016). Evaluation of the impact of National HIV Testing Day: United States, 2011–2014. *Morbidity and Mortality Weekly Report, 65*(24), 613–618. doi:10.15585/mmwr.mm6524a2

LeGrand, S., Muessig, K. E., McNulty, T., Soni, K., Knudtson, K., Lemann, A.,...Hightow-Weidman, L. B. (2016). Epic Allies: Development of a gaming app to improve antiretroviral therapy adherence among young HIV-positive men who have sex with men. *JMIR Serious Games, 4*(1), e6. doi:10.2196/games.5687

Lehman, J. S., Carr, M. H., Nichol, A. J., Ruisanchez, A., Knight, D. W., Langford, A. E.,...Mermin, J. H. (2014). Prevalence and public health implications of state laws that criminalize potential HIV exposure in the United States. *AIDS and Behavior, 18*(6), 997–1006. doi:10.1007/s10461-014-0724-0

Leibowitz, A. A., Harawa, N., Sylla, M., Hallstrom, C. C., & Kerndt, P. R. (2013). Condom distribution in jail to prevent HIV infection. *AIDS and Behavior, 17*(8), 2695–2702. doi:10.1007/s10461-012-0190-5

Lelutiu-Weinberger, C., Pachankis, J. E., Golub, S. A., Walker, J. J., Bamonte, A. J., & Parsons, J. T. (2013). Age cohort differences in the effects of gay-related stigma, anxiety and identification with the gay community on sexual risk and substance use. *AIDS and Behavior, 17*(1), 340–349. doi:10.1007/s10461-011-0070-4

Lewis, M. A., Uhrig, J. D., Bann, C. M., Harris, J. L., Furberg, R. D., Coomes, C., & Kuhns, L. M. (2013). Tailored text messaging intervention for HIV adherence: A proof-of-concept study. *Health Psychology, 32*(3), 248–253. doi:10.1037/a0028109

Liu, A. Y., Cohen, S. E., Vittinghoff, E., Anderson, P. L., Doblecki-Lewis, S., Bacon, O.,...Kolber, M. A. (2016). Preexposure prophylaxis for HIV infection integrated with municipal- and community-based sexual health services. *JAMA Internal Medicine, 176*(1), 75–84. doi:10.1001/jamainternmed.2015.4683

Liu, A. Y., Glidden, D. V., Anderson, P. L., Amico, K. R., McMahan, V., Mehrotra, M.,...Grant, R. (2014). Patterns and correlates of PrEP drug detection among MSM and transgender women in the Global iPrEx Study. *Journal of Acquired Immune Deficiency Syndromes, 67*(5), 528–537. doi:10.1097/qai.0000000000000351

Liu, A. Y., Hessol, N. A., Vittinghoff, E., Amico, K. R., Kroboth, E., Fuchs, J.,...Buchbinder, S. P. (2014). Medication adherence among men who have sex with men at risk for HIV infection in the United States: Implications for pre-exposure prophylaxis implementation. *AIDS Patient Care STDs, 28*(12), 622–627. doi:10.1089/apc.2014.0195

Lloyd, S., & Operario, D. (2012). HIV risk among men who have sex with men who have experienced childhood sexual abuse: Systematic review and meta-analysis. *AIDS Education and Prevention, 24*(3), 228–241. doi:10.1521/aeap.2012.24.3.228

Martin, L., Knight, V., Ryder, N., Lu, H., Read, P. J., & McNulty, A. (2013). Client feedback and satisfaction with an express sexually transmissible infection screening service at an inner-city sexual health center. *Sexually Transmitted Diseases, 40*(1), 70–74. doi:10.1097/OLQ.0b013e318275343b

Mayer, K. H. (2011). Sexually transmitted diseases in men who have sex with men. *Clinical Infectious Diseases, 53*(Suppl. 3), S79–S83. doi:10.1093/cid/cir696

Melendez-Torres, G. J., Nye, E., & Bonell, C. (2016). Is location of sex associated with sexual risk behaviour in men who have sex with men? Systematic review of within-subjects studies. *AIDS and Behavior, 20*(6), 1219–1227. doi:10.1007/s10461-015-1093-z

Meyer, I. H. (2003). Prejudice, social stress, and mental health in lesbian, gay, and bisexual populations: Conceptual issues and research evidence. *Psychological Bulletin, 129*(5), 674–697.

Millett, G. A., Flores, S. A., Peterson, J. L., & Bakeman, R. (2007). Explaining disparities in HIV infection among Black and White men who have sex with men: A meta-analysis of HIV risk behaviors. *AIDS, 21*(15), 2083–2091. doi:10.1097/QAD.0b013e3282e9a64b

Mitchell, J. W., & Horvath, K. J. (2013). Factors associated with regular HIV testing among a sample of US MSM with HIV-negative main partners. *Journal of Acquired Immune Deficiency Syndromes, 64*(4), 417–423. doi:10.1097/QAI.0b013e3182a6c8d9

Mojola, S. A., & Everett, B. (2012). STD and HIV risk factors among US young adults: Variations by gender, race, ethnicity and sexual orientation. *Perspectives on Sexual and Reproductive Health, 44*(2), 125–133. doi:10.1363/4412512

Moskowitz, D. A., Seal, D. W., Rintamaki, L., & Rieger, G. (2011). HIV in the leather community: Rates and risk-related behaviors. *AIDS and Behavior, 15*(3), 557–564. doi:10.1007/s10461-009-9636-9

Mugavero, M. J., Amico, K. R., Horn, T., & Thompson, M. A. (2013). The state of engagement in HIV care in the United States: From cascade to continuum to control. *Clinical Infectious Diseases, 57*(8), 1164–1171. doi:10.1093/cid/cit420

Mustanski, B., Garofalo, R., Herrick, A., & Donenberg, G. (2007). Psychosocial health problems increase risk for HIV among urban young men who have sex with men: Preliminary evidence of a syndemic in need of attention. *Annals of Behavioral Medicine, 34*(1), 37–45. doi:10.1080/08836610701495268

National Alliance to End Homelessness. (2006). Fact sheet: Homelessness and HIV/AIDS. Retrieved from http://www.endhomelessness.org/library/entry/fact-sheet-homelessness-and-hiv-aids

Nemoto, T., Operario, D., Keatley, J., Han, L., & Soma, T. (2004). HIV risk behaviors among male-to-female transgender persons of color in San Francisco. *American Journal of Public Health, 94*(7), 1193–1199.

Office of Women's Health, U.S. Department of Health and Human Services (2009). Lesbian and bisexual health fact sheet. Retrieved from https://www.womenshealth.gov/publications/our-publications/fact-sheet/lesbian-bisexual-health.html

Operario, D., Yang, M.-F., Reisner, S. L., Iwamoto, M., & Nemoto, T. (2014). Stigma and the syndemic of HIV–related health risk behaviors in a diverse sample of transgender women. *Journal of Community Psychology, 42*(5), 544–557. doi:10.1002/jcop.21636

Oster, A. M., Pieniazek, D., Zhang, X., Switzer, W. M., Ziebell, R. A., Mena, L. A., . . . Heffelfinger, J. D. (2011). Demographic but not geographic insularity in HIV transmission among young Black MSM. *AIDS, 25*(17), 2157–2165. doi:10.1097/QAD.0b013e32834bfde9

Pathela, P., Jamison, K., Braunstein, S. L., Schillinger, J. A., Varma, J. K., & Blank, S. (2017). Incidence and predictors of HIV infection among men who have sex with men attending public sexually transmitted disease clinics, New York City, 2007–2012. *AIDS and Behavior, 21*(5), 1444–1451. doi:10.1007/s10461-016-1499-2

Patton, M. E., Kidd, S., Llata, E., Stenger, M., Braxton, J., Asbel, L., . . . Weinstock, H. (2014). Extragenital gonorrhea and chlamydia testing and infection among men who have sex with men: STD Surveillance Network, United States, 2010–2012. *Clinical Infectious Diseases, 58*(11), 1564–1570. doi:10.1093/cid/ciu184

Patton, M. E., Su, J. R., Nelson, R., & Weinstock, H. (2014). Primary and secondary syphilis: United States, 2005–2013. *Morbidity and Mortality Weekly Report, 63*(18), 402–406.

Phillips-Guzman, C. M., Martinez-Donate, A. P., Hovell, M. F., Blumberg, E. J., Sipan, C. L., Rovniak, L. S., & Kelley, N. J. (2011). Engaging local businesses in HIV prevention efforts: The consumer perspective. *Health Promotion Practice, 12*(4), 620–629. doi:10.1177/1524839909343166

Przybyla, S. M., Golin, C. E., Widman, L., Grodensky, C. A., Earp, J. A., & Suchindran, C. (2013). Serostatus disclosure to sexual partners among people living with HIV: Examining the roles of partner characteristics and stigma. *AIDS Care, 25*(5), 566–572.

Reisner, S. L., Mimiaga, M., Case, P., Grasso, C., O'Brien, C. T., Harigopal, P.,...Mayer, K. H. (2010). Sexually transmitted disease (STD) diagnoses and mental health disparities among women who have sex with women screened at an urban community health center, Boston, Massachusetts, 2007. *Sexually Transmitted Diseases, 37*(1), 5–12. doi:10.1097/OLQ.0b013e3181b41314

Reisner, S. L., Perkovich, B., & Mimiaga, M. J. (2010). A mixed methods study of the sexual health needs of New England transmen who have sex with nontransgender men. *AIDS Patient Care and STDs, 24*(8), 501–513.

Reisner, S. L., Poteat, T., Keatley, J., Cabral, M., Mothopeng, T., Dunham, E.,...Baral, S. D. (2016). Global health burden and needs of transgender populations: A review. *Lancet, 388*(10042), 412–436. doi:10.1016/s0140-6736(16)00684-x

Reisner, S. L., Vetters, R., White, J. M., Cohen, E. L., LeClerc, M., Zaslow, S.,..., Mimiaga, M. J. (2015). Laboratory-confirmed HIV and sexually transmitted infection seropositivity and risk behavior among sexually active transgender patients at an adolescent and young adult urban community health center. *AIDS Care, 27*(8), 1031–1036. doi:10.1080/09540121.2015.1020750

Reisner, S. L., White, J. M., Mayer, K. H., & Mimiaga, M. J. (2014). Sexual risk behaviors and psychosocial health concerns of female-to-male transgender men screening for STDs at an urban community health center. *AIDS Care, 26*(7), 857–864. doi:10.1080/09540121.2013.855701

Reiter, P. L., & McRee, A. L. (2017). HPV infection among a population-based sample of sexual minority women from USA. *Sexually Transmitted Infections, 93*(1), 25–31.

Renaud, T. C., Bocour, A., Irvine, M. K., Bernstein, K. T., Begier, E. M., Sepkowitz, K. A.,...Weglein, D. (2009). The free condom initiative: Promoting condom availability and use in New York City. *Public Health Reports, 124*(4), 481–489.

Rhodes, S. D., Vissman, A. T., Stowers, J., Miller, C., McCoy, T. P., Hergenrather, K. C.,...Eng, E. (2011). A CBPR partnership increases HIV testing among men who have sex with men (MSM): Outcome findings from a pilot test of the CyBER/testing internet intervention. *Health Education & Behavior, 38*(3), 311–320. doi:10.1177/1090198110379572

Rodger, A. J., Cambiano, V., Bruun, T., Vernazza, P., Collins, S., van Lunzen, J.,...Lundgren, J. (2016). Sexual activity without condoms and risk of HIV transmission in serodifferent couples when the HIV-positive partner is using suppressive antiretroviral therapy. *Journal of the American Medical Association, 316*(2), 171–181. doi:10.1001/jama.2016.5148

Rothman, R. E., Ketlogetswe, K. S., Dolan, T., Wyer, P. C., & Kelen, G. D. (2003). Preventive care in the emergency department: Should emergency departments conduct routine HIV screening? A systematic review. *Academic Emergency Medicine, 10*(3), 278–285.

Rovniak, L. S., Hovell, M. F., Hofstetter, C. R., Blumberg, E. J., Sipan, C. L., Batista, M. F.,...Ayala, G. X. (2010). Engaging community businesses in human immunodeficiency virus prevention: A feasibility study. *American Journal of Health Promotion, 24*(5), 347–353. doi:10.4278/ajhp.080721-ARB-129

Rowniak, S., & Chesla, C. (2013). Coming out for a third time: Transmen, sexual orientation, and identity. *Archives of Sexual Behavior, 42*(3), 449–461. doi:10.1007/s10508-012-0036-2

Sayles, J. N., Wong, M. D., Kinsler, J. J., Martins, D., & Cunningham, W. E. (2009). The association of stigma with self-reported access to medical care and antiretroviral therapy adherence in persons living with HIV/AIDS. *Journal of General Internal Medicine, 24*(10), 1101–1108. doi:10.1007/s11606-009-1068-8

Scott, H. M., Vittinghoff, E., Irvin, R., Sachdev, D., Liu, A., Gurwith, M., & Buchbinder, S. P. (2014). Age, race/ethnicity, and behavioral risk factors associated with per contact risk of HIV infection among men who have sex with men in the United States. *Journal of Acquired Immune Deficiency Syndromes, 65*(1), 115–121. doi:10.1097/QAI.0b013e3182a98bae

Sevelius, J. (2009). "There's no pamphlet for the kind of sex I have": HIV-related risk factors and protective behaviors among transgender men who have sex with nontransgender men. *Journal of the Association of Nurses in AIDS Care, 20*(5), 398–410. doi:10.1016/j.jana.2009.06.001

Sidibé, M. (2016). Charting a path to end the AIDS epidemic. *Bulletin of the World Health Organization, 94*(6), 408. doi:10.2471/blt.16.176875

Singh, D., Fine, D. N., & Marrazzo, J. M. (2011). Chlamydia trachomatis infection among women reporting sexual activity with women screened in Family Planning Clinics in the Pacific Northwest, 1997 to 2005. *American Journal of Public Health, 101*(7), 1284–1290. doi:10.2105/AJPH.2009.169631

Skarbinski, J., Rosenberg, E., Paz-Bailey, G., Hall, H. I., Rose, C. E., Viall, A. H.,...Mermin, J. H. (2015). Human immunodeficiency virus transmission at each step of the care continuum in the United States. *JAMA Internal Medicine, 175*(4), 588–596. doi:10.1001/jamainternmed.2014.8180

Smit, P. J., Brady, M., Carter, M., Fernandes, R., Lamore, L., Meulbroek, M.,...Thompson, M. (2012). HIV-related stigma within communities of gay men: A literature review. *AIDS Care, 24*(3–4), 405–412. doi:10.1080/09540121.2011.613910

Smith, A. M., Grierson, J., Wain, D., Pitts, M., & Pattison, P. (2004). Associations between the sexual behaviour of men who have sex with men and the structure and composition of their social networks. *Sexually Transmitted Infections, 80*(6), 455–458. doi:10.1136/sti.2004.010355

Snowden, J. M., Chen, Y. H., McFarland, W., & Raymond, H. F. (2017). Prevalence and characteristics of users of pre-exposure prophylaxis (PrEP) among men who have sex with men, San Francisco, 2014 in a cross-sectional survey: Implications for disparities. *Sexually Transmitted Infections, 93*(1), 52–55. doi:10.1136/sextrans-2015-052382

Subhrajit, C. (2014). Problems faced by LGBT people in the mainstream society: Some recommendations. *International Journal of Interdisciplinary and Multidisciplinary Studies, 1*(5), 317–331.

Sun, C. J., Stowers, J., Miller, C., Bachmann, L. H., & Rhodes, S. D. (2015). Acceptability and feasibility of using established geosocial and sexual networking mobile applications to promote HIV and STD testing among men who have sex with men. *AIDS and Behavior, 19*(3), 543–552. doi:10.1007/s10461-014-0942-5

Taylor, M. M., Aynalem, G., Olea, L. M., He, P., Smith, L. V., & Kerndt, P. R. (2008). A consequence of the syphilis epidemic among men who have sex with men (MSM): Neurosyphilis in Los Angeles, 2001–2004. *Sexually Transmitted Diseases, 35*(5), 430–434. doi:10.1097/OLQ.0b013e3181644b5e

Ubrihien, A., Davies, S. C., & Driscoll, T. (2016). Is cost a structural barrier preventing men who have sex with men accessing condoms? A systematic review. *AIDS Care, 28*(11), 1473–1480. doi:10.1080/09540121.2016.1189999

UNAIDS. (2016). Global AIDS update, 2016. Retrieved from http://www.who.int/hiv/pub/arv/global-AIDS-update-2016_en.pdf?ua=1

UNAIDS Special Analysis. (2016). AIDS by the numbers: AIDS is not over, but it can be. Retrieved from http://www.unaids.org/en/resources/documents/2016/AIDS-by-the-numbers

van de Laar, T. J., Matthews, G. V., Prins, M., & Danta, M. (2010). Acute hepatitis C in HIV-infected men who have sex with men: An emerging sexually transmitted infection. *AIDS, 24*(12), 1799–1812. doi:10.1097/QAD.0b013e32833c11a5

Van Handel, M., & Mulatu, M. S. (2014). Effectiveness of the U.S. national HIV testing day campaigns in promoting HIV testing: Evidence from CDC-funded HIV testing sites, 2010. *Public Health Reports, 129*(5), 446–454.

Volk, J. E., Marcus, J. L., Phengrasamy, T., Blechinger, D., Nguyen, D. P., Follansbee, S., & Hare, C. B. (2015). No new HIV infections with increasing use of HIV preexposure prophylaxis in a clinical practice setting. *Clinical Infectious Diseases, 61*(10), 1601–1603. doi:10.1093/cid/civ778

White Hughto, J. M., Reisner, S. L., & Pachankis, J. E. (2015). Transgender stigma and health: A critical review of stigma determinants, mechanisms, and interventions. *Social Science & Medicine, 147*, 222–231. doi:10.1016/j.socscimed.2015.11.010

Women's Institute (2009). *HIV risk for lesbians, bisexuals, & other women who have sex with women.* New York, NY: Women's Institute at Gay Men's Health Crisis. Retrieved from http://www.gmhc.org/files/editor/file/GMHC_lap_whitepaper_0609.pdf

Wong, C. F., Schrager, S. M., Chou, C. P., Weiss, G., & Kipke, M. D. (2013). Changes in developmental contexts as predictors of transitions in HIV-risk behaviors among young men who have sex with men (YMSM). *American Journal of Community Psychology, 51*(3–4), 439–450. doi:10.1007/s10464-012-9562-2

Wong, W., Chaw, J. K., Kent, C. K., & Klausner, J. D. (2005). Risk factors for early syphilis among gay and bisexual men seen in an STD clinic: San Francisco, 2002–2003. *Sexually Transmitted Diseases, 32*(7), 458–463.

Workowski, K. A., & Bolan, G. A. (2015). Sexually transmitted diseases treatment guidelines, 2015. *MMWR Recommendations and Reports, 64*(3), 1–137.

World Health Organization. (2013). Global update on HIV treatment 2013: Results, impact, and opportunities. Retrieved from http://www.unaids.org/sites/default/files/sub_landing/files/20130630_treatment_report_en_3.pdf

World Health Organization. (2015). Global summary of the AIDS epidemic, 2015. Retrieved from http://www.who.int/hiv/data/epi_core_2016.png?ua=1

World Health Organization. (2016). Consolidated guidelines on the use of antiretroviral drugs for treating and preventing HIV infection: Recommendations for a public health approach. Retrieved from http://apps.who.int/iris/bitstream/10665/208825/1/9789241549684_eng.pdf?ua=1

Xu, F., Sternberg, M. R., & Markowitz, L. E. (2010a). Men who have sex with men in the United States: Demographic and behavioral characteristics and prevalence of HIV and HSV-2 infection: Results from National Health and Nutrition Examination Survey 2001–2006. *Sexually Transmitted Diseases, 37*(6), 399–405. doi:10.1097/OLQ.0b013e3181ce122b

Xu, F., Sternberg, M. R., & Markowitz, L. E. (2010b). Women who have sex with women in the United States: Prevalence, sexual behavior and prevalence of herpes simplex virus type 2 infection: Results from National Health and Nutrition Examination Survey 2001–2006. *Sexually Transmitted Diseases, 37*(7), 407–413. doi:10.1097/OLQ.0b013e3181db2e18

Young, S. D., Swendeman, D., Holloway, I. W., Reback, C. J., & Kao, U. (2015). Use of technology to address substance use in the context of HIV: A systematic review. *Current HIV/AIDS Reports, 12*(4), 462–471. doi:10.1007/s11904-015-0295-3

SECTION ▌▌▌

SPECIAL CONSIDERATIONS FOR SPECIFIC GROUPS

CHAPTER **14**

Gender Minority Health: Affirmative Care for the Community

lore m. dickey and Colt Keo-Meier

Health care is typically considered to be a basic human right; however, there are many groups of people who are not able to avail themselves of this right. One such group is transgender and gender diverse people, referred to throughout this chapter as "gender minority people" (see Chapter 1 for an in-depth discussion of terminology; we acknowledge variations in terms used for gender diverse individuals exist and have selected terminology consistent with the remainder of this text). As the gender and sexual minority (GSM) group that faces the highest levels of discrimination and even violence, gender minority people face magnified pressures that impact a variety of health behaviors and outcomes even beyond their cisgender sexual minority counterparts (Conron, Mimiaga, & Landers, 2010; dickey, Budge, Katz-Wise, & Garza, 2016). In this chapter we will explore the health care needs of gender minority adolescents and adults, address the ways in which providers can engage in competent care, discuss the known health risks for gender minority people, and elucidate additional health care concerns such as insurance coverage.

This chapter is not intended to provide basic information about the identities of gender minority people; there are other resources that cover this material in detail (American Psychological Association, 2015; Carroll, 2010; Lev, 2004; Singh & dickey, 2017; Vanderburgh, 2007). However, it is important to cover several terms to assure understanding for the reader. We use the term *gender minority* to be as broadly inclusive as possible to capture all people for whom their gender identity or gender expression varies from the binary sex they were assigned at birth. This includes people who identify as transgender, transsexual, cross-dresser, nonbinary, genderqueer, and gender fluid. The last terms may be unfamiliar to some readers and merit further attention. Historically, gender minority people were expected to either live life as the sex assigned at birth or to transition that sex to their "true" binary gender (e.g., male to female). These expectations relate in large part to the majority of U.S. society assuming that there are only two gender or sex options (e.g., masculine and feminine or male and female). However, we know that gender minority people do not necessarily identify with the gender binary and may use terms like *genderqueer* to affirm their[1] nonbinary identity (i.e., an identification with aspects of both binary genders, or a fluid gender identity that at times may be more in line with one gender, but at times with the other). We also know that although these terms may seem new, "out of the binary" identities have existed throughout history in many different cultures (Herdt, 1996).

We recognize that the health and health care needs of gender minority individuals extend well beyond the transition process, and also recognize that many gender minority individuals either have not yet or never will engage in medically assisted transitioning. Unfortunately, there is very little known regarding the larger health needs of gender minority individuals, as the field of gender minority health is still in its infancy. As a result, throughout this chapter we will address primarily the needs of gender minority people who are making a medical transition (involving some combination of hormone treatment and/or surgical care). We will also attempt to summarize the limited literature regarding the broader health care needs of gender minority individuals, again with the caveat that the literature is still quite undeveloped.

A final concept that we would like to define is the meaning of "affirmative care." Singh and dickey (2017) define affirmative care as care which is "culturally-relevant for [gender minority] clients and their multiple social identities, addresses the influence of social inequities on the lives of [gender minority] clients, enhances the [gender minority] client resilience and coping, advocates to reduce systemic barriers to [gender minority] mental and physical health, and leverages [gender minority] client strengths" (p. 4). The Gender Affirmative Model (Hidalgo et al., 2013) presents premises including that gender variations are not disorders and, if there is pathology, it commonly stems from the culture's reaction to the person rather than from within the person. Many gender minority individuals have reported horrific and traumatizing experiences with their health care providers (Grant et al., 2011), to the point that some gender minority people have refused to access care due to fear of stigmatization (dickey, Budge, et al., 2016). If health care is intended to be a basic human right, then much work is needed to assure that providers are clinically and culturally competent to work with their gender minority patients.

---

[1] We will use "their" as a pronoun for singular or plural purposes. The singular use of 'their' acknowledges that some TGD people do not identify with the gender binary and therefore use pronouns that do not reify it (American Psychological Association, 2015).

■ GENDER MINORITY ADOLESCENT HEALTH

The experiences of gender minority adolescents are unique in their gender and sexual orientation identity development processes, medical transition options available to them, and open school attendance. Many gender minority youth disclose their gender identity in early childhood, the same time that cisgender youth's gender identities develop (early onset gender dysphoria; J. Olson, Forbes, & Belzer, 2011). However, some do not discover their gender minority identity until puberty (pubertal-onset gender dysphoria). Gender diverse and transgender youth are not part of a "new" phenomenon. History suggests that they have existed in a wide range of cultures for thousands of years (Herdt, 1996). Youth's sense of their internal gender is not caused by anything a family member did or did not do (Substance Abuse and Mental Health Services Administration [SAMHSA], 2015). Importantly, by adolescence, one's gender identity is resistant to any type of environmental intervention (American Psychological Association, 2013a; 2013b; SAMHSA, 2015).

Sexual orientation is thought to develop between childhood and adolescence, around ages 7 and 9 years (Savin-Williams & Cohen, 2007), typically after gender identity (J. Olson et al., 2011). When providers meet with gender minority youth, they assess both gender and sexual orientation development as well as the youth's understanding of these concepts as separate, but interrelated (American Psychological Association, 2015). A small group of researchers studying the persistence of gender minority identities through childhood claims that the majority of these youth will not persist with their gender minority identities from childhood through adolescence and adulthood (Steensma, McGuire, Kreukels, Beekman, & Cohen-Kettenis, 2013). Their data, based on youth who meet *DSM-IV-TR's* Gender Identity Disorder criteria (American Psychiatric Association, 2000), finds that youth who meet these criteria in childhood are more likely to identify as cisgender gay and bisexual adults. One of the many problems with their methodology is that they measured both nonconforming gender expression and gender identity and they did not follow up with the participants to measure diverse gender expression in adulthood (Ehrensaft, 2016). Additionally, they assumed that if a person did not return for care after initial consultation, they did not maintain a gender diverse identity (American Psychological Association, 2015); therefore, they were classified as "desisters."

If adolescents' gender dysphoria and/or gender minority identity persists through the beginning of puberty and their sexual orientation development process, they are much more likely to continue identifying as transgender through adulthood (Edwards-Leeper, 2017; Edwards-Leeper, Leibowitz, & Sangganjanavanich, 2016). Initial clinical observations have noticed that youth who do not have a history of childhood nonconforming gender expressions and discover their gender minority identity at the onset of puberty are also more likely to identify as sexual minorities (e.g., queer, pansexual, lesbian, gay, bisexual) than youth with early onset gender dysphoria who identify mostly as heterosexual (Keo-Meier, 2015). This can be very confusing to parents and untrained providers. It is common for parents to ask providers questions similar to the following: "My 15-year-old daughter who has never shown the signs of being transgender just told me that she is a gay male; is that even possible?" It is possible and more common than most would expect. The adolescent may very well have a male gender identity and be sexually attracted to men.

Pubertal Suppression

Pubertal suppression is a unique medical option that may be appropriate for some gender minority adolescents. This intervention has been used in children with pre-cocious puberty who showed signs of puberty in young childhood (J. Olson et al., 2011). The medication is a gonadotropin-releasing hormone (GnRH) agonist that works by pausing the process of puberty. This intervention in transgender youth began to be used in a Dutch gender clinic (Delemarre-van de Waal & Cohen-Kettenis, 2008). Candidates for this treatment are periadolescents who have recently shown the first signs of puberty. Medical providers can determine this by examining the patient's Tanner stage (Hembree et al., 2009; Spack et al., 2012). All people start out at Tanner stage 1; once initial pubic hairs appear, breast buds develop, and penis and testicles begin to grow, adolescents start moving through the Tanner stages, one at a time (Erickson-Scroth, Gilbert, & Smith, 2014). Once they reach Tanner stage 5, they are said to have completed puberty. The ideal time to begin pubertal suppression is once the initial signs of puberty occur, Tanner stage 2. Once an adolescent is through puberty, pubertal suppression is no longer an option.

Pubertal suppression is completely reversible and can be a life-saving intervention (e.g., reduced risk for anxiety, depression, and substance abuse; Edwards-Leeper & Spack, 2012; J. Olson, Schrager, Belzer, Simons, & Clark, 2015; Steensma, Kreukels, de Vries, & Coehn-Kettenis, 2013). Once adolescents begin pubertal suppression, they are followed up by their provider(s) to assess their gender identity and ideas about which puberty they desire to go through (i.e., feminizing or masculinizing; Deutsch, 2016). This can be a challenging task for youth who identify outside of the gender binary, as everyone has to go through at least one puberty. Youth with early onset gender dysphoria whose gender minority identity persists through the initial stages of puberty are more likely than not to persist in their identity and desire a puberty different than their endogenous puberty (Edwards-Leeper et al., 2016; Steensma, Kreukels, et al., 2013; Steensma, McGuire, et al., 2013). Medical providers work with the youth and family to determine when to begin hormone therapy. If the youth's gender minority identity desists, they have the option to stop the puberty blocking medication and resume their endogenous puberty (Edwards-Leeper et al., 2016). Recent research indicates that once transgender youth begin blocking medication, they almost always later begin hormone therapy and go through the puberty congruent with their affirmed gender identity (Carmichael, 2016).

The benefits of pubertal suppression followed by hormone treatment (e.g., going through only one puberty) are numerous and supported in the literature (Edwards-Leeper et al., 2016; Hidalgo et al., 2013; Steensma, Kreukels, et al., 2013; Steensma, McGuire, et al., 2013). This treatment stops unwanted endoge-nous pubertal development, thereby limiting the experience of going through an incongruent puberty. It also brings a sense of reassurance to youth who dread going through their endogenous puberty. Gender minority boys and transmasculine youth undergoing pubertal suppression will not experience breast growth and will therefore not need to undergo chest surgery (e.g., top surgery). Gender minority girls and transfeminine youth will not experience masculinization associated with testosterone (e.g., facial and body hair growth, increased muscle mass, lowering the pitch of one's voice, and protrusion of the Adam's apple), which can be debilitating and complicates being seen as they would like to be seen in society. They may also gain the same amount of breast development as they would have if they were a cisgender girl (Deutsch, 2016).

Pubertal suppression followed by hormone therapy typically does not allow for a person to become fertile (dickey, Ducheny, & Ehrbar, 2016). This typically gives parents pause. Most gender minority youth will say that they are not worried about their fertility, that they will consider adoption. They are typically more concerned with their own immediate survival rather than their future ability to have biological children (Ehrensaft, 2016). Youth who begin puberty-blocking medication and decide that they would like to preserve their fertility may decide to discontinue pubertal suppression to continue their endogenous puberty until their egg or sperm development is mature (dickey, Ducheny, & Ehrbar, 2016). For gender minority girls, sperm preservation is typically achieved by obtaining sperm samples through masturbation; however, if gender minority girls are not physically mature enough and/or are too uncomfortable or distressed by the thought of having to masturbate, sperm cells can be surgically retrieved directly from the testes (i.e., testicular sperm extraction [TESE]; Johnson & Finlayson, 2016). The process of harvesting eggs from transgender boys involves major hormone treatment, vaginal ultrasounds, and invasive retrieval processes (dickey, Ducheny, & Ehrbar, 2016). It is also very costly (i.e., upward of $20,000) and insurance rarely covers this process, especially for young patients who are not infertile (dickey, Ducheny, & Ehrbar, 2016).

There are several barriers to accessing puberty-blocking medication. The first is the parental support necessary for consenting for treatment. In some cases, one parent is further along in their support and acceptance of their child than the other is (American Psychological Association, 2015; Edwards-Leeper et al., 2016). Unfortunately, some youth have no parental support and are not legally able to consent for this treatment. Some become eligible for treatment before the age of 10, well before they are able to consent for medical treatment in any state (D. L. Coleman & Rosoff, 2013). Next, many medical providers lack training in pubertal suppression in transgender youth and are either hesitant to prescribe or are unaware that this is a potential treatment option. Another barrier is that many youth and families are not aware of this option, or are aware but do not have a full understanding of the associated benefits, effects, and risks (J. Olson et al., 2011). Finally, the cost of pubertal suppression is rarely covered by health insurance for gender minority youth (J. Olson et al., 2011). Puberty-suppressing implants can range up to $20,000 annually; this includes the cost of the medication and surgical procedure to implant it (Edwards-Leeper & Spack, 2012). There are therefore many barriers to pubertal suppression even beyond willingness, consent, and acceptance which in-and-of themselves are significant barriers for many gender minority adolescents.

Other options exist for gender minority adolescents who are not eligible for pubertal suppression or who cannot access it. Transgender boys who have already started their menstrual cycle may have the option of suppressing it as they are determining if and when to start testosterone treatment (i.e., the menstrual cycle can be suppressed with a different medication that does not block puberty; Deutsch, 2016). This can be particularly useful, especially if the adolescent experiences distress related to the menstrual cycle. Clinical observations by the authors include gender minority boys using nontraditional methods (e.g., bandanas) for managing their menstrual cycle instead of "feminine" hygiene products, not using any methods to catch their blood resulting in blood-stained underwear, and exacerbation of mental health symptoms including self-harm during the menstrual cycle. Transgender girls may have the option of starting an antiandrogen medication, most commonly Spironolactone, to block further masculinization from endogenous testosterone (Hembree et al., 2009). Spironolactone suppresses testosterone, which is not the same as puberty suppression with GnRH treatments. Both of these options can provide a great sense of relief. However, neither treatment option provides the feminization or masculinization that many gender minority adolescents desire.

There is controversy surrounding the age at which gender minority adolescents are allowed to access hormone therapy and surgeries. The Endocrine Society Guidelines (Hembree et al., 2009) recommend waiting until 16 years of age to start hormone therapy. The World Professional Association for Transgender Health (WPATH) Standards of Care (E. Coleman et al., 2012) recommend waiting until age 18 (or age of majority in any given country) before accessing surgical treatment. However, these age restrictions are hotly debated by some of the leading providers in the United States. They argue that there should not be a set age limit that applies to all cases. Rather, they suggest that several factors be taken into account when determining when to start hormone therapy and recommend surgeries in an adolescent. Some of the most important factors frequently discussed include developmental level, severity of gender dysphoria, the patient's desire for particular intervention, as well as relation to the timing of pubertal onset in their peer adolescents at school (J. Olson et al., 2011). Sixteen is very late to start puberty, especially as the average age for onset of puberty among cisgender girls is between 10 and 14 years and among cisgender boys is between 12 and 16 years (MedicineNet, 2016). Considering the strong positive effects of hormone therapy on the health and well-being of transgender people (Keo-Meier et al., 2015), coupled with the great suffering associated with gender dysphoria, withholding hormone therapy based on age may not be in the best interests of many gender minority adolescents. Therefore, it is becoming common practice to start hormone therapy before the age of 16 in gender minority adolescents who understand the effects and risks of hormone therapy and whose parents consent to this treatment. Some surgeons are also beginning to treat adolescents, especially for chest masculinization surgery, which the authors have observed some transgender boys accessing as young as 12 years of age. This is offering extreme relief from attempting to live as a boy with breasts. Although the Endocrine Society and WPATH provide guidelines on age restrictions for treatment, individual providers have the responsibility of assisting families to make treatment decisions with the patient's well-being at the forefront of the decision-making process.

Gender minority adolescents are unique from adults who come out later in life in that they make gender transitions while attending middle and high school. Unfortunately, the majority of transgender youth experience verbal harassment in school from other students as well as teachers and school staff, with few experiences of anyone intervening on their behalf (Kosciw, Greytak, Palmer, & Boesen, 2014; Toomey, Ryan, Diaz, & Russell, 2011). If a student has a trusted staff member on campus, the staff member may be able to address any student concerns, stop experiences of harassment, and bring about consequences for harmful behaviors. Some high schools have Gender Sexuality Alliances (GSAs, more commonly known as Gay Straight Alliances) for students to connect with and receive support from one another and an identified faculty member. However, these groups do not exist in most schools and are even rarer in middle schools, when gender identity has developed and sexuality is in development in the students (GLSEN, 2016).

Only recently, the federal government provided guidance to schools on how to respond when students identify themselves to their school representative(s) (e.g., teacher, counselor, nurse) as transgender (Department of Justice and Department of Education, 2016); however, such guidelines are subject to political pressure and were subsequently rescinded. Comprehensive planning resources for schools exist (Orr & Baum, 2015) to help schools and families come together to make decisions regarding name and pronoun usage, disclosure of transgender identity, school uniforms, sports and extracurricular groups, and bathroom usage. Recently, bathrooms have become the focus of antitransgender legislation, with attempts to force gender minority people to use restrooms incongruent with who they are. Even youth who have plans with their school to use the bathroom aligned with their gender may avoid using the restroom at school. This can lead to infections and kidney problems and should be assessed by physical and mental health providers. At the time of publication of this book, the issue has not been decided at the federal level, following the U.S. Supreme Court's decision to send the *Gloucester County School Board v. G. G.* (2016) case back to the Court of Appeals and thus not guarantee federal protections for bathroom use by gender minority adolescents or adults.

Parental acceptance, support, and understanding of their child's gender minority identity are some of the strongest predictors of positive mental health outcomes (K. Olson, Durwood, DeMeules, & McLaughlin, 2016). Mental health and medical providers play a crucial role in the education of parents regarding negative health outcomes associated with actual and perceived rejection of youths' gender minority identities. These include higher likelihood of HIV, homelessness, problematic substance use, depression, self-injury, and suicidality (dickey, Reisner, & Juntunen, 2015). Providers should also normalize gender minority identities and gender identity and expression exploration in childhood as well as provide resources in their local communities including support groups where families can meet others with similar experiences.

Providers should work with the parents wherever they are on their journey to acceptance. Parents can be their youth's best advocate, even those who initially respond with rejection. They can demand respect for their youth in all environments, such as the home, school, and extracurricular activities. Respect includes consistent use of only the names and pronouns requested by the gender minority adolescent and inclusion in activities as consistent with other youth who share the same gender identity. In the authors' experience, it is more common for adults to resist respectful treatment of gender minority youth than for other youth, especially young children who seem to be particularly unphased by gender minority identities.

Even with parental acceptance, gender minority youth experience physical health and mental health disparities. The experience of gender minority stress (Hendricks & Testa, 2012), including internalized transphobia, negative expectations about the future, and lack of acceptance, takes a toll on the physical and mental health of gender minority adolescents. Gender minority adolescents are the most at-risk group for suicidal ideation and suicide attempts (Grossman & D'Augelli, 2007), even with supportive parents. The need for appropriate and supportive mental health care is great, as recent studies have shown that 41% of transgender adults have a history of suicide attempt, a rate that is over 25 times higher than their cisgender counterparts (Grant et al., 2011). Mental health providers can play an important role in gender minority adolescent health. They can provide culturally competent assessment and interventions designed at building resilience within youth in addition to ensuring youth are referred for gender affirming medical treatment, which may include pubertal suppression, hormone therapy, and/or surgical interventions. Mental health treatment can be very helpful, especially for youth who are engaging in self-injurious behaviors and coping with suicidality. Counseling, including individual, group, and family counseling, can be helpful for a host of experiences unique to gender minority youth including further identity exploration, processing rejection by family members or friends with a therapist, decisions about medical interventions, and thinking through the disclosure process. Ideally, mental health providers and medical providers collaborate in the treatment of gender minority adolescents for best outcomes (Ducheny, Hendricks, & Keo-Meier, 2017).

ADULT HEALTH

In this section, we will focus on the health care needs of gender minority adults. We begin by addressing hormone treatments and follow this with surgical options that a gender minority person may choose to complete. It is important to keep in mind that there is no singular way in which a gender minority person may make a medical transition (American Psychological Association, 2015; E. Coleman et al., 2012). Some gender minority people may want affirming surgical procedures without any hormone treatment; others may want only a low dose of hormones; and still others may choose to initiate hormones and undergo gender affirming surgical procedures. Others still may elect to have no medical intervention as part of their transition. Providers should not foreclose on a proscribed script to which patients must adhere. This manner of thinking is outdated and can lead to psychological distress on the part of the patient (American Psychological Association, 2015).

Diagnosis

There continues to be controversy about the usefulness of diagnosing gender minority people with an "official" psychiatric disorder. Gender Dysphoria—the current officially recognized related psychiatric disorder—first appeared in the fifth edition of the *Diagnostic and Statistical Manual of Mental Disorders, fifth edition* (*DSM-5*; American Psychiatric Association, 2013). For some, the presence of the diagnosis makes it possible for people to access care (Ehrbar, 2010), as insurance coverage of medical intervention is often linked to a formal diagnosis indicating medical necessity. As such, the formal diagnosis of Gender Dysphoria supports access to care among jail and prison inmates, military veterans, and people who are disabled or living in poverty (dickey, 2017). For others, the diagnosis represents unnecessary pathologization of a normal human variation (Winters, 2008)—the corollary among sexual minority individuals being the removal of same-sex attraction from the *DSM* upon publication of the *DSM-IV* (American Psychiatric Association, 1994). A number of changes were made to the Gender Dysphoria diagnosis in *DSM-V* that merit attention. The diagnosis no longer includes sexual orientation specifiers. Additionally, activists held great concerns about the previous diagnosis of Gender Identity Disorder (*DSM-IV-TR*; American Psychiatric Association, 2000) because there was no exit clause. The Gender Dysphoria diagnosis allows that a person is "diagnosable" only when experiencing distress (American Psychiatric Association, 2013). It also allows that a person may decide later in life to seek additional medical treatments (typically surgery).

It is important to separate an individual's experiences of gender dysphoria (not capitalized) with the diagnosis Gender Dysphoria. The lowercase gender dysphoria is generally used to describe feelings that "something is not quite right" with their gender or body as well as the impact of internalized transphobia and worries about personal safety. This phenomenon is not experienced by all transgender people (E. Coleman et al., 2012); however, it can be devastating to those whom it impacts. Many symptoms that appear to be depression, anxiety, or paranoia may actually be secondary to the experience of gender dysphoria (Keo-Meier et al., 2015). These secondary symptoms can be alleviated by the treatment of gender dysphoria, which is largely medical (Keo-Meier et al., 2015).

The decision to formally diagnose a person is ultimately the responsibility of the health care provider, be it physical or mental. It is important that the provider and the client have a frank, open discussion about the usefulness of a diagnosis. To the extent that a diagnosis increases a person's access to care, it might be useful. If diagnosing a patient with Gender Dysphoria would limit or preclude access to care (e.g., insurance denials), then the diagnosis should not be made, especially if the patient is opposed to such information being included in their health record.

Hormone Treatment

Hormone treatment is one of the most basic medical transition-related aspects of gender minority health care. In this section we will address the types of care a person might seek; however, this is not intended as a medical guideline for treatment. Readers are referred to the work of Gorton, Buth, and Spade (2005) and the Center of Excellence for Transgender Health (Deutsch, 2016) for information about medical administration of hormones.

Hormones for Nonbinary Patients

Providers might be under the assumption that nonbinary gender minority people have little to no interest in accessing hormones that would lead to masculinization or feminization. This may be the case for some people, but is likely not the case for others. Providers are encouraged to work closely with their patients to understand their medical goals, keeping in mind that these may change over time. The fact that goals change over time does not indicate that a person does not have a stable gender identity (American Psychological Association, 2015). Nonbinary people may choose to take a lower dose of hormones than binary gender minority individuals. In some cases, this may be for the purpose of how the hormones can lead to changes in their body. It may also be a means of stabilizing their emotional well-being (Keo-Meier et al., 2015). Providers will need to attend to the same monitoring of hormones regardless of the dosage a patient utilizes (Deutsch, 2016).

Masculinizing Hormones

Most often, testosterone is taken by gender minority male-identified people (e.g., transgender men). The results of the use of testosterone can be quite profound in a relatively short period of time for some and may take a more significant amount of time for others (Deutsch, 2016). Transgender men might expect some or all of the following effects: cessation of menses, clitoral growth, changes in body fat and muscle mass, increase in facial and body hair, male pattern baldness, lowering of vocal pitch, and increases in libido (E. Coleman et al., 2012). Treatment with masculinizing hormones can result in side effects—some of which mirror male puberty (e.g., acne), and others that may have more serious medical implications (e.g., elevated hematocrit levels; Deutsch, 2016).

Feminizing Hormones

For feminizing hormones to be effective, transgender women typically need to first counteract the effects of endogenous testosterone (Deutsch, 2016). This is accomplished by antiandrogen medication, most commonly Spironolactone. Typically, transgender women take both an antiandrogen medication and estrogen. Some also take a cyclical regimen of progesterone, believing that it increases breast growth (Deutsch, 2016). However, no conclusive benefits of progesterone have been demonstrated (Wierckx, Gooren, & T'Sjoen, 2014). Similar to testosterone, there are some desired and undesired effects. Desired effects include softening of the skin, thinning and slowed growth of body hair, loss of muscle tone, and breast growth. For some, a less desirable effect is a decrease in libido (Deutsch, 2016). Further, there is some concern regarding the established risks associated with estrogen use in cisgender women (e.g., heart disease, breast cancer; Deutsch, 2016); however, long-term outcome studies to examine this effect are not available among transgender women undergoing feminizing hormone treatment.

Surgical Treatment

There are several surgical procedures that a gender minority person may want to obtain. Colloquially in gender minority communities, these are often referred to as "top" or "bottom" surgery. Although it is necessary for health care providers to refer to these procedures as their formal names in training and consultation, when with patients, reflecting the language they use is preferable for building rapport. Facial surgeries are most commonly accessed by those wanting to feminize facial features and may include rhinoplasty, brow lift, tracheal shave, jaw contouring, and cheek enhancement. Chest surgeries include chest masculinization (e.g., mastectomy) or breast augmentation. Genital surgeries include hysterectomy (removal of the uterus and potentially the ovaries), orchiectomy (removal of the testes), metoidioplasty (enhancement of the clitoris), phalloplasty (construction of a penis), scrotoplasty (construction of a scrotum), and vaginoplasty (construction of a vagina).

Nonbinary Surgical Care

Some nonbinary individuals will seek to access surgical procedures that will feminize or masculinize their bodies. Providers should not assume that because a person is nonbinary they have no interest in surgical interventions. As outlined in the WPATH Standards of Care (E. Coleman et al., 2012), gender minority people may have different goals for how they will reach their affirmed gender identity. Nonbinary people may specifically seek a surgical intervention that helps them to attain a gender presentation that moves them away from being perceived as either male or female.

Feminizing Surgical Procedures

Some gender minority women may be interested in facial feminization surgery in order to reverse the masculinizing effects endogenous testosterone has had on their face and neck. They may seek breast augmentation if they did not achieve the amount of breast growth that they had hoped for through hormone treatment. The WPATH SOCv7 recommends waiting at least 12 months after starting hormone treatment before undergoing breast augmentation in order for the patient and surgeon to determine how much breast growth will result in that time frame (E. Coleman et al., 2012). Breast augmentation is a relatively straightforward procedure, which is performed routinely. Unfortunately, both facial feminization surgery and breast augmentation surgery are often not covered by health insurance as these procedures are viewed by insurance carriers as being "cosmetic" or "elective" surgery. However, for a gender minority woman's emotional well-being, these procedures may be medically necessary in the broader sense (E. Coleman et al., 2012; WPATH, 2016). Unfortunately, there appears to be little support within the insurance community for the medical necessity of these procedures.

Genital surgeries have become somewhat routine for those providers who specialize in this medical practice. Some gender minority women will seek to have an orchiectomy to remove their testes. This removes the source of endogenous testosterone. Once this surgery has been completed, a gender minority woman may no longer need to take antiandrogen medication. Another procedure that some gender minority women access is a vaginoplasty. This procedure is used to create a vulva and neovagina. Women who have this procedure are required to use dilators on a regular basis for at least 1 year to ensure that the new vagina remains intact and does not collapse on itself (Deutsch, 2016).

Masculinizing Surgical Procedures

Similar to the procedures for gender minority women, there are both chest and genital surgery options available for gender minority men. Chest masculinization surgery is an outpatient procedure that many gender minority men complete. There are different types of surgeries that may be specific to the surgeon performing the surgery or related to the size of a gender minority person's chest. A double incision procedure with nipple grafts is the most common procedure and works for all breast sizes. A periareolar (colloquially, "keyhole") procedure is ideal for those with A cup size breasts. Similar to breast augmentation, this procedure may be considered to be cosmetic by some insurance companies, rather than a medically necessary procedure. However, for a gender minority man's emotional well-being, these procedures are often medically necessary (Davis & Meier, 2013) even if not viewed as such by insurance companies.

Some gender minority men choose to have genital surgery. This may include a hysterectomy, metoidioplasty, scrotoplasty, and/or phalloplasty. Hysterectomies are performed routinely for cisgender women and may be a prerequisite to other genital surgeries, depending on the surgeon and/or the patient's fertility goals (National Women's Health Network, 2015). One option to preserve fertility is to leave one ovary, while removing the uterus and the other ovary. The main goal of metoidioplasty and phalloplasty is to create a larger, more apparent phallus. Both of these procedures have the option of a urethral extension and re-rerouting through the phallus, which allows the patient to urinate from a standing position. However, complications may result requiring one or more revisions. The metoidioplasty, commonly referred to as the "clitoral release," is a much simpler procedure than the phalloplasty, as it makes use of the genital enlargement from testosterone treatment and enhances the tissue that already exists. A phalloplasty typically requires a skin graft, which has the potential to leave significant scarring at the donor site. Common sources of skin grafts are the radial forearm, abdomen, and thigh (Deutsch, 2016). Phalloplasty procedures are done in multiple stages, typically including three stages, each with several weeks of recovery required in between (Deutsch, 2016). In addition to the metoidioplasty and the phalloplasty, a gender minority man may also have a scrotoplasty. In this procedure, a scrotal sac is created from the existing labia. A final procedure a person might complete is a vaginectomy. In this procedure, the vagina is surgically removed and the vaginal opening is closed. Gender minority individuals may have the option to leave their vagina open. This has benefits for those who use it for sexual activity (i.e., maintaining the G-spot for pleasure) as well as those who may want to access their ovaries for egg donation at a later time.

Decisions about undergoing gender affirming surgical procedures can be complicated by a variety of factors. There may be medical contraindications that prevent a person from being a good surgical candidate (e.g., heart or lung disease; Boyd & Jackson, 2005). The cost of procedures, most of which are rarely covered by health insurance, can be very prohibitive. A final challenge that gender minority people face is that many of these procedures require specialized training. As a result, it can be difficult to find a competent provider whom the gender minority person can access without significant travel costs.

■ HEALTH RISKS RELATED TO TRANSITIONING

In general, medical and surgical interventions involved in gender transition were originally created for cisgender people. Pubertal suppression was designed to treat precocious puberty. Facial feminization and breast augmentation are routinely sought out by cisgender women. Chest masculinization surgery was developed from mastectomy procedures designed for the removal of breast cancers and from breast reduction surgeries, both of which were originally applied in cisgender women. Hysterectomies have been performed on cisgender women for decades. Vaginoplasties and phalloplasties were designed to treat malformations, incomplete formations, and/or cancer treatment in cisgender people. They were modified for use in gender minority people. As such, while the risks and outcomes among gender minority individuals have not been extensively examined, much can also be gleaned from existing literature on the use of these procedures among cisgender individuals.

Puberty Suppression and Fertility

Pubertal suppression is a safe treatment with minimal side effects (Cohen-Kettenis & van Goozen, 1998). However, long-term outcome data are lacking. The effects of pubertal suppression are completely reversible and temporary (Carel, Eugster, Rogol, Ghizzoni, & Palmert, 2009). The use of this treatment in gender minority periadolescents has been well documented and researched since the early 2000s (Cohen-Kettenis & Pfäfflin, 2003). No untoward risks have been reported as a result of pubertal suppression (Carel et al., 2009), and gender minority adolescents experience significant relief by undergoing this treatment (J. Olson et al., 2015).

Discussions around loss and/or preservation of fertility associated with pubertal suppression immediately followed by hormone therapy are some of the most difficult and require collaborative effort, and both the therapist and the medical provider need to be skilled in talking about fertility preservation (dickey, Ducheny, & Ehrbar, 2016). If a youth begins blockers early in puberty, before the body develops mature eggs or sperm, and then moves directly to hormone treatment, that youth will forfeit the opportunity to build a family with gametes of their own. If a youth has already begun to produce mature eggs or sperm, they can cryopreserve gametes to use through assisted reproductive procedures later in life (dickey, Ducheny, & Ehrbar, 2016). Providers need to describe these processes, which may induce dysphoria resulting from the requirement of masturbation for sperm donation or use of a vaginal ultrasound probe to monitor ovarian follicular development, in addition to the use of high doses of hormones (dickey, Ducheny, & Ehrbar, 2016).

Hormone Treatment

Hormone therapy is associated with undesired effects and risks. Most of the risks involve moving from a "male" risk level to a "female" risk level, or vice versa, for health outcomes such as heart disease and breast cancer (Deutsch, 2016). Although gender minority men develop a higher risk for heart disease, theoretically, they are not at a higher risk than if they had a twin brother; in essence, the risk is simply matching their true gender. In fact, they may be at a lower risk than a twin brother if they have not been exposed to as much testosterone for as long a period of time (Deutsch, 2016). Risks associated with testosterone treatment include: increased hematocrit levels (polycythemia), increased risk of heart disease, acne, weight gain, and sleep apnea (E. Coleman et al., 2012). Medical risks associated with estrogen treatment include deep vein thrombosis, gallstones, weight gain, elevated liver enzymes, and hypertriglyceridemia (E. Coleman et al., 2012).

Routine monitoring and selecting the method of administration can help to reduce and treat negative side effects resulting from hormone therapy. Testosterone should not be given orally and is most commonly used in injectable forms (subcutaneously and intramuscular) on a weekly basis (Deutsch, 2016). Transdermal testosterone is available for daily use, yet in the authors' experience is over 10 times more expensive than injectable testosterone. Feminizing hormone therapy (estrogen and antiandrogen) is most commonly prescribed in a daily oral or pill form, although some patients prefer injections (Deutsch, 2016), and in studies of cisgender women, dermally delivered estrogen (patch) is associated with a lower risk of heart disease than oral estrogen (Simon et al., 2016).

Few longitudinal studies have been completed that explore the long-term health risks of hormone treatment. There is a great need for funding to support this type of research. Gender minority people have the right to understand the implications of beginning hormone treatment, and the cautions that providers are able to give to their gender minority patients are often based on the experiences of cisgender patients. This type of information is woefully inadequate in helping gender minority people navigate the challenges associated with hormone treatment.

Surgical Complications and Risks

Any time a person undergoes a surgical procedure there is a risk of complications. In some cases these complications are minor concerns; in others, the complications may be life threatening. Surgeons typically require a surgical candidate to acquire a release from their primary care physician prior to final clearance for surgery.

Feminizing Surgical Risks

There are a number of risks associated with a vaginoplasty. These include fistula, granulation tissue, urinary tract infections, and issues with sensation and orgasm (Meltzer, 2016). Transgender women must be prepared to talk frankly with their surgeon about these risks and the best means of avoiding and/or recognizing these complications. It is important to have access to care to ensure that these potential complications are addressed with appropriate care. For individuals who travel a significant distance, or even outside the country, it is important to ensure that there is a provider near one's home who has the knowledge and skills necessary to address any complications.

Masculinizing Surgical Risks

Similar to transgender women, transgender men also are at risk for complications following genital procedures. These include: wound infection, urinary catheter difficulties, flap loss, hematomas, and urethral stricture (Crane, 2016). Depending on the severity of the complications, it is possible that additional surgeries will be required. Transgender men also need to have frank discussions with their surgeon about these complications and the ways to reduce the risk of occurrence, and need to have a local provider able to provide competent postsurgical follow-up care.

■ TREATING THE ORGAN SYSTEMS THAT ARE PRESENT

Little has been written on the topic of the importance of treating the organ systems that are present in a gender minority person's body. This is an important part of affirming and competent care (Roberts & Fantz, 2014). Some gender minority people may be reluctant to talk about organ systems that are associated with the sex they were assigned at birth. For many, this is a major cause of the distress a person feels about their body. However, as long as these organ systems are present, the patient may need associated medical treatment. It is incumbent on the provider to create a climate that allows for open and safe discussions with the gender minority patient.

Another area of possible complication concerns the use of electronic health records (EHRs). EHRs are typically designed in a way that allows for the coding of a patient's sex as either male or female. This coding then aligns with the various procedure codes that are consistent with a person's stated sex (Deutsch & Buchholtz, 2015; Deutsch, Green, Keatley, Mayer, Hastings, & Hall, 2013). However, if a transgender man has been diagnosed with ovarian cancer, it is important to document that he received care for the condition. Providers may need to advocate on behalf of their patients to assure they have access to the care they need based on their organ systems, not on the choices provided by an EHR.

■ BROADER HEALTH CONSIDERATIONS

Until now, this chapter has focused primarily on the transition-related health care concerns of gender minority people, as that is the area of research that is furthest in its development. Although the literature on the broader health concerns (i.e., beyond transitioning) of gender minority people is somewhat limited, there is emerging evidence that they face a variety of disparities in health risk behaviors and even health outcomes well beyond the medical transition. Although many of these are discussed in more detail throughout this text (e.g., gender minority disparities in substance use are discussed in Chapter 12), in the following we provide a brief summary of the evidence emerging in the literature.

Largely due to experiences of systematic and social oppression, gender minority groups face a multitude of psychosocial vulnerabilities and barriers to health care that increase their risk for a variety of mental and physical health concerns. More specifically, gender minority individuals encounter significant discrimination across multiple domains including employment, housing, health care, and public accommodations/services (i.e., restaurants, hotels, public transportation, and government agencies), with 63% of a national sample of gender minority individuals reporting at least one major experience of discrimination that significantly impacted their financial and/or emotional functioning and overall quality of life (Grant et al., 2011). As a result, rates of unemployment, poverty, and homelessness are significantly higher among gender minority individuals when compared to the general population (Conron, Scott, Stowell, & Landers, 2012; Grant et al., 2011).

In addition to experiences of discrimination, gender minority individuals report alarmingly high rates of harassment and victimization that significantly increase their risk for serious harm, injury, or even death. For example, 26% of participants in the National Transgender Discrimination Survey reported that they had been physically assaulted because of their gender identity/expression, with 10% having been the victim of transphobia-related sexual assault (Grant et al., 2011). Other psychosocial vulnerabilities experienced with greater severity by gender minority individuals (when compared to their cisgender sexual minority and/or heterosexual counterparts) include lower levels of social support, self-esteem, feelings of community belongingness, and overall quality of life and higher levels of internalized stigma and identity concealment (Dargie, Blair, Pukall, & Coyle, 2014; Factor & Rothblum, 2008; Fredriksen-Goldsen et al., 2013; Grant et al., 2011; Newfield, Hart, Dibble, & Kohler, 2006; Warren, Smalley, & Barefoot, 2016a).

Gender minority individuals also experience significant structural and psychosocial barriers to appropriate and ongoing health care. For example, in comparison to the general population, gender minority individuals are less likely to have access to employee-sponsored health insurance and more likely to depend on public programs such as Medicare or Medicaid for health care coverage, with an estimated 19% lacking health insurance altogether (dickey, Budge et al., 2016; Grant et al., 2011). Furthermore, 50% of gender minority individuals report that they have had to teach their health care providers about transgender health because they were uninformed, 28% have experienced harassment in a health care setting, 48% have postponed needed health care due to an inability to pay, 28% have postponed care due to fears of discrimination, 19% have been denied medical care due to their gender identity/expression, and 2% have been victims of violence within a health care setting (Grant et al., 2011). Additionally, recent research suggests that gender minority individuals, especially transgender women, may be less likely than their cisgender sexual minority counterparts to seek needed medical care and follow medical advice (Smalley, Warren, & Barefoot, 2015), while transgender men may be less likely to engage in routine preventive health care (including Pap tests; Peitzmeier, Khullar, Reisner, & Potter, 2014; Reisner, et al., 2015).

Overall, these psychosocial vulnerabilities and barriers to health care translate into a variety of health disparities for gender minority individuals. Namely, emerging research suggests that, in comparison to their cisgender sexual minority and/or heterosexual counterparts, gender minority individuals may be more likely to experience higher rates of the following mental and physical health risk factors and outcomes: psychological distress (i.e., depression, anxiety, and stress) and a history of mental health concerns (Bockting, Miner, Swinburne Romine, Hamilton,

& Coleman, 2013; Budge, Adelson, & Howard, 2013; Dargie et al., 2014; Fredriksen-Goldsen et al., 2013; Su et al., 2016; Warren et al., 2016a); self-harm and suicidality (with approximately 41% of gender minority individuals reporting a lifetime history of nonsuicidal self-injury and/or suicide attempt; dickey et al., 2015; Grant et al., 2011); self-perceived need for mental health care (Warren et al., 2016a); alcohol and illicit drug use (Benotsch et al., 2013; Keuroghlian, Reisner, White, & Weiss, 2015; Reisner, Greytak, Parsons, & Ybarra, 2015; Reback & Fletcher, 2014; Santos et al., 2014); HIV infection (Grant et al., 2011; Herbst et al., 2008; Poteat, Reisner, & Radix, 2014); poor diet and exercise habits (i.e., eating fewer fruits/vegetables, drinking more caloric beverages, eating when not hungry, and exercising less than 3 days/week), especially among transgender women (Smalley et al., 2015); obesity (with the highest prevalence among transgender men; Conron et al., 2012; Fredriksen-Goldsen et al., 2013; VanKim et al., 2014; Warren Smalley, & Barefoot, 2016b); and poor physical health and disability among older adults (Fredriksen-Goldsen et al., 2013). The need for additional research into the broader health needs of gender minority populations is sorely needed, as well as research focused on developing culturally tailored and gender-affirming intervention programs.

◼ CONCLUSION

All people deserve the right to access competent and timely medical care. In this chapter, we have explored a variety of concerns that impact the use of health care services by gender minority patients, explored the medical aspects of the transitioning process, and presented emerging evidence of broader health disparities faced by gender minority groups. Because of the critical role that positive interactions with medical providers play in future pursuit of health care (American Psychological Association, 2015), physical and mental health providers are strongly encouraged to examine their own values and the ways in which their practice is designed to be a welcoming place for gender minority patients. In addition, the broader public health community should take strides to consider the health needs and health disparities faced by gender minority individuals, and develop programming and other intervention programs designed to meet their unique health needs.

◼ REFERENCES

American Psychiatric Association. (1994). *Diagnostic and statistical manual of mental disorders (4th ed.)*. Washington, DC: Author.

American Psychiatric Association. (2000). *Diagnostic and statistical manual of mental disorders (4th ed., text revision)*. Washington, DC: Author.

American Psychiatric Association. (2013). *Diagnostic and statistical manual of mental disorders (5th ed.)*. Arlington, VA: American Psychiatric Publishing.

American Psychological Association. (2013a). Fact sheet: Gender diversity and transgender identity in children. Retrieved from http://www.apadivisions.org/division-44/resources/advocacy/transgender-children.pdf

American Psychological Association. (2013b). Fact Sheet: Gender Diversity and Transgender Identity in Adolescents. Retrieved from http://www.apadivisions.org/division-44/resources/advocacy/transgender-adolescents.pdf

American Psychological Association. (2015). Guidelines for psychological practice with transgender and gender nonconforming people. *American Psychologist, 70,* 832–864. doi:10.1037/a0039906

Benotsch, E. G., Zimmerman, R., Cathers, L., McNulty, S., Pierce, J., Heck, T.,... Snipes, D. (2013). Non-medical use of prescription drugs, polysubstance use, and mental health in transgender adults. *Drug and Alcohol Dependence, 132,* 391–394. doi:10.1016/j.drugalcdep.2013.02.027

Bockting, W., Miner, M., Swinburne Romine, R., Hamilton, A., & Coleman, E. (2013). Stigma, mental health, and resilience in an online sample of the US transgender population. *American Journal of Public Health, 103,* 943–951. doi:10.2105/AJPH.2013.301241

Boyd, O., & Jackson, N. (2005). How is risk defined in high-risk surgical patient management? *Critical Care, 9*(4), 390–396. doi:10.1186/cc3057

Budge, S. L., Adelson, J. L., & Howard, K. S. (2013). Anxiety and depression in transgender individuals: The roles of transition status, loss, social support, and coping. *Journal of Consulting and Clinical Psychology, 81,* 545–557. doi:10.1037/a0031774

Carel, J.-C., Eugster, E. A., Rogol, A., Ghizzoni, L., & Palmert, M. R. (2009). Consensus statement on the use of gonadotropin-releasing hormone analogs in children. *Pediatrics, 123,* e752–e762. doi:10.1542/peds.2008-1783

Carmichael, P. (2016, June). Time to reflect: Gender dysphoria in children and adolescents, defining best practice in a fast changing context. Plenary session presented at the World Professional Association for Transgender Health Biennial Symposium, Amsterdam, The Netherlands.

Carroll, L. (2010). *Counseling Sexual and Gender Minorities.* Boston, MA: Pearson.

Cohen-Kettenis, P. T., & Pfäfflin, F. (2003). *Transgenderism and intersexuality in childhood and adolescence: Making choices (Vol. 46).* Thousand Oaks, CA: Sage.

Cohen-Kettenis, P. T., & van Goozen, S. H. (1998). Puberty delay as an aid in the diagnosis and treatment of a transsexual adolescent. *European Child and Adolescent Psychiatry, 7*(4), 246–248.

Coleman, D. L., & Rosoff, P. M. (2013). The legal authority of mature minors to consent to general medical treatment. *Pediatrics, 131*(4), 786–793. doi:10.1542/peds.2012-2470

Coleman, E., Bockting, W., Botzer, M., Cohen-Kettenis, P., DeCuypere, G., Feldman, J.,...Zucker, K. (2012). Standards of care for the health of transsexual, transgender, and gender nonconforming people, version 7. *International Journal of Transgenderism, 13*(4), 165–232. doi:10.1080/15532739.2011.700873

Conron, K. J., Mimiaga, M. J., & Landers, S. J. (2010). A population-based study of sexual orientation identity and gender differences in adult health. *American Journal of Public Health, 100*(10), 1953–1960. doi:10.2105/AJPH.2009.174169

Conron, K. J., Scott, G., Stowell, G. S., & Landers, S. J. (2012). Transgender health in Massachusetts: Results from a household probability sample of adults. *American Journal of Public Health, 102*(1), 118–122. doi:10.2105/AJPH.2011.300315

Crane, C. (2016). Phalloplasty and metaoidioplasty: Overview and postoperative considerations. Retrieved from http://transhealth.ucsf.edu/trans?page=guidelines-phalloplasty

Dargie, E., Blair, K. L., Pukall, C. F., & Coyle, S. M. (2014). Somewhere under the rainbow: Exploring the identities and experiences of trans persons. *Canadian Journal of Human Sexuality, 23,* 60–74. doi:10.3138/cjhs.2378

Davis, S. A., & Meier, C. (2013). Effects of testosterone treatment and chest reconstruction surgery in mental health and sexuality in female-to-male transgender people. *International Journal of Sexual Health, 26,* 113–128. doi:10.1080/19317644.2013.833152

Delemarre-van de Waal, H. & Cohen-Kettenis, P. (2008). Clinical management of gender identity disorder in adolescents: A protocol on psychological and paediatric endocrinology aspects. *European Journal of Endocrinology, 155,* S131–S137. doi:10.1530/eje.1.02231

Deutsch, M. B. (Ed.) (2016). *Guidelines for the primary and gender-affirming care of transgender and gender nonbinary people (2nd ed.)*. San Francisco: Center for Excellence in Transgender Health, Department of Family and Community Medicine, University of California, San Francisco. Retrieved from http://transhealth.ucsf.edu/trans?page=guidelines-home

Deutsch, M. B., & Buchholz, D. (2015). Electronic health records and transgender patients: Practical recommendations for the collection of gender identity data. *Journal of General Internal Medicine, 30*, 834–847. doi:10.1007/s11606-014-3148-7

Deutsch, M. B., Green, J., Keatley, J., Mayer, G., Hastings, J., & Hall, A. M. (2013). Electronic medical records and the transgender patient: Recommendations from the world professional association for transgender health EMR Working Group. *Journal of the American Medical Informatics Association, 20*, 700–703. doi:10.1136/amiajnl-2012-001472

dickey, l. m. (2017). Toward developing clinical competence: Improving health care of gender diverse people. *American Journal of Public Health, 107*(2), 222–223. doi:10.2105/AJPH.2016.303581

dickey, l. m., Budge, S. A., Katz-Wise, S., & Garza, M. V. (2016). Health disparities in the transgender community: Exploring differences in insurance coverage. *Psychology of Sexual Orientation and Gender Diversity, 3*(3), 275–282. doi:10.1037/sgd0000169

dickey, l. m., Ducheny, K., & Ehrbar, R. D. (2016). Family creation options for transgender and gender nonconforming people. *Psychology of Sexual Orientation and Gender Diversity, 3*, 173–179. doi:10.1037/sgd0000178

dickey, l. m., Reisner, S. L., & Juntunen, C. L. (2015). Non-suicidal self-injury in a large online sample of transgender adults. *Professional Psychology: Research & Practice, 46*(1), 3–11. doi:10.1037/a0038803

Ducheny, K., Hendricks, M. L., & Keo-Meier, C. L. (2017). TGNC-affirmative interdisciplinary collaborative care. In A. A. Singh & l. m. dickey (Eds.), *Affirmative counseling and psychological practice with transgender and gender nonconforming clients* (pp. 69–93). Washington, DC: American Psychological Association.

Edwards-Leeper, L. (2017). Affirmative care of TGNC children and adolescents. In A. A. Singh & l. m. dickey (Eds.), *Affirmative counseling and psychological practice with transgender and gender nonconforming clients* (pp. 119–141). Washington, DC: American Psychological Association.

Edwards-Leeper, L., Leibowitz, S., & Sangganjanavanich, V. F. (2016). Affirmative practice with transgender and gender nonconforming youth: Expanding the model. *Psychology of Sexual Orientation and Gender Diversity, 3*, 165–172. doi:10.1037/sgd0000167

Edwards-Leeper, L., & Spack, N. P. (2012). Psychological evaluation and medical treatment of transgender youth in an interdisciplinary "Gender Management Service" (GeMS) in a major pediatric center. *Journal of Homosexuality, 59*, 321–336. doi:10.1080/00918369.2012.653302

Ehrbar, R. D. (2010). Consensus from differences: Lack of professional consensus on the retention of the gender identity disorder diagnosis. *International Journal of Transgenderism, 12*, 60–74. doi:10.1080/15532729.2010.513928

Ehrensaft, D. (2016). *The gender creative child: Pathways for nurturing and supporting children who live outside gender boxes*. New York, NY: The Experiment.

Erickson-Scroth, L. Gilbert, M. A., & Smith, T. E. (2014). Sex and gender development. In L. Erickson-Scroth (Ed.) *Trans bodies, trans selves: A resource for the transgender community* (pp. 80–101). New York, NY: Oxford University Press.

Factor, R. J., & Rothblum, E. D. (2008). A study of transgender adults and their non-transgender siblings on demographic characteristics, social support, and experiences of violence. *Journal of LGBT Health Research, 3*, 11–30. doi:10.1080/15574090802092879

Fredriksen-Goldsen, K. I., Cook-Daniels, L., Kim, H.-J., Erosheva, E. A., Emlet, C. A., Hoy-Ellis, C., … Muraco, A. (2013). Physical and mental health of transgender older adults:

An at-risk and underserved population. *The Gerontologist, 54,* 488–500. doi:10.1093/geront/gnt021

Gloucester County School Board v. G. G. (2016). Case 16-273.

GLSEN. (2016). The 2015 National School Climate Survey: The experiences of lesbian, gay, bisexual transgender, and queer youth in our nation's schools. Retrieved from https://www.glsen.org/sites/default/files/GLSEN%202015%20National%20School%20Climate%20Survey%20%28NSCS%29%20-%20Executive%20Summary.pdf

Gorton, R. N., Buth, J., & Spade, D. (2005). Medical therapy and health maintenance for transgender men: A guide for health care providers. Retrieved from http://www.nickgorton.org/Medical%20Therapy%20and%20HM%20for%20Transgender%20Men_2005.pdf

Grant, J. M., Mottet, L. A., Tanis, J., Harrison, J., Herman, J. L., & Keisling, M. (2011) Injustice at every turn: A report of the national transgender discrimination survey. Retrieved from http://endtransdiscrimination.org/PDFs/NTDS_Report.pdf

Grossman, A. & D'Augelli, A. (2007). Transgender youth and life-threatening behaviors. *Suicide & Life-threatening Behavior, 37*(5), 527–537.

Hembree, W., Cohen-Kettenis, P., Delemarre-van de Waal, H., Gooren, L., Meyer, W., III, Spack, N.,…Montori, V. (2009). Endocrine treatment of transsexual persons: An Endocrine Society clinical practice guideline. *Journal of Clinical Endocrinology and Metabolism, 94,* 3132–3154. doi:10.1210/jc.2009-0345

Hendricks, M. L., & Testa, R. J. (2012). A conceptual framework for clinical work with transgender and gender nonconforming clients: An adaptation of the minority stress model. *Professional Psychology: Research & Practice, 43,* 460–467. doi:10.1037/a0029597

Herbst, J. H., Jacobs, E. D., Finlayson, T. J., McKleroy, V. S., Neumann, M. S., & Crepaz, N. (2008). Estimating HIV prevalence and risk behaviors of transgender persons in the United States: A systematic review. *AIDS and Behavior, 12*(1), 1–17. doi:10.1007/s10461-007-9299-3

Herdt, G. (1996). *Third sex, third gender: Beyond sexual dimorphism in culture and history.* New York, NY: Zone Books.

Hidalgo, M. A., Ehrensaft, D., Tishelman, A. C., Clark, L. F., Garofalo, R., Rosenthal, S. M.,…Olson, J. (2013). The gender affirmative model: What we know and what we aim to learn. *Human Development, 56*(5), 285–290.

Johnson, E. K., & Finlayson, C. (2016). Preservation of fertility potential for gender and sex diverse individuals. *Transgender Health, 1*(1), 41–44. doi:10.1089/trgh.2015.0010

Keo-Meier, C. (2015, October). *Development of gender identity and sexual orientation.* Oral presentation presented at Gender Infinity, Houston, TX.

Keo-Meier, C., Herman, L., Reisner, S., Pardo, S., Sharp, C., & Babcock, J. (2015). Testosterone treatment and MMPI-2 improvement in transgender men: A prospective controlled study. *Journal of Consulting and Clinical Psychology, 83,* 143–156. doi:10.1037/a0037599

Keuroghlian, A. S., Reisner, S. L., White, J. M., & Weiss, R. D. (2015). Substance use and treatment of substance use disorders in a community sample of transgender adults. *Drug and Alcohol Dependence, 152,* 139–146. doi:10.1016/j.drugalcdep.2015.04.008

Kosciw, J. G., Greytak, E. A., Palmer, N. A., & Boesen, M. J. (2014). *The 2013 National School Climate Survey: The experiences of lesbian, gay, bisexual, and transgender youth in our nation's schools.* New York, NY: Gay, Lesbian, and Straight Education Network.

Lev, A. I. (2004). *Transgender emergence: Therapeutic guidelines for working with gender-variant people and their families.* New York, NY: Haworth Clinical Press.

MedicineNet. (2016). Puberty. Retrieved from http://www.medicinenet.com/puberty/article.htm

Meltzer, T. (2016). Vaginoplasty procedures, complications and aftercare. Retrieved from http://transhealth.ucsf.edu/trans?page=guidelines-vaginoplasty

National Women's Health Network. (2015). Hysterectomy. Retrieved from https://www.nwhn.org/hysterectomy/

Newfield, E., Hart, S., Dibble, S., & Kohler, L. (2006). Female-to-male transgender quality of life. *Quality of Life Research, 15*, 1447–1457. doi:10.1007/s11136-006-0002-3

Olson, J., Forbes, C., & Belzer, M. (2011). Management of the transgender adolescent. *Archives of Pediatric Adolescent Medicine, 165*, 171–176. doi:10.1001/archpediatrics.2010.275

Olson, J., Schrager, S. M., Belzer, M., Simons, L. K., & Clark, L. F. (2015). Baseline physiologic and psychosocial characteristics of transgender youth seeking care for gender dysphoria. *Journal of Adolescent Health, 57*(4), 374–380. doi:10.1016/j.jadohealth.2015.04.027

Olson, K., Durwood, L., DeMeules, M., & McLaughlin, K. (2016). Mental health of transgender children who are supported in their identities. *Pediatrics, 137*, e20153223. doi:10.1542/peds.2015-3223

Orr, A., & Baum, J. (2015). Schools in transition: A guide for supporting transgender students in K–12 schools. Retrieved from https://www.nea.org/assets/docs/Schools_in_Transition_2015.pdf

Peitzmeier, S. M., Khullar, K., Reisner, S. L., & Potter, J. (2014). Pap test use is lower among female-to-male patients than non-transgender women. *American Journal of Preventive Medicine, 47*(6), 808–812. doi:10.1016/j.amepre.2014.07.031

Poteat, T., Reisner, S. L., & Radix, A. (2014). HIV epidemics among transgender women. *Current Opinion in HIV and AIDS, 9*(2), 168–173. doi:10.1097/COH.0000000000000030

Reback, C. J., & Fletcher, J. B. (2014). HIV prevalence, substance use, and sexual risk behaviors among transgender women recruited through outreach. *AIDS and Behavior, 18*(7), 1359–1367. doi:10.1007/s10461-013-0657-z

Reisner, S. L., Greytak, A., Parsons, J. P., & Ybarra, M. (2015). Gender minority social stress in adolescence: Disparities in adolescent bullying and substance use by gender identity. *Journal of Sex Research, 52*, 243–256. doi:10.1080/00224499.2014.886321

Reisner, S. L., Pardo, S. T., Gamarel, K. E., Hughto, J. M., Pardee, D. J., & Keo-Meier, C. L. (2015). Substance use to cope with stigma in healthcare among U.S. female-to-male trans masculine adults. *LGBT Health, 2*(4), 324–332. doi:10.1089/lgbt.2015.0001

Roberts, T. K., & Fantz, C. R. (2014). Barriers to quality health care for the transgender population. *Clinical Biochemistry, 47*, 983–987. doi:10.1016/j.clinbiochem.2014.02.009

Santos, G. M., Rapues, J., Wilson, E. C., Macias, O., Packer, T., Colfax, G., & Raymond, H. F. (2014). Alcohol and substance use among transgender women in San Francisco: Prevalence and association with human immunodeficiency virus infection. *Drug and Alcohol Review, 33*, 287–295. doi:10.1111/dar.12116

Savin-Williams, R., & Cohen, K. (2007). Development of same-sex attracted youth. In I. H. Meyer & M. E. Northridge (Eds.), *Public health perspectives on lesbian, gay, bisexual and transgender populations* (pp. 27–47). New York, NY: Springer Publishing.

Simon, J. A., Laliberté, F., Duh, M. S., Pilon, D., Kahler, K. H., Nyirady, J.,…Lefebvre, P. (2016). Venous thromboembolism and cardiovascular disease complications in menopausal women using transdermal versus oral estrogen therapy. *Menopause, 23*(6), 600–610. doi:10.1097/GME.0000000000000590

Singh, A. A., & dickey, l. m. (2017). *Affirmative counseling and psychological practice with transgender and gender nonconforming clients.* Washington, DC: American Psychological Association.

Smalley, K. B., Warren, J. C., & Barefoot, K. N. (2015). Differences in health risk behaviors across understudied LGBT subgroups. *Health Psychology, 35*(2), 103–114. doi:10.1037/hea0000231

Spack, N. P., Edwards-Leeper, L., Feldman, H. A., Leibowitz, S., Mandel, F., Diamond, D. A., & Vance, S. R. (2012). Children and adolescents with gender identity disorder referred to a pediatric medical center. *Pediatrics, 129*, 418–425. doi:10.1542/peds.2011-0907

Steensma, T. D., Kreukels, B. P., de Vries, A. L., & Cohen-Kettenis, P. T. (2013). Gender identity development in adolescence. *Hormones and Behavior, 64*(2), 288–297. doi:10.1016/j.yhbeh.2013.02.020

Steensma, T. D., McGuire, J. K., Kreukels, B. P., Beekman, A. J., & Cohen-Kettenis, P. T. (2013). Factors associated with desistence and persistence of childhood gender dysphoria: A quantitative follow-up study. *Journal of the American Academy of Child and Adolescent Psychiatry, 52*, 582–590. doi:10.1016/j.jaac.2013.03.016

Su, D., Irwin, J. A., Fisher, C., Ramos, A., Kelley, M., Mendoza, D. A. R., & Coleman, J. D. (2016). Mental health disparities within the LGBT population: A comparison between transgender and nontransgender individuals. *Transgender Health, 1*(1), 12–20. doi:10.1089/trgh.2015.0001

Substance Abuse and Mental Health Services Administration. (2015). *Ending conversion therapy: Supporting and affirming LGBTQ youth (HHS Publication No. SMA 15-4928)*. Rockville, MD: Author.

Toomey, R. B., Ryan, C., Diaz, R. M., & Russell, S. T. (2011). High school gay-straight alliances (GSAs) and young adult well-being: An examination of GSA presence, participation, and perceived effectiveness. *Applied Developmental Science, 15*(4), 175–185. doi:10.1080/10888691.2011.607378

U.S. Department of Justice and U.S. Department of Education. (2016). Dear colleague letter on transgender students. Retrieved from www2.ed.gov/about/offices/list/ocr/letters/colleague-201605-title-ix-transgender.pdf

Vanderburgh, R. (2007). *Transition and Beyond: Observations on Gender Identity*. Portland, OR: Q Press.

VanKim, N. A., Erickson, D. J., Eisenberg, M. E., Lust, K. E., Simon Rosser, B. R., & Laska, M. N. (2014). Weight-related disparities for transgender college students. *Health Behavior and Policy Review, 1*(2), 161–171. doi:10.14485/HBPR.1.2.8

Warren, J. C., Smalley, K. B., & Barefoot, K. N. (2016a). Psychological well-being among transgender and genderqueer individuals. *International Journal of Transgenderism, 17*(3–4), 114–123. doi:10.1080/15532739.2016.1216344

Warren, J. C., Smalley, K. B., & Barefoot, K. N. (2016b). Differences in psychosocial predictors of obesity among LGBT subgroups. *LGBT Health, 3*(4), 283–291. doi:10.1089/lgbt.2015.0076

Wierckx, K., Gooren, L., & T'Sjoen, G. (2014). Clinical review: Breast development in trans women receiving cross-sex hormones. *Journal of Sexual Medicine, 11*, 1240–1247. doi:10.1111/jsm.12487

Winters, K. (2008). *Gender madness in psychiatry: Essays from the struggle for dignity*. Dillon, CO: GID Reform Advocates.

World Professional Association for Transgender Health. (2016). Position statement on medical necessity of treatment, sex reassignment, and insurance coverage in the U.S.A. Retrieved from http://www.wpath.org/site_page.cfm?pk_association_webpage_menu=1352&pk_association_webpage=3947

CHAPTER **15**

The Health of Racial and Ethnic Minority Gender and Sexual Minority Populations

Jacob C. Warren, K. Bryant Smalley, and K. Nikki Barefoot

As in the non–lesbian, gay, bisexual, and transgender (LGBT) community, gender and sexual minority (GSM) individuals who are also members of one or more racial/ethnic minority populations face unique sociocultural dynamics that impact the ability to achieve and maintain health. Given the field of health disparities itself was originally developed in response to unexplained health differences between racial/ethnic majority and minority groups, it is surprising the extent to which the intersection of sexual orientation/gender identity and race/ethnicity is understudied. While gains are being made, the field remains in need of substantial further investigation. The literature on racial/ethnic minority GSM groups has been described as focusing primarily on outcomes rather than processes, and largely ignoring the intersectionality of sexual orientation and race/ethnicity as an investigated factor (Toomey, Huynh, Jones, Lee, & Revels-Macalinao, 2016; Wade & Harper, 2015). In essence, while the literature regarding racial/ethnic minority GSM health is growing, the literature that actually examines the interplay of racial/ethnic identity and GSM identity, and the associated impact on health, is still lacking.

As a result, this chapter focuses primarily on describing the literature that has examined racial/ethnic disparities in a variety of outcomes, attempting to describe what is known regarding the actual impact of intersectionality whenever possible. Reflective of the current literature, the majority of the content in this chapter

269

centers on the African American and Hispanic sexual minority male population, and HIV, substance use, and mental health as outcomes. As echoed throughout this book, the need for expansion of the focal areas of research is sorely needed—even more so among the underrepresented populations discussed within this chapter. We begin with an exploration of barriers to health that reach across outcomes and populations, then discuss four specific outcomes with more developed bodies of literature (HIV/sexual health, substance use, mental health/suicide, and victimization), and then summarize the initial evidence from three emerging lines of inquiry (chronic conditions, incarceration, and women's health).

■ BARRIERS TO HEALTH

One of the clearest and most salient barriers to health for racial/ethnic minority GSM is prejudice due to both sexual orientation/gender identity and racial/ethnic identity. For racial/ethnic minority GSM, stigma regarding sexual orientation is perceived from families, religious communities, and racial/ethnic communities (Balaji et al., 2012). From early in the history of the field, African American sexual minority men have reported perceiving members of their own racial community as being less accepting of diverse sexual orientations than the majority White community (Stokes & Peterson, 1998). This also manifests for African American sexual minority women, with the majority of women reporting some degree of social isolation as a result of disclosing their sexual orientation (Jackson & Brown, 1996). These perceptions (and realities) can impact the identity development and disclosure process. For instance, African American and Hispanic sexual minority women have substantially different timing and disclosure of identity when compared to White women (Parks, Hughes, & Matthews, 2004), potentially delaying disclosure due to fears of cultural reactions.

When considering disclosure, family support appears critical for racial/ethnic minority GSM youth, particularly given the centrality of family in many racial/ethnic minority cultures. Rejection by family can lead to a host of negative effects. For example, Asian sexual minority youth who perceive lower levels of caring from their family report lower self-esteem and greater psychological distress, which places them at heightened risk for many of the outcomes discussed later in this chapter (Homma & Saewyc, 2007). Unfortunately, there appear to be substantial differences in family acceptance across racial/ethnic groups. Hispanic sexual minority young adults are more likely than their White counterparts to report negative family reactions to disclosure of sexual orientation, which in turn significantly predicts poorer health (Ryan, Huebner, Díaz, & Sanchez, 2009). Because of the often matriarchal structure of African American families, acceptance by African American women may be particularly important for African American GSM; however, African American women have been shown to have more negative attitudes toward sexual minority men and women than White women, and in particular have more negative attitudes toward gay men than lesbians (Vincent, Peterson, & Parrott, 2009). While the vast majority (68%) of Hispanic sexual minority men report feeling closely connected to their ethnic community, over 40% of Hispanic sexual minority men report having experienced both homophobia and racism within the past 12 months (Mizuno et al., 2012; L. O'Donnell et al., 2002). Because of similar experiences, African American sexual minority men are less likely than their White counterparts to report disclosure of their sexual orientation (Kennamer, Honnold, Bradford, & Hendricks, 2000; Millett, Flores, Peterson, & Bakeman, 2007; Moradi et al., 2010), as are Hispanic and African American youth (Rosario, Schrimshaw, & Hunter, 2004).

Religious discrimination may be particularly impactful for racial/ethnic minority GSM, with African American sexual minority men in particular often describing the importance of maintaining connections even with nonaffirming churches in order to stay connected to family and community (Quinn, Dickson-Gomez, & Kelly, 2016). Interestingly, Hispanic sexual minority men frequently break from their childhood religion (often Catholicism) in favor of a different religious group in adulthood (García, Gray-Stanley, & Ramirez-Valles, 2008); therefore, the experience is not identical across groups, and Hispanic GSM appear to seek social support in other areas. Among older adults, African American sexual minority men and women report feelings of alienation both from the African American community and from organized religion (Woody, 2014), but are also highly likely to conceal their sexual minority identity (Jimenez, 2003), impacting their ability to find connection to the broader LGBT community.

While understanding the dynamics of acceptance within an individual's immediate family and racial/ethnic community is important, it is equally important to recognize that racist experiences occur even within the LGBT community. In fact, two out of three racial/ethnic minority sexual minority men report being stressed as a result of racism experienced directly from within the LGBT community (Han et al., 2015), and intergroup racism has been found to lead to a sense of "invisibility" among racial/ethnic minority GSM within the LGBT community (Giwa & Greensmith, 2012). Racial/ethnic minority GSM often feel forced to deny certain important aspects of their identity to receive support from their racial/ethnic community, and certain other important aspects to receive support within the LGBT community, adding even further layers of oppression (Nabors et al., 2001). This is sometimes expressed via code-switching or role flexing, where racial/ethnic minority individuals alter their behaviors based upon the context of the social group they are in (Balaji et al., 2012). At the extreme, this can manifest in the concept of long-term "passing" within the lived community, wherein individuals attempt to be continually perceived as straight/cisgender (Brooks, 2016).

One of the most fundamental systemic barriers to achieving and maintaining health for racial/ethnic minority GSM centers on access to care and issues of health care discrimination. While a major concern across the spectrum of GSM individuals, limited access to appropriate and affirming care has been repeatedly shown to disproportionately impact GSM who identify as members of a racial/ethnic minority group. Racial/ethnic minority GSMs are less likely to have health insurance than their White GSM counterparts, even when in a relationship (Gonzales & Ortiz, 2015; Macapagal, Bhatia, & Greene, 2016). Unfortunately, the barriers to access are not just focused on financial access. Among both African American and Asian/Pacific Islander GSM, both sexual orientation and gender identity have been identified by patients as negatively impacting the patient/provider relationship and, ultimately, the ability to engage in appropriate shared decision-making regarding medical care (Peek et al., 2016; Tan et al., 2016). While data are largely unavailable regarding the prevalence of health care discrimination experienced by minority GSM, Eaton et al. (2015) found that, among their sample of African American sexual minority men, 29% reported feeling stigmatized by their providers and nearly half (48%) reported a mistrust of medical establishments. A similar study by Irvin et al. (2014) found that nearly 20% of African American sexual minority men had specifically experienced racial health care discrimination toward a family member, friend, or self, and of all racial/ethnic minority groups, African American gender minority men and women are at highest risk for actual physical attack in a doctor's office (Grant et al., 2011).

These experiences of health care discrimination directly impact care-seeking, with reduced health care utilization found after negative experiences in both African American sexual minority men (Eaton et al., 2015) and women (Li, Matthews, Aranda, Patel, & Patel, 2015). Although similar data are largely unavailable for other racial/ethnic groups, Asian sexual minority women report a greater unmet need for health care services than their non-sexual minority Asian female counterparts (Hahm, Lee, Chiao, Valntine, & Lê Cook, 2016), likely reflecting a similar pattern of avoidance of care. To help prevent the effects of negative health care experiences, a number of models have been developed to facilitate appropriate patient/provider interactions with racial/ethnic minority GSM, with a particular focus on shared decision making (DeMeester, Lopez, Moore, Cook, & Chin 2016; Peek et al., 2016; Tan et al., 2016; see also Chapter 22).

■ HIV/SEXUAL HEALTH

As with much of the work that has been done regarding the health of GSM groups, there is a significant focus within the literature on HIV prevention and sexual health among racial/ethnic minority GSM, particularly sexual minority men (see Chapter 13 for a comprehensive discussion of HIV and other STIs). African American and Hispanic sexual minority men face disparities in both prevalence and outcomes related to HIV—both groups have elevated prevalence in comparison to White sexual minority men, and African American sexual minority men have lower 3-year survival rates after AIDS diagnosis than either White or Hispanic sexual minority men (Hall, Byers, Ling, & Espinoza, 2007). The magnitude of the disparity is shocking—the Centers for Disease Control and Prevention (2017) predicts that, should current trends continue, 50% of all African American and 25% of all Hispanic sexual minority men will be diagnosed with HIV in their lifetimes, contrasted with less than 10% of White sexual minority men. Even beyond HIV, in comparison to White sexual minority men, African American sexual minority men also have 50% higher seroprevalence of herpes simplex virus type 2 (Okafor et al., 2015), elevated rates of HPV infection, and higher rates of HPV-related anal dysplasia (Walsh, Bertozzi-Villa, & Schneider, 2015).

Overall, the magnitude of the impact of the HIV epidemic in African American and Hispanic sexual minority men has been attributed largely to factors *other* than individual behavior—that is, the disparity is maintained largely due to the already high prevalence, increased likelihood of unknown serostatus, lower condom use self-efficacy, diagnosis later in the course of disease, inadequate access to culturally competent services, health care stigma and discrimination, and histories of specific risk factors such as childhood sexual abuse (Díaz, Morales, Bein, Dilán, & Rodríguez, 1999; Feldman, 2010; Levy et al., 2014; Mannheimer et al., 2014; Rhodes, Yee, & Hergenrather, 2006). In fact, sexual minority African American men report having fewer sex partners than heterosexual African American men (MacCarthy et al., 2015). Thus, the dynamics of the disparity go far beyond individual sexual behavior.

The effect of racism has direct implications for sexual risk: stress from racism has been shown to have a significant effect on unprotected sex among African American sexual minority men (Han et al., 2015). Internalized homophobia is also a risk factor for unprotected sex for African American sexual minority men (Crosby, Salazar, Mena, & Geter, 2016), as is socioeconomic distress (Huebner et al., 2014). The effects of socioeconomic stress may be particularly important—in a comparative study, young African American sexual minority men who had recently missed meals due to lack of money (found in 22% of participants) were more likely to have multiple concurrent partners, have partners who were at least 5 years older, not have used condoms at first encounter with current sexual partner, and depend on sexual partners for food, money, and shelter (Mena, Crosby, & Geter, 2016).

Although not the dominant factor in the presence of the HIV disparity, it is still helpful to understand the dynamics of condom use in racial/ethnic minority sexual minority men. Among African American and Hispanic sexual minority men, predictors of unprotected sex with a serodiscordant or sero-unknown partner include experiences of homophobia, racism, financial hardship, and lack of social support (Ayala, Bingham, Kim, Wheeler, & Millett, 2012; Mizuno et al., 2012). The impact of alcohol on sexual decision making appears to vary by sexual orientation—bisexual African American men are more likely to report unprotected sex with men while under the influence of alcohol than are gay African American men (Dyer, Regan, Wilton, Harawa, Wang, & Shoptaw, 2013). Predictors of unprotected sex for young sexual minority men also appear to vary by racial/ethnic group. For African American youth, being in a long-term relationship, having been kicked out of the home due to sexual orientation, and younger age at sexual debut are predictors of unprotected sex, whereas for Hispanic youth, higher degree of ethnic identification and older age at sexual debut are associated with unprotected sex (Warren et al., 2008).

The role and importance of ethnic identity in sexual risk-taking appear complex and vary between racial/ethnic groups. While ethnic exploration appears to enhance the protective effect of sexual identity pride on unprotected sex among young Hispanic men, it weakens the effect for African American men (Corsbie-Massay et al., 2016). Further, young African American sexual minority men have been shown to be less likely to engage in unprotected sex with partners who are also African American than with partners of another race (Clerkin, Newcomb, & Mustanski, 2011). Among Hispanic sexual minority men, community involvement serves as a buffer in the relationship between sexual orientation/racial stigma and sexual risk behaviors (Ramirez-Valles, Kuhns, Campbell, & Díaz, 2010), despite the fact that gender norms, such as machismo, have been directly tied to risky sexual behaviors (Estrada, Rigali-Oiler, Arciniega, & Tracey, 2011). Among Hispanic sexual minority men, immigration status also plays into cultural influences on HIV risk. The relationship between immigrant status and HIV prevalence varies by geographic location for Hispanic sexual minority men—for example, HIV prevalence is higher in San Franciscan U.S.–born residents, but in Chicago, the opposite has been found (Ramirez-Valles, Garcia, Campbell, Díaz, & Heckathorn, 2008). Furthermore, in South Florida, Spanish-only speaking Hispanic sexual minority men are less likely than their bilingual or English-only speaking counterparts to report having been tested for HIV (Spadafino et al., 2016). The role of racial/ethnic identity is therefore strongly related to sexual decision making, and merits further investigation.

Much less is known regarding HIV risk among sexual minority men of other racial/ethnic groups and among racial/ethnic minority sexual minority women and gender minority individuals. Native American sexual minority men and women are more likely to report early sexual debut with opposite-sex partners; thus, sexual risk-taking even among sexual minority Native American youth may be more related to opposite-sex rather than same-sex encounters (Saewyc, Skay, Bearinger, Blum, & Resnick, 1998). Regardless, HIV prevalence estimates in Native American GSM samples are highest in sexual minority men (34%) and are higher in sexual minority women (15%) than White sexual minority men (Cassels, Pearson, Walters, Simoni, & Morris, 2010), and therefore speak to a largely ignored component of the HIV epidemic. When considering cisgender women, bisexual African American women are more likely than gay African American women to report a history of an STD (Muzny, Austin, Harbison, & Hook, 2014), and Asian sexual minority women are more likely to report engaging in sexual behaviors that place them at risk for the acquisition of HIV (Lee & Hahm, 2012).

Among gender minority individuals, there are profound disparities related to HIV prevalence, with 25% of African American gender minority men and women reporting HIV infection, as compared to only 11% of Hispanic, 7% of Native American, and 4% of Asian gender minority men and women (Grant et al., 2011). Predictors of high-risk behaviors in racial/ethnic minority transgender women include higher rates of depression, low self-esteem, less social support, poorer sex communication skills, and history of incarceration (Garofalo, Osmer, Sullivan, Doll, & Harper, 2007). Little else is known, however, regarding the HIV risk of these understudied groups and more research is strongly needed.

■ SUBSTANCE USE

Due to its frequent association with HIV prevention research, substance use among racial and ethnic minority GSM is comparatively well-studied, again particularly among sexual minority men. When considering alcohol abuse, experiences of racism and homophobia are related to binge drinking among Hispanic sexual minority men (Mizuno et al., 2012), with prevalence of heavy episodic drinking estimated at 35% (Rhodes et al., 2012). Among African American sexual minority men, problematic drinking has been associated with depression and unprotected sex, although the direction of association is unclear (Reisner et al., 2010). Overall, rates of alcohol use and abuse appear comparable among racial and ethnic minority sexual minority women (Hughes et al., 2006; Parks & Hughes, 2005). Among gender minority populations, half of Native American two-spirit individuals meet criteria for past-year alcohol dependence (Yuan, Duran, Walters, Pearson, & Evans-Campbell, 2014), and nearly half of Hispanic transgender women report high-risk alcohol consumption within the past 30 days (Martinez et al., 2016).

Tobacco use is also a concern among racial/ethnic minority GSM, with racial/ethnic disparities in smoking rates among GSM beginning in adolescence (Corliss et al., 2014). Within all racial/ethnic groups, GSM are more likely to report cigarette smoking than their heterosexual counterparts (Blosnich, Jarrett, & Horn, 2011). Among Hispanic sexual minority men, prevalence of smoking every day is 6.5% (Rhodes et al., 2012), and general tobacco use is higher in the Puerto Rican LGBT community (20.8%) than the general Puerto Rican population (14.8%; Cabrera-Serrano, Felici-Giovanini, Díaz-Toro, & Cases-Rosario, 2014). When considering racial/ethnic differences in smoking, both African American and Asian gender minority men are less likely to smoke than White gender minority men (Ortiz, Duncan, Blosnich, Salloum, & Battle, 2015). Native American two-spirit individuals report high rates of smoking (45%), with racial discrimination found to be a significant predictor of tobacco use (Johnson-Jennings, Belcourt, Town, Walls, & Walters, 2014). Interestingly, among smokers, while African American GSM are more likely to report that they are trying to quit smoking than White GSM, they are less likely to succeed (Jordan, Everett, Ge, & McElroy, 2015).

There are substantially more variations across race/ethnicity when examining illicit drug use. Overall, contrary to many social stereotypes, African American sexual minority men report less substance use than White sexual minority men (Harawa et al., 2004; Millett et al., 2007). However, racial/ethnic sexual minority women have a greater risk of lifetime substance use than both heterosexual women and White sexual minority women (Mereish & Bradford, 2014). Hispanic sexual minority adolescents report more cigarette consumption and illegal drug use than non-sexual minority Hispanic adolescents (Ocasio, Feaster, & Prado, 2016), and urban samples of Hispanic sexual minority men have demonstrated very high rates of club drug use, with more than half reporting recent use (Fernández et al., 2005). However, gay male Native American youth have been shown to have comparable rates of substance use with their heterosexual peers (Barney, 2003), and Native American two-spirit individuals have comparable marijuana and alcohol use, but are more likely to use drugs other than marijuana (Balsam, Huang, Fieland, Simoni, & Walters, 2004). On the whole, Asian sexual minority men report the lowest levels of substance use (Grov, Bimbi, Bimbi, & Parsons, 2006).

Variations in risk factors for substance use across groups have not been as well studied. As with other findings throughout this chapter, while discrimination related to sexual orientation/gender identity is positively associated with illicit drug use, discrimination related to racism is not as clearly related (Drazdowski et al., 2016). When considering variations among sexual orientations, being bisexually identified appears to amplify substance use risk across racial/ethnic groups: among racial/ethnic minority GSM, bisexual men and women are more likely to have substance use problems in comparison to their gay counterparts (Meyer, Dietrich, & Schwartz, 2008). Due to its association with acquisition of HIV, motivations for methamphetamine use have been specifically investigated. For Hispanic sexual minority men, often-cited benefits of methamphetamine use include enhanced energy, improved work and sexual performance, increased social connections, and use as an alternative coping strategy (Díaz, Heckert, & Sánchez, 2005). When considering culturally specific risk factors, lower attachment to Hispanic identity has been demonstrated to increase the risk of methamphetamine use among this subpopulation (Fernández et al., 2007).

■ MENTAL HEALTH

Overall Psychological Health

There are several mental health outcomes and risk factors that disproportionately impact the lives of racial/ethnic minority GSM individuals. When considering overall mental health and well-being, Hispanic sexual minority men and women report lower levels of mental health quality of life than their non-Hispanic sexual minority peers, with the difference attributed to strong effects of socioeconomic status, experiences of discrimination, and lower social connectedness (Kim & Fredriksen-Goldsen, 2016). Other mental health factors are directly related to social and cultural norms. African American sexual minority men frequently report experiencing rigid, antigay gender norms from family, peers, and their racial community—when combined with conflict about adhering to those norms, the effect has been associated with psychological distress (E. L. Fields et al., 2015). These effects appear more closely tied to sexual orientation than race—internalized heterosexism, but not internalized racism, is a significant predictor of psychological distress for African American sexual minority men (Szymanski & Gupta, 2009). For Asian sexual minority men and women, psychological distress has been tied to both racism and outness, with the combination of racist experiences and a high degree of outness having the highest levels of psychological distress (Sandil, Robinson, Brewster, Wong, & Geiger, 2015).

Racial and ethnic minority transgender youth have increased vulnerabilities for mental health concerns even in comparison to their racial/ethnic minority sexual minority peers, with lower levels of education, employment, and residential stability linked with overall higher symptoms of depression and anxiety (Bauermeister, Goldenberg, Connochie, Jadwin-Cakmak, & Stephenson, 2016). The same holds for African American transgender adult women, who show increased vulnerabilities beyond their African American sexual minority counterparts such as lower educational attainment and greater likelihood of homelessness (Siembida, Eaton, Maksut, Driffin, & Baldwin, 2016). For gender minority adults, affirming social circles play a very important role in bolstering mental health; among African American transgender women in particular, greater social affirmation of true gender identity is associated with more positive mental health outcomes (Crosby, Salazar, & Hill, 2016).

Even in the face of the increased need just described, racial/ethnic minority groups are more likely to go without needed mental health care. Despite increased need, young African American and Asian/Pacific Islander sexual minority men are less likely to access mental health counseling/treatment (Storholm et al., 2013), and Hispanic sexual minority women exhibit a higher degree of unmet mental health care needs than do African American or White sexual minority women (Jeong, Veldhuis, Aranda, & Hughes, 2016). The main exception is for Asian sexual minority women, who are more likely than heterosexual Asian women to have received mental health care within the past year (Hahm et al., 2016).

Depression and Anxiety

Two of the most-investigated mental health conditions among racial/ethnic minority GSM are depression and anxiety. Nearly half (43.8%) of African American sexual minority men report depressive symptomatology (Williams et al., 2015). In addition, there are high rates of anxiety and depression among Hispanic sexual minority men, with 44% of men reporting anxious symptoms and 80% reporting depressed mood within the past 6 months (Díaz, Ayala, Bein, Henne, & Marin, 2001). The prevalence of depressive symptoms is similarly high among Hispanic sexual minority immigrants, with an estimated 69% to 75% exhibiting significant depressive symptoms (Rhodes et al., 2013). For cisgender women, Hispanic and Asian sexual minority women exhibit an elevated risk of positive 1-year and lifetime history of depressive disorders in comparison to their heterosexual counterparts (Cochran, Mays, Alegria, Ortega, & Takeuchi, 2007).

The factors leading to depression specifically in racial/ethnic minority GSM are highly understudied. Across racial and ethnic minority sexual minority men, recent experiences of racism and homophobia have been tied to both depression and anxiety symptoms (Choi, Paul, Ayala, Boylan, & Gregorich, 2013). In fact, over half of the variance in anxiety and over 60% of the variance in depression among African American sexual minority men has been shown to be explained by the combination of discrimination, harassment, and internalized homophobia (Graham, Aronson, Nichols, Stephens, & Rhodes, 2011). Correspondingly, among African American sexual minority men, the size of a man's emotional, financial, and medical support network is significantly associated longitudinally with fewer depressive symptoms (Latkin et al., 2016). Predictors of depression in Hispanic sexual minority men include low social support and, interestingly, high self-esteem (Rhodes et al., 2013). Experiences of discrimination are also related to clinically significant depressive symptoms among Hispanic sexual minority men and transgender women (Sun et al., 2016).

Suicide

Unfortunately, the impact of mental health concerns appears to combine in ways that also increase the risk of suicide among some racial/ethnic minority GSM. The impact of societal stigma on suicide appears to occur from an early age—sexual minority youth consistently report more experiences of sadness; suicidal ideation, plan, and intent; suicide attempts; and other intentional self-harm behaviors when compared to heterosexual youth, and this effect has been demonstrated within each major racial/ethnic group (Lytle, De Luca, & Blosnich, 2014). Native American gay male youth are twice as likely as Native American heterosexual male youth to have thought about or attempted suicide (Barney, 2003). Hispanic and Asian sexual minority men are also more likely to report a history of a recent suicide attempt than Hispanic and Asian heterosexual men (Cochran et al., 2007), with prevalence of suicidal ideation within the past 6 months in Hispanic sexual minority men at 17% (Díaz et al., 2001). Similar findings occur when considering women. Asian sexual minority women are two to three times more likely to report experiencing suicidal ideation than Asian heterosexual women (Lee & Hahm, 2012), with initial research showing that among Vietnamese sexual minority women, negative treatment from family members related to higher odds of attempted suicide (Nguyen et al., 2016). While comparison rates are not readily available, over one-third of Hispanic transgender women report suicidal ideation or self-harm within the preceding 2 weeks (Bazargan & Galvan, 2012).

When comparing across racial/ethnic groups, some studies have found Asian and African American GSM youth exhibit lower frequency of suicidal behavior than White youth, with Native American, Hispanic, Pacific Islander, and multiracial GSM youth reporting higher frequency (Bostwick et al., 2014; Lytle, De Luca, Blosnich, & Brownson, 2015). Similar effects are seen in adults—as in the adult non-GSM population, African American sexual minority adults are less likely to have a history of suicide attempts than are Hispanic and White sexual minority adults (Meyer et al., 2008). These racial/ethnic variations have been shown to not be linked to excess rates of depression or substance use (S. O'Donnell, Meyer, & Schwartz, 2011), and may therefore reflect the effects of much deeper cultural factors. Interestingly, while discrimination related to sexual orientation and gender identity has been shown to impact risk of suicidal ideation indirectly through an impact on overall mental health among racial/ethnic minority GSM, discrimination based upon race has not been shown to have an effect on suicidal ideation (Sutter & Perrin, 2016). As with the other outcomes discussed in this chapter, research into specific reasons for these disparities is needed.

■ VICTIMIZATION

Another area with a fair amount of recent research is that of victimization, including discrimination, harassment, interpersonal violence, and sexual abuse. A history of harassment appears nearly universal for racial and ethnic minority GSM due to their presence at the intersection of (at least) two marginalized populations (Dang & Vianney, 2007; Díaz, Ayala, & Bein, 2004; Van Sluytman et al., 2015). Of note, Dang and Vianney (2007) found that experiences of verbal harassment among Asian GSM were comparable for harassment based upon ethnic background (77%) and GSM status (74%). Thus, both racial/ethnic and GSM identity are associated with significant risk of experiences of outward hostility. While victimization is possible in any location, for African American GSM, risks for discrimination, harassment, and violence are particularly heightened within the school system (Graham, 2014). Among Native American sexual minority youth, differences by gender have been demonstrated. While both sexual minority male and female youth have been shown to be more likely to have run away from home than their heterosexual counterparts, only sexual minority male youth have demonstrated an elevated risk of associated abuse (Saewyc et al., 1998). Thus, while abuse may play a role for sexual minority male youth in risk of running away, the reasons for Native American sexual minority female youth may be more complex.

There are other substantial variations in likelihood of victimization, particularly among sexual minority women. Consistently, Native American sexual minority women report the highest rates of victimization, followed by Hispanic women, African American women, Asian women, and then White women (Morris & Balsam, 2003). Among transgender women, however, African American women had the highest rates of physical assault (with nearly one-quarter of transgender women reporting being physically assaulted, and nearly 10% reporting a history of being assaulted in a public place; Grant et al., 2011). These experiences of harassment are ever-present fears that can have substantial emotional impact. To illustrate, one-quarter of Hispanic transgender women report experiencing discrimination multiple times per week (Bazargan & Galvan, 2012).

When considering physical assault, Native American populations are particularly impacted. Two-spirit individuals report an increased likelihood of childhood physical abuse and of historical trauma in the family (Balsam et al., 2004), gay male Native American youth have been shown to be twice as likely to have a lifetime history of physical abuse as their heterosexual peers (Barney, 2003), and over three-quarters of Native American GSM women report a history of physical assault (Lehavot, Walters, & Simoni, 2009). Across genders, a greater proportion of Hispanic and Asian sexual minority adults report a history of childhood physical abuse in comparison to other racial/ethnic groups (Balsam, Lehavot, Beadnell, & Circo, 2010). For intimate partner violence (IPV), both African American and Hispanic sexual minority men report a history of IPV in excess of that found in nonminority sexual minority men. The magnitude of IPV is substantial—a history of IPV has been found in 52% of both African American and Hispanic sexual minority men (Feldman, Díaz, Ream, & El-Bassel, 2008; Williams et al., 2015; for additional discussion of IPV, please see Chapter 8).

Beyond the immediate emotional impact of harassment and physical assault experiences, bullying among youth related to sexual orientation has been tied to depressive symptomatology, suicide attempts, and an increased risk of parental abuse among sexual minority men of color (Hightow-Weidman et al., 2011). Other aftereffects of abuse appear to vary by racial/ethnic group, with emotional abuse tied more strongly to posttraumatic stress disorder (PTSD) among African American than White sexual minority adults, and physical abuse tied more strongly to PTSD and anxiety for Hispanic than White sexual minority adults (Balsam et al., 2010). A history of discrimination experiences is also a particular risk for depression and anxiety among Hispanic sexual minority men (Díaz et al., 2001) and Hispanic transgender women (Sun et al., 2016). A history of victimization is very high among Native American two-spirit individuals with alcohol abuse problems, with 63% reporting a history of physical abuse and 72% a history of emotional abuse (Yuan et al., 2014).

There are also stark disparities with respect to histories of childhood sexual abuse. Overall, both Hispanic and African American sexual minority adults report the highest history of childhood sexual abuse (Balsam et al., 2010). When compared to White sexual minority men, Hispanic sexual minority men are twice as likely to report a history of sexual abuse before the age of 13 (22% vs. 11%; Arreola, Neilands, Pollack, Paul, & Catania, 2005). Rates of early childhood sexual abuse are even higher for African American sexual minority men, with estimates over 30% in multiple studies (S. D. Fields, Malebranche, & Feist-Price, 2008; Williams et al., 2015). The burden of sexual abuse and assault appears to continue in other ages, with 30% of African American sexual minority men reporting unwanted sexual encounters from the ages of 12 to 16 (Williams et al., 2015). Native American gay male youth have also been found to have very high rates of childhood sexual abuse that are more than five times that found in Native American heterosexual youth (i.e., 13.3% vs. 2.4%; Barney, 2003). Disturbingly, the vast majority (85%) of Native American lesbian, bisexual, and two-spirit women report a history of sexual assault (Lehavot et al., 2009), and significant differences in history of childhood sexual assault and forcible rape have been found among racial/ethnic minority GSM women, with African American sexual minority women having a greater prevalence of childhood sexual assault when compared to their White counterparts (48.1% vs. 35.8%, respectively; Balsam et al., 2015).

The long-term effects of childhood sexual abuse are many, and may contribute to increased levels of internalized homophobia, a major risk factor for many other outcomes. S. D. Fields et al. (2008) found that African American sexual minority men who experienced childhood sexual abuse often "blame" their same-sex attraction on their abuse history, which may significantly alter their ability to form an integrated and affirming GSM identity. Among sexual minority Hispanic men, childhood sexual abuse has been shown to negatively impact adherence to regimens of antiretroviral therapy, with the relationship mediated by depression (Sauceda, Wiebe, & Simoni, 2016). One of the darkest long-term effects of a history of victimization is risk for incarceration, discussed in more detail later in this chapter—African American GSM with a history of incarceration are significantly more likely to report a history of childhood violence or sexual experience (Brewer et al., 2014a).

■ CHRONIC CONDITIONS

Research into the burden of chronic medical conditions on the overall LGBT community is very limited, and there is correspondingly no cohesive body of research literature that has examined chronic diseases among racial/ethnic minority GSM. Given the documented disparities in chronic disease outcomes affecting the overall racial/ethnic minority community (Russell, 2010), it is highly likely that minority GSM similarly face higher prevalence and worse outcomes related to chronic conditions. The literature, however, is in its early infancy. Very recent biomarker studies hold much promise for elucidating disparities—for instance, African American sexual minority men have been shown to have elevated evening cortisol levels (a physiological indicator of stress response) in comparison to White sexual minority men, showing that racial stress continues to place excess physiological burden even beyond the discrimination experienced by the LGBT community as a whole (Cook, Juster, Calebs, Heinze, & Miller, 2017). However, there is substantial work to be done to more fully understand chronic disease disparities.

What work has been done has focused largely on risk factors for chronic conditions rather than outcomes themselves, focused predominantly on cisgender sexual minority women. These studies have shown that while prevalence of chronic conditions appears to be similar across racial/ethnic minority GSM women, they demonstrate higher behavioral risks and lower engagement in preventive care than racial/ethnic minority non-GSM women (Mays, Yancey, Cochran, Weber, & Fielding, 2002). For instance, studies have demonstrated that when compared to non-GSM women of the same race/ethnicity, White and African American lesbian and bisexual women are more likely than non-GSM women to be overweight by the age of 18 years and to maintain an overweight status during adulthood, but these findings do not appear to hold for Hispanic or Asian women (Deputy & Boehmer, 2014). When comparing across racial/ethnic groups within GSM women, African American women have been shown to have higher BMIs than White women, while Asian and Pacific Islander GSM women have lower BMIs (Yancey, Cochran, Corliss, & Mays, 2003). For African American sexual minority women, high rates of obesity-linked chronic conditions have been demonstrated, including back pain (23%), high cholesterol (15.3%), hypertension (19%), heart disease (12%), and type 2 diabetes (5%), with infrequent exercise and poor dietary habits cited as common obesity risk factors (Matthews, Li, McConnell, Aranda, & Smith, 2016). Additional studies have also shown African American sexual minority women to be more likely to report low fruit and vegetable intake, limited physical activity, a higher BMI, and a history of high blood pressure and/or diabetes (Molina, Lehavot, Beadnell, & Simoni, 2014).

■ INCARCERATION

As with cisgender heterosexual African American men, incarceration is a major sociopolitical factor impacting health for African American GSM, one that can be difficult to escape due to a vicious cycle of recidivism. In their study of incarceration and HIV risk among sexual minority African American GSM, Brewer and colleagues (2014b) found that 1-year incidence of incarceration among previously incarcerated sexual minority men and transgender women was a shocking 35%. Beyond the effect of previous history of incarceration, having a transgender identity (Brewer et al., 2014a) and experiencing higher levels of perceived racism (Brewer et al., 2014b) have also been shown to be independently associated with an increased risk of incarceration. Troublingly, the length of time spent incarcerated also appears to vary by race/ethnicity. While 15% of previously incarcerated African American transgender men and women spent 5 or more years imprisoned, only 4% of non-African American transgender men and women spent 5 or more years imprisoned (Grant et al., 2011). This becomes particularly upsetting when considering that nearly half of transgender women report being victimized while incarcerated (Reisner, Bailey, & Sevelius, 2014). Additional research into the factors predicting and protecting against incarceration for racial/ethnic minority GSM groups is sorely needed.

WOMEN'S HEALTH

When considering women's health issues, disparities between sexual orientations exist and have sometimes opposite implications for health risk. For instance, while African American lesbians are less likely than African American bisexual women to have ever been pregnant, they are also less likely to have had a Pap test within the past year and the past 3 years (Agénor, Austin, Kurt, Austin, & Muzny, 2016). While this reflects similar findings for Caucasian lesbians and bisexual women, Hispanic women do not demonstrate a difference in Pap tests between sexual orientations (Agénor, Krieger, Austin, Hanes, & Gottlieb, 2014). The finding regarding Pap screening is particularly concerning and reflects assumptions regarding the prior sexual history of lesbians discussed in more detail in Chapter 7. Specific barriers related to racial and ethnic minority sexual minority women's experiences with preventive cancer screening include fear and experience of discrimination within the health care setting, heteronormative provider assumptions, and provider communication style (Agénor, Bailey, Krieger, Austin, & Gottlieb, 2015).

CONCLUSION

Racial/ethnic minority GSM individuals represent a vulnerable subpopulation of the LGBT community. Most notably, due to their intersecting (and oftentimes conflicting) cultural identities, racial/ethnic minority GSM appear to be at heightened risks for rejection and discrimination from within the LGBT community, their racial/ethnic and religious communities, and society at large, as well as other psychosocial risk factors including increased barriers to medical and mental health care, lower levels of outness, lower quality of life, increased rates of incarceration, and greater experiences of physical and sexual assault across the life span. Furthermore, emerging research suggests that the intersection between being a racial/ethnic minority and a gender and/or sexual minority may exacerbate the risks for a multitude of physical and mental health risk factors and outcomes among GSM individuals, including HIV/STDs, problematic drinking, tobacco and illicit drug use, depression and anxiety, suicidality, poor diet and exercise habits, overweight/obesity, and other risky health behaviors.

Because the field is so young, there is very little theory-driven work that has been completed to explain the direct and intersectional impact of racial/ethnic identity beyond that experienced by GSM as a whole. Minority stress theory— discussed throughout this book—has been initially expanded to incorporate dual minority stress, and helps provide an informative perspective on the experiences of GSM from racial/ethnic minority backgrounds (Meyer, 2010); however, much more work in this area is needed to identify factors that are potential targets for intervention programs. As researchers expand their focus on the study of intersectionality itself, it will be important to also examine additional intersecting identities. For example, early work has shown that women who have a racial/ ethnic and sexual minority identity must navigate a context of triple oppression wherein intersectional stigma (based on gender, race, and sexual orientation) is encountered on a daily basis (Greene, 2000; Logie & Rwigema, 2014). Overall, it is important for health care providers working with racial/ethnic minority GSM individuals to be aware of the unique health risks and needs of these patients in order to provide them with affirming, patient-centered care that takes into consideration their intersecting cultural identities and incorporates aspects of shared decision making between the patient and provider.

■ REFERENCES

Agénor, M., Austin, S. B., Kort, D., Austin, E. L., & Muzny, C. A. (2016). Sexual orientation and sexual and reproductive health among African American sexual minority women in the US South. *Women's Health Issues, 26*(6), 612–621. doi:10.1016/j.whi.2016.07.004

Agénor, M., Bailey, Z., Krieger, N., Austin, S. B., & Gottlieb, B. R. (2015). Exploring the cervical cancer screening experiences of Black lesbian, bisexual, and queer women: The role of patient-provider communication. *Women & Health, 55*(6), 717–736. doi:10.1080/ 03630242.2015.1039182

Agénor, M., Krieger, N., Austin, S. B., Haneuse, S., & Gottlieb, B. R. (2014). At the intersection of sexual orientation, race/ethnicity, and cervical cancer screening: Assessing Pap test use disparities by sex of sexual partners among Black, Latina, and White US women. *Social Science & Medicine, 116*, 110–118. doi:10.1016/j.socscimed.2014.06.039

Arreola, S. G., Neilands, T. B., Pollack, L. M., Paul, J. P., & Catania, J. A. (2005). Higher prevalence of childhood sexual abuse among Latino men who have sex with men than non-Latino men who have sex with men: Data from the Urban Men's Health Study. *Child Abuse & Neglect, 29*(3), 285–290. doi:10.1016/j.chiabu.2004.09.003

Ayala, G., Bingham, T., Kim, J., Wheeler, D. P., & Millett, G. A. (2012). Modeling the impact of social discrimination and financial hardship on the sexual risk of HIV among Latino and Black men who have sex with men. *American Journal of Public Health, 102*(S2), S242–S249.

Balaji, A. B., Oster, A. M., Viall, A. H., Heffelfinger, J. D., Mena, L. A., & Toledo, C. A. (2012). Role flexing: How community, religion, and family shape the experiences of young Black men who have sex with men. *AIDS Patient Care and STDs, 26*(12), 730–737.

Balsam, K. F., Huang, B., Fieland, K. C., Simoni, J. M., & Walters, K. L. (2004). Culture, trauma, and wellness: A comparison of heterosexual and lesbian, gay, bisexual, and two-spirit Native Americans. *Cultural Diversity and Ethnic Minority Psychology, 10*(3), 287–301.

Balsam, K. F., Lehavot, K., Beadnell, B., & Circo, E. (2010). Childhood abuse and mental health indicators among ethnically diverse lesbian, gay, and bisexual adults. *Journal of Consulting and Clinical Psychology, 78*(4), 459–468. doi:10.1037/a0018661

Balsam, K. F., Molina, Y., Blayney, J. A., Dillworth, T., Zimmerman, L., & Kaysen, D. (2015). Racial/ethnic differences in identity and mental health outcomes among young sexual minority women. *Cultural Diversity and Ethnic Minority Psychology, 21*(3), 380–390. doi:10.1037/a0038680

Barney, D. D. (2003). Health risk-factors for gay American Indian and Alaska Native adolescent males. *Journal of Homosexuality, 46*(1–2), 137–157.

Bauermeister, J. A., Goldenberg, T., Connochie, D., Jadwin-Cakmak, L., & Stephenson, R. (2016). Psychosocial disparities among racial/ethnic minority transgender young adults and young men who have sex with men living in Detroit. *Transgender Health, 1*(1), 279–290. doi:10.1089/trgh.2016.002

Bazargan, M., & Galvan, F. (2012). Perceived discrimination and depression among low-income Latina male-to-female transgender women. *BMC Public Health, 12*(1), 663. doi:10.1186/1471-2458-12-663

Blosnich, J. R., Jarrett, T., & Horn, K. (2011). Racial and ethnic differences in current use of cigarettes, cigars, and hookahs among lesbian, gay, and bisexual young adults. *Nicotine & Tobacco Research, 13*(6), 487–491. doi:10.1093/ntr/ntq261

Bostwick, W. B., Meyer, I., Aranda, F., Russell, S., Hughes, T., Birkett, M., & Mustanski, B. (2014). Mental health and suicidality among racially/ethnically diverse sexual minority youths. *American Journal of Public Health, 104*(6), 1129–1136. doi:10.2105/AJPH.2013.301749

Brewer, R. A., Magnus, M., Kuo, I., Wang, L., Liu, T. Y., & Mayer, K. H. (2014a). The high prevalence of incarceration history among Black men who have sex with men in the United States: Associations and implications. *American Journal of Public Health, 104*(3), 448–454.

Brewer, R. A., Magnus, M., Kuo, I., Wang, L., Liu, T. Y., & Mayer, K. H. (2014b). Exploring the relationship between incarceration and HIV among Black men who have sex with men in the United States. *Journal of Acquired Immune Deficiency Syndromes 65*(2), 218–225. doi:10.1097/01.qai.0000434953.65620.3d

Brooks, S. (2016). Staying in the hood: Black lesbian and transgender women and identity management in North Philadelphia. *Journal of Homosexuality, 63*(12), 1573–1593. doi:10.1080/00918369.2016.1158008

Cabrera-Serrano, A., Felici-Giovanini, M. E., Díaz-Toro, E. C., & Cases-Rosario, A. L. (2014). Disproportionate tobacco use in the Puerto Rico lesbian, gay, bisexual, and transgender community of 18 years and over: A descriptive profile. *LGBT Health, 1*(2), 107–112. doi:10.1089/lgbt.2013.0011

Cassels, S., Pearson, C. R., Walters, K., Simoni, J. M., & Morris, M. (2010). Sexual partner concurrency and sexual risk among gay, lesbian, bisexual, and transgender American Indian/Alaska Natives. *Sexually Transmitted Diseases, 37*(4), 272–278. doi:10.1097/OLQ.0b013e3181c37e3e

Centers for Disease Control and Prevention. (2017). HIV among African American Gay and Bisexual Men. Retrieved from https://www.cdc.gov/hiv/group/msm/bmsm.html

Choi, K. H., Paul, J., Ayala, G., Boylan, R., & Gregorich, S. E. (2013). Experiences of discrimination and their impact on the mental health among African American, Asian and Pacific Islander, and Latino men who have sex with men. *American Journal of Public Health, 103*(5), 868–874. doi:10.2105/AJPH.2012.301052

Clerkin, E. M., Newcomb, M. E., & Mustanski, B. (2011). Unpacking the racial disparity in HIV rates: the effect of race on risky sexual behavior among Black young men who have sex with men (YMSM). *Journal of Behavioral Medicine, 34*(4), 237–243. doi:10.1007/s10865-010-9306-4

Cochran, S., Mays, V., Alegria, M., Ortega, A., & Takeuchi, D. (2007). Mental health and substance use disorders among Latino and Asian American lesbian, gay, and bisexual adults. *Journal of Consulting and Clinical Psychology, 75*(5), 785–794.

Cook, S. H., Juster, R. P., Calebs, B. J., Heinze, J., & Miller, A. L. (2017). Cortisol profiles differ by race/ethnicity among young sexual minority men. *Psychoneuroendocrinology, 75*, 1–4. doi:10.1016/j.psyneuen.2016.10.006

Corliss, H. L., Rosario, M., Birkett, M. A., Newcomb, M. E., Buchting, F. O., & Matthews, A. K. (2014). Sexual orientation disparities in adolescent cigarette smoking: Intersections with race/ethnicity, gender, and age. *American Journal of Public Health, 104*(6), 1137–1147. doi:10.2105/AJPH.2013.301819

Corsbie-Massay, C. L. P., Miller, L. C., Christensen, J. L., Appleby, P. R., Godoy, C., & Read, S. J. (2016). Identity conflict and sexual risk for Black and Latino YMSM. *AIDS and Behavior*. Advance online publication. doi:10.1007/s10461-016-1522-7

Crosby, R. A., Salazar, L. F., & Hill, B. J. (2016). Gender affirmation and resiliency among Black transgender women with and without HIV infection. *Transgender Health, 1*(1), 86–93. doi:10.1089/trgh.2016.0005

Crosby, R. A., Salazar, L. F., Mena, L., & Geter, A. (2016). Associations between internalized homophobia and sexual risk behaviors among young Black men who have sex with men. *Sexually Transmitted Diseases, 43*(10), 656–660. doi:10.1097/OLQ.0000000000000505

Dang, A., & Vianney, C. (2007). *Living in the margins: A national survey of lesbian, gay, bisexual and transgender Asian and Pacific Islander Americans.* New York, NY: The National Gay and Lesbian Task Force Policy Institute. Retrieved from http://www.thetaskforce.org/static_html/downloads/reports/reports/API_ExecutiveSummaryEnglish.pdf

DeMeester, R. H., Lopez, F. Y., Moore, J. E., Cook, S. C., & Chin, M. H. (2016). A model of organizational context and shared decision making: Application to LGBT racial and ethnic minority patients. *Journal of General Internal Medicine, 31*(6), 651–662.

Deputy, N. P., & Boehmer, U. (2014). Weight status and sexual orientation: Differences by age and within racial and ethnic subgroups. *American Journal of Public Health, 104*(1), 103–109. doi:10.2105/AJPH.2013.301391

Díaz, R. M., Ayala, G., & Bein, E. (2004). Sexual risk as an outcome of social oppression: Data from a probability sample of Latino gay men in three US cities. *Cultural Diversity and Ethnic Minority Psychology, 10*(3), 255–267. doi:10.1037/1099-9809.10.3.255

Díaz, R. M., Ayala, G., Bein, E., Henne, J., & Marin, B. V. (2001). The impact of homophobia, poverty, and racism on the mental health of gay and bisexual Latino men: Findings from 3 US cities. *American Journal of Public Health, 91*(6), 927–932.

Díaz, R. M., Heckert, A. L., & Sánchez, J. (2005). Reasons for stimulant use among Latino gay men in San Francisco: A comparison between methamphetamine and cocaine users. *Journal of Urban Health, 82*(Suppl 1), i71–i78. doi:10.1093/jurban/jti026

Díaz, R. M., Morales, E. S., Bein, E., Dilán, E., & Rodríguez, R. A. (1999). Predictors of sexual risk in Latino gay/bisexual men: The role of demographic, developmental, social cognitive, and behavioral variables. *Hispanic Journal of Behavioral Sciences, 21*(4), 480–501.

Drazdowski, T. K., Perrin, P. B., Trujillo, M., Sutter, M., Benotsch, E. G., & Snipes, D. J. (2016). Structural equation modeling of the effects of racism, LGBTQ discrimination, and internalized oppression on illicit drug use in LGBTQ people of color. *Drug and Alcohol Dependence, 159*, 255–262. doi:10.1016/j.drugalcdep.2015.12.029

Dyer, T. P., Regan, R., Wilton, L., Harawa, N. T., Wang, L., & Shoptaw, S. (2013). Differences in substance use, psychosocial characteristics and HIV-related sexual risk behavior between Black men who have sex with men only (BMSMO) and Black men who have sex with men and women (BMSMW) in six US cities. *Journal of Urban Health, 90*(6), 1181–1193. doi:10.1007/s11524-013-9811-1

Eaton, L. A., Driffin, D. D., Kegler, C., Smith, H., Conway-Washington, C., White, D., & Cherry, C. (2015). The role of stigma and medical mistrust in the routine health care engagement of Black men who have sex with men. *American Journal of Public Health, 105*(2), e75–e82. doi:10.2105/AJPH.2014.302322

Estrada, F., Rigali-Oiler, M., Arciniega, G. M., & Tracey, T. J. (2011). Machismo and Mexican American men: An empirical understanding using a gay sample. *Journal of Counseling Psychology, 58*(3), 358–367. doi:10.1037/a0023122

Feldman, M. B. (2010). A critical literature review to identify possible causes of higher rates of HIV infection among young Black and Latino men who have sex with men. *Journal of the National Medical Association, 102*(12), 1206–1221.

Feldman, M. B., Díaz, R. M., Ream, G. L., & El-Bassel, N. (2008). Intimate partner violence and HIV sexual risk behavior among Latino gay and bisexual men. *Journal of LGBT Health Research, 3*(2), 9–19.

Fernández, M. I., Bowen, G. S., Varga, L. M., Collazo, J. B., Hernandez, N., Perrino, T., & Rehbein, A. (2005). High rates of club drug use and risky sexual practices among Hispanic men who have sex with men in Miami, Florida. *Substance Use & Misuse, 40*(9–10), 1347–1362.

Fernández, M. I., Bowen, G. S., Warren, J. C., Ibañez, G. E., Hernandez, N., Harper, G. W., & Prado, G. (2007). Crystal methamphetamine: A source of added sexual risk for Hispanic men who have sex with men? *Drug and Alcohol Dependence, 86*(2), 245–252. doi:10.1016/j.drugalcdep.2006.06.016

Fields, E. L., Bogart, L. M., Smith, K. C., Malebranche, D. J., Ellen, J., & Schuster, M. A. (2015). "I always felt I had to prove my manhood": Homosexuality, masculinity, gender role strain, and HIV risk among young Black men who have sex with men. *American Journal of Public Health, 105*(1), 122–131. doi:10.2105/AJPH.2013.301866

Fields, S. D., Malebranche, D., & Feist-Price, S. (2008). Childhood sexual abuse in Black men who have sex with men: Results from three qualitative studies. *Cultural Diversity and Ethnic Minority Psychology, 14*(4), 385–390. doi:10.1037/1099-9809.14.4.385

García, D. I., Gray-Stanley, J., & Ramirez-Valles, J. (2008). "The priest obviously doesn't know that I'm gay": The religious and spiritual journeys of Latino gay men. *Journal of Homosexuality, 55*(3), 411–436. doi:10.1080/00918360802345149

Garofalo, R., Osmer, E., Sullivan, C., Doll, M., & Harper, G. (2007). Environmental, psychosocial, and individual correlates of HIV risk in ethnic minority male-to-female transgender youth. *Journal of HIV/AIDS Prevention in Children & Youth, 7*(2), 89–104. doi:10.1300/J499v07n02_06

Giwa, S., & Greensmith, C. (2012). Race relations and racism in the LGBTQ community of Toronto: Perceptions of gay and queer social service providers of color. *Journal of Homosexuality, 59*(2), 149–185. doi:10.1080/00918369.2012.648877

Gonzales, G., & Ortiz, K. (2015). Health insurance disparities among racial/ethnic minorities in same-sex relationships: An intersectional approach. *American Journal of Public Health, 105*(6), 1106–1113. doi:10.2105/AJPH.2014.302459

Graham, L. F. (2014). Navigating community institutions: Black transgender women's experiences in schools, the criminal justice system, and churches. *Sexuality Research and Social Policy, 11*(4), 274–287. doi:10.1007/s13178-014-0144-y

Graham, L. F., Aronson, R. E., Nichols, T., Stephens, C. F., & Rhodes, S. D. (2011). Factors influencing depression and anxiety among Black sexual minority men. *Depression Research and Treatment.* Online publication. doi:10.1155/2011/587984

Grant, J. M., Mottet, L. A., Tanis, J., Harrison, J., Herman, J. L., & Keisling, M. (2011) Injustice at every turn: A report of the National Transgender Discrimination Survey. Retrieved from http://endtransdiscrimination.org/PDFs/NTDS_Report.pdf

Greene, B. (2000). African American lesbian and bisexual women. *Journal of Social Issues, 56*(2), 239–249.

Grov, C., Bimbi, D. S., Bimbi, J. E., & Parsons, J. T. (2006). Exploring racial and ethnic differences in recreational drug use among gay and bisexual men in New York City and Los Angeles. *Journal of Drug Education, 36*(2), 105–123.

Hahm, H. C., Lee, J., Chiao, C., Valentine, A., & Lê Cook, B. (2016). Use of mental health care and unmet needs for health care among lesbian and bisexual Chinese-, Korean-, and Vietnamese-American women. *Psychiatric Services, 67*(12), 1380–1383. doi:10.1176/appi.ps.201500356

Hall, H. I., Byers, R. H., Ling, Q., & Espinoza, L. (2007). Racial/ethnic and age disparities in HIV prevalence and disease progression among men who have sex with men in the United States. *American Journal of Public Health, 97*(6), 1060–1066. doi:10.2105/AJPH.2006.087551

Han, C. S., Ayala, G., Paul, J. P., Boylan, R., Gregorich, S. E., & Choi, K. H. (2015). Stress and coping with racism and their role in sexual risk for HIV among African American,

Asian/Pacific Islander, and Latino men who have sex with men. *Archives of Sexual Behavior, 44*(2), 411–420. doi:10.1007/s10508-014-0331-1

Harawa, N. T., Greenland, S., Bingham, T. A., Johnson, D. F., Cochran, S. D., Cunningham, W. E.,... McFarland, W. (2004). Associations of race/ethnicity with HIV prevalence and HIV-related behaviors among young men who have sex with men in 7 urban centers in the United States. *Journal of Acquired Immune Deficiency Syndromes, 35*(5), 526–536.

Hightow-Weidman, L. B., Phillips, G., Jones, K. C., Outlaw, A. Y., Fields, S. D., & Smith, J. C. (2011). Racial and sexual identity-related maltreatment among minority YMSM: Prevalence, perceptions, and the association with emotional distress. *AIDS Patient Care and STDs, 25*(S1), S39–S45. doi:10.1089/apc.2011.9877

Homma, Y., & Saewyc, E. M. (2007). The emotional well-being of Asian-American sexual minority youth in school. *Journal of LBGT Health Research, 3*(1), 67–78.

Huebner, D. M., Kegeles, S. M., Rebchook, G. M., Peterson, J. L., Neilands, T. B., Johnson, W. D., & Eke, A. N. (2014). Social oppression, psychological vulnerability, and unprotected intercourse among young Black men who have sex with men. *Health Psychology, 33*(12), 1568–1578. doi:10.1037/hea0000031

Hughes, T. L., Wilsnack, S. C., Szalacha, L. A., Johnson, T., Bostwick, W. B., Seymour, R.,... Kinnison, K. E. (2006). Age and racial/ethnic differences in drinking and drinking-related problems in a community sample of lesbians. *Journal of Studies on Alcohol, 67*(4), 579–590.

Irvin, R., Wilton, L., Scott, H., Beauchamp, G., Wang, L., Betancourt, J.,... Buchbinder, S. (2014). A study of perceived racial discrimination in Black men who have sex with men (MSM) and its association with healthcare utilization and HIV testing. *AIDS and Behavior, 18*(7), 1272–1278. doi:10.1007/s10461-014-0734-y

Jackson, K., & Brown, L. B. (1996). Lesbians of African heritage: Coming out in the straight community. *Journal of Gay & Lesbian Social Services, 5*(4), 53–68.

Jeong, Y. M., Veldhuis, C. B., Aranda, F., & Hughes, T. L. (2016). Racial/ethnic differences in unmet needs for mental health and substance use treatment in a community-based sample of sexual minority women. *Journal of Clinical Nursing, 25*(23–24), 3557–3569. doi:10.1111/jocn.13477

Jimenez, A. D. (2003). Triple jeopardy: Targeting older men of color who have sex with men. *Journal of Acquired Immune Deficiency Syndromes, 33*(S2), S222–S225.

Johnson-Jennings, M. D., Belcourt, A., Town, M., Walls, M. L., & Walters, K. L. (2014). Racial discrimination's influence on smoking rates among American Indian Alaska Native two-spirit individuals: Does pain play a role? *Journal of Health Care for the Poor and Underserved, 25*(4), 1667–1678. doi:10.1353/hpu.2014.0193

Jordan, J. N., Everett, K. D., Ge, B., & McElroy, J. A. (2015). Smoking and intention to quit among a large sample of Black sexual and gender minorities. *Journal of Homosexuality, 62*(5), 604–620. doi:10.1080/00918369.2014.987569

Kennamer, J., Honnold, J., Bradford, J., & Hendricks, M. (2000). Differences in disclosure of sexuality among African American and White gay/bisexual men: Implications for HIV/AIDS prevention. *AIDS Education and Prevention, 12*(6), 519–531.

Kim, H. J., & Fredriksen-Goldsen, K. I. (2016). Disparities in mental health quality of life between Hispanic and non-Hispanic White LGB midlife and older adults and the influence of lifetime discrimination, social connectedness, socioeconomic status, and perceived stress. *Research on Aging.* Advance online publication. doi:10.1177/0164027516650003

Latkin, C. A., Van Tieu, H., Fields, S., Hanscom, B. S., Connor, M., Hanscom, B.,... Magnus, M. (2016). Social network factors as correlates and predictors of high depressive symptoms among Black men who have sex with men in HPTN 061. *AIDS and Behavior.* Advance online publication. doi:10.1007/s10461-016-1493-8

Lee, J., & Hahm, H. C. (2012). HIV risk, substance use, and suicidal behaviors among Asian American lesbian and bisexual women. *AIDS Education and Prevention, 24*(6), 549–563. doi:10.1521/aeap.2012.24.6.549

Lehavot, K., Walters, K. L., & Simoni, J. M. (2009). Abuse, mastery, and health among lesbian, bisexual, and two-spirit American Indian and Alaska Native women. *Cultural Diversity and Ethnic Minority Psychology, 15*(3), 275–284. doi:10.1037/a0013458

Levy, M. E., Wilton, L., Phillips, G., Glick, S. N., Kuo, I., Brewer, R. A.,... Magnus, M. (2014). Understanding structural barriers to accessing HIV testing and prevention services among Black men who have sex with men (BMSM) in the United States. *AIDS and Behavior, 18*(5), 972–996.

Li, C. C., Matthews, A. K., Aranda, F., Patel, C., & Patel, M. (2015). Predictors and consequences of negative patient-provider interactions among a sample of African American sexual minority women. *LGBT Health, 2*(2), 140–146. doi:10.1089/lgbt.2014.0127

Logie, C. H., & Rwigema, M. J. (2014). "The normative idea of queer is a White person": Understanding perceptions of White privilege among lesbian, bisexual, and queer women of color in Toronto, Canada. *Journal of Lesbian Studies, 18*(2), 174–191. doi:10.1080/10894160.2014.849165

Lytle, M. C., De Luca, S. M., & Blosnich, J. R. (2014). The influence of intersecting identities on self-harm, suicidal behaviors, and depression among lesbian, gay, and bisexual individuals. *Suicide and Life-Threatening Behavior, 44*(4), 384–391.

Lytle, M. C., De Luca, S. M., Blosnich, J. R., & Brownson, C. (2015). Associations of racial/ethnic identities and religious affiliation with suicidal ideation among lesbian, gay, bisexual, and questioning individuals. *Journal of Affective Disorders, 178*, 39–45. doi:10.1016/j.jad.2014.07.039

Macapagal, K., Bhatia, R., & Greene, G. J. (2016). Differences in health care access, use, and experiences within a community sample of racially diverse lesbian, gay, bisexual, transgender, and questioning emerging adults. *LGBT Health, 3*(6), 434–442. doi10.1089/lgbt.2015.0124

MacCarthy, S., Mena, L., Chan, P. A., Rose, J., Simmons, D., Riggins, R.,... Nunn, A. (2015). Sexual network profiles and risk factors for STIs among African American sexual minorities in Mississippi: A cross-sectional analysis. *LGBT Health, 2*(3), 276–281. doi:10.1089/lgbt.2014.0019

Mannheimer, S., Wang, L., Wilton, L., Tieu, H. V., Del Rio, C., Buchbinder, S.,... Koblin, B. (2014). Infrequent HIV testing and late HIV diagnosis are common among a cohort of Black men who have sex with men (BMSM) in six US cities. *Journal of Acquired Immune Deficiency Syndromes, 67*(4), 438–445. doi:10.1097/QAI.0000000000000334

Martinez, O., Wu, E., Levine, E. C., Muñoz-Laboy, M., Spadafino, J., Dodge, B.,... Fernández, M. I. (2016). Syndemic factors associated with drinking patterns among Latino men and Latina transgender women who have sex with men in New York City. *Addiction Research & Theory, 24*(6), 466–476. doi:10.3109/16066359.2016.1167191

Matthews, A. K., Li, C. C., McConnell, E., Aranda, F., & Smith, C. (2016). Rates and predictors of obesity among African American sexual minority women. *LGBT Health, 3*(4), 275–282. doi:10.1089/lgbt.2015.0026

Mays, V. M., Yancey, A. K., Cochran, S. D., Weber, M., & Fielding, J. E. (2002). Heterogeneity of health disparities among African American, Hispanic, and Asian American women: Unrecognized influences of sexual orientation. *American Journal of Public Health, 92*(4), 632–639.

Mena, L., Crosby, R. A., & Geter, A. (2016). A novel measure of poverty and its association with elevated sexual risk behavior among young Black MSM. *International Journal of STD & AIDS*. Advance online publication. doi:10.1177/0956462416659420

Mereish, E. H., & Bradford, J. B. (2014). Intersecting identities and substance use problems: Sexual orientation, gender, race, and lifetime substance use problems. *Journal of Studies on Alcohol and Drugs, 75*(1), 179–188.

Meyer, I. H. (2010). Identity, stress, and resilience in lesbians, gay men, and bisexuals of color. *The Counseling Psychologist, 38*(3), 442–454. doi:10.1177/0011000009351601

Meyer, I. H., Dietrich, J., & Schwartz, S. (2008). Lifetime prevalence of mental disorders and suicide attempts in diverse lesbian, gay, and bisexual populations. *American Journal of Public Health, 98*(6), 1004–1006.

Millett, G. A., Flores, S. A., Peterson, J. L., & Bakeman, R. (2007). Explaining disparities in HIV infection among Black and White men who have sex with men: A meta-analysis of HIV risk behaviors. *AIDS, 21*(15), 2083–2091. doi:10.1097/QAD.0b013e3282e9a64b

Mizuno, Y., Borkowf, C., Millett, G. A., Bingham, T., Ayala, G., & Stueve, A. (2012). Homophobia and racism experienced by Latino men who have sex with men in the United States: Correlates of exposure and associations with HIV risk behaviors. *AIDS and Behavior, 16*(3), 724–735. doi:10.1007/s10461-011-9967-1

Molina, Y., Lehavot, K., Beadnell, B., & Simoni, J. (2014). Racial disparities in health behaviors and conditions among lesbian and bisexual women: The role of internalized stigma. *LGBT Health, 1*(2), 131–139. doi:10.1089/lgbt.2013.0007

Moradi, B., Wiseman, M. C., DeBlaere, C., Goodman, M. B., Sarkees, A., Brewster, M. E., & Huang, Y. P. (2010). LGB of color and White individuals' perceptions of heterosexist stigma, internalized homophobia, and outness: Comparisons of levels and links. *The Counseling Psychologist, 38*(3), 397–424.

Morris, J. F., & Balsam, K. F. (2003). Lesbian and bisexual women's experiences of victimization: Mental health, revictimization, and sexual identity development. *Journal of Lesbian Studies, 7*(4), 67–85. doi:10.1300/J155v07n04_05.

Muzny, C. A., Austin, E. L., Harbison, H. S., & Hook III, E. W. (2014). Sexual partnership characteristics of African American women who have sex with women: Impact on sexually transmitted infection risk. *Sexually Transmitted Diseases, 41*(10), 611–617. doi:10.1097/OLQ.0000000000000194

Nabors, N. A., Hall, R. L., Miville, M. L., Nettles, R., Pauling, M. L., & Ragsdale, B. L. (2001). Multiple minority group oppression: Divided we stand? *Journal of the Gay and Lesbian Medical Association, 5*(3), 101–105.

Nguyen, T. Q., Bandeen-Roche, K., German, D., Nguyen, N. T. T., Bass, J. K., & Knowlton, A. R. (2016). Negative treatment by family as a predictor of depressive symptoms, life satisfaction, suicidality, and tobacco/alcohol use in Vietnamese sexual minority women. *LGBT Health, 3*(5), 357–365. doi:10.1089/lgbt.2015.0017

Ocasio, M. A., Feaster, D. J., & Prado, G. (2016). Substance use and sexual risk behavior in sexual minority Hispanic adolescents. *Journal of Adolescent Health, 59*(5), 599–601. doi:10.1016/j.jadohealth.2016.07.008

O'Donnell, L., Agronick, G., San Doval, A., Duran, R., Myint-U, A., & Stueve, A. (2002). Ethnic and gay community attachments and sexual risk behaviors among urban Latino young men who have sex with men. *AIDS Education and Prevention, 14*(6), 457–471.

O'Donnell, S., Meyer, I., & Schwartz, S. (2011). Increased risk of suicide attempts among Black and Latino lesbians, gay men, and bisexuals. *American Journal of Public Health, 101*(6), 1055–1059. doi:10.2105/AJPH.2010.300032

Okafor, N., Rosenberg, E. S., Luisi, N., Sanchez, T., Rio, C. D., Sullivan, P. S., & Kelley, C. F. (2015). Disparities in herpes simplex virus type 2 infection between Black and White men who have sex with men in Atlanta, GA. *International Journal of STD & AIDS, 26*(10), 740–745. doi:10.1177/0956462414552814

Ortiz, K. S., Duncan, D. T., Blosnich, J. R., Salloum, R. G., & Battle, J. (2015). Smoking among sexual minorities: Are there racial differences? *Nicotine & Tobacco Research, 17*(11), 1362–1368. doi:10.1093/ntr/ntv001

Parks, C. A., & Hughes, T. L. (2005). Alcohol use and alcohol-related problems in self-identified lesbians: An historical cohort analysis. *Journal of Lesbian Studies, 9*(3), 31–44. doi:10.1300/J155v09n03_04

Parks, C. A., Hughes, T. L., & Matthews, A. K. (2004). Race/ethnicity and sexual orientation: Intersecting identities. *Cultural Diversity and Ethnic Minority Psychology, 10*(3), 241–254. doi:10.1037/1099-9809.10.3.241

Peek, M. E., Lopez, F. Y., Williams, H. S., Xu, L. J., McNulty, M. C., Acree, M. E., & Schneider, J. A. (2016). Development of a conceptual framework for understanding shared decision making among African American LGBT patients and their clinicians. *Journal of General Internal Medicine, 31*(6), 677–687. doi:10.1007/s11606-016-3616-3

Quinn, K., Dickson-Gomez, J., & Kelly, J. A. (2016). The role of the Black church in the lives of young Black men who have sex with men. *Culture, Health & Sexuality, 18*(5), 524–537. doi:10.1080/13691058.2015.1091509

Ramirez-Valles, J., Garcia, D., Campbell, R. T., Díaz, R. M., & Heckathorn, D. D. (2008). HIV infection, sexual risk behavior, and substance use among Latino gay and bisexual men and transgender persons. *American Journal of Public Health, 98*(6), 1036–1042. doi:10.2105/AJPH.2006.102624

Ramirez-Valles, J., Kuhns, L. M., Campbell, R. T., & Díaz, R. M. (2010). Social integration and health: Community involvement, stigmatized identities, and sexual risk in Latino sexual minorities. *Journal of Health and Social Behavior, 51*(1), 30–47.

Reisner, S. L., Bailey, Z., & Sevelius, J. (2014). Racial/ethnic disparities in history of incarceration, experiences of victimization, and associated health indicators among transgender women in the US. *Women & Health, 54*(8), 750–767. doi:10.1080/03630242.2014.932891

Reisner, S. L., Mimiaga, M. J., Bland, S., Skeer, M., Cranston, K., Isenberg, D.,... Mayer, K. H. (2010). Problematic alcohol use and HIV risk among Black men who have sex with men in Massachusetts. *AIDS Care, 22*(5), 577–587. doi:10.1080/09540120903311482

Rhodes, S. D., Martinez, O., Song, E. Y., Daniel, J., Alonzo, J., Eng, E.,... Miller, C. (2013). Depressive symptoms among immigrant Latino sexual minorities. *American Journal of Health Behavior, 37*(3), 404–413. doi:10.5993/AJHB.37.3.13

Rhodes, S. D., McCoy, T. P., Hergenrather, K. C., Vissman, A. T., Wolfson, M., Alonzo, J.,... Eng, E. (2012). Prevalence estimates of health risk behaviors of immigrant Latino men who have sex with men. *The Journal of Rural Health, 28*(1), 73–83. doi:10.1111/j.1748-0361.2011.00373.x

Rhodes, S. D., Yee, L. J., & Hergenrather, K. C. (2006). A community-based rapid assessment of HIV behavioural risk disparities within a large sample of gay men in southeastern USA: a comparison of African American, Latino and White men. *AIDS Care, 18*(8), 1018–1024. doi:10.1080/09540120600568731

Rosario, M., Schrimshaw, E. W., & Hunter, J. (2004). Ethnic/racial differences in the coming-out process of lesbian, gay, and bisexual youths: A comparison of sexual identity development over time. *Cultural Diversity and Ethnic Minority Psychology, 10*(3), 215–228.

Russell, L. (2010). Fact Sheet: Health Disparities by Race and Ethnicity. Center for American Progress. Retrieved from https://cdn.americanprogress.org/wp-content/uploads/issues/2010/12/pdf/disparities_factsheet.pdf

Ryan, C., Huebner, D., Díaz, R. M., & Sanchez, J. (2009). Family rejection as a predictor of negative health outcomes in White and Latino lesbian, gay, and bisexual young adults. *Pediatrics, 123*(1), 346–352. doi:10.1542/peds.2007-3524

Saewyc, E. M., Skay, C. L., Bearinger, L. H., Blum, R. W., & Resnick, M. D. (1998). Sexual orientation, sexual behaviors, and pregnancy among American Indian adolescents. *Journal of Adolescent Health, 23*(4), 238–247.

Sandil, R., Robinson, M., Brewster, M. E., Wong, S., & Geiger, E. (2015). Negotiating multiple marginalizations: Experiences of South Asian LGBQ individuals. *Cultural Diversity and Ethnic Minority Psychology, 21*(1), 76–88. doi:10.1037/a0037070

Sauceda, J. A., Wiebe, J. S., & Simoni, J. M. (2016). Childhood sexual abuse and depression in Latino men who have sex with men: Does resilience protect against nonadherence to antiretroviral therapy? *Journal of Health Psychology, 21*(6), 1096–1106. doi:10.1177/1359105314546341

Siembida, E. J., Eaton, L. A., Maksut, J. L., Driffin, D. D., & Baldwin, R. (2016). A comparison of HIV-related risk factors between Black transgender women and Black men who have sex with men. *Transgender Health, 1*(1), 172–180. doi:10.1089/trgh.2016.0003

Spadafino, J. T., Martinez, O., Levine, E. C., Dodge, B., Muñoz-Laboy, M., & Fernández, M. I. (2016). Correlates of HIV and STI testing among Latino men who have sex with men in New York City. *AIDS Care, 28*(6), 695–698. doi:10.1080/09540121.2016.1147017

Stokes, J. P., & Peterson, J. L. (1998). Homophobia, self-esteem, and risk for HIV among African American men who have sex with men. *AIDS Education and Prevention, 10*(3), 278–292.

Storholm, E. D., Siconolfi, D. E., Halkitis, P. N., Moeller, R. W., Eddy, J. A., & Bare, M. G. (2013). Sociodemographic factors contribute to mental health disparities and access to services among young men who have sex with men in New York City. *Journal of Gay & Lesbian Mental Health, 17*(3), 294–313. doi:10.1080/19359705.2012.763080

Sun, C. J., Ma, A., Tanner, A. E., Mann, L., Reboussin, B. A., Garcia, M., ... Rhodes, S. D. (2016). Depressive symptoms among Latino sexual minority men and Latina transgender women in a new settlement state: The role of perceived discrimination. *Depression Research and Treatment*. Online publication. doi:10.1155/2016/4972854

Sutter, M., & Perrin, P. B. (2016). Discrimination, mental health, and suicidal ideation among LGBTQ people of color. *Journal of Counseling Psychology, 63*(1), 98–105. doi:10.1037/cou0000126

Szymanski, D. M., & Gupta, A. (2009). Examining the relationship between multiple internalized oppressions and African American lesbian, gay, bisexual, and questioning persons' self-esteem and psychological distress. *Journal of Counseling Psychology, 56*(1), 110–118. doi:10.1037/a0013317

Tan, J. Y., Xu, L. J., Lopez, F. Y., Jia, J. L., Pho, M. T., Kim, K. E., & Chin, M. H. (2016). Shared decision making among clinicians and Asian American and Pacific Islander sexual and gender minorities: An intersectional approach to address a critical care gap. *LGBT Health, 3*(5), 327–334. doi:10.1089/lgbt.2015.0143

Toomey, R. B., Huynh, V. W., Jones, S. K., Lee, S., & Revels-Macalinao, M. (2016). Sexual minority youth of color: A content analysis and critical review of the literature. *Journal of Gay & Lesbian Mental Health, 21*(1), 3–31. doi:10.1080/19359705.2016.1217499

Van Sluytman, L., Spikes, P., Nandi, V., Van Tieu, H., Frye, V., Patterson, J., & Koblin, B. (2015). Ties that bind: Community attachment and the experience of discrimination among Black men who have sex with men. *Culture, Health & Sexuality, 17*(7), 859–872. doi:10.1080/13691058.2015.1004762

Vincent, W., Peterson, J. L., & Parrott, D. J. (2009). Differences in African American and White women's attitudes toward lesbians and gay men. *Sex Roles, 61*(9–10), 599–606. doi:10.1007/s11199-009-9679-4

Wade, R. M., & Harper, G. W. (2015). Young Black gay/bisexual and other men who have sex with men: A review and content analysis of health-focused research between 1988 and 2013. *American Journal of Men's Health*. Advance online publication. doi:10.1177/1557988315606962

Walsh, T., Bertozzi-Villa, C., & Schneider, J. A. (2015). Systematic review of racial disparities in human papillomavirus–associated anal dysplasia and anal cancer among men who have sex with men. *American Journal of Public Health, 105*(4), e34–e45. doi:10.2105/AJPH.2014.302469

Warren, J. C., Fernández, M. I., Harper, G. W., Hidalgo, M. A., Jamil, O. B., & Torres, R. S. (2008). Predictors of unprotected sex among young sexually active African American, Hispanic, and White MSM: The importance of ethnicity and culture. *AIDS and Behavior, 12*(3), 459–468. doi:10.1007/s10461-007-9291-y

Williams, J. K., Wilton, L., Magnus, M., Wang, L., Wang, J., Dyer, T. P.,...Cummings, V. (2015). Relation of childhood sexual abuse, intimate partner violence, and depression to risk factors for HIV among Black men who have sex with men in 6 US cities. *American Journal of Public Health, 105*(12), 2473–2481. doi:10.2105/AJPH.2015.302878

Woody, I. (2014). Aging out: A qualitative exploration of ageism and heterosexism among aging African American lesbians and gay men. *Journal of Homosexuality, 61*(1), 145–165. doi:10.1080/00918369.2013.835603

Yancey, A. K., Cochran, S. D., Corliss, H. L., & Mays, V. M. (2003). Correlates of overweight and obesity among lesbian and bisexual women. *Preventive Medicine, 36*(6), 676–683. doi:10.1016/S0091-7435(03)00020-3

Yuan, N. P., Duran, B. M., Walters, K. L., Pearson, C. R., & Evans-Campbell, T. A. (2014). Alcohol misuse and associations with childhood maltreatment and out-of-home placement among urban two-spirit American Indian and Alaska native people. *International Journal of Environmental Research and Public Health, 11*(10), 10461–10479.

CHAPTER **16**

Bisexual Health

Jacob C. Warren, K. Bryant Smalley, and K. Nikki Barefoot

Despite representing a substantial portion of the adult gender and sexual minority (GSM) population, research into the specific health needs of bisexual individuals has lagged behind research into other GSM groups. In fact, the landmark Institute of Medicine (IOM) Committee on Lesbian, Gay, Bisexual, and Transgender Health Issues and Research Gaps and Opportunities (2011) report on lesbian, gay, bisexual, and transgender (LGBT) health referred to throughout this text specifically identifies bisexually-identified individuals as being distinctly understudied in terms of health and well-being. This occurs despite estimates of bisexuality of 2.6% in adult men and 3.6% in adult women, as well as 1.5% of male youth and 8.4% of female youth (Herbenick et al., 2010). Even in studies that incorporate a focus on bisexuality specifically, fewer than 20% separately analyze bisexual individuals in a way that allows for contrasts with their gay/lesbian counterparts (Kaestle & Ivory, 2012).

Although still in its early stages, the literature on bisexual health has consistently found that bisexual men and women appear to exhibit more health disparities when compared to heterosexual men and women than when comparing gay men and women to heterosexual men and women (Dilley, Simmons, Boysun, Pizacani, & Stark, 2010). This chapter will lay the groundwork for the reasons bisexual men and women face unique pressures related to their health; discuss the dynamics of stigma, discrimination, and victimization that they experience; and then examine specific health outcomes for which there is emerging evidence of particular need within the bisexual community.

As a note, in preparing this chapter, and in assessing the overall state of the literature, one of the challenges in identifying research that examines the health of bisexual men in particular is the tendency for studies to group gay and bisexual men under the umbrella of "men who have sex with men." While this methodological decision harkens back to the origins of GSM health research in the HIV epidemic, the persistence of this research categorization tends to perpetuate a lack of research that specifically investigates bisexual men, and even more so that examines them in contrast to both heterosexual and gay men. As such, much of the literature reviewed in this chapter focuses on sexual minority women, as the tendency to combine lesbians and bisexual women is not as ingrained in research heritage.

■ ACCESS TO AND UTILIZATION OF MEDICAL CARE

To frame the rest of the chapter, it is helpful to first understand the specific barriers that bisexual individuals face in accessing affirming care. When describing barriers to care, bisexual men and women often report perceptions that medical providers are not welcoming to or affirming of bisexual identities (Dobinson, MacDonnell, Hampson, Clipsham, & Chow, 2005). Bisexual men and women also report feeling that providers make judgments regarding their sexual behavior, pathologize bisexuality, and at times focus on their bisexual identity to the exclusion of issues they consider more relevant to their care (Eady, Dobinson, & Ross, 2011). Even "LGBT-friendly" services often fail to meet the needs of bisexual patients, as bisexual men and women frequently feel that LGBT-friendly services are actually tailored to gay men and lesbians (Dobinson et al., 2005).

As a natural result of the intersection of these challenges, bisexual men and women are less likely than gay men and lesbians to feel comfortable discussing issues related to their sexual orientation with their primary health care provider (Smalley, Warren, & Barefoot, 2015a), and are more likely than both their gay/lesbian and heterosexual counterparts to avoid and/or delay care due to an inability to pay (with bisexual women 2.5 times as likely to do so; Blosnich, Farmer, Lee, Silenzio, & Bowen, 2014; Jackson, Agénor, Johnson, Austin, & Kawachi, 2016; Ward et al., 2014). As a result of these barriers, bisexual adults are more likely than both heterosexual and gay/lesbian adults to not have a regular source of medical care and to identify the limited availability of providers as a barrier to care (Smalley et al., 2015a; Ward, Dahlhamer, Galinsky, & Joestl, 2014; Wheldon & Kirby, 2013).

The effects of this avoidance of care can be clearly seen in bisexual women, who despite being equally likely as heterosexual women to have had a recent gynecological examination are less likely to use preventive services overall, to have obtained a Pap test within the past 3 years, and to have received age-appropriate mammography (Agénor et al., 2015; Dilley et al., 2010; D. L. Kerr, Ding, & Thompson, 2013; Koh, 2000). In terms of vaccination, while bisexual women are more likely than heterosexual women to both initiate and complete HPV vaccination, bisexual and heterosexual men have comparable HPV vaccination rates (Agénor et al., 2016).

■ STIGMA, DISCRIMINATION, AND VICTIMIZATION

One of the most robust areas of bisexual health research relates to stigma, discrimination, and the associated victimization experienced by bisexual men and women. There is a well-documented cultural stigma against bisexual individuals that impacts men and women, increasing the risk of a variety of outcomes (Bostwick, 2012; Dodge et al., 2016). The issue of stigma is widespread, as one-third of bisexual men and women report experiencing stigma or biased treatment due specifically to their sexual orientation (Page, 2004).

Attitudes toward bisexual individuals appear to vary by gender of the bisexual person. Not only are overall attitudes more negative toward bisexual men than bisexual women, they are more negative toward bisexual men than all other sexual orientations (Helms & Waters, 2016). These anti-bisexual attitudes also appear to vary by gender on the part of the stereotype-holder, with women having comparable attitudes toward bisexual men and women, but men having worse attitudes toward bisexual men than bisexual women (Yost & Thomas, 2012). Yost and Thomas (2012) argue that this increased acceptance of bisexual women by heterosexual men is at least partially explained by the eroticization of female same-sex sexual activity. Anti-bisexual attitudes have also been related to age, education, income, geography (i.e., Southern and rural areas), religiosity, conservativism, and hegemonic gender norms (Casazza, Ludwig, & Cohn, 2015; Herek, 2002).

The source of stigma is not just from the broader society, however. When describing their relationship with family members, bisexual men and women often describe experiencing invalidation and even hostility from family members and a perception by their family members that they are sexually irresponsible (Todd, Oravecz, & Vejar, 2016). Consequently, bisexual men and women report having lower levels of parental attachment than heterosexual and gay men and women (Wilson, Zeng, & Blackburn, 2011). For bisexual female youth, this can have a direct effect on help-seeking behaviors; for them, stigma from within the family is associated with a lower degree of openness regarding sexual orientation with medical providers (Arbeit, Fisher, Macapagal, & Mustanski, 2016).

One prevailing stigma toward bisexual individuals, despite overwhelming evidence to the contrary, is that bisexuality is simply a "transitional phase" between identifying as heterosexual and eventually identifying as gay (Cahill, 2005), which inherently delegitimizes bisexual identities. This false belief appears to permeate more than just society at large—bisexual men and women specifically report feeling discrimination not only from outside, but also from within the LGBT community (Dodge, Schnarrs, Reece, Goncalves, et al., 2012; Dodge, Schnarrs, Reece, Martinez, et al., 2012). Bisexual men and women report that some members of the gay and lesbian community perceive that bisexuality is not a "genuine" sexual orientation, while also stereotyping bisexual individuals as promiscuous (Hequembourg & Brallier, 2009). Bisexual-specific microaggressions experienced from a variety of sources include hostility, dismissal of sexual orientation or pressure to change it, dating exclusion, and being stereotyped as hypersexual (Bostwick & Hequembourg, 2014). As a result, bisexual individuals often report disguising their sexual orientation both in dominantly heterosexual and dominantly gay/lesbian social situations to avoid "double discrimination" (Hequembourg & Brallier, 2009; Mulick & Wright, 2002). While double discrimination is a true challenge, bisexual individuals report experiencing the most stigma overall from heterosexual individuals (Hertlein, Hartwell, & Munns, 2016; Roberts, Horne, & Hoyt, 2015).

Potentially because of the stigma from within and outside of the LGBT community, bisexual men and women report lower levels of commitment to their sexual minority identity and less community identification and involvement than gay men and lesbians (Herek, Norton, Allen, & Sims, 2010). Bisexual men and women also report a greater degree of identity confusion and lower levels of self-disclosure and general community connection when compared to their gay and lesbian counterparts (Balsam & Mohr, 2007; Lewis, Derlega, Brown, Rose, & Henson, 2009). The social effects of stigma are so strong that rural bisexual young adults are less likely than other sexual orientation groups to even view social support as being helpful to them at all (Whiting, Boone, & Cohn, 2012).

There is wide diversity in the paths that bisexual adults have taken in acknowledging and accepting their sexual orientation, with concealment another major effect of stigma (Goetstouwers, 2006). When compared to their cisgender gay and lesbian counterparts, bisexual men and women express less comfort with disclosure of sexual orientation, even within the context of research studies (Hottes et al., 2016; Smalley et al., 2015a). For bisexual men, concealment is higher among individuals with higher income and those living with an opposite-sex partner (Schrimshaw, Siegel, Downing, & Parsons, 2013). Other effects of stigma are more insidious—bisexual men and women exhibit greater levels of internalized heterosexism and homonegativity than gay men and lesbians (Costa, Pereira, & Leal, 2013; Puckett, Surace, Levitt, & Horne, 2016), placing them at risk for a host of negative outcomes including substance use and self-harm (Cabaj, Gorman, Pellicio, Ghindia, & Neisen, 2012).

Parental abuse appears to be a particular threat for bisexual men and women. When comparing rates of parental physical abuse, there is a larger gap between bisexual men/women and heterosexual men/women than between gay men/lesbians and heterosexual men/women (Friedman et al., 2011). Sexual violence is also a pressing concern for bisexual women, who are more likely to have been raped, to have experienced sexual violence other than rape, and to have been stalked by an intimate partner than both lesbians and heterosexual women (Walters, Chen, & Breiding, 2013).

■ SUBSTANCE USE

Bisexual individuals also show elevated risk of use of several substances. Bisexual men and women are more likely than heterosexual men and women to be current smokers (Blosnich et al., 2014), and bisexual women are more likely to have ever smoked (Valanis et al., 2000). An examination of potential risk factors revealed that lower access to health care and income level are both tied to increased risk of smoking among bisexual men and women (Balsam, Beadnell, & Riggs, 2012).

While there is general consensus regarding the elevated use of alcohol among bisexual men and women, there have been studies that have not replicated this finding in specific demographic subgroups—for instance, college-enrolled bisexual women have been found to not drink in excess of their heterosexual counterparts; however, this may have more to do with the overall rates of alcohol consumption in college-enrolled women than a lack of consistency of findings (Bostwick et al.,

2007). In general, when compared to heterosexual men and women, bisexual men and women are more likely to report binge drinking (Jackson et al., 2016). Further, bisexual women are more likely to report any use of alcohol and report drinking more when they do drink when compared to heterosexual women (Valanis et al., 2000). Compared to heterosexual women, bisexual women are also less likely to completely abstain from alcohol and have higher odds of alcohol-related social consequences, alcohol dependence, and a history of alcohol-related help seeking (Drabble, Midanik, & Trocki, 2005). Although not consistent across studies, some researchers have found elevated risk of alcohol consumption when comparing bisexual women to lesbians (Burgard, Cochran, & Mays, 2005). Interestingly, while some studies have suggested that bisexual women are less likely to frequent bars, bisexual women are more likely to drink heavily both in bars and in party contexts when compared to heterosexual women (Drabble & Trocki, 2005).

Older studies found that use of illicit drugs was higher in bisexual women than in heterosexual women, but comparable to lesbians (Koh, 2000); however, more recent studies have found that cisgender bisexual men and women demonstrate notably increased risk of substance use in comparison to even their gay, lesbian, and transgender counterparts (Smalley, Warren, & Barefoot, 2015b). While specific rates are largely unavailable, bisexual women are more likely than exclusively heterosexual women to report marijuana use (Trocki, Drabble, & Midanik, 2009), with past-year usage rates estimated at 33.6% and 13.8% of bisexual women reporting using marijuana twice or more per week (Robinson, Sanches, MacLeod, 2016).

■ MENTAL HEALTH

One area that has been more widely researched relates to the mental health of bisexual men and women. Across mood and anxiety disorders, bisexual men and women report the greatest risk when compared to all other sexual orientations (Bostwick, Boyd, Hughes, & McCabe, 2010; Dodge & Sandfort, 2007; Persson & Pfaus, 2015). Bisexual men and women are more likely to report feelings of sadness than both heterosexual and gay counterparts and have lower levels of self-esteem (Conron, Mimiaga, & Landers, 2010; Wilson et al., 2011). Further, bisexual women are more likely to report frequent mental distress and overall poor mental health than heterosexual women and lesbians (Fredriksen-Goldsen, Kim, Barkan, Balsam, & Mincer, 2010; D. D. Kerr, Santurri, & Peters, 2013).

When considering estimates of rates, bisexual women are twice as likely as lesbians to report severe to extremely severe levels of depression (31.2% vs. 15.6%) and stress (24.5% vs. 11.7%), while bisexual men are significantly more likely than gay men to report severe to extremely severe anxiety (27.3% vs. 18.6%; Smalley, Warren, & Barefoot, 2016). Interestingly, unlike in the non-LGBT community, there do not appear to be gender differences in traditional mental health outcomes such as depression and anxiety; rather, differences are found based on sexual orientation. For example, bisexual men and women have similar levels of depression, stress, and anxiety symptoms to each other, but bisexual women have higher levels of each outcome when compared to lesbians, and bisexual men have higher levels of anxiety when compared to gay men (Smalley et al., 2015a).

When considering suicide and self-injury, bisexual men and women are more likely to report a 12-month history of suicidal ideation than heterosexual men and women, with bisexual men also reporting a higher lifetime prevalence of suicidality (Brennan, Ross, Dobinson, Veldhuizen, & Steele, 2010; Conron et al., 2010; Koh & Ross, 2006). While specific risk factors are largely uninvestigated, bisexual women who are not out about their sexual orientation are at greater risk for attempting suicide (Conron et al., 2010), and bisexual women have been found to have higher suicidal intent than bisexual men (Mathy, Lehmann, & Kerr, 2003). Whatever the reason, there appears to be a particularly elevated stressor in place, as bisexual individuals report engaging in more self-injurious behaviors than even lesbians and gay men (Balsam, Beauchaine, Mickey, & Rothblum, 2005; D. D. Kerr et al., 2013).

The disparities in mental health outcomes are even more troubling when considered in light of differences in help-seeking behavior. Not only do bisexual men and women seek help for mental health issues related to sexual orientation less frequently than gay men and lesbians, when they do seek out help they are less likely to feel comfortable discussing their sexual orientation with their mental health care provider (Smalley et al., 2015a) and more likely to feel that the care that they received was not helpful (Page, 2004). This could in part be due to the fact that counselors have been shown to automatically perceive bisexual clients as having a lower level of psychosocial functioning (Mohr, Israel, & Sedlacek, 2001), impacting their ability to provide unbiased care. Young bisexual women report that biphobia presents a significant challenge to their mental health, and potentially as a result, bisexual women are less likely to use psychotherapy for depression than lesbians (Flanders, Dobinson, & Logie, 2015; Koh & Ross, 2006).

■ SEXUAL HEALTH

While sexual health is one of the best-studied areas of GSM health, the evidence is uneven in terms of bisexual men and women. While bisexual men and women are more likely than heterosexual men and women to report multiple sexual partners within the preceding month (King & Nazareth, 2006), there is less literature than may otherwise be anticipated with regard to the unique sexual health of bisexual individuals. As discussed in Chapter 13, there is a prevailing notion that sexual minority women are not at risk for sexually transmitted diseases (STDs), and bisexual men are frequently combined with gay men under the umbrella "men who have sex with men" for the purposes of research on sexual behavior. However, there is a growing body of literature that has begun to specifically examine the sexual health of bisexual individuals.

When considering women, bisexual women are more likely than both heterosexual women and lesbians across the developmental spectrum to report risky sexual behaviors, including substance use in the context of sexual encounters, and are more likely than lesbians to have been previously diagnosed with an STD (Bostwick, Hughes, & Everett, 2015; Herrick, Kuhns, Kinsky, Johnson, & Garofalo, 2013; D. L. Kerr et al., 2013; Koh, Gomez, Shade, & Rowley, 2005). Perhaps reflective of this risk, bisexual women are more likely to have received an STD and

HIV test than heterosexual women (Agénor et al., 2015; D. L. Kerr et al., 2013). Bisexual women are also more likely to report a history of childhood sexual experiences than heterosexual women (King & Nazareth, 2006).

Studies of sexual health in bisexual men have focused heavily on HIV. Bisexually identified men report similar rates of condom use as gay men with male partners, and higher rates of condom use with women than heterosexual men (Jeffries & Dodge, 2007). However, studies of the sexual behaviors of bisexuality may not be fully reflective of the experiences of bisexually active individuals, as sexual behaviors vary based on typology (e.g., bisexually identified, down-low, MSM; Dodge, Schick, et al., 2012). In terms of actual HIV risk, bisexual men appear to be both less likely than gay men and more likely than heterosexual men to be HIV positive (Zule, Bobashev, Wechsberg, Costenbader, & Coomes, 2009); however, it is unclear if part of the gay/bisexual disparity is due to undiagnosed HIV, as bisexual men are less likely than gay men to have a history of being tested for HIV (Fredriksen-Goldsen, Kim, Barkan, Muraco, & Hoy-Ellis, 2013).

CHRONIC DISEASE RISK

There is growing evidence that bisexual men and women are disproportionately impacted by a variety of risk factors for chronic diseases, and for chronic disease outcomes themselves. Chronic diseases may impact bisexual women more than men—while lesbians are more likely than heterosexual women to report a high number of poor mental health days, bisexual women are more likely to report a high number of poor physical health days, appearing to have an overall increased likelihood of poor general health (Diamant & Wold, 2003; Fredriksen-Goldsen et al., 2010).

The majority of chronic disease risk factor research has focused on obesity-related risk factors, which appear to operate in multiple directions. Bisexual men and women are less likely to report physical inactivity when compared to their heterosexual counterparts (Jackson et al., 2016), and bisexual men have lower rates of obesity and overweight than heterosexual men (Brennan et al., 2010). Bisexual women, however, appear to be particularly impacted by other obesity risks. In addition to being more likely to be overweight and/or obese (Dilley et al., 2010; Laska et al., 2015), bisexual women are more likely than heterosexual women to weight cycle, to have an overall increasing BMI trajectory, and to engage in unhealthy weight control practices (e.g., skipping meals; Jun et al., 2012; Polimeni, Austin, & Kavanah, 2009). They are also more than twice as likely as lesbians to report a history of an eating disorder (Koh & Ross, 2006). In terms of prevention, predictors of obesity appear to vary between bisexual individuals and other GSM groups. For bisexual women, age, relationship status, and employment status are all related to obesity risk; however, while age, employment status, depression, anxiety, and stress are all predictive of obesity for gay men, none of these factors predict obesity for bisexual men (Warren, Smalley, & Barefoot, 2016).

There is also a growing body of information regarding outcomes themselves. While bisexual men and women appear to have risk for high blood pressure comparable to heterosexual men and women (Everett & Mollborn, 2013), and bisexual women appear to have a lower risk of heart disease than lesbians, bisexual men and women appear to be at higher risk for heart disease and diabetes than heterosexual men and women (Conron et al., 2010; Diamant & Wold, 2003; Dilley et al., 2010; Fredriksen-Goldsen et al., 2013). Bisexual women are also more likely to report having a history of cancer (17.6% vs. 11.9% in heterosexual women), with elevations appearing to relate mainly to breast and cervical cancer (Valanis et al., 2000). In addition, bisexual men and women are more likely than heterosexual men and women to report a history of asthma (Blosnich et al., 2014; Dilley et al., 2010).

■ CONCLUSION

Overall, bisexual men and women represent a highly stigmatized and often ignored subgroup of the LGBT community, sometimes referred to as "bisexual invisibility" or "bisexual erasure" (San Francisco Human Rights Commission, LGBT Advisory Committee, 2011). Most concerning is the fact that bisexual men and women are subject to experiences of discrimination and microaggressions from not only cisgender heterosexuals, but also their GSM peers (i.e., "double discrimination"; Mulick & Wright, 2002). Despite these added vulnerabilities, the health and well-being of bisexual men and women have been largely neglected within the realm of GSM health research, with bisexual participants traditionally being collapsed into single groups with their lesbian and gay male counterparts (IOM, 2011), further perpetuating their invisibility. However, emerging research on the unique health risks and needs of bisexual men and women reveals alarming mental and physical health disparities beyond those experienced by sexual minorities as a whole. Most notably, in comparison to their gay/lesbian counterparts, bisexual men and women have been found to have lower levels of outness, self-esteem, and community identification and involvement and higher levels of internalized heterosexism/homonegativity and psychological distress. Furthermore, research suggests that bisexual individuals also engage in several health risks behaviors at higher rates, including substance use, self-injurious behavior, sexual risk-taking, and unhealthy weight control practices, in addition to being at greater risk for asthma, diabetes, heart disease, cancer, and poor overall health. Future research is needed to better understand and address the unique health disparities faced by bisexual men and women separate from their gay and lesbian counterparts.

■ REFERENCES

Agénor, M., Peitzmeier, S. M., Gordon, A. R., Charlton, B. M., Haneuse, S., Potter, J., & Austin, S. B. (2016). Sexual orientation identity disparities in human papillomavirus vaccination initiation and completion among young adult US women and men. *Cancer Causes & Control, 27*(10), 1187–1196. doi:10.1007/s10552-016-0796-4

Agénor, M., Peitzmeier, S., Gordon, A. R., Haneuse, S., Potter, J. E., & Austin, S. B. (2015). Sexual orientation identity disparities in awareness and initiation of the human papillomavirus vaccine among U.S. women and girls: A national survey. *Annals of Internal Medicine, 163*(2), 99–106. doi:10.7326/M14-2108

Arbeit, M. R., Fisher, C. B., Macapagal, K., & Mustanski, B. (2016). Bisexual invisibility and the sexual health needs of adolescent girls. *LGBT Health, 3*(5), 342–349. doi:10.1089/lgbt.2016.0035

Balsam, K., Beadnell, B., & Riggs, K. (2012). Understanding sexual orientation health disparities in smoking: A population-based analysis. *The American Journal of Orthopsychiatry, 82*(4), 482–493. doi:10.1111/j.1939-0025.2012.01186.x

Balsam, K. F., Beauchaine, T. P., Mickey, R. M., & Rothblum, E. D. (2005). Mental health of lesbian, gay, bisexual, and heterosexual siblings: Effects of gender, sexual orientation, and family. *Journal of Abnormal Psychology, 114*(3), 471–476. doi:10.1037/0021-843X.114.3.471

Balsam, K. F., & Mohr, J. J. (2007). Adaptation to sexual orientation stigma: A comparison of bisexual and lesbian/gay adults. *Journal of Counseling Psychology, 54*(3), 306–319.

Blosnich, J. R., Farmer, G. W., Lee, J. L., Silenzio, V. B., & Bowen, D. J. (2014). Health inequalities among sexual minority adults: Evidence from ten U.S. states, 2010. *American Journal of Preventive Medicine, 46*(4), 337–349. doi:10.1016/j.amepre.2013.11.010

Bostwick, W. B. (2012). Assessing bisexual stigma and mental health status: A brief report. *Journal of Bisexuality, 12*(2), 214–222. doi:10.1080/15299716.2012.674860

Bostwick, W. B., Boyd, C., Hughes, T., & McCabe, S. (2010). Dimensions of sexual orientation and the prevalence of mood and anxiety disorders in the United States. *American Journal of Public Health, 100*(3), 468–475. doi:10.2105/AJPH.2008.152942

Bostwick, W. B., & Hequembourg, A. (2014). 'Just a little hint': Bisexual-specific microaggressions and their connection to epistemic injustices. *Culture, Health & Sexuality, 16*(5), 488–503. doi:10.1080/13691058.2014.889754

Bostwick, W. B., Hughes, T. L., & Everett, B. (2015). Health behavior, status, and outcomes among a community-based sample of lesbian and bisexual women. *LGBT Health, 2*(2), 121–126. doi:10.1089/lgbt.2014.0074

Bostwick, W. B., McCabe, S. E., Horn, S., Hughes, T., Johnson, T., & Valles, J. R. (2007). Drinking patterns, problems, and motivations among collegiate bisexual women. *Journal of American College Health, 56*(3), 285–292. doi:10.3200/JACH.56.3.285-292

Brennan, D., Ross, L., Dobinson, C., Veldhuizen, S., & Steele, L. (2010). Men's sexual orientation and health in Canada. *Canadian Journal of Public Health, 101*(3), 255–258.

Burgard, S. A., Cochran, S. D., & Mays, V. M. (2005). Alcohol and tobacco use patterns among heterosexually and homosexually experienced California women. *Drug & Alcohol Dependence, 77*(1), 61–70. doi:10.1016/j.drugalcdep.2004.07.007

Cabaj, R. P., Gorman, M., Pellicio, W. J., Ghindia, D. J. & Neisen, J. H. (2012). An overview for providers treating LGBT clients. In *A provider's introduction to substance abuse treatment for lesbian, gay, bisexual, and transgender individuals* (pp. 1–14). HHS Publication No. (SMA) 12-4104. Rockville, MD: U.S. Department of Health and Human Services. Retrieved from https://store.samhsa.gov/shin/content/SMA12-4104/SMA12-4104.pdf

Cahill, S. (2005). Bisexuality: Dispelling the myths. National Gay and Lesbian Task Force. Retrieved from http://www.thetaskforce.org/static_html/downloads/reports/BisexualityDispellingtheMyths.pdf

Casazza, S. P., Ludwig, E., & Cohn, T. J. (2015). Heterosexual attitudes and behavioral intentions toward bisexual individuals: Does geographic area make a difference? *Journal of Bisexuality, 15*(4), 532–553. doi:10.1080/15299716.2015.1093994

Conron, K., Mimiaga, M., & Landers, S. (2010). A population-based study of sexual orientation identity and gender differences in adult health. *American Journal of Public Health, 100*(10), 1953–1960. doi:10.2105/AJPH.2009.174169

Costa, P. A., Pereira, H., & Leal, I. (2013). Internalized homonegativity, disclosure, and acceptance of sexual orientation in a sample of Portuguese gay and bisexual men, and lesbian and bisexual women. *Journal of Bisexuality, 13*(2), 229–244. doi:10.1080/15299716.2013.782481

Diamant, A. L., & Wold, C. (2003). Sexual orientation and variation in physical and mental health status among women. *Journal of Women's Health, 12*(1), 41–49.

Dilley, J., Simmons, K., Boysun, M., Pizacani, B., & Stark, M. (2010). Demonstrating the importance and feasibility of including sexual orientation in public health surveys: Health disparities in the Pacific Northwest. *American Journal of Public Health, 100*(3), 460–467. doi:10.2105/AJPH.2007.130336

Dobinson, C., MacDonnell, J., Hampson, E., Clipsham, J., & Chow, K. (2005). Improving the access and quality of public health services for bisexuals. *Journal of Bisexuality, 5*(1), 39–77. doi:10.1300/J159v05n01_05

Dodge, B., Herbenick, D., Friedman, M. R., Schick, V., Fu, T. J., Bostwick, W.,... Sandfort, T. G. M. (2016). Attitudes toward bisexual men and women among a nationally representative probability sample of adults in the United States. *PLOS ONE, 11*(10), e0164430. doi:10.1371/journal.pone.0164430

Dodge, B., & Sandfort, T. G. M. (2007). A review of mental health research on bisexual individuals when compared to homosexual and heterosexual individuals. In B. A. Firestein (Ed.), *Becoming visible* (pp. 28–51). New York, NY: Columbia University Press.

Dodge, B., Schick, V., Rosenberger, J., Reece, M., Herbenick, D., & Novak, D.S. (2012). Beyond "risk": Exploring sexuality among diverse typologies of bisexual men in the United States. *Journal of Bisexuality, 12*(1), 13–34. doi:10.1080/15299716.2012.645696

Dodge, B., Schnarrs, P. W., Reece, M., Goncalves, G., Martinez, O., Nix, R.,...Fortenberry, J. D. (2012). Community involvement among behaviourally bisexual men in the Midwestern USA: Experiences and perceptions across communities. *Culture, Health & Sexuality, 14*(9), 1095–1110. doi:10.1080/13691058.2012.721136

Dodge, B., Schnarrs, P. W., Reece, M., Martinez, O., Goncalves, G., Malebranche, D.,...Fortenberry, J. D. (2012). Individual and social factors related to mental health concerns among bisexual men in the Midwestern United States. *Journal of Bisexuality, 12*(2), 223–245. doi:10.1080/15299716.2012.674862

Drabble, L. L., Midanik, L. T., & Trocki, K. K. (2005). Reports of alcohol consumption and alcohol-related problems among homosexual, bisexual and heterosexual respondents: Results from the 2000 National Alcohol Survey. *Journal of Studies on Alcohol, 66*(1), 111–120.

Drabble, L., & Trocki, K. (2005). Alcohol consumption, alcohol-related problems, and other substance use among lesbian and bisexual women. *Journal of Lesbian Studies, 9*(3), 19–30. doi: 10.1300/J155v09n03_03

Eady, A., Dobinson, C., & Ross, L. l. (2011). Bisexual people's experiences with mental health services: A qualitative investigation. *Community Mental Health Journal, 47*(4), 378–389.

Everett, B., & Mollborn, S. (2013). Differences in hypertension by sexual orientation among U.S. young adults. *Journal of Community Health, 38*(3), 588–596. doi:10.1007/s10900-013-9655-3

Flanders, C. E., Dobinson, C., & Logie, C. (2015). "I'm never really my full self": Young bisexual women's perceptions of their mental health. *Journal of Bisexuality, 15*(4), 454–480. doi:10.1080/15299716.2015.1079288

Fredriksen-Goldsen, K. I., Kim, H. J., Barkan, S. E., Balsam, K. F., & Mincer, S. L. (2010). Disparities in health-related quality of life: A comparison of lesbians and bisexual women. *American Journal of Public Health, 100*(11), 2255–2261. doi:10.2105/AJPH.2009.177329

Fredriksen-Goldsen, K. I., Kim, H.-J., Barkan, S. E., Muraco, A., & Hoy-Ellis, C. P. (2013). Health disparities among lesbian, gay, and bisexual older adults: Results from a population-based study. *American Journal of Public Health, 103*(10), 1802–1809. doi:10.2105/AJPH.2012.301110

Friedman, M. S., Marshal, M. P., Guadamuz, T. E., Wei, C., Wong, C. F., Saewyc, E. M., & Stall, R. (2011). A meta-analysis of disparities in childhood sexual abuse, parental physical abuse, and peer victimization among sexual minority and sexual nonminority individuals. *American Journal of Public Health, 101*(8), 1481–1494. doi:10.2105/AJPH.2009.190009

Goetstouwers, L. (2006). Affirmative psychotherapy with bisexual men. *Journal of Bisexuality, 6*(1–2), 27–49. doi:10.1300/J159v06n01_03

Helms, J. L., & Waters, A. M. (2016). Attitudes toward bisexual men and women. *Journal of Bisexuality, 16*(4), 454–467. doi:10.1080/15299716.2016.1242104

Hequembourg, A. L., & Brallier, S. A. (2009). An exploration of sexual minority stress across the lines of gender and sexual identity. *Journal of Homosexuality, 56*(3), 273–298. doi:10.1080/00918360902728517

Herbenick, D., Reece, M., Schick, V., Sanders, S. A., Dodge, B., & Fortenberry, J. D. (2010). An event–level analysis of the sexual characteristics and composition among adults ages 18 to 59: Results from a national probability sample in the United States. *The Journal of Sexual Medicine, 7*(S5), 346–361. doi:10.1111/j.1743-6109.2010.02020

Herek, G. M. (2002). Heterosexuals' attitudes toward bisexual men and women in the United States. *Journal of Sex Roles, 39*(4), 264–274.

Herek, G. M., Norton, A. T., Allen, T. J., & Sims, C. L. (2010). Demographic, psychological, and social characteristics of self-identified lesbian, gay, and bisexual adults in a US probability sample. *Sexuality Research & Social Policy, 7*(3), 176–200. doi:10.1007/s13178-010-0017-y

Herrick, A., Kuhns, L., Kinsky, S., Johnson, A., & Garofalo, R. (2013). Demographic, psychosocial, and contextual factors associated with sexual risk behaviors among young sexual minority women. *Journal of the American Psychiatric Nurses Association, 19*(6), 345–355. doi:10.1177/1078390313511328

Hertlein, K. M., Hartwell, E. E., & Munns, M. E. (2016). Attitudes toward bisexuality according to sexual orientation and gender. *Journal of Bisexuality, 16*(3), 339–360. doi:10.1080/15299716.2016.1200510

Hottes, T. S., Gesink, D., Ferlatte, O., Brennan, D. J., Rhodes, A. E., Marchand, R., & Trussler, T. (2016). Concealment of sexual minority identities in interviewer-administered government surveys and its impact on estimates of suicide ideation among bisexual and gay men. *Journal of Bisexuality, 16*(4), 427–453. doi:10.1080/15299716.2016.1225622

Institute of Medicine, Committee on Lesbian, Gay, Bisexual, and Transgender Health Issues and Research Gaps and Opportunities. (2011). *The health of lesbian, gay, bisexual, and transgender people: Building a foundation for better understanding.* Washington, DC: National Academies Press.

Jackson, C. L., Agénor, M., Johnson, D. A., Austin, S. B., & Kawachi, I. (2016). Sexual orientation identity disparities in health behaviors, outcomes, and services use among men and women in the United States: A cross-sectional study. *BMC Public Health, 16*, 807. doi:10.1186/s12889-016-3467-1

Jeffries, W. L., & Dodge, B. (2007). Male bisexuality and condom use at last sexual encounter: Results from a national survey. *The Journal of Sex Research, 44*(3), 278–289. doi:10.1080/00224490701443973

Jun, H., Corliss, H., Nichols, L., Pazaris, M., Spiegelman, D., & Austin, S. (2012). Adult body mass index trajectories and sexual orientation: The Nurses' Health Study II. *American Journal of Preventive Medicine, 42*(4), 348–354. doi:10.1016/j.amepre.2011.11.011

Kaestle, C. E., & Ivory, A. H. (2012). A forgotten sexuality: Content analysis of bisexuality in the medical literature over two decades. *Journal of Bisexuality, 12*(1), 35–48. doi:10.1080/15299716.2012.645701

Kerr, D. D., Santurri, L., & Peters, P. (2013). A comparison of lesbian, bisexual, and heterosexual college undergraduate women on selected mental health issues. *Journal of American College Health, 61*(4), 185–194. doi:10.1080/07448481.2013.787619

Kerr, D. L., Ding, K., & Thompson, A. J. (2013). A comparison of lesbian, bisexual, and heterosexual female college undergraduate students on selected reproductive health screenings and sexual behaviors. *Women's Health Issues, 23*(6), e347–e355. doi:10.1016/j.whi.2013.09.003

King, M., & Nazareth, I. (2006). The health of people classified as lesbian, gay and bisexual attending family practitioners in London: A controlled study. *BMC Public Health, 6*(1), 127. doi:10.1186/1471-2458-6-127

Koh, A. (2000). Use of preventive health behaviors by lesbian, bisexual, and heterosexual women: Questionnaire survey. *The Western Journal of Medicine, 172*(6), 379–384.

Koh, A. S., Gomez, C. A., Shade, S., & Rowley, E. (2005). Sexual risk factors among self-identified lesbians, bisexual women, and heterosexual women accessing primary care settings. *Sexually Transmitted Diseases, 32*(9), 563–569.

Koh, A. S., & Ross, L. K. (2006). Mental health issues: A comparison of lesbian, bisexual and heterosexual women. *Journal of Homosexuality, 51*(1), 33–57.

Laska, M. N., VanKim, N. A., Erickson, D. J., Lust, K., Eisenberg, M. E., & Rosser, B. R. (2015). Disparities in weight and weight behaviors by sexual orientation in college students. *American Journal of Public Health, 105*(1), 111–121. doi:10.2105/AJPH.2014.302094

Lewis, R. J., Derlega, V. J., Brown, D., Rose, S., & Henson, J. M. (2009). Sexual minority stress, depressive symptoms, and sexual orientation conflict: Focus on the experiences of bisexuals. *Journal of Social and Clinical Psychology, 28*, 971–992. doi:10.1521/jscp.2009.28.8.971

Mathy, R. M., Lehmann, B. A., & Kerr, D. L. (2003). Bisexual and transgender identities in a nonclinical sample of North Americans: Suicidal intent, behavioral difficulties, and mental health treatment. *Journal of Bisexuality, 3*(3–4), 93–109. doi:10.1300/J159v03n03_07

Mohr, J. J., Israel, T., & Sedlacek, W. (2001). Counselors' attitudes regarding bisexuality as predictors of counselors' clinical responses: An analogue study of a female bisexual client. *Journal of Counseling Psychology, 48*, 212–222. doi: 10.1037/0022-0167.48.2.212

Mulick, P. S., & Wright Jr, L. W. (2002). Examining the existence of biphobia in the heterosexual and homosexual populations. *Journal of Bisexuality, 2*(4), 45–64. doi:10.1300/J159v02n04_03

Page, E. H. (2004). Mental health services experiences of bisexual women and bisexual men: An empirical study. *Journal of Bisexuality, 4*(1/2), 137–160. doi:10.1300/J159v04n01_11

Persson, T. J., & Pfaus, J. G. (2015). Bisexuality and mental health: Future research directions. *Journal of Bisexuality, 15*(1), 82–98. doi:10.1080/15299716.2014.994694

Polimeni, A., Austin, S., & Kavanagh, A. M. (2009). Sexual orientation and weight, body image, and weight control practices among young Australian women. *Journal of Women's Health, 18*(3), 355–362. doi:10.1089/jwh.2007.0765

Puckett, J. A., Surace, F. I., Levitt, H. M., & Horne, S. G. (2016). Sexual orientation identity in relation to minority stress and mental health in sexual minority women. *LGBT Health, 3*(5), 350–356. doi:10.1089/lgbt.2015.0088

Roberts, T. S., Horne, S. G., & Hoyt, W. T. (2015). Between a gay and a straight place: Bisexual individuals' experiences with monosexism. *Journal of Bisexuality, 15*(4), 554–569. doi:10.1080/15299716.2015.1111183

Robinson, M., Sanches, M., & MacLeod, M. A. (2016). Prevalence and mental health correlates of illegal cannabis use among bisexual women. *Journal of Bisexuality, 16*(2), 181–202. doi:10.1080/15299716.2016.1147402

San Francisco Human Rights Commission, LGBT Advisory Committee. (2011). Bisexual invisibility: Impacts and recommendations. Retrieved from http://sf-hrc.org/sites/default/files/Documents/HRC_Publications/Articles/Bisexual_Invisiblity_Impacts_and_Recommendations_March_2011.pdf

Schrimshaw, E. W., Siegel, K., Downing, M. R., & Parsons, J. T. (2013). Disclosure and concealment of sexual orientation and the mental health of non-gay-identified, behaviorally bisexual men. *Journal of Consulting and Clinical Psychology, 81*(1), 141–153. doi:10.1037/a0031272

Smalley, K. B., Warren, J. C., & Barefoot, K. N. (2015a). Barriers to care and psychological distress differences between bisexual and gay men and women. *Journal of Bisexuality, 15*(2), 230–247. doi:10.1080/15299716.2015.1025176

Smalley, K. B., Warren, J. C., & Barefoot, K. N. (2015b). Differences in health risk behaviors across understudied LGBT subgroups. *Health Psychology, 35*(2), 103–114. doi:10.1037/hea0000231

Smalley, K. B., Warren, J. C., & Barefoot, K. N. (2016). Variations in psychological distress between gender and sexual minority groups. *Journal of Gay and Lesbian Mental Health, 20*(2), 99–115. doi:10.1080/19359705.2015.1135843

Todd, M. E., Oravecz, L., & Vejar, C. (2016). Biphobia in the family context: Experiences and perceptions of bisexual individuals. *Journal of Bisexuality, 16*(2), 144–162. doi:10.1080/15299716.2016.1165781

Trocki, K. F., Drabble, L. A., & Midanik, L. T. (2009). Tobacco, marijuana, and sensation seeking: Comparisons across gay, lesbian, bisexual, and heterosexual groups. *Psychology of Addictive Behaviors, 23*(4), 620–631. doi:10.1037/a0017334

Valanis, B. G., Bowen, D. J., Bassford, T., Whitlock, E., Charney, P., & Carter, R. A. (2000). Sexual orientation and health: Comparisons in the women's health initiative sample. *Archives of Family Medicine, 9*(9), 843–853.

Walters, M. L., Chen, J., & Breiding, M. J. (2013). *The National Intimate Partner and Sexual Violence Survey (NISVS): 2010 findings on victimization by sexual orientation.* Atlanta, GA: National Center for Injury Prevention and Control, Centers for Disease Control and Prevention. Retrieved from https://www.cdc.gov/violenceprevention/pdf/nisvs_sofindings.pdf

Ward, B. W., Dahlhamer, J. M., Galinsky, A. M., & Joestl, S. S. (2014). Sexual orientation and health among US adults: National Health Interview Survey, 2013. *National Health Statistics Report, 77*, 1–12. Retrieved from https://www.cdc.gov/nchs/data/nhsr/nhsr077.pdf

Warren, J. C., Smalley, K. B., & Barefoot, K. N. (2016). Differences in psychosocial predictors of obesity among LGBT subgroups. *LGBT Health, 3*(4), 283–291. doi:10.1089/lgbt.2015.0076

Wheldon, C. W., & Kirby, R. S. (2013). Are there differing patterns of health care access and utilization among male sexual minorities in the United States? *Journal of Gay & Lesbian Social Services, 25*(1), 24–36. doi:10.1080/10538720.2013.751886

Whiting, E. L., Boone, D. N., & Cohn, T. J. (2012). Exploring protective factors among college-aged bisexual students in rural areas: An exploratory study. *Journal of Bisexuality, 12*(4), 507–518. doi:10.1080/15299716.2012.729431

Wilson, G. A., Zeng, Q., & Blackburn, D. G. (2011). An examination of parental attachments, parental detachments and self-esteem across hetero-, bi-, and homosexual individuals. *Journal of Bisexuality, 11*(1), 86–97. doi:10.1080/15299716.2011.545312

Yost, M. R., & Thomas, G. D. (2012). Gender and binegativity: Men's and women's attitudes toward male and female bisexuals. *Archives of Sexual Behavior, 41*(3), 691–702. doi:10.1007/s10508-011-9767-8

Zule, W. A., Bobashev, G. V., Wechsberg, W. M., Costenbader, E. C., & Coomes, C. M. (2009). Behaviorally bisexual men and their risk behaviors with men and women. *Journal of Urban Health, 86*(1), 48–62. doi:10.1007/s11524-009-9366-3

CHAPTER **17**

Advances in Research With Gender and Sexual Minority Youth in the 21st Century

Nicholas C. Heck, Lucas A. Mirabito, and Juan P. Zapata

When behavioral health scientists of the future look back upon the beginning of the 21st century, how will they describe this era of research as it relates to the health and well-being of gender and sexual minority (GSM) identified people? Will it be viewed as a golden age of research with GSM populations, where advancements are viewed as groundbreaking and paradigm shattering? Will our current theories about GSM health disparities stand the test of time, or will they fade away only to be viewed as an anachronistic artifact of a society that stigmatized sexual orientation and gender diversity? Given how far we as GSM health scientists have come, our hope is that, with time, both of these perspectives will eventually ring true.

At present, significant gains with respect to marriage equality, the repeal of *Don't Ask, Don't Tell*, and the passage of the Affordable Care Act are undoubtedly advancing the health and well-being of GSM people. While sexual orientation diversity is more accepted today than ever before (Meyer, 2016; Pew Research Center, 2014), gender diversity and those who embody it are facing an ardent backlash that threatens the safety and well-being of transgender people in our society (e.g., Grant et al., 2011; Human Rights Campaign & Trans People of Color Coalition, 2015; Kopan & Scott, 2016; Sanchez, 2016). And once again, lost in the mix and perpetually left behind is a relatively powerless demographic that exists without the social and financial capital necessary to influence the political climate in meaningful ways to improve their lives—GSM youth.

Using Bronfenbrenner's Ecological Systems Theory (1979) the present chapter highlights the unique strengths and challenges faced by GSM youth, while high-lighting future directions for research that we believe hold promise in promoting the health and well-being of this special population. First, however, we begin with a review of the research as applied to physical and mental health disparities that impact GSM youth. We then discuss the two dominant psychosocial models that explain the origins of and contributing factors to these disparities.

■ MENTAL AND PHYSICAL HEALTH DISPARITIES IMPACTING GSM YOUTH

One major challenge to identifying health disparities among GSM youth has involved the failure of large-scale epidemiologic studies and health-reporting sys-tems to ask about sexual orientation and gender minority identities. Thus, early research (and still a great deal of research today) relied heavily upon convenience samples to study health outcomes among GSM people. In fact, the first attempt to study GSM youth focused on the experiences of 60 gay men between the ages of 16 and 22 years (Roesler & Deisher, 1972). Many of the men had or were actively engaged in sex work, they reported high levels of psychological distress, and almost half of the sample had sought professional help.

Unfortunately, this study was fairly typical of the early investigations into the lives of GSM youth, which focused on health risk behaviors, especially substance use, risky sexual behavior, and suicide among young gay men (Savin-Williams, 2006). Today, however, topics like these are still studied, yet methodologies have improved and researchers are interested in contextualizing findings within the broad diversity that exists among GSM youth. There is now an improved balance between studying risks and resilience (Meyer, 2015).

An increasing number of nationally representative longitudinal databases and health-reporting systems are asking about sexual minority identities, and some state-level reporting systems have started to ask about gender minority identities. Unfortunately, with respect to transgender and other gender minority youth, much of our knowledge is limited by our own professions, which routinely fail to give trans-gender people opportunities to identify themselves within research settings (Flentje, Bacca, & Cochran, 2015; Heck, Mirabito, LeMaire, Livingston, & Flentje, 2017).

Mental Health, Substance Use, and Sexual Minority Youth

The prevalence rates of specific mental health disorders among GSM youth in the United States are not well established because most large-scale studies that have asked about GSM identities do not include diagnostic interviews, while similar studies of adolescents that have included diagnostic interviews have not often que-ried sexual orientation or provided options for gender minority self-identification. However, data from a New Zealand birth cohort showed that sexual minority youth and young adults were at elevated risk for major depressive disorder (odds ratio [OR] = 4.0), generalized anxiety disorder (OR = 2.8), nicotine dependence (OR = 5.0), and substance abuse/dependence (OR = 1.9), relative to their cisgender heterosexual counterparts (Fergusson, Horwood & Beautrais, 1999).

In the United States, Mustanski, Garofalo, and Emerson (2010) administered structured diagnostic interviews to an urban, community sample of GSM youth (*n* = 246) living in Chicago. Results revealed that 33% of youth met criteria for at least one mental health disorder, 17% for conduct disorder, 15% for major depression, 9% for posttraumatic stress disorder, and 1% for anorexia nervosa. Notable differences revealed that racial/ethnic minority youth were at elevated risk for conduct disorder (OR = 7.75) relative to White youth, and bisexual youth were at lower risk for meeting criteria for any disorder (OR = 0.52) relative to gay/lesbian youth. Finally, age was significantly associated with increased odds of major depressive disorder.

Along these lines, Diemer, Grant, Munn-Chernoff, Patterson, and Duncan (2015) found that rates of past-year, self-reported eating disorder diagnoses and past-month use of diet pills and laxatives/self-induced vomiting were highest among transgender college students and lowest among cisgender heterosexual men. Their findings are based on data from 289,024 college students participating in the American College Health Association-National College Health Assessment, conducted between 2008 and 2011. Notably, cisgender sexual minority men (but not cisgender sexual minority women) also evidenced increased risk for past-year, self-reported eating disorder diagnoses relative to cisgender heterosexual women; however, cisgender sexual minority women (but not cisgender sexual minority men) evidenced significantly lower risk for past-month diet pill use and self-induced vomiting/laxative use.

Aside from the aforementioned studies, much of what we know about risks for mental health disorders among GSM youth is based on indicators of disorders (e.g., having depressed mood, feeling anxious, or engaging in heavy drinking). Further, many studies pertaining to the health of GSM youth are based upon state- and city-level data collected through the Centers for Disease Control and Prevention's (CDC) Youth Risk Behavior Surveillance System (YRBSS; Kann et al., 2016). Additionally, two longitudinal studies with nationally representative samples, the National Longitudinal Study of Adolescent Health (Add Health; Mullan, 2009) and the Growing Up Today Study (GUTS; e.g., Berlan, Corliss, Field, Goodman, & Austin, 2010; Ziyadeh et al., 2007), have contributed substantially to the knowledge base.

That being said, meta-analytic and longitudinal studies consistently show that sexual minority youth evidence higher rates of anxiety, depression, and substance use relative to their cisgender heterosexual counterparts (Corliss et al., 2010; Fergusson et al., 1999; Marshal et al., 2008; Ziyadeh et al., 2007). However, important differences in risk for various mental health and substance use outcomes emerge depending upon the way sexual orientation is operationalized. For example, the earliest research using YRBSS data from Massachusetts found that youth who reported ever having a same-sex sexual partner reported more alcohol use, binge drinking, marijuana use, cocaine use, and injection drug use when compared to peers who reported only opposite-sex sexual behavior (Faulkner & Cranston, 1998). Of note, the authors were required to combine youth with same-sex and both-sex sexual behavior histories and were unable to control for possible confounds due to the limited size of the same-sex/both-sex samples (Faulkner & Cranston, 1998).

Using Wave 1 Add Health data, Russell and Joyner (2001) combined youth who reported same-sex attraction and those reporting same-sex sexual relationships and compared them with youth who reported only opposite-sex attractions and relationships. The results revealed that those in the same-sex orientation group were more likely to report suicidal thoughts and a past suicide attempt. While there may have been gender-by-sexual orientation effects in relation to these suicide outcomes, data from the GUTS study revealed that females identifying as "mostly heterosexual" and females identifying as lesbian and bisexual were at elevated risk for past-month alcohol use, past-year binge drinking, and early age of alcohol initiation (i.e., before 12 years of age), in addition to reporting significantly more depressive symptoms than their exclusively heterosexual peers (Ziyadeh et al., 2007). Among males, those identifying as "mostly heterosexual" reported significantly more depressive symptoms and were at elevated risk for past-year binge drinking and for having friends who drink alcohol; gay/bisexual identified males did not evidence increased risk for any of the alcohol-related outcomes under investigation nor were their depression scores significantly different from their exclusively heterosexual counterparts.

Based on data from Waves 1–4 of the Add Health study, Needham (2012) compared mental health and substance use outcomes in accordance with sexual attraction stability (or change) over time. Participants reporting consistent same-sex attractions at Waves 1 and 4, along with those participants who reported opposite-sex attraction at Wave 1 and same-sex attraction at Wave 4 (labeled "transition to LGB attraction"), were compared to participants who reported consistent opposite-sex attraction at Waves 1 and 4. Notably, females reporting consistent lesbian/bisexual attractions (i.e., from adolescence to adulthood) evidenced greater depressive symptomatology, suicidality, and risks for smoking, heavy drinking and marijuana use at Wave 1, relative to females consistently reporting opposite-sex attractions. Females who transition to lesbian/bisexual attractions by Wave 4 had higher levels of depression and suicidal ideation and increased risk for smoking and marijuana use at Wave 1. In relation to males with a consistent opposite-sex attraction, those with consistent same-sex attraction had greater depressive symptomatology and suicidality (but did not evidence increased risk for smoking, heavy drinking, or marijuana use), while males who transitioned to same-sex attraction were found to evidence only an increased risk for smoking. Notably, Marshal, Friedman, Stall, and Thompson (2009) examined trajectories of substance use over time using data from Waves 1–3 of the Add Health study and determined that sexual minority youth reported higher rates of substance use than their heterosexual peers, and that sexual minority adolescents' use of substances tended to increase at a faster rate than their heterosexual peers.

Mental Health, Substance Use, and Transgender Youth

Although there are still many improvements that could be made to ensure appropriate representation of sexual minority youth in behavioral health research, the experiences and health of gender minority youth remain understudied and even less well understood. There are numerous factors contributing to this gap in our knowledge. First, there are simply fewer gender minority people than there are sexual minority people, with roughly 3.5% of Americans identifying as a sexual minority and 0.3% identifying as transgender (Gates, 2011). Second, historically, the sexual minority and gender minority communities have often been united in their efforts to combat the power structures that marginalize their community members. This has resulted in a societal conflation of sexual minority– and gender minority–related concerns that permeate the research enterprise. In other words, researchers and research studies often study GSM youth together, yet there is hardly equal or even proportional representation of gender minority youth relative to sexual minority youth in the existing literature. Third, social acceptance of gender minority groups has been slower to come about and this is, not surprisingly, reflected in research and public policy. For example, questions about sexual orientation and sexual behavior were first included on the national and standard versions of the Youth Risk Behavior Surveillance Survey in 2015; however, assessments of gender identity and expression within this survey are still not inclusive of gender minority identities (Baker & Hughes, 2016; Conron, Landers, Reisner, & Sell, 2014). Thus, much of what we know about the health of transgender youth is derived from cross-sectional studies that often rely on convenience sampling methods.

From the available data, it is clear that gender minority youth are at elevated risk for experiencing depression, posttraumatic stress disorder, and suicidality (Grossman & D'Augelli, 2007; Roberts, Rosario, Corliss, Koenenn, & Austin, 2012; Roberts, Rosario, Slopen, Calzo, & Austin, 2013). For example, Roberts and colleagues (2012) analyzed data from the GUTS study to evaluate associations among childhood gender nonconformity, childhood abuse, and posttraumatic stress disorder symptoms. The authors found that youth in the top decile of gender nonconformity before 11 years of age evidenced increased risk for posttraumatic stress disorder and a range of childhood abuse outcomes; notably, childhood abuse partially mediated the relationship between gender nonconformity and posttraumatic stress. A similar finding for depression was detected in the GUTS study, with 26% of participants in the top decile of gender nonconformity reporting mild or moderate depression by 23 to 30 years of age, compared to 18% for those lower in gender nonconformity; again, abuse and bullying accounted for almost half of this increased risk in mediation models (Roberts et al., 2013).

Using electronic health records data from 180 transgender youth and young adults (aged 12–29 years) receiving services at a community health clinic in Boston, Reisner and colleagues (2015) compared 106 transgender male and 74 transgender female patients with matched samples of cisgender controls and found that transgender youth had two to three times the risk for anxiety (27% vs. 10%), depression (51% vs. 21%), suicidal ideation (31% vs. 11%), suicide attempts (17% vs. 6%), and self-injurious behavior (17% vs. 4%). Transgender patients also accessed inpatient (23% vs. 11%) and outpatient (46% vs. 16%) mental health services at significantly higher rates than their cisgender counterparts. Notably, significant differences in mental health outcomes between the two samples of transgender participants were not observed.

Physical Health

While a large and ever-growing body of research exists to document the mental health of GSM youth, less appears to be known about their physical health (Institute of Medicine [IOM], 2011). Of the research that does exist, there appears to be increased risk for pregnancy among sexual minority adolescents relative to their heterosexual peers (Charlton et al., 2013; Saewyc, Poon, Homma, & Skay, 2008). This elevated risk may be attributable to sexual minority youth reporting greater numbers of sexual partners, earlier ages of sexual initiation, and less consistent use of contraceptives (Goodenow, Szalacha, Robin, & Westheimer, 2008; Ybarra, Rosario, Saewyc, & Goodenow, 2016). Correspondingly, GSM youth are also at elevated risk for sexually transmitted infections including HIV, which disproportionately impacts young sexual minority men, especially those who are members of ethnic/racial minority communities (CDC, 2016). Data from the CDC show that from 2005 to 2014, new HIV diagnoses increased by more than 20% among Latino and Black sexual minority men, but decreased by 18% among White sexual minority men. Youth aged 13 to 24 years accounted for approximately 22% of new HIV diagnoses in 2014, with sexual minority men accounting for nearly 80% of these diagnoses (CDC, 2016). Less is known about the prevalence of HIV among gender minority youth; however, systematic reviews and meta-analyses indicate that adult transgender women are disproportionately impacted by HIV (Baral et al., 2013; Herbst et al., 2008) and it is inevitable that transmission occurs for some transgender people during youth.

Fortunately, the advent of preexposure prophylaxis (PrEP), a daily medication taken to prevent HIV infection, may reduce the transmission of HIV and curtail the epidemic. Clinical trials with high-risk populations (e.g., serodiscordant couples, sex workers) show that PrEP can dramatically reduce the risk for HIV infection, especially when adherence to the medication regimen is high (Anderson et al., 2012; Grant et al., 2010; Karim et al., 2010). While the first clinical trial of PrEP for adolescents in the United States is still underway, initial findings indicate that youth can be enrolled into PrEP trials; however, as with adults, adherence to the medication declines over time, indicating that counseling and regular monitoring are necessary to promote adherence and screen for other sexually transmitted infections (STIs; Hosek et al., 2013).

In addition to sexual health outcomes, researchers have documented disparities in obesity on the basis of sexual orientation using YRBS data, with bisexual male (OR = 2.10) and female (OR = 2.25) youth evidencing elevated risk in comparison to their same-gender, heterosexual peers (Austin, Nelson, Birkett, Calzo, & Everett, 2013). Based on GUTS data from the 1998 to 2005 waves, Austin and colleagues (2009) found that sexual minority females consistently had higher body mass indices throughout adolescence than their heterosexual counterparts. Among males, however, sexual minority youth evidenced higher body mass indices than their heterosexual counterparts at younger ages (i.e., 12–14 years), but strikingly lower body mass indices than their heterosexual peers at older ages (i.e., 19–20 years). With respect to gender, among female youth, nonconformity or greater masculinity is linked to higher body mass indices; however, among male youth, conformity or greater masculinity is also associated with higher body mass indices (Austin et al., 2016).

In summary, GSM youth evidence risk for a range of mental and physical health conditions relative to their heterosexual and cisgender peers. Clearly additional research is needed to better understand the full scope of these risks, especially for transgender youth. Yet, while awaiting the advancement of the literature, as a field we are also fortunate to have strong theoretical models that can guide our future research and inform interventions and policies in order to reduce health disparities and promote the well-being of GSM youth in our society.

▪ PSYCHOSOCIAL MODELS TO EXPLAIN GSM YOUTH HEALTH DISPARITIES

Minority Stress

Meyer's (1995, 2003) highly influential and pioneering Minority Stress Model explains why sexual minority populations experience higher rates of mental disorders when compared to heterosexual populations. Using the concept of minority stress, Meyer (2003) demonstrated how stigma, prejudice, expectations of rejection, internalized homophobia, and maladaptive coping processes can lead to increased risk for mental health problems. Meyer (2003) explains that identification as a member of a minority group leads to increased stress, expectations of rejection, and internalized homophobia as one learns to identify as a stigmatized and devalued minority.

According to the model, a unique factor affecting GSM youth is the fact that they are not "born in" to a minority community, but come to identify with the community later in life. This may prevent them from experiencing the protective benefit of growing up in the minority identity, which can provide validating experiences and a form of group cohesion and strength (Meyer, 2003). In contrast to other minority groups, GSM youth are more heterogeneous, are less likely to be born into a family that identifies as the same minority group, and are not readily identifiable visually; as a result, they may go through adolescence without other GSM youth providing validation and support. As a result, GSM youth struggling with identity in adolescence may feel extremely isolated.

Research has generally supported the minority stress model for lesbian, gay, and bisexual youth by showing that lack of social support related to sexual minority identity, awareness of sexual orientation–related discrimination and stigma, and internalized homophobia are the greatest predictors of poorer mental health outcomes (Berghe, Dewaele, Cox, & Vincke, 2010). In addition, a meta-analysis conducted by Fedawa and Ahn (2011) supports a link between increased bullying and victimization experienced by GSM youth and their increased risk of suicidal ideation, suicide attempts, mental health, and substance use problems. The increased risk of victimization and bullying may not be universal for GSM youth, however. Sexual minority women may face less stigma and threats of physical harm for violating traditional gender roles than their male counterparts (Bostwick,

Boyd, Hughes, & McCabe, 2009). In addition, D'Augelli (2002) found that lesbian, gay, and bisexual adolescents who self-reported being more "readily identifiable" as a gender and/or sexual minority reported more mental health symptoms. Males who were unsure of the "label" for their sexual orientation were at higher risk for mood disorders, while females who were unsure were not. Interestingly, those who identify as bisexual (regardless of gender) face the highest risk of mood disorders over their lifetimes (Bostwick et al., 2009). As with adults (see Chapter 16), youth who identify as bisexual may face dual stigma from the heterosexual community and from the lesbian and gay communities, which both continue to harbor harmful stereotypes about bisexuality (Bostwick et al., 2009). This shows that a blanket statement that all individuals who engage in same-sex sexual behavior face the same level of risk of mental health disorder is too reductive and supports the need for intergroup comparisons within the lesbian, gay, bisexual, and transgender (LGBT) community.

Unique to GSM youth, individuals who come out at an early age may not be able to cope as effectively with the resulting stigma and bullying as those who come out later in adolescence or early adulthood (Corliss et al., 2010). This may partially explain the increased risk of substance use in sexual minority adolescents, which may in turn correlate with the increased risk of substance use disorder in GSM adults (Corliss et al., 2010). Supporting this hypothesis is research that connects drinking and substance use in lesbian and gay youth with internalized stigma, coming out, and feelings of connectedness to the gay community (Baiocco, D'Alessio, & Laghi, 2010). Research has shown that lesbian and gay youth binge drink at higher rates than their heterosexual peers, and this higher alcohol use is associated with higher internalized homophobia, supporting the minority stress model (Baiocco et al., 2010). Other research has also shown that perceived discrimination accounts for more than half of the variance in depressive symptoms and suicidal ideation in gay male adolescents (Almeida, Johnson, Corliss, Molnar, & Azrael, 2009). The prevailing explanation for increased alcohol and illicit drug use in sexual minority adolescents is that individuals use alcohol to cope with stress and for its anxiety-reducing (and therefore reinforcing) effects (Khantzian, 1997). This is certainly consistent with the context of Meyer's (2003) minority stress model, where the multiplicative effects of minority stress, on top of the already high stress of adolescence, may certainly increase the odds that GSM teens will turn to alcohol to relieve stress and anxiety. Minority stress resulting from experiences of discrimination may be the most important explanation for the increased rates of depression observed among GSM youth. Research has shown that GSM youth who do not report experiences of discrimination have comparable levels of depressive symptoms when compared to cisgender heterosexual students (Almeida et al., 2009).

Meyer (2003) theorizes that there may be generational differences in the experience of minority stress. Notably, public opinion has been shifting toward greater acceptance and inclusion of the LGBT community, and the 21st century has seen a large increase in the number of protections and rights afforded to GSM individuals (Meyer, 2016). Future research should continue to examine and replicate the impact of minority stress in more recent cohorts of GSM adolescents to determine whether improvements in the social environment result in decreases in health disparities.

Syndemic Theory

The concept of a health syndemic comes from the anthropologist Merrill Singer (2009), who cleverly combined the meanings of the Greek words *synergos*, referring to two or more agents that work simultaneously to create a product that is greater than the sum of each agent working alone, and *demos*, referring to people. Thus, "the concentration and deleterious interaction of two or more diseases or other health conditions in a population, especially as a consequence of social inequity and the unjust exercise of power" (Singer, 2009, p. XV) defines a syndemic. At the heart of syndemic theories is the notion that cultural marginalization dynamics can produce multiple health epidemics that coalesce and comprise a single syndemic, and the notion that impoverished minority groups are especially vulnerable to syndemic situations (Stall, Friedman, & Catania, 2008).

Building on the work of Meyer (1995, 2003) and Díaz (1998), Stall and colleagues (2008) offered a syndemic theory to explain elevated rates of disease, morbidity, and mortality found among sexual minority men. The central assumptions of this theory are that: (a) the cluster of interacting health epidemics observed for this population is largely socially produced; (b) the conditions that give rise to syndemics can evolve over time and across populations; and (c) some proportion of men in each generation exhibit same-sex attractions and behaviors and that some, but certainly not all of these men, demonstrate gender nonconformity at early ages. Stall and colleagues (2008) go on to specify that early-adolescent socialization among sexual minority men who do not conform to masculine ideals results in early life adversity, followed by efforts to escape adverse environments via migration (e.g., moving to larger cities). This dynamic process and the associated stress it causes set the stage for the onset of a health syndemic among sexual minority men.

Recently, Mustanski, Andrews, Herrick, Stall, and Schnarrs (2014) pooled data from the 2005 and 2007 YRBSS from 11 jurisdictions to examine syndemic production in young men who have sex with only men (MSM) and men who have sex with men and women (MSMW), relative to men who have sex with only women (MSW). The researchers sought to determine whether health syndemics are a general phenomenon or whether they occur and are linked with negative health outcomes that are specific to select subpopulations (e.g., MSM and MSMW). The authors hypothesized and tested three syndemic drivers: (a) being attacked with a weapon; (b) having personal property stolen/damaged; and (c) being physically forced to have sex. The relationships between syndemic drivers and syndemic indicators (i.e., depressive symptoms, binge drinking, marijuana use, cocaine use, risky sexual behavior, and intimate partner violence) were then modeled in relation to having a past-year suicide attempt that required medical attention. Consistent with syndemic theory (Stall et al., 2008), the results revealed that a stable, latent health syndemic could be derived from the interrelations of the syndemic indicators, with the strongest correlations among the indicators being detected among MSMW. As expected, the syndemic drivers increased syndemic burden for all participants; however, these drivers accounted for more than three times the variance in syndemic burden among MSM (38%) and MSMW (44%) relative to the MSW (10%). Finally, syndemic burden significantly increased the odds of a serious suicide attempt among MSM (OR = 5.75) and MSMW (OR = 5.08); the final model including syndemic drivers and indicators explained approximately 60% of the variance in suicide attempts for MSM and MSMW, but only 34% of the variance in this outcome for MSW.

■ ECOLOGICAL SYSTEMS, STRESS, AND RESILIENCE

Bronfenbrenner's (1979) ecological systems theory provides a useful framework for organizing research relevant to understanding potential mediating and moderating factors that link individuals' experience of stress with their subsequent health and well-being. Briefly, Bronfrenbrenner (1979) proposed that in addition to the individual, there are five systems that influence human development (in order of increasing size: microsystem, mesosystem, exosystem, macrosystem, and chronosystem). With respect to GSM youth, a great deal of research has focused on how individual development is influenced by factors at the microsystem level (e.g., family, peers, school). However, there is also a growing body of research examining the degree to which general psychological processes are similar or distinct for GSM people (Livingston et al., 2015; Livingston, Oost, Heck, & Cochran, 2015). While there is perhaps less research focused on the ways in which various microsystems interact at the mesosystem and exosystem levels, this is clearly an area ripe for greater exploration and study. Finally, at the macrosystem and chronosystem levels, there are recent studies evaluating the impact of social policies and climate on health outcomes for GSM youth.

Individual

At the individual level are general psychological processes that confer risk or promote resilience in relation to health and well-being. For example, a significant body of research indicates that rumination, "a maladaptive emotion regulation strategy in which an individual passively and repetitively focuses on his/her symptoms of distress and the circumstances surrounding these symptoms" (Hatzenbuehler, 2009, p. 716), is a consistent and robust predictor of internalizing forms of psychopathology (Nolen-Hoeksema, Wisco, & Lyubomirsky, 2008). Whether this finding generalizes to GSM adolescents was unexplored until Hatzenbuehler, McLaughlin, and Nolen-Hoeksema (2008) found that, indeed, rumination does appear to mediate the relationship between sexual orientation and internalizing symptoms.

Such studies are important because they can suggest possible targets for intervention. Hatzenbuehler (2009) proposed a psychological mediation framework, identifying general psychological processes (e.g., coping motives, expectancies, and negative self-schemas) that mediate the relationship between experiencing prejudice events and subsequent psychopathology. Using this model, Pachankis (2014) and Heck (2015) have described how cognitive behavioral intervention strategies can be used to target mediators that link prejudice with psychopathology and thereby promote positive mental health outcomes among GSM youth and young adults. Notably, the study of general psychological processes as they relate to health outcomes among GSM populations is an area that is ripe for future research, as there are a number of general processes that confer risk or promote resilience that have yet to be explored using GSM samples.

Microsystem

Bronfrenbrenner (1979) specified that the microsystem is made of the people and groups that most directly impact an individual's development. These include parents, peers, schools, and religious institutions. There is a fairly substantial body of research examining how the microsystem influences health outcomes for GSM youth. Notably, when GSM youth first disclose their sexual orientation or gender identity to other people, it is often their heterosexual peers, and not their parents, who have the first chance to provide support and affirmation (Beals & Peplau, 2006). Receiving support after disclosing one's GSM identity is an important predictor of adjustment, and the experience of losing friends following such a disclosure is associated with increased distress and substance use (D'Augelli, 2002; Rosario, Schrimshaw, & Hunter, 2004). Studies have also found that GSM youth report experiencing lower levels of parental support than their cisgender heterosexual counterparts (Eisenberg & Resnick, 2006; Saewyc et al., 2009), and lower levels of parental support are associated with risk for depression, suicide, and drug use (Needham & Austin, 2010).

Beyond parents and peers, schools are important settings that shape the health and development of GSM youth. Unfortunately, school settings are often hostile environments for GSM youth, rather than institutions that promote the acquisition of knowledge and foster social development. School-based bullying and victimization of GSM youth are significant public health concerns associated with poor school performance, psychological distress, suicide, substance use, and sexual risk behavior (Birkett, Russell, & Corliss, 2014; Bontempo & D'Augelli, 2002; Fedawa & Ahn, 2011; Russell, Ryan, Toomey, Díaz & Sanchez, 2011). Data from the 2013 National School Climate Survey, comprising 7,898 GSM students from 2,770 unique school districts, show that school-based victimization is highly prevalent, with nearly three out of four GSM youth reporting that they experienced verbal harassment because of their sexual orientation. Further, one out of three and one out of six students in the survey reported physical harassment and physical assaults based upon their sexual orientation, respectively (Kosciw, Greytak, Palmer, & Boesen, 2014). More than half of those who were harassed or assaulted in school did not report the incident and two-thirds of those who did report an incident of harassment or assault said that school staff did nothing in response. Clearly, schools in our nation can do better to ensure the safety and well-being of GSM students.

One method to help address bullying and support GSM students involves the provision of gay-straight alliances (GSAs), which are school-based clubs for GSM students and their allies that provide members with opportunities to receive support, socialize, engage in advocacy, and acquire information about GSM-related issues (Gay, Lesbian, & Straight Education Network, n.d.; Griffin, Lee, Waugh, & Beyer, 2004). Numerous cross-sectional studies suggest that GSM youth who attend schools with GSAs report experiencing more school belongingness, less school victimization, and lower levels of depression and psychological distress (Goodenow, Szalacha, & Westheimer, 2006; Heck, Flentje & Cochran, 2011; Poteat, Sinclair, DiGiovanni, Koenig, & Russell, 2013; Toomey, Ryan, Díaz, & Russell, 2011). Attending schools with GSAs has also been associated with lower levels of alcohol use, drug use, and suicide attempts (Goodenow et al., 2006; Heck et al., 2011, 2014). The first prospective study on GSAs confirmed that the presence of a GSA is associated with greater feelings of safety at school and fewer experiences of homophobic bullying, and the addition of a GSA to a school further enhances feelings of safety for sexual minority students (Ioverno, Belser, Baiocco, Grossman, & Russell, 2016). Recently, Davis, Royne Stafford, and Pullig (2014) analyzed data from the California Healthy Kids Survey and found that the presence of a GSA within a school reduces the strength of the relationship between victimization and suicide attempts by reducing feelings of hopelessness. Davis and colleagues (2014) estimate between 4,800 and 12,800 suicide attempts (per 1 million adolescents) could be prevented by establishing GSA-like clubs within schools in our nation.

Finally, participation in religious organizations is typically associated with favorable health outcomes among adolescents in the general population (e.g., Kim-Spoon, Farley, Holmes, Longo, & McCullough, 2014). However, the existing research suggests that the protective benefits associated with participating in religious organizations may not extend to GSM youth and young adults, and in fact may have the opposite effect. For example, Rostosky, Danner, and Riggle (2007, 2008) analyzed Add Health data and found that adolescent religiosity (measured at Wave 1) serves as a protective factor against binge drinking, marijuana use, and cigarette smoking (measured at Wave 3 in young adulthood), but this was true only among heterosexual adolescents. This effect appears strongest for females. Among heterosexual females (but not lesbians), religiosity appears to reduce risk for binge drinking; however, religiosity was associated with increased risk for binge drinking behavior among bisexual females (Rostosky, Danner & Riggle, 2010). As adolescents, heterosexual females and gay males reported significantly higher levels of religiosity than heterosexual males and bisexual females, while lesbian adolescents were not significantly different in terms of their level of religiosity from their heterosexual and bisexual peers of either gender. While religiosity was found to decline across all sexual orientation groups from adolescence to young adulthood, the greatest reductions were detected among sexual minority participants (Rostosky et al., 2008).

Mesosystem

At the mesosystem are the interactions between components of the microsystem (i.e., interaction between parents and teachers of GSM youth). While this system has historically not been studied, there is emerging research at the mesosystem level; however, much of this research is focused on the experiences of same-sex parents navigating the workplace and school systems (Goldberg & Smith, 2013, 2014). For example, Goldberg and Smith (2014) investigated the school selection process and school-related experiences of 30 gay, 35 lesbian, and 40 heterosexual couples with preschool age children who were adopted. Notably, gay and lesbian parents had somewhat different school considerations (e.g., gay-friendliness of a school; presence of other adoptive or mixed-race families in a school) than their heterosexual counterparts. Furthermore, while heterosexual couples were more likely to attribute mistreatment from school personnel to their adoptive status than gay/lesbian couples, gay/lesbian couples living in less affirming communities were more likely to attribute mistreatment to their sexual orientation than gay/lesbian couples living in more gay-friendly communities. Clearly additional research is needed to understand the experiences of parents, siblings, peers, and teachers of GSM youth as they interact with one another within the mesosystem. Additional information on same-sex parenting can be found in Chapter 7.

Exosystem, Macrosystem, and Chronosystem

For GSM individuals living in the United States, a lot has changed since the 20th century. Sodomy laws are now ruled as unconstitutional, *Don't Ask, Don't Tell* has been repealed, and marriage equality for same-sex couples exists in all 50 states. Nationally and globally, GSM people are making monumental advances toward achieving equal rights (Meyer, 2016). Despite this, there is currently no federal law that explicitly prohibits employment discrimination based on sexual orientation or gender identity, nor are there legislative protections for GSM students.

The social environment, culture(s), and economics of nations influence the health and well-being of people, including GSM youth. Hatzenbuehler (2011) showed that sexual minority youth are 20% more likely to have a past-year suicide attempt when they live in social environments that are more hostile toward GSM people, even after controlling for demographic variables and common suicide risk factors. GSM adolescents living in neighborhoods with a higher prevalence of hate crimes targeting GSM people also exhibit greater risk for suicidal ideation and suicide attempts (Duncan & Hatzenbuehler, 2014). Collectively then, it is unsurprising but deeply troubling that sexual minority individuals who live in communities with high levels of antigay prejudice have a shorter life expectancy—by a full 12 years—than those living in areas of low levels of antigay prejudice (Hatzenbuehler et al., 2014). On the bright side, data at the chronosystem level suggest that we are seeing improvements in the social conditions that give rise to health disparities among GSM youth. For example, Goodenow and colleagues (2016) analyzed data from the Massachusetts YRBSS from 1999 to 2013 and found that school-based bullying is on the decline for sexual minority students; however, disparities in health outcomes have yet to diminish between heterosexual and LGB youth, suggesting that greater efforts are still needed to promote mental health outcomes among sexual minority students.

▪ CONCLUSION

As we have shown, GSM youth evidence a number of health disparities in relation to their cisgender and heterosexual peers. Over time, research methodologies have improved and in turn led to greater specificity in what we now understand about the health and experiences of GSM youth. Theoretical advances have helped guide an ever-expanding field of behavioral health researchers that span anthropology, medicine, psychology, public health, sociology, and other allied disciplines. Time will tell if we are in an era of promise with a steadfast commitment to eliminating disparities that disproportionately impact GSM youth. It is our hope that society is quick to eliminate the prejudices that undermine the health of GSM people; however, only time will tell if such a hope will come to fruition in the years to come.

▪ REFERENCES

Almeida, J., Johnson, R. M., Corliss, H. L., Molnar, B. E., & Azrael, D. (2009). Emotional distress among LGBT youth: The influence of perceived discrimination based on sexual orientation. *Journal of Youth and Adolescence, 38*, 1001–1014. doi:10.1007/s10964-009-9397-9

Anderson, P. L., Glidden, D. V., Liu, A., Buchbinder, S., Lama, J. R., Guanira, J. V.,...Grant, R. M. (2012). Emtricitabine-tenofovir exposure and pre-exposure prophylaxis efficacy in men who have sex with men. *Science Translational Medicine, 4*(151), 151ra125. doi:10.1126/scitranslmed.3004006

Austin, S. B., Nelson, L. A., Birkett, M. A., Calzo, J. P., & Everett, B. (2013). Eating disorder symptoms and obesity at the intersections of gender, ethnicity and sexual orientation in U.S. high school students. *American Journal of Public Health, 103*(2), e16–e22. doi:10.2105/AJPH.2012.301150

Austin, S. B., Ziyadeh, N. J., Calzo, J. P., Sonneville, K. R., Kennedy, G. A., Roberts, A. L.,...Scherer, E. A. (2016). Gender expression associated with BMI in a prospective cohort study of US adolescents. *Obesity, 24*(2), 506–515. doi:10.1002/oby.21338

Austin, S. B., Ziyadeh, N. J., Corliss, H. L., Haines, J., Rockett, H. R., Wypij, D., & Field, A. E. (2009). Sexual orientation disparities in weight status in adolescence: Findings from a prospective study. *Obesity, 17*(9), 1776–1782. doi:10.1038/oby.2009.72

Baiocco, R., D'Alessio, M., & Laghi, F. (2010). Binge drinking among gay, and lesbian youths: The role of internalized sexual stigma, self-disclosure, and individuals' sense of connectedness to the gay community. *Addictive Behaviors, 35*(10), 896–899. doi:10.1016/j.addbeh.2010.06.004

Baker, K., & Hughes, M. (2016). *Sexual orientation and gender identity data collection in the behavioral risk factor surveillance system.* Washington, DC: Center for American Progress. Retrieved from https://cdn.americanprogress.org/content/uploads/2016/03/05064109/BRFSSdatacollect-brief-04.05.17.pdf

Baral, S., Poteat, T., Stromdahl, S., Wirtz, A., Guadamuz, T., & Beyrer, C. (2013). Worldwide burden of HIV in transgender women: A systematic review and meta-analysis. *Lancet Infectious Diseases, 13*, 214–222. doi:10.1016/S1473-3099(12)70315-8

Beals, K. P., & Peplau, L. A. (2006). Disclosure patterns within social networks of gay men and lesbians. *Journal of Homosexuality, 51*(2), 101–120.

Berghe, W., Dewaele, A., Cox, N., & Vincke, J. (2010). Minority-specific determinants of mental well-being among lesbian, gay, and bisexual youth. *Journal of Applied Social Psychology, 40*, 153–166. doi:10.1111/j.1559-1816.2009.00567.x

Berlan, E. D., Corliss, H. L., Field, A. E., Goodman, E., & Austin, S. B. (2010). Sexual orientation and bullying among adolescents in the Growing Up Today Study. *Journal of Adolescent Health, 46*(4), 366–371. doi:10.1016/j.jadohealth.2009.10.015

Birkett, M., Russell, S. T., & Corliss, H. L. (2014). Sexual-orientation disparities in school: The mediational role of indicators of victimization in achievement and truancy because of feeling unsafe. *American Journal of Public Health, 104*(6), 1124–1128. doi:10.2105/AJPH.2013.301785

Bontempo, D. E., & D'Augelli, A. R. (2002). Effects of at-school victimization and sexual orientation on lesbian, gay, or bisexual youths' health risk behavior. *Journal of Adolescent Health, 30*(5), 364–374.

Bostwick, W. B., Boyd, C. J., Hughes, T. L., & McCabe, S. E. (2009). Dimensions of sexual orientation and the prevalence of mood and anxiety disorders in the United States. *American Journal of Public Health, 99*, 1–8. doi:10.2105/AJPH.2008.152942

Bronfenbrenner, U. (1979). *The ecology of human development: Experiments by nature and design.* Cambridge, MA: Harvard University Press.

Centers for Disease Control and Prevention (2016). HIV among African Americans, 2016. *HIV Surveillance Report, 26.* Retrieved from https://www.cdc.gov/nchhstp/news room/docs/factsheets/cdc-hiv-aa-508.pdf

Charlton, B. M., Corliss, H. L., Missmer, S. A., Rosario, M., Spiegelman, D., & Austin, S. B. (2013). Sexual orientation differences in teen pregnancy and hormonal contraceptive use: An examination across generations. *American Journal of Obstetrics and Gynecology, 209*(3), 204.e1–204.e8. doi:10.1016/j.ajog.2013.06.036

Conron, K. J., Landers, S. J., Reisner, S. L., & Sell, R. L. (2014). Sex and gender in the US Health Surveillance System: A call to action. *American Journal of Public Health, 104*(6), 970–976. doi:10.2105/AJPH.2013.301831

Corliss, H. L., Rosario, M., Wypij, D., Wylie, S. A., Frazier, A. L., & Austin, S. B. (2010). Sexual orientation and drug use in a longitudinal cohort study of U.S. adolescents. *Addictive Behaviors, 35*(5), 517–521. doi:10.1016/j.addbeh.2009.12.019

D'Augelli, A. R. (2002). Mental health problems among lesbian, gay, and bisexual youths ages 14 to 21. *Clinical Child Psychology and Psychiatry, 7*, 433–456. doi:10.1177/1359104502007003010

Davis, B., Royne Stafford, M. B., & Pullig, C. (2014). How gay-straight alliance groups mitigate the relationship between gay-bias victimization and adolescent suicide attempts. *Journal of the American Academy of Child & Adolescent Psychiatry, 53*(12), 1271–1278. doi:10.1016/j.jaac.2014.09.010

Díaz, R. (1998) *Latino gay men and HIV: Culture, sexuality, and risk behavior.* New York, NY: Routledge.

Diemer, E. W., Grant, J. D., Munn-Chernoff, M. A., Patterson, D. A., & Duncan, A. E. (2015). Gender identity, sexual orientation, and eating-related pathology in a national sample of college students. *Journal of Adolescent Health, 57*(2), 144–149. doi:10.1016/j.jadohealth.2015.03.003

Duncan, D. T., & Hatzenbuehler, M. L. (2014). Lesbian, gay, bisexual, and transgender hate crimes and suicidality among a population-based sample of sexual-minority adolescents in Boston. *American Journal of Public Health, 104*(2), 272–278. doi:10.2105/AJPH.2013.30142

Eisenberg, M., & Resnick, M. (2006). Suicidality among gay, lesbian and bisexual youth: The role of protective factors. *Journal of Adolescent Health, 39*, 662–668. doi:10.1016/j.jadohealth.2006.04.024

Faulkner, A. H., & Cranston, K. (1998). Correlates of same-sex sexual behavior in a random sample of Massachusetts high school students. *American Journal of Public Health, 88*(2), 262–266.

Fedawa, A. L., & Ahn, S. (2011). The effects of bullying and peer victimization on sexual minority and heterosexual youths: A quantitative meta-analysis of the literature. *Journal of GLBT Family Studies, 7*, 398–418. doi:10.1080/1550428X.2011.592968

Fergusson, D. M., Horwood, L. J., & Beautrais, A. L. (1999). Is sexual orientation related to mental health problems and suicidality in young people? *Archives of General Psychiatry, 56*(10), 876–880.

Flentje, A., Bacca, C. L., & Cochran, B. N. (2015). Missing data in substance abuse research? Researchers' reporting practices of sexual orientation and gender identity. *Drug and Alcohol Dependence, 147,* 280–284. doi:10.1016/j.drugalcdep.2014.11.012

Gates, G. (2011). *How many people are lesbian, gay, bisexual and transgender?* Los Angeles, CA: The Williams Institute, UCLA School of Law. Retrieved from: http://escholarship.org/uc/item/09h684x2

Gay, Lesbian, and Straight Education Network. (n.d.). Gay-straight alliances. Retrieved from http://www.glsen.org/participate/student-action/gsa

Goldberg, A. E., & Smith, J. Z. (2013). Predictors of psychological adjustment in early placed adopted children with lesbian, gay, and heterosexual parents. *Journal of Family Psychology, 27*(3), 431–442. doi:10.1037/a0032911

Goldberg, A., & Smith, J. (2014). Preschool selection considerations and experiences of school mistreatment among lesbian, gay, and heterosexual adoptive parents. *Early Childhood Research Quarterly, 29,* 64–75. doi:10.1016/j.ecresq.2013.09.006

Goodenow, C., Szalacha, L. A., Robin, L. E., & Westheimer, K. (2008). Dimensions of sexual orientation and HIV-related risk among adolescent females: Evidence from a statewide survey. *American Journal of Public Health, 98*(6), 1051–1058. doi:10.2105/AJPH.2005.080531

Goodenow, C., Szalacha, L., & Westheimer, K. (2006). School support groups, other school factors, and the safety of sexual minority adolescents. *Psychology in the Schools, 43*(5), 573–589.

Goodenow, C., Watson, R., Adjei, J., Homma, Y., Doull, M. & Saewyc, E. (2016). Sexual orientation trends and disparities in school bullying and violence-related experiences 1999–2013. *Psychology of Sexual Orientation and Gender Diversity, 3*(4), 386–396. doi:10.1037/sgd0000188

Grant, J. M., Mottet, L. A., Tanis, J., Harrison, J., Herman, J. L., & Keisling, M. (2011) Injustice at every turn: A report of the national transgender discrimination survey. Retrieved from http://endtransdiscrimination.org/PDFs/NTDS_Report.pdf

Grant, J. M., Mottet, L. A., Tanis, J., Herman, J. L., Harrison, J., & Keisling, M. (2010). *National Transgender Discrimination Survey Report on health and health care.* Washington, DC: National Center for Transgender Equality and the National Gay and Lesbian Task Force.

Griffin, P., Lee, C., Waugh, J., & Beyer, C. (2004). Describing roles that gay-straight alliances play in schools: From individual support to social change. *Journal of Gay & Lesbian Issues in Education, 1*(3), 7–22.

Grossman, A. H., & D'Augelli, A. R. (2007). Transgender youth and life-threatening behaviors. *Suicide and Life-Threatening Behavior, 37*(5), 527–537. doi:10.1521/suli.2007.37.5.527

Hatzenbuehler, M. L. (2009). How does sexual minority stigma "get under the skin"? A psychological mediation framework. *Psychological Bulletin, 135*(5), 707–730. doi:10.1037/a0016441

Hatzenbuehler, M. L. (2011). The social environment and suicide attempts in lesbian, gay, and bisexual youth. *Pediatrics, 127*(5), 896–903. doi:10.1542/peds.2010-3020

Hatzenbuehler, M. L., Bellatorre, A., Lee, Y., Finch, B. K., Muennig, P., & Fiscella, K. (2014). Structural stigma and all-cause mortality in sexual minority populations. *Social Science & Medicine, 103,* 33–41. doi:10.1016/j.socscimed.2013.06.005

Hatzenbuehler, M. L., McLaughlin, K. A., & Nolen-Hoeksema, S. (2008). Emotion regulation and internalizing symptoms in a longitudinal study of sexual minority and heterosexual adolescents. *Journal of Child Psychology and Psychiatry, and Allied Disciplines, 49*(12), 1270–1278. doi:10.1111/j.1469-7610.2008.01924.x

Heck, N. C. (2015). The potential to promote resilience: Piloting a minority stress-informed, GSA-based, mental health promotion program for LGBTQ youth. *Psychology of Sexual Orientation and Gender Diversity, 2*(3), 225–231. doi:10.1037/sgd0000110

Heck, N. C., Flentje, A., & Cochran, B. (2011). Offsetting risks: High school gay-straight alliances and lesbian, gay, bisexual, and transgender (LGBT) youth. *School Psychology Quarterly, 26*, 161–174. doi:10.1037/a0023226.

Heck, N. C., Livingston, N. A., Flentje, A., Oost, K., Stewart, B. T., & Cochran, B. N. (2014). Reducing risk for illicit drug use and prescription drug misuse: High school gay-straight alliances and lesbian, gay, bisexual, and transgender youth. *Addictive Behaviors, 39*(4), 824–828. doi:10.1016/j.addbeh.2014.01.007

Heck, N. C., Mirabito, L. A., LeMaire, K., Livingston, N. A., & Flentje, A. (2017). Omitted data in randomized controlled trials for anxiety and depression: A systematic review of the inclusion of sexual orientation and gender identity. *Journal of Consulting and Clinical Psychology, 85*(1), 72–76. doi:10.1037/ccp0000123

Herbst, J. H., Jacobs, E. D., Finlayson, T. J., McKleroy, V. S., Neumann, M. S., & Crepaz, N. (2008). Estimating HIV prevalence and risk behaviors of transgender persons in the United States: A systematic review. *AIDS and Behavior, 12*(1), 1–17. doi:10.1007/s10461-007-9299-3

Hosek, S., Green, K., Siberry, G., Lally, M., Balthazar, C., Serrano, P., & Kapogiannis, B. (2013). Integrating behavioral HIV interventions into biomedical prevention trials with youth: Lessons from Chicago's Project PrEPare. *Journal of HIV/AIDS & Social Services, 12*, 333–348. doi:10.1080/15381501.2013.773575

Human Rights Campaign & Trans People of Color Coalition. (2015). Addressing anti-transgender violence: Exploring realities, challenges, and solutions for policymakers and community advocates. Retrieved from http://hrc-assets.s3-website-us-east-1.amazonaws.com//files/assets/resources/HRC-AntiTransgenderViolence-0519.pdf

Institute of Medicine, Committee on Lesbian, Gay, Bisexual, and Transgender Health Issues and Research Gaps and Opportunities. (2011). *The health of lesbian, gay, bisexual, and transgender people: Building a foundation for better understanding.* Washington, DC: National Academies Press.

Ioverno, S., Belser, A., Baiocco, R., Grossman, A., & Russell, S. (2016). The protective role of gay-straight alliances for lesbian, gay, bisexual, and questioning students: A prospective analysis. *Psychology of Sexual Orientation and Gender Diversity, 3*(4), 397–406. doi:10.1037/sgd0000193

Kann, L., McManus, T., Harris, W. A., Shanklin, S. L., Flint, K. H., Hawkins, J., . . . Zaza, S. (2016). Youth risk behavior surveillance—United States, 2015. *MMWR Surveillance Summaries, 65*, 1–174.

Karim, Q., Karim, S., Frohlich, J., Grobler, A., Baxter, C., Mansoor, L., . . . Taylor, D. (2010). Effectiveness and safety of Tenofovir Gel, an antiretroviral microbicide, for the prevention of HIV infection in women. *Science, 329*, 1168–1174. doi:10.1126/science.1193748

Khantzian, E. K. (1997). The self-medication hypothesis of substance use disorders: A reconsideration and recent applications. *Harvard Review of Psychiatry, 4*(5), 231–244.

Kim-Spoon, J., Farley, J. P., Holmes, C., Longo, G. S., & McCullough, M. E. (2014). Processes linking parents' and adolescents' religiousness and adolescent substance use: Monitoring and self-control. *Journal of Youth and Adolescence, 43*(5), 745–756. doi:10.1007/s10964-013-9998-1

Kopan, T. & Scott, E. (2016, March). North Carolina governor signs controversial transgender bill. *CNN Politics.* Retrieved from http://www.cnn.com/2016/03/23/politics/north-carolina-gender-bathrooms-bill/

Kosciw, J. G., Greytak, E. A., Palmer, N. A., & Boesen, M. J. (2014). *The 2013 National School Climate Survey: The experiences of lesbian, gay, bisexual and transgender youth in our nation's schools.* New York, NY: Gay, Lesbian and Straight Education Network.

Livingston, N., Heck, N., Flentje, A., Gleason, H., Oost, K., & Cochran, B. (2015). Sexual minority stress and suicide risk: Identifying resilience through personality profile analysis. *Psychology of Sexual Orientation and Gender Diversity, 2*(3), 321–328. doi:10.1037/sgd0000116

Livingston, N. A., Oost, K. M., Heck, N. C., & Cochran, B. N. (2015). The role of personality in predicting drug and alcohol use among sexual minorities. *Psychology of Addictive Behaviors, 29*(2), 414–419. doi:10.1037/adb0000034

Marshal, M. P., Friedman, M. S., Stall, R., King, K. M., Miles, J., Gold, M. A.,…Morse, J. Q. (2008). Sexual orientation and adolescent substance use: A meta-analysis and methodological review. *Addiction, 103*(4), 546–556.

Marshal, M. P., Friedman, M. S., Stall, R., & Thompson, A. L. (2009). Individual trajectories of substance use in lesbian, gay and bisexual youth and heterosexual youth. *Addiction, 104*(6), 974–981. doi:10.1111/j.1360-0443.2009.02531.x

Meyer, I. H. (1995). Minority stress and mental health in gay men. *Journal of Health and Social Behavior, 36*(1), 38–56. doi:10.2307/2137286

Meyer, I. H. (2003). Prejudice, social stress, and mental health in lesbian, gay, and bisexual populations: Conceptual issues and research evidence. *Psychological Bulletin, 129*(5), 674–697. doi:10.1037/0033-2909.129.5.674

Meyer, I. H. (2015). Resilience in the study of minority stress and health of sexual and gender minorities. *Psychology of Sexual Orientation and Gender Diversity, 2*(3), 209–213. doi:10.1037/sgd0000132

Meyer, I. H. (2016). The elusive promise of LGBT equality. *American Journal of Public Health, 106*(8), 1356–1358. doi:10.2105/AJPH.2016.303221

Mullan, H. K. (2009). *The National Longitudinal Study of Adolescent to Adult Health (Add Health) waves I & II, 1994–1996; wave III, 2001–2002; wave IV, 2007–2009* [Machine-readable data file and documentation]. Chapel Hill: Carolina Population Center, University of North Carolina at Chapel Hill. doi:10.3886/ICPSR27021.v9

Mustanski, B., Andrews, R., Herrick, A., Stall, R., & Schnarrs, P. W. (2014). A syndemic of psychosocial health disparities and associations with risk for attempting suicide among young sexual minority men. *American Journal of Public Health, 104*(2), 287–294. doi:10.2105/AJPH.2013.301744

Mustanski, B. S., Garofalo, R., & Emerson, E. M. (2010). Mental health disorders, psychological distress, and suicidality in a diverse sample of lesbian, gay, bisexual, and transgender youths. *American Journal of Public Health, 100*(12), 2426–2432. doi:10.2105/AJPH.2009.178319

Needham, B. L. (2012). Sexual attraction and trajectories of mental health and substance use during the transition from adolescence to adulthood. *Journal of Youth and Adolescence, 41*(2), 179–190. doi:10.1007/s10964-011-9729-4

Needham, B. L., & Austin, E. L. (2010). Sexual orientation, parental support, and health during the transition to young adulthood. *Journal of Youth and Adolescence, 39*(10), 1189–1198. doi:10.1007/s10964-010-9533-6.

Nolen-Hoeksema, S., Wisco, B. E., & Lyubomirsky, S. (2008). Rethinking rumination. *Perspectives on Psychological Science, 3*(5), 400–424. doi:10.1111/j.17456924.2008.00088.x

Pachankis, J. E. (2014). Uncovering clinical principles and techniques to address minority stress, mental health, and related health risks among gay and bisexual men. *Clinical Psychology, 21*(4), 313–330. doi:10.1111/cpsp.12078

Pew Research Center. (2014). Changing attitudes on gay marriage. Retrieved from http://www.pewforum.org/2014/09/24/graphics-slideshow-changing-attitudes-on-gay-marriage

Poteat, V. P., Sinclair, K. O., DiGiovanni, C. D., Koenig, B. W., & Russell, S. T. (2013). Gay-straight alliances are associated with student health: A multischool comparison of

LGBTQ and heterosexual youth. *Journal of Research on Adolescence, 23*(2), 319–330. doi:10.1111/j.1532-7795.2012.00832.x

Reisner, S. L., Vetters, R., Leclerc, M., Zaslow, S., Wolfrum, S., Shumer, D., & Mimiaga, M. J. (2015). Mental health of transgender youth in care at an adolescent urban community health center: A matched retrospective cohort study. *Journal of Adolescent Health, 56*(3), 274–279. doi:10.1016/j.jadohealth.2014.10.264

Roberts, A. L., Rosario, M., Corliss, H. L., Koenen, K. C., & Austin, S. B. (2012). Elevated risk of posttraumatic stress in sexual minority youths: Mediation by childhood abuse and gender nonconformity. *American Journal of Public Health, 102*(8), 1587–1593. doi:10.2105/AJPH.2011.300530

Roberts, A. L., Rosario, M., Slopen, N., Calzo, J. P., & Austin, S. B. (2013). Childhood gender nonconformity, bullying victimization, and depressive symptoms across adolescence and early adulthood: An 11-year longitudinal study. *Journal of the American Academy of Child and Adolescent Psychiatry, 52*(2), 143–152. doi:10.1016/j.jaac.2012.11.006

Roesler, T., & Deisher, R. W. (1972). Youthful male homosexuality. Homosexual experience and the process of developing homosexual identity in males aged 16 to 22 years. *Journal of the American Medication Association, 219*(8), 1018–1023. doi:10.1001/jama.1972.03190340030006

Rosario, M., Schrimshaw, E. W., & Hunter, J. (2004). Predictors of substance use over time among gay, lesbian, and bisexual youths: An examination of three hypotheses. *Addictive Behaviors, 29*(8), 1623–1631. doi:10.1016/j.addbeh.2004.02.032

Rostosky, S. S., Danner, F., & Riggle, E. D. (2007). Is religiosity a protective factor against substance use in young adulthood? Only if you're straight! *Journal of Adolescent Health, 40*(5), 440–447.

Rostosky, S. S., Danner, F., & Riggle, E. D. B. (2008). Religiosity and alcohol use in sexual minority and heterosexual youth and young adults. *Journal of Youth and Adolescence, 37*, 552–563. doi:10.1007/s10964-007-9251-x

Rostosky, S. S., Danner, F., & Riggle, E. D. (2010). Religiosity as a protective factor against heavy episodic drinking (HED) in heterosexual, bisexual, gay, and lesbian young adults. *Journal of Homosexuality, 57*(8), 1039–1050. doi:10.1080/00918369.2010.503515

Russell, S. T., & Joyner, K. (2001). Adolescent sexual orientation and suicide risk: Evidence from a national study. *American Journal of Public Health, 91*(8), 1276–1281. doi:10.2105/AJPH.91.8.1276

Russell, S. T., Ryan, C., Toomey, R. B., Diaz, R. M., & Sanchez, J. (2011). Lesbian, gay, bisexual, and transgender adolescent school victimization: Implications for young adult health and adjustment. *Journal of School Health, 81*(5), 223–230. doi:10.1111/j.17461561.2011.00583.x

Saewyc, E. M., Homma, Y., Skay, C. L., Bearinger, L. H., Resnick, M. D., & Reis, E. (2009). Protective factors in the lives of bisexual adolescents in North America. *American Journal of Public Health, 99*(1), 110–117. doi:10.2105/AJPH.2007.123109

Saewyc, E. M., Poon, C. S., Homma, Y., & Skay, C. L. (2008). Stigma management? The links between enacted stigma and teen pregnancy trends among gay, lesbian, and bisexual students in British Columbia. *Canadian Journal of Human Sexuality, 17*(3), 123–139.

Sanchez, R. (2016, May). Feds' transgender guidance provokes fierce backlash. *CNN Politics.* Retrieved from http://www.cnn.com/2016/05/14/politics/transgender-bathrooms-backlash

Savin-Williams, R. C. (2006). Who's gay? Does it matter? *Current Directions in Psychological Science, 15*(1), 40–44. doi:10.1111/j.0963-7214.2006.00403.x

Singer, M. (2009). *Introduction to syndemics.* San Francisco, CA: Jossey-Bass.

Stall, R., Friedman, M., & Catania, J. (2008). Interacting epidemics and gay men's health: A theory of syndemic production among urban gay men. In R. Wolitski, R. Stall,

& R. O. Valdiserri (Eds.), *Unequal opportunity: Health disparities affecting gay and bisexual men in the United States*. New York: Oxford University Press.

Toomey, R. B., Ryan, C., Diaz, R. M., & Russell, S. T. (2011). High school gay-straight alliances (GSAs) and young adult well-being: An examination of GSA presence, participation, and perceived effectiveness. *Applied Developmental Science, 15*(4), 175–185. doi:10.1080/10888691.2011.607378

Ybarra, M. L., Rosario, M., Saewyc, E., & Goodenow, C. (2016). Sexual behaviors and partner characteristics by sexual identity among adolescent girls. *Journal of Adolescent Health, 58*(3), 310–316. doi:10.1016/j.jadohealth.2015.11.001

Ziyadeh, N. J., Prokop, L. A., Fisher, L. B., Rosario, M., Field, A. E., Camargo, C. A., & Austin, S. B. (2007). Sexual orientation, gender, and alcohol use in a cohort study of U.S. adolescent girls and boys. *Drug and Alcohol Dependence, 87*(2–3), 119–130. doi:10.1016/j.drugalcdep.2006.08.004

CHAPTER **18**

Rural Gender and Sexual Minority Health

K. Bryant Smalley, Jacob C. Warren, Amanda Rickard, and K. Nikki Barefoot

Rural areas have unique health problems, resource shortages, demographic characteristics, cultural behaviors, and economic concerns that combine to impact the health of its residents in systematic and persistent ways. Unfortunately, rural areas are remarkably understudied—particularly given the fact that approximately one out of five Americans lives in a rural area (U.S. Census Bureau, 2010) and 75% of the nation's counties are designated as rural (Hart, Larson, & Lishner, 2005). Although limited and largely based on cross-sectional research, the literature does agree that rural areas have unique health considerations that ultimately result in persistent health disparities in outcomes ranging from diabetes to suicide (Warren & Smalley, 2014).

When considering the source of rural health disparities, rural areas have a unique cultural background and heritage that can impact health behaviors and outcomes in strong and surprising ways—both for the overall population and for subpopulations within rural areas. This culture is shaped by many key factors, including remoteness and isolation, lower income, lower educational levels, increased religiosity, unique behavioral norms, increased health care stigma, increased transportation burdens, and additional distance to care (Smalley & Warren, 2012; Smalley et al., 2010; Ziller, 2014). These factors combine to impact not only potential need for health care, but also the ways in which residents will seek out care, and ultimately their outcomes as well. Unfortunately, despite the recognition of the breadth of challenges faced in rural health, there has been remarkably little progress in eliminating rural health disparities. Much health research makes the assumption that theories, practices, and programs developed in urban settings will be, for the most part, translatable into rural settings, leaving a distinct lack of rural-focused research and care models to improve the health of rural populations. This lack of rural consideration unfortunately impacts not only rural residents at large, but particularly also minority groups within rural areas (e.g., gender and sexual minority, or GSM, groups), which remains a virtually unstudied branch of rural health.

The broader health of GSM individuals who reside in rural areas is virtually unstudied, despite the fact that being either a rural resident or a gender and/or sexual minority places them within a dual-minority context that increases the risk of health risk factors and outcomes including diabetes, hypertension, depression, substance use, sexually transmitted diseases (STDs), reproductive cancers, smoking, alcohol abuse, poor diet, medication adherence, and physical inactivity (Harvey & Housel, 2014; Institute of Medicine [IOM], Committee on Lesbian, Gay, Bisexual, and Transgender Health Issues and Research Gaps and Opportunities, 2011; Meit et al., 2014; Warren & Smalley, 2014). A PubMed search conducted in preparation for this chapter revealed fewer than 50 articles published since 1987 with a titular focus on rural GSM individuals (outside of our own work), several of which were conducted outside of the United States. As a result, the subfield is still rapidly evolving. Within this chapter, we summarize the existing literature and discuss ways in which existing knowledge regarding general rural health can be extended into a deeper understanding of the health needs of rural GSM residents.

■ THE DYNAMICS OF RURAL COMMUNITIES

While there is an overall lack of knowledge regarding the health outcomes of rural GSM groups, there is a robust level of knowledge regarding the specific intrapersonal, interpersonal, and cultural factors that influence health in rural communities, generated largely from qualitative investigations. Specifically, factors related to heterosexism, invisibility, discrimination, isolation, and lack of social support all directly impact the ability of rural GSM individuals to achieve and maintain both physical and mental health. The majority of the literature summarized below focuses on sexual minority residents of rural communities, as research investigating rural gender minority individuals is functionally nonexistent and is sorely needed.

Heterosexism and Homophobia

Rural living is associated with conservatism, religiosity, uniformity, gossip, social conformity, and heteronormative culture (Barefoot, Rickard, Smalley, & Warren, 2015; Hastings & Hoover-Thompson, 2011; Preston & D'Augelli, 2013; Rosenkrantz, Black, Abreu, Aleshire, & Fallin-Bennett, 2016; Smalley & Warren, 2012; Swank, Frost, & Fahs, 2012; Williams, Bowen, & Horvath, 2005). Residing in a rural area has been shown to increase negative attitudes toward sexual minority individuals (i.e., heterosexism and/or homophobia), which is largely influenced by fear of HIV/AIDS, fundamental religiosity, conservative political ideologies, and less contact with GSM individuals (Barton, 2010; Dillon & Savage, 2006; Eldridge, Mack, & Swank, 2006; Gottschalk & Newton, 2009; Herek, 2002; Hopwood & Connors, 2002; Neely, 2005; Preston & D'Augelli, 2013; Rosenkrantz et al., 2016; Snively, Kreuger, Stretch, Watt, & Chadha, 2004; Swank, Fahs, Frost, 2013). These effects are not just at the interpersonal level—rural social institutions are also perceived as heterosexist; schools in particular have been identified by GSM youth and adults as hostile climates fraught with high levels of heterosexism- and homophobia-related microaggressions, harassment, discrimination, and victimization (Kosciw, Greytak, & Diaz, 2009; Leedy & Connolly, 2007; Palmer, Kosciw, & Bartkiewicz, 2012). This heightened level of heterosexism and homophobia in rural areas translates into greater experiences of felt stigma (i.e., perceiving one's immediate environment as unaffirming of and/or hostile toward gay men/lesbians) among rural sexual minority individuals when compared to their urban peers both within the workplace and the larger local community (Swank et al., 2012).

As a result, rural areas can be more dangerous environments for GSM individuals to navigate. Exposure to heterosexism and stigma from others can create internalized homophobia and/or transphobia (i.e., negative or prejudiced thoughts against themselves and others based on one's sexual orientation/gender identity) among rural GSM individuals. This effect was demonstrated by Kennedy (2010) who found that gay men in rural Ontario, Canada, harbored negative feelings, guilt, and low self-esteem as adults stemming from their childhood experiences of discrimination and religious guilt. As a result, many of these men had since rejected organized religion altogether, which is a frequent source of social interaction and support in rural areas. Similar results were found in an earlier study of gay men living in rural areas of New England, wherein there was a high degree of internalization of negative oppressive messages from parents, teachers, members of the clergy, and peers (Cody & Welch, 1997). As a result of these experiences, some rural gay men reported seeking mental health services to change their sexual orientation (so-called "conversion therapies"). Other studies have also suggested that a number of sexual minority individuals in rural areas conceal their sexual identity in public to be accepted within their communities (Lee & Quam, 2013; Leedy & Connolly, 2007; Lyons, Hosking, & Rozbroj, 2014; McCarthy, 2000; Oswald & Culton, 2003; Swank et al., 2013), further perpetuating issues of isolation and invisibility discussed in more detail later. Some researchers suggest that such an admission of feelings of shame and guilt or lack of indignation about experienced oppression by sexual minority individuals residing in rural areas may be evidence of internalized heterosexism; however, it is also important to recognize that due to the even more oppressive culture encountered by rural GSM individuals, concealment may be a genuine act of self-preservation and safety (Swank et al., 2013).

Invisibility and "Don't Ask, Don't Tell"

As discussed earlier, some sexual minority individuals seek to conceal their sexual orientation within the rural environment. In fact, recent research suggests that rural sexual minority individuals have lower levels of outness and are more guarded about their sexual orientation in comparison to their nonrural counterparts (Lee & Quam, 2013; Lyons et al., 2014). Rural sexual minority individuals have consistently reported to researchers that they fear coming out to their rural neighbors because they may be victimized, discriminated against, or ostracized from their community (Bell & Valentine, 1995; Cody & Welch, 1997; Lee & Quam, 2013; McCarthy, 2000; Oswald & Culton, 2003). In one study, sexual minority individuals who lacked confidence and a sense of belongingness in their rural New Mexico communities reported experiencing fear of disclosure as a major stressor (Willging, Salvador, & Kano, 2006a). Those same sexual minority individuals reported being fearful of disclosing their sexual or gender identity to health providers for fear of bias, discrimination, and negative response (Willging et al., 2006a). Unfortunately, emerging research with rural sexual minority individuals has found evidence that being out about one's sexual orientation in rural communities may in fact make them more vulnerable to discrimination and victimization. For example, Swank et al. (2013) found that higher levels of outness and visibility were associated with increased experiences of enacted stigma (i.e., harassment, discrimination, and victimization) in one's community for rural, but not urban, sexual minority adults.

Boulden (2001) discovered an unspoken "don't ask, don't tell" mentality between rural gay men and their neighbors. More specifically, a hyperawareness of surroundings and others was a common theme in the interviews Boulden (2001) conducted, and rural gay men reported guarding against purposefully revealing their sexual orientation in front of their neighbors in order to be accepted in the community. Participants described how they were careful to be on guard in public and not engage in behaviors such as holding hands with their partners, referring to their partners by pet names, or acting in ways that could be perceived as effeminate (Boulden, 2001). Similar findings regarding concealment were found by Oswald and Culton (2003) in rural Illinois and by Leedy and Connolly (2007) in rural Wyoming. Interestingly, the sexual minority men in Leedy and Connolly's (2007) rural Wyoming study described developing "public personas" to improve their quality of life and ease of existence in rural culture, with these personas especially present in community and work settings.

Leedy and Connolly (2007) posited that the rural sexual minority men in their study may have been selective about coming out to coworkers, friends, and neighbors based on the nature of anticipated response, because many respondents rated the actual reactions of their friends, coworkers, and neighbors postdisclosure as neutral or generally positive. This anticipatory planning regarding to whom to reveal their sexual identity seems consistent with the caution reported by sexual minority individuals residing in rural areas concerning how to navigate the heterosexist landscape of rural community life. However, many of the rural gay men interviewed by Boulden (2001) believed that many of their neighbors knew of or suspected their sexual orientation and reported that others in the community would avoid socializing with them or would not come to their homes for fear that association with them would imply that they were also GSM. Thus, despite efforts to hide sexual orientation in public, most felt that many people in the community were actually silently aware. Thus, the dynamic at play for many rural sexual minority residents can be likened to "don't ask, don't tell" (Boulden, 2001), which clearly can impact one's ability to achieve and maintain health and mental well-being.

Victimization and Discrimination

One consistent finding in the literature is that, despite increased attempts to remain invisible, GSM youth and adults residing in rural areas experience harassment, discrimination, and violence at levels higher than their nonrural counterparts (Kosciw et al., 2009; Palmer et al., 2012; Swank et al., 2012, 2013). Most notably, a very high proportion (i.e., 71%–87%) of rural GSM individuals have experienced some form of enacted stigma (i.e., harassment, discrimination, and/or victimization) in their lifetime (Leedy & Connolly, 2007; Palmer et al., 2012). Examples of enacted stigma experienced by rural gender and/or sexual minority youth and adults include: being exposed to homophobic statements and slurs and receiving threatening telephone calls; being discriminated against in credit and banking decisions, tax benefits, entry into community groups, housing options, employment opportunities and benefits, and termination of employment; having their property destroyed or damaged; and being verbally threatened, chased or followed, and/or physically or sexually attacked (Boulden, 2001; Leedy & Connolly, 2007; Palmer et al., 2012; Swank et al., 2012, 2013). Reflecting the gradient of risk present within rural communities, sexual minority individuals residing in the least densely populated counties—presumably with the highest level of adherence to rural cultural norms—have been found to experience the highest levels of discrimination at the personal, community, and institutional levels (Leedy & Connolly, 2007).

Isolation

Rural GSM individuals living in rural areas may be more susceptible to negative effects from victimization and discrimination because they feel isolated and have fewer opportunities to socialize with other GSM individuals through lesbian, gay, bisexual and transgender (LGBT)-affirming organizations and events (King & Dabelko-Schoeny, 2009; Li, Hubach, & Dodge, 2015; Rosenberger, Schick, Schnarrs, Novak, & Reece, 2014). For instance, among a large, nationally diverse sample of rural sexual minority men ($N = 5,357$), the majority had never been to or had access to an LGBT community center (77%), a social group specifically for sexual minority men (69%), an LGBT-owned restaurant/coffee shop, and/or a gay pride event (60%; Rosenberger et al., 2014). It is well-documented that LGBT community support relieves feelings of isolation and psychological distress (Li et al., 2015; Waldo, Hesson-McInnis, & D'Augelli, 1998); however, the general lack of community-based LGBT organizations and resources in rural areas heightens feelings of social isolation among rural-residing individuals (King & Dabelko-Schoeny, 2009; Lyons et al., 2014; McCarthy, 2000; Willging, Salvador, & Kano, 2006b), with rural sexual minority individuals significantly less likely than their urban counterparts to feel connected to LGBT communities (Swank et al., 2012). To illustrate, Oswald and Culton (2003) found that rural GSM residents of Illinois identified the lack of a community as the "worst thing" about living in a rural area, and described the

LGBT community as being small, hidden, fragmented, and lacking in resources. These feelings of isolation are likely exacerbated by other structural and cultural aspects of rural living including geographic isolation, greater travel distances, limited sources of transportation, smaller population sizes, and the previously discussed conservative and heteronormative climate of rural areas.

Some sexual minority individuals find a small group of gay or lesbian friends with whom to socialize in their rural areas, which functions as a small LGBT community (Boulden, 2001; Leedy & Connolly, 2007; McCarthy, 2000). The groups go to dinner, socialize at each other's houses, go to the theater together, and share other small group social activities. Yet, even these small groups tend to be kept secret and underground to minimize the risk of being "exposed," and the small groups tend not to socialize with one another. Therefore, to find and become an invited member of such a group can be quite challenging (Boulden, 2001; Leedy & Connolly, 2007; McCarthy, 2000). Despite these small informal groups, there remains a paucity of LGBT-affirming services and organizations in rural communities, which in itself raises the risk for GSM individuals to feel isolated, vulnerable, and psychologically distressed.

Lack of Support

In addition to the lack of structural support, rural GSM individuals can also lack support and acceptance from family and friends, with rural sexual minority individuals being found to have lower levels of social support than their rural heterosexual peers (Lyons et al., 2014). For example, half of the gay men previously interviewed by Cody and Welch (1997) who were living in rural New England indicated they experienced some sort of censorship by their families regarding their sexual orientation. Their families responded to the men's coming out with silence, disinterest, ambivalence, or a lack of support. Some of the men had not verbally come out to their families, and instead had developed an unspoken understanding about their sexual orientation (Cody & Welch, 1997). Waldo et al. (1998) found that unsupportive family and friends were more likely to victimize or enable victimization of a GSM individual. On the other hand, supportive family and friends were found to be more likely to protect a gender or sexual minority individual from victimization and offer resources to help avoid victimization. Qualitative interviews with midlife and older sexual minority men and women living in rural areas also revealed themes of limited social support from family, friends, and the community that heightens feelings of social isolation and a lack of community belongingness (King & Dabelko-Schoeny, 2009).

Cody and Welch (1997) found that rural sexual minority individuals dealt with family censorship and lack of support by developing a family of choice from a group of close gay and ally friends within their communities; however, as described previously this community can be difficult to find and maintain. Given the findings that rural sexual minority individuals are more likely to conceal their sexual orientation due to fears of rejection and/or discrimination, experience higher levels of both felt and enacted stigma, feel less connected to LGBT communities, and have lower levels of social support, Swank and colleagues (2012) have suggested that these proximal and distal vulnerabilities translate into a higher prevalence of overall minority stress among rural-residing sexual minorities. Furthermore, given that the community coping resources available to rural sexual minorities are further limited by their location, Swank and colleagues (2012) postulate that the negative impact that minority stress exposure has on the health of sexual minority individuals is likely exacerbated by rural location.

■ PHYSICAL HEALTH OUTCOMES AND PROVIDERS

The context just described creates an extremely challenging environment in which rural GSM individuals must navigate multiple layers of barriers and oppression while attempting to achieve and maintain physical and mental health. Unfortunately, given the scarcity of research focused on rural GSM populations, there is very little information regarding actual health outcomes, and researchers are left largely to combine what is known about both communities separately to draw inferences. The literature base regarding mental health among rural GSM individuals (discussed in more detail later) is more developed than that focusing on physical health, but two areas that have received the most research attention in physical health are the dynamics of receipt of care in rural environments and emerging information regarding differences in health risk behaviors.

Access to Physical Health Care and Experiences With Providers

Because of the dynamics described earlier and a general history of negative experiences within the health care system, GSM individuals (both urban and rural) are often hesitant to disclose their sexual orientation or gender identity to providers, particularly when not queried in an affirming way (Brotman, Ryan, Jalbert, & Rowe, 2002; Daley, 1998, 2010; Durso & Meyer, 2013; Klitzman & Greenberg, 2002; St Pierre, 2012). Within rural areas, this becomes even more problematic—having an open discussion regarding sexual orientation or gender identity with what may be the only health care provider in a person's hometown (or even county) could have significant implications regarding access to care. Similarly, concerns over confidentiality—often cited by rural residents in general (Bourke et al., 2004; Larson, Corrigan, & Cothran, 2012; Smalley & Warren, 2012; Warner et al., 2005)—may also impede open discussions with providers regarding sexual orientation and gender identity. Such hesitance to disclose to health providers can significantly impact both the quality of care they receive and even health outcomes (Bonvicini & Perlin, 2003; Brotman et al., 2002; IOM, 2011; Klitzman & Greenberg, 2002; Petroll & Mosack, 2011; St Pierre, 2012; Whitehead, Shaver, & Stephenson, 2016), and this may be contributing substantially to health disparities within rural GSM populations.

The few studies that have been conducted and that have focused on interactions with health care providers reveal that rural GSM residents often avoid disclosing their sexual orientation in personal, professional, and medical situations, which directly impacts their ability to receive culturally competent care (Austin, 2013; Barefoot, Smalley, & Warren, 2017; Lee & Quam, 2013; Lyons et al., 2014;

Petroll & Mosack, 2011; Preston, D'Augelli, Kassab, & Starks, 2007; Rosenkrantz et al., 2016). Rural GSM residents express concerns that if their sexual orientation is disclosed to their provider and they are rejected or discriminated against, they will be unable to access safe and appropriate care given the scarcity of providers in rural areas (Tiemann, Kennedy, & Haga, 1998). This places an extreme amount of stress upon the population in their decision to be open with their medical provider and, in turn, complicates care. Further complicating this decision-making process is the fact that rural areas have substantial limitations in the availability of LGBT-affirming health care services (Barefoot, Smalley, & Warren, 2015; IOM, 2011; Warren et al., 2014; Whitehead et al., 2016; Willging et al., 2006b). To illustrate, among a large, nationally diverse sample of rural GSM individuals (N = 1,014), only 4% had received services from a clinic specifically specializing in LGBT health in the past year (Whitehead et al., 2016).

In terms of experiences with rural health care providers, a recent quantitative comparison of the health care disclosure–related experiences of rural and nonrural lesbians revealed that not only did rural lesbians endorse fewer attitudes/beliefs that promote health care disclosure, communicate less about their sexual orientation to their providers, and experience fewer health care opportunities that facilitate disclosure, but also when rural lesbians have decided to come out to their providers, they were more likely than their nonrural counterparts to experience negative reactions to their disclosure (Barefoot, Smalley, & Warren, 2017). Furthermore, when accessing women's health care services, the majority of rural lesbians reported receiving inadequate care from providers; namely, 61.2% had not been asked about their sexual orientation, 78.6% had not been provided appropriate safe-sex education, and 43.5% felt that their women's health care provider did not seem knowledgeable about lesbian health concerns (Barefoot, Warren, & Smalley, 2017). Additional barriers to ongoing and appropriate medical care cited by rural GSMs include being uninsured and/or other financial limitations (Farmer, Blosnich, Jabson, Matthews, 2015; Whitehead et al., 2016). Most notably, rural sexual minority women have been found to report significantly greater cost barriers to care than rural heterosexual women (Farmer et al., 2015). Taken together, this emerging research suggests that rural GSMs likely face unique obstacles and vulnerabilities when attempting to access appropriate and affirming health care services.

Health Risk Behaviors

As discussed throughout this book, GSM groups are at elevated risk for engaging in a variety of health risk behaviors, including alcohol and tobacco use, binge drinking, sexual risk taking, self-injury, poor diet, and lack of exercise (Harvey & Housel, 2014; IOM, 2011). Similarly, rural residents are known to be at increased risk of alcohol and tobacco use and dependence, sedentary lifestyle, poor diet, avoidance of care, self-injury and suicide, domestic violence, and aggression (Meit et al., 2014; Warren & Smalley, 2014). Thus, simply by being members of either group, rural GSM residents face substantial elevated risk of a multitude of health risk behaviors.

Sexual minority individuals may be particularly vulnerable to engaging in health risk behaviors as a means of maladaptive coping with the previously discussed stressors and problems associated with rural life. While the evidence regarding rural/urban differences in health risk behaviors specifically within GSM groups is limited, initial evidence suggests that rural GSM residents have unique health behavior profiles. For example, a study of sexual minority men in rural Pennsylvania found that sexual sensation seeking and related sexual risk behaviors may be a maladaptive coping response to experiences of discrimination, rejection, and victimization (Preston et al., 2007). Similarly, other studies have found that rural sexual minority men and women both have a greater prevalence of overall HIV risk (i.e., unprotected sex, giving or receiving money or drugs for sex, intravenous drug use, and having a current or previous STD diagnosis) than their rural heterosexual counterparts (Farmer et al., 2015). Rural sexual minority men are especially at risk for engaging in unsafe sexual behaviors (i.e., unprotected anal intercourse) associated with using the Internet to meet sexual partners when compared to their urban counterparts (Horvath, Bowen, & Williams, 2006; Kakietek, Sullivan, & Heffelfinger, 2011).

In terms of substance use, Whitehead and colleagues (2016) found that 40% of their sample of rural GSM adults were current smokers and 14% reported heavy alcohol use, with available comparison studies suggesting that rural sexual minority youth engage in greater substance use than their urban peers (Poon & Saewyc, 2009), while rural sexual and gender minority adults have significantly higher odds of smoking than their rural cisgender/heterosexual peers (Bennett, McElroy, Johnson, Munk, & Everett, 2015). While another study of transgender adults found no significant rural/nonrural differences in either substance use or sexual risk behaviors, the rates of marijuana use among transgender men and the rates of sexual risk taking among transgender women were relatively high across locations (Horvath, Iantaffi, Swinburne-Romine, & Bockting, 2014). Extending on these findings, our own prior work has shown that nationally diverse samples of rural residents who identify as a gender and/or sexual minority are more likely to have unhealthy diets, to engage in elevated motor vehicle risk behaviors, to engage in aggressive behaviors, to smoke, and to have more risky health care engagement behaviors (e.g., not taking prescriptions, not seeking medical care, and not following medical advice) when compared to their urban counterparts (Warren, Smalley, & Barefoot, 2016). Furthermore, lesbians residing in rural areas were found to be more likely than their urban-residing counterparts to report that they never engage in exercise (Barefoot, Warren, & Smalley, 2015). Sadly, these health risk behaviors can lead to serious negative health consequences including HIV/STDs, cancer, heart disease, pulmonary disease, stroke, renal disease, vascular disease, ulcers, liver disease, obesity, blood pressure, diabetes, injury, and even death (Fagerström, 2002; Foster & Marriott, 2006). Additional research is needed to focus on the underlying reasons for these elevations, and if they represent rural-only or compounded risk (i.e., are these behaviors comparable to non-GSM rural residents, or do they represent additive/intersectional risk even beyond simply being a rural resident?).

Engagement in Preventive Care

Whitehead and colleagues' (2016) recent survey of rural sexual and gender minority adults from across the United States provides some preliminary descriptive data on the preventive behavior of this population. Most notably, rates of engagement in a variety of preventive services were relatively low for the total sample of rural GSM individuals, with 43% not being up-to-date on HIV testing (i.e., within the past 12 months or selecting a legitimate reason for not being tested); 55% having never been tested for gonorrhea/chlamydia; 59% not receiving the influenza vaccine in the past year; and 74% not being vaccinated for human papilloma virus (HPV; ages 18–34 only). Furthermore, among the participants assigned female at birth and currently with a cervix, 31% were not up-to-date on their cervical cancer screenings (i.e., within the last 3 years for ages 21–30 years or in the last 5 years for ages 30–65 years) and 38% of participants assigned female at birth and currently with breast tissue were not up-to-date on mammogram screenings (i.e., within the past 2 years for ages 50–75 years). Our own research on the preventive behavior of rural lesbians reveals that they have similarly low rates of HPV vaccination (22.8% and 29.0%, respectively) and/or being screened for HIV/sexually transmitted infection (STI; 43.0% and 47.8%) or cervical cancer (62.0% and 64.5%) in the past 3 years as their urban counterparts, with rural lesbians significantly less likely than urban lesbians to have received an age-appropriate (i.e., older than 40 years) mammogram within the past 3 years (63.2% vs. 83.2%; Barefoot, Warren, & Smalley, 2017). Overall, this research suggests that engagement in regular preventive care is a significant health concern for rural GSM residents and future efforts are needed to better understand and address the preventive health care needs of this vulnerable population.

Physical Health Outcomes and Disparities

As previously noted, much less is known about the actual health outcomes of rural GSM individuals. What we do know about the physical health outcomes and disparities faced by this population comes from Whitehead et al.'s (2016) survey of the health needs of rural GSMs and our own research. Most notably, Whitehead and colleagues (2016) estimated that approximately 35% of rural GSM adults have been diagnosed with at least one chronic disease, with subgroup rates as follows: 38% of sexual minority women, 32% of sexual minority men, and 35% of transgender and nonbinary persons. In terms of rural disparities, our recent survey of rural and urban lesbians from across the United States reveals that current rural residence (but not previous rural background) appears to exacerbate the risk for obesity among sexual minority women (Barefoot, Warren, & Smalley, 2015). More specially, we found that, after controlling for age, race/ethnicity, and educational background, not only did rural-residing lesbians have higher body mass indexes (BMIs) than their urban dwelling counterparts, their average BMI was in the obese range (i.e., 30.6), whereas the average BMI for the urban sample was only in the overweight range (i.e., 28.5). Future research is needed to better understand the physical health outcomes and disparities experienced by rural and gender sexual minorities, in addition to their unique experiences and barriers to care related to chronic disease and other health outcomes.

■ MENTAL HEALTH OUTCOMES AND PROVIDERS

Mental Health Disparities and Outcomes

Given the unique psychosocial vulnerabilities and added sources of minority stress associated with rural living that are discussed throughout this chapter, it is not surprising that research consistently finds higher levels of psychological distress among rural GSM youth and adults when compared to either their nonrural GSM counterparts and/or their rural cisgender/heterosexual peers (Barefoot, Smalley, & Warren, 2015; Cohn & Leake, 2012; Horvath et al., 2014; Lyons et al., 2014). In terms of suicidiality, Poon and Saewyc (2009) found that rural sexual minority boys are more likely to report suicidal behavior than their urban peers. In addition, Horvath and colleagues (2014) found that, when compared to their nonrural counterparts, rural transgender women and men endorsed greater somatization symptoms, with transgender men also endorsing greater depression and anxiety symptoms, lower self-esteem, and higher global symptom severity. The mental health needs of this population are further highlighted by the fact that 50% of Whitehead and colleagues' (2016) sample of rural GSMs scored in the clinically depressed range (i.e., greater than 9) on the Center for Epidemiologic Studies Depression Scale (CESD).

Access to Mental Health Care and Experiences With Providers

Unfortunately, despite being at risk for greater psychological distress (i.e., depression, anxiety, and stress) due to heterosexism, victimization, discrimination, invisibility, isolation, and lack of familial and social support, LGBT-affirming mental health services may not be readily available in many rural areas. Willging et al. (2006b) found that rural mental health providers: lacked appropriate training to treat GSM individuals; reported individual and institutional forms of bias in institutions providing mental health services in rural areas; assumed clients were heterosexual; isolated GSM individuals in treatment facilities; discouraged sexual orientation or gender identity disclosure in group therapy; and indicated many observed examples of fellow colleagues mistreating GSM individuals. Some mental health providers compensated for their biases by attempting to treat GSM individuals as no different from other clients (Willging et al., 2006b). This attempt at therapeutic neutrality is problematic because the mental health provider neglects confronting lack of training in GSM issues, as well as failing to consider the impact sexual orientation and gender identity issues may have on the client's mental health problems (Willging et al., 2006b). Additionally, given the cultural realities, even mental health providers knowledgeable about GSM issues struggle with whether to encourage individuals to live more openly or continue to hide their identity in their rural communities, when both options could have detrimental effects (Willging et al., 2006b).

Even if care is available, there remains an underlying dynamic that serves as a barrier to seeking care in rural communities. A lack of social networks, fear of discrimination based on sexual orientation or gender identity, misconceptions of mental illness and substance abuse, and financial concerns are some factors reported by rural GSM individuals as preventing them from seeking mental health services (Willging et al., 2006a). Many rural GSM individuals indicate that they have previously experienced discrimination, inappropriate care, or premature discontinuation of care due to their sexual orientation or gender identity when they sought mental health services in their communities. Several individuals in the Willging et al. (2006a) study reported turning to religious institutions for treatment of emotional distress and substance abuse issues due to financial concerns, yet many of those individuals kept their sexual or gender identities secret while seeking religious assistance. Participants from Latino and Native American families in particular reported that their family influenced their decision to utilize religious treatment options (Willging et al., 2006a).

While it is natural to assume that seeking treatment is a beneficial endeavor, rural GSM individuals sometimes report significantly *harmful* treatment from mental health professionals based on their sexual orientation or gender identities, such as humiliation, laughter, and disparaging remarks (Willging et al., 2006a). Misconceptions about mental illness and substance abuse that prevent GSM individuals in rural areas from seeking mental health treatment include believing that mental illness is a sign of personal weakness that can be overcome by perseverance and hard work (Willging et al., 2006a). Access to LGBT-affirming mental health services is limited in rural areas, and financial concerns as well as lack of referrals to such services prevent many individuals from traveling to LGBT-affirming providers in urban areas (Willging et al., 2006a). Rural sexual minority individuals sometimes assume that seeking mental health services will require either a suppression of the topic of their sexual orientation or that their sexual orientation will be treated with either therapeutic neutrality or hostility (Oswald & Culton, 2003).

To illustrate the unique vulnerabilities and barriers to mental health care faced by rural sexual minority individuals, a comparison of the reasons cited for their inability to access needed mental health care in the past 2 years between rural and nonrural lesbians reveals that rural lesbians were more likely to endorse the following barriers: a lack of mental health care coverage/financial limitations (51.4% vs. 36.2%, respectively); a limited availability of mental health care providers in one's area (24.6% vs. 15.4%, respectively); and avoidance of needed mental health care due to fears of discrimination and/or mistreatment (22.3% vs. 13.2%, respectively). Furthermore, almost one-fourth of rural lesbians indicated that they had forgone needed mental health care due to the lack of LGBT-friendly providers in their community (Barefoot, Smalley, & Warren, 2015). Overall, these research findings expose a critical area in which mental health practitioners need further specialized training, continuing education, and mandated practice standards to improve the care provided to GSM individuals, especially those residing in rural areas.

CONCLUSION

Taken as a whole, we currently know very little about the dynamics of health experienced by GSM individuals who reside in rural areas. Sitting at the intersection of two vulnerable and underserved groups intuitively places rural-residing GSM individuals at elevated levels of risk for a variety of health risk behaviors and outcomes; however, there is very little evidence regarding the best ways to counteract these negative effects and work to improve their physical and mental health. Cultural competency training is highly needed, as is additional research to elucidate both the barriers and facilitators of health and to accurately describe what disparities are present. At the same time, it is important for researchers to remember the positive aspects of rural culture (e.g., sense of community, strength of family relationships) and to examine ways in which those aspects can be directed toward benefiting the GSM residents of those communities.

■ NOTE

Portions of this chapter are adapted from material that previously appeared in *Rural Mental Health* (2012), Springer Publishing.

■ REFERENCES

Austin, E. L. (2013). Sexual orientation disclosure to health care providers among urban and nonurban southern lesbians. *Women & Health, 53*(1), 41–55. doi:10.1080/03630242.2012.743497

Barefoot, K. N., Rickard, A., Smalley, K. B., & Warren, J. C. (2015). Rural lesbians: Unique challenges and implications for mental health providers. *Journal of Rural Mental Health, 39*(1), 22–33. doi:10.1037/rmh0000014

Barefoot, K. N., Smalley, K. B., & Warren, J. C. (2015). Psychological distress and perceived barriers to care for rural lesbians. *Journal of Gay and Lesbian Mental Health, 19*(4), 347–369. doi:10.1080/19359705.2015.1041629

Barefoot, K. N., Smalley, K. B., & Warren, J. C. (2016). A quantitative comparison of the health-care disclosure experiences of rural and nonrural lesbians. *Stigma and Health, 2*(3), 195–207. doi:10.1037/sah0000052

Barefoot, K. N., Warren, J. C., & Smalley, K. B. (2015). An examination of past and current influences of rurality on lesbians' overweight/obesity risks. *LGBT Health, 2*(2), 154–161. doi:10.1089/lgbt.2014.0112

Barefoot, K. N., Warren, J. C., & Smalley, K. B. (2017). Women's healthcare: The experiences and behaviors of rural and urban lesbians in the US. *Rural and Remote Health, 17*(1), 3875.

Barton, B. (2010). "Abomination" life as a bible-belt gay. *Journal of Homosexuality, 57*(4), 464–484. doi:10.1080/00918361003608558

Bell, D. D. & Valentine, G. G. (1995). Queer country: Rural lesbian and gay lives. *Journal of Rural Studies, 11*(2), 113–122.

Bennett, K., McElroy, J. A., Johnson, A. O., Munk, N., & Everett, K. D. (2015). A persistent disparity: Smoking in rural sexual and gender minorities. *LGBT Health, 2*(1), 62–70. doi:10.1089/lgbt.2014.0032

Bonvicini, K. A., & Perlin, M. J. (2003). The same but different: Clinician–patient communication with gay and lesbian patients. *Patient Education and Counseling, 51*(2), 115–122. doi:10.1016/s0738-3991(02)00189-1

Boulden, W. T. (2001). Gay men living in a rural environment. *Journal of Gay & Lesbian Social Services, 12*(3–4), 63–75. doi:10.1300/J041v13n01_06

Bourke, L., Sheridan, C., Russell, U., Jones, G., DeWitt, D., & Liaw, S. T. (2004). Developing a conceptual understanding of rural health practice. *Australian Journal of Rural Health, 12*(5), 181–186.

Brotman, S., Ryan, B., Jalbert, Y., & Rowe, B. (2002). The impact of coming out on health and health care access: The experiences of gay, lesbian, bisexual and two-spirit people. *Journal of Health & Social Policy, 15*(1), 1–29.

Cody, P. J., & Welch, P. L. (1997). Rural gay men in northern New England: Life experiences and coping styles. *Journal of Homosexuality, 33*(1), 51–67. doi:10.1300/J082v33n01_04

Cohn, T. J., & Leake, V. S. (2012) Affective distress among adolescents who endorse same-sex sexual attraction: Urban versus rural differences and the role of protective factors. *Journal of Gay & Lesbian Mental Health, 16*(4), 291–305. doi:10.1080/19359705.2012.690931

Daley, A. (1998). Lesbian invisibility in health care services: Heterosexual hegemony and strategies for change. *Canadian Social Work Review, 15*(1), 57–71.

Daley, A. (2010). Being recognized, accepted, and affirmed: Self-disclosure of lesbian/queer sexuality within psychiatric and mental health service settings. *Social Work in Mental Health, 8*(4), 336–355. doi:10.1080/15332980903158202

Dillon, M., & Savage, S. (2006). Values and religion in rural America: Attitudes toward abortion and same-sex relations. In *The Carsey Institute Reports on Rural America* (Issue Brief No. 1). Durham: Carsey Institute, University of New Hampshire.

Durso, L. E., & Meyer, I. H. (2013). Patterns and predictors of disclosure of sexual orientation to healthcare providers among lesbians, gay men, and bisexuals. *Sexuality Research & Social Policy, 10*(1), 35–42. doi:10.1007/s13178-012-0105-2

Eldridge, V. L., Mack, L., & Swank, E. (2006). Explaining comfort with homosexuality in rural America. *Journal of Homosexuality, 51*(2), 39–56. doi:10.1300/j082v51n02_03

Fagerström, K. (2002). The epidemiology of smoking: Health consequences and benefits of cessation. *Drugs, 62*(Suppl. 2), 1–9. doi:10.2165/00003495-200262002-00001

Farmer, G. W., Blosnich, J. R., Jabson, J. M., & Matthews, D. D. (2016). Gay acres: Sexual orientation differences in health indicators among rural and nonrural individuals. *Journal of Rural Health, 32*(3), 321–331. doi:10.1111/jrh.12161

Foster, R. K., & Marriott, H. E. (2006). Alcohol consumption in the new millennium: Weighing up the risks and benefits for our health. *Nutrition Bulletin, 31*(4), 286–331. doi:10.1111/j.1467-3010.2006.00588.x

Gottschalk, L., & Newton, J. (2009). Rural homophobia: Not really gay. *Gay and Lesbian Issues and Psychology Review, 5*(3), 153–159.

Hart, L. G., Larson, E. H., & Lishner, D. M. (2005). Rural definitions for health policy and research. *American Journal of Public Health, 95*(7), 1149–1155. doi:10.2105/AJPH.2004.042432

Harvey, V. L., & Housel, T. H. (2014). *Health Disparities and the LGBT Population.* Lanham, MD: Lexington Books.

Hastings, S. L., & Hoover-Thompson, A. (2011). Effective support for lesbians in rural communities: The role of psychotherapy. *Journal of Lesbian Studies, 15*(2), 197–204. doi:10.1080/10894160.2011.521104

Herek, G. M. (2002). Heterosexuals' attitudes toward bisexual men and women in the United States. *Journal of Sex Research, 39*(4), 264–274. doi:10.1080/00224490209552150

Hopwood, M., & Connors, J. (2002). Heterosexual attitudes to homosexuality: Homophobia at a rural Australian university. *Journal of Gay & Lesbian Social Services, 14*(2), 79–94. doi:10.1300/J041v14n02_07

Horvath, K. J., Bowen, A. M., & Williams, M. L. (2006). Virtual and physical venues as contexts for HIV risk among rural men who have sex with men. *Health Psychology, 25*(2), 237–242. doi:10.1037/0278-6133.25.2.237

Horvath, K. J., Iantaffi, A., Swinburne-Romine, R., & Bockting, W. (2014). A comparison of mental health, substance use, and sexual risk behaviors between rural and nonrural transgender persons. *Journal of Homosexuality, 61*(8), 1117–1130. doi:10.1080/00918369.2014.872502

Institute of Medicine, Committee on Lesbian, Gay, Bisexual, and Transgender Health Issues and Research Gaps and Opportunities (2011). *The health of lesbian, gay, bisexual, and transgender people: Building a foundation for better understanding.* Washington, DC: National Academies Press.

Kakietek, J., Sullivan, P. S., & Heffelfinger, J. D. (2011). You've got male: Internet use, rural residence, and risky sex in men who have sex with men recruited in 12 U.S. cities. *AIDS Education and Prevention, 23*(2), 118–127. doi:10.1521/aeap.2011.23.2.118

Kennedy, M. (2010). Rural men, sexual identity and community. *Journal of Homosexuality, 57*(8), 1051–1091. doi:10.1080/00918369.2010.507421

King, S., & Dabelko-Schoeny, H. (2009). "Quite frankly, I have doubts about remaining": Aging-in-place and health care access for rural midlife and older lesbian, gay, and bisexual individuals. *Journal of LGBT Health Research, 5*(1/2), 10–21. doi:10.1080/15574090903392830

Klitzman, R. L., & Greenberg, J. D. (2002). Patterns of communication between gay and lesbian patients and their health care providers. *Journal of Homosexuality, 42*(4), 65–75.

Kosciw, J. G., Greytak, E. A., & Diaz, E. M. (2009). Who, what, where, when, and why: Demographic and ecological factors contributing to hostile school climate for lesbian, gay, bisexual, and transgender youth. *Journal of Youth and Adolescence, 38*(7), 976–988. doi:10.1007/s10964-009-9412-1

Larson, J. E., Corrigan, P. W., & Cothran, T. P. (2012). The impact of mental health stigma on clients from rural settings. In K. B. Smalley, J. C. Warren, & J. P. Rainer (Eds.), *Rural mental health: Issues, policies, and best practices* (pp. 267–280). New York, NY: Springer Publishing.

Lee, M. G., & Quam, J. K. (2013). Comparing supports for LGBT aging in rural versus urban areas. *Journal of Gerontological Social Work, 56*(2), 112–126. doi:10.1080/01634372.2012.747580

Leedy, G., & Connolly, C. (2007). Out of the cowboy state: A look at lesbian and gay lives in Wyoming. *Journal of Gay & Lesbian Social Services, 19*(1), 17–34. doi:10.1300/J041v19n01_02

Li, M. J., Hubach, R. D., & Dodge, B. (2015). Social milieu and mediators of loneliness among gay and bisexual men in rural Indiana. *Journal of Gay & Lesbian Mental Health, 19*(4), 331–345. doi:10.1080/19359705.2015.1033798

Lyons, A., Hosking, W., & Rozbroj, T. (2015). Rural-urban differences in mental health, resilience, stigma, and social support among young Australian gay men. *Journal of Rural Health, 31*(1), 89–97. doi:10.1111/jrh.12089

McCarthy, L. (2000). Poppies in a wheat field: Exploring the lives of rural lesbians. *Journal of Homosexuality, 39*(1), 75–94. doi:10.1300/J082v39n01

Meit, M., Knudson, A., Gilbert, T., Yu, A. T. C., Tanenbaum, E., Ormson, E., ... Popat, M. S. (2014). The 2014 update of the rural-urban chartbook. Rural Health Reform Policy Research Center. Retrieved from https://ruralhealth.und.edu/projects/health-reform-policy-research-center/pdf/2014-rural-urban-chartbook-update.pdf

Neely, C. (2005). Gay men and lesbians in rural areas: Acknowledging, valuing, and empowering this stigmatized invisible people. In N. Lohmann & R. A. Lohmann (Eds.), *Rural social work practice* (pp. 232–254). New York: Columbia University Press.

Oswald, R., & Culton, L. S. (2003). Under the rainbow: Rural gay life and its relevance for family providers. *Family Relations, 52*(1), 72–81. doi:10.1111/j.1741-3729.2003.00072.x

Palmer, N. A., Kosciw, J. G., & Bartkiewicz, M. J. (2012). *Strengths and silences: The experiences of lesbian, gay, bisexual and transgender students in rural and small town schools.* New York, NY: Gay, Lesbian, & Straight Education Network. Retrieved from https://www.glsen.org/sites/default/files/Strengths%20%26%20Silences.pdf

Petroll, A. E., & Mosack, K. E. (2011). Physician awareness of sexual orientation and preventive health recommendations to men who have sex with men. *Sexually Transmitted Diseases, 38*(1), 63–67. doi:10.1097/OLQ.0b013e3181ebd50f

Poon, C. S., & Saewyc, E. M. (2009). Out yonder: Sexual-minority adolescents in rural communities in British Columbia. *American Journal of Public Health, 99*(1), 118–124. doi:10.2105/AJPH.2007.122945

Preston, D. B., & D'Augelli, A. R. (2013). *The challenges of being a rural gay man: Coping with stigma.* New York, NY: Routledge.

Preston, D. B., D'Augelli, A. R., Kassab, C. D., & Starks, M. T. (2007). The relationship of stigma to the sexual risk behavior of rural men who have sex with men. *AIDS Education and Prevention, 19*(3), 218–230. doi:10.1521/aeap.2007.19

Rosenberger, J. G., Schick, V., Schnarrs, P., Novak, D. S., & Reece, M. (2014). Sexual behaviors, sexual health practices, and community engagement among gay and bisexually identified men living in rural areas of the United States. *Journal of Homosexuality, 61*(8), 1192–1207. doi:10.1080/00918369.2014.872525

Rosenkrantz, D. E., Black, W. W., Abreu, R. L., Aleshire, M. E., & Fallin-Bennett, K. (2017). Health and health care of rural sexual and gender minorities: A systematic review. *Stigma and Health, 2*(3), 229–243. doi:10.1037/sah0000055

Smalley, K. B., & Warren, J. C. (2012). Rurality as a diversity issue. In K. B. Smalley, J. C. Warren, & J. P. Rainer (Eds.), *Rural mental health: Issues, policies, and best practices* (pp. 37–48). New York, NY: Springer Publishing.

Smalley, K. B., Yancey, C. T., Warren, J. C., Naufel, K., Ryan, R., & Pugh, J. L. (2010). Rural mental health and psychological treatment: A review for practitioners. *Journal of Clinical Psychology, 66*(5), 479–489. doi:10.1002/jclp.20688

Snively, C. A., Kreuger, L., Stretch, J. J., Watt, J., & Chadha, J. (2004). Understanding homophobia: Preparing for practice realities in urban and rural settings. *Journal of Gay & Lesbian Social Services, 17*(1), 59–81. doi:10.1300/J041v17n01_05

St. Pierre, M. (2012). Under what conditions do lesbians disclose their sexual orientation to primary healthcare providers? A review of the literature. *Journal of Lesbian Studies, 16*(2), 199–219. doi:10.1080/10894160.2011.604837

Swank, E., Fahs, B., & Frost, D. (2013). Region, social identities, and disclosure practices as predictors of heterosexist discrimination against sexual minorities in the United States. *Sociological Inquiry, 83*(2), 238–258.

Swank, E., Frost, D. M., & Fahs, B. (2012). Rural location and exposure to minority stress among sexual minorities in the United States. *Psychology & Sexuality, 3*(3), 226–243. doi:10.1080/19419899.2012.700026

Tiemann, K. A., Kennedy, S. A., & Haga, M. P. (1998). Rural lesbians' strategies for coming out to health care professionals. *Journal of Lesbian Studies, 2*(1), 61–75. doi:10.1300/J155v02n01_05

U.S. Census Bureau (2010). American FactFinder. Retrieved from http://factfinder.census .gov/servlet/DCGeoSelectServlet?ds_name=DEC_2000_SF1_U

Waldo, C. R., Hesson-McInnis, M. S., & D'Augelli, A. R. (1998). Antecedents and consequences of victimization of lesbian, gay, and bisexual young people: A structural model comparing rural university and urban samples. *American Journal of Community Psychology, 26*(2), 307–334. doi:10.1023/A:1022184704174

Warner, T. D., Monaghan-Geernaert, P., Battaglia, J., Brems, C., Johnson, M. E., & Roberts, L. W. (2005). Ethical considerations in rural health care: A pilot study of clinicians in Alaska and New Mexico. *Community Mental Health Journal, 41*(1), 21–33. doi:10.1007/s10597-006-2597-1

Warren, J. C., & Smalley, K. B. (2014). *Rural public health: Best practices and prevention models.* New York, NY: Springer Publishing.

Warren, J. C., Smalley, K. B., & Barefoot, K. N. (2016). Rural/urban differences in health risk behaviors among gender and sexual minorities. *Health Behavior and Policy Review, 3*(1), 43–53. doi:10.14485/HBPR.3.1.5

Warren, J., Smalley, K. B., Rimando, M., Barefoot, K. N., Hatton, A., & LeLeux-LaBarge, K. (2014). Rural minority health: Race, ethnicity, and sexual orientation. In J. Warren & K. B. Smalley (Eds.), *Rural public health: Best practice and preventive models* (pp. 203–226). New York, NY: Springer Publishing.

Whitehead, J., Shaver, J., & Stephenson, R. (2016). Outness, stigma, and primary health care utilization among rural LGBT populations. *PlOS ONE, 11*(1), e0146139. doi:10.1371/journal.pone.0146139

Willging, C. E., Salvador, M., & Kano, M. (2006a). Pragmatic help seeking: How sexual and gender minority groups access mental health care in a rural state. *Psychiatric Services, 57*(6), 871–874. doi:10.1176/appi.ps.57.6.871

Willging, C. E., Salvador, M., & Kano, M. (2006b). Unequal treatment: Mental health care for sexual and gender minority groups in a rural state. *Psychiatric Services, 57*(6), 867–870. doi:10.1176/appi.ps.57.6.867

Williams, M. L., Bowen, A. M., & Horvath, K. J. (2005). The social/sexual environment of gay men residing in a rural frontier state: Implications for the development of HIV prevention programs. *Journal of Rural Health, 21*(1), 48–55. doi:10.1111/j.1748-0361.2005.tb00061.x

Ziller, E. (2014). Access to medical care in rural American. In J. C. Warren & K. B. Smalley (Eds.), *Rural public health: Best practices and preventive models* (pp. 11–28). New York, NY: Springer Publishing.

CHAPTER **19**

Gender and Sexual Minority Military Personnel and Veterans

Nicholas Grant and Jeri Muse

Gender and sexual minority (GSM) individuals have been part of the U.S. military personnel and veteran populations throughout history; however, research related to the health and well-being of these service members has been lacking until recent years. There are many factors that have contributed to the difficulty in studying these groups, including but not limited to issues related to serving in silence, policies such as Don't Ask, Don't Tell (DADT), and lack of access to culturally competent health care focused on addressing GSM-specific health disparities. Recent sociopolitical movements and advances in health care culture have shed some light on the health needs of GSM military personnel and veterans; however, there is still much more to do both to document and to meet their health needs.

It is estimated that the Veterans Health Administration (VHA) is the largest health care provider to GSM individuals across the globe, providing care to about 250,000 out of an estimated 1 million GSM veterans in the United States (Kauth & Shipherd, 2016). The majority of existing research has focused on gay and bisexual men with HIV, leaving little known about non-HIV-infected males (Mattocks, Kauth, et al., 2013). Sexual minority women service members and veterans have been studied even less, but research has shown they experience increased odds of poor physical health when compared to sexual minority women without a military history (Blosnich, Foynes, & Shipherd, 2013). Although there have been recent advances in the study of transgender health, the unique health care needs of trans-gender veterans are even more understudied, and thus even less understood by health care providers (Lutwak et al., 2014).

As discussed throughout this book, precise prevalence rates are difficult to establish in research with GSM populations due to a variety of factors, including the need for and variations of disclosure of a GSM identity. This is exacerbated in the military and veteran populations in part due to the history of persecution of GSM service members, including differences in discharge status, loss of benefits, and other forms of discrimination (Miller & Cray, 2013). These forms of gender/sexual identity stigma, whether overt, felt, or internalized (Herek, Gillis, & Cogan, 2009), all play an important role in health disparities experienced by GSM military personnel and veterans.

■ A HISTORY OF SERVING IN SILENCE

In order to gain a thorough understanding of the impact that military service can have on the health of GSM individuals, it is important to review motivations for service and the history related to serving while being required to conceal certain components of one's identity ("serving in silence"). Military policies related to GSM individuals serving in the Armed Forces have changed over time, with the first written policies banning their service being developed during World War II. Adherence to such policies was inconsistent through 1982, when the Department of Defense (DoD) put forth a directive banning sexual minority men and women from serving in the military (Evans, 2001). It is important to note that the impact of such policies on GSM service members varies widely and that factors, including the era and branch of service in which one serves, contributes to service members' experiences (Evans, 2001).

Similar to the continuing changes of these policies over time, the impact they have had, including motivations to serve, have continued to develop. There is a wide range of motivating factors for any individual to enlist with the Armed Services, including tradition, desire to improve quality of life, and wanting to serve one's country (Kane, 2006); however, for GSM individuals, there are additional factors that may motivate this decision. For example, some individuals may be motivated by a desire to escape a rejecting or discriminatory environment, such as is seen in situations of family or community rejection (Anderson & Smith, 1993). Others may be motivated by a desire to engage with a system, such as the military, that is often considered traditionally hypermasculine as a means of avoiding thoughts and feelings related to same-sex attractions or experiences of gender dysphoria (Anderson & Smith, 1993; Brown, 1988; Brown & Jones, 2016). As such, GSM individuals often have diverse motivating factors that are not experienced by their heterosexual counterparts when joining the Armed Forces (Anderson & Smith, 1993).

GSM military personnel often share similar experiences with GSM civilians but are additionally subject to institutional factors that impact military person-nel long after they leave the military. Serving in the military and being forced to conceal one's identity, information about meaningful life events, and daily information about whom they love can take a tremendous toll over time. Living in fear of others knowing about one's GSM identity and the potential costs of being harassed, discharged from the military, and potentially losing benefits as a veteran can result in ongoing anxiety and fear. This concealment and mistrust carries over into health care visits where concealment can then become a risk factor for increased rates of disease and other health conditions secondary to inadequate care. When providers are educated on appropriate communication with service members and veterans around sexual orientation and gender identity, which includes providing explanations of how these factors relate to a patient's health, they have the opportunity to improve the patient's health care experience (Sherman, Kauth, Shipherd, & Street, 2014b).

The impact of serving in silence, including concealment of one's GSM identity, has generally shown negative outcomes on health and well-being. Research has shown that GSM veterans' perceptions of the relationship between military cohesion and concealment of one's sexual orientation is related to increased isolation and work-related stress (Moradi, 2009), two factors known to negatively impact overall health (Sears & Mallory, 2011). When considering the significance of military cohesion, individuals who are concealing their GSM identity can experience increased rates of stress, decreases in social support, and increased risk of both physical and mental health disparities (Moradi, 2009). Victimization and lack of social support have also been shown to be important risk factors related to suicide risk among GSM military personnel and veterans (Matarazzo et al., 2014).

■ THE IMPACT OF DADT

DADT is the common name for the policy signed into law by President Bill Clinton in 1993 that, in theory, lifted the ban on sexual minority individuals serving in the military. President Clinton had initially hoped to completely eradicate the ban; however, after being met with much opposition, he compromised and agreed to the DADT policy which prevented the military from asking about sexual orientation and sexual behavior (Connell, 2015). Once signed into law, the policy allowed for sexual minorities to serve in the military so long as they did not disclose any information related to their sexual orientation or same-sex relationships while serving. Additionally, it specified that investigations on a service member's sexual orientation, in some cases referred to as "witch hunts," could not be initiated without having directly witnessed related behaviors (Connell, 2015).

Perhaps one of the most researched GSM-related topics for service members and veterans has been the repeal of DADT in 2011. Although this change in policy specifically allowed sexual minority members to serve openly in the military, the impact on gender minority members has been studied as well. Overall, research findings have varied, with some focusing on improved health outcomes due to not having to serve in silence and others focusing on risks that may arise for GSM service members and veterans after the repeal, including, but not limited to, increased rates of victimization and decreases in victim reporting and help seeking (Burks, 2011). Since its repeal, the DoD and VHA have continued to make steps toward providing GSM service members and veterans with competent and affirming care (L. Johnson, Shipherd & Walton, 2016; Kauth & Shipherd, 2016; Sharpe & Uchendu, 2014).

Some of the concerns that arose during the repeal of DADT involved the possibility that health care providers, including both mental health and medical providers, may not be prepared to deliver culturally competent care to GSM service members due to a lack of training and exposure to "out" patients (L. Johnson & Federman, 2014; Sherman et al., 2014). Additional concerns arose around the safety of "out" service members due to possible increases in harassment and victimization, including sexual/gender identity stigma and prejudice (Burks, 2011). Concern around how leadership within the military would manage issues around disclosure, adjust towards a less heterosexist culture, and view the repeal also arose (W. B. Johnson, Rosenstein, Buhrke, & Haldeman, 2015). These issues continue to be investigated, and only after more time has passed will the true effects be fully assessable.

HEALTH DISPARITIES AMONG GSM MILITARY PERSONNEL AND VETERANS

While the military has historically collected considerable data on the health of its personnel, there is very little research about the health care needs of GSM service members and veterans. There are unique challenges that a gender and/or sexual minority service member experiences that compound the civilian experiences of discrimination, marginalization, and bias (Sherman, Kauth, Shipherd, & Street, 2014a). Studies on GSM civilians demonstrate a number of health disparities discussed throughout this text, including but not limited to increased rates of cancer, tobacco, substance use and abuse, depression, anxiety, and posttraumatic stress disorder (PTSD; Goldbach & Castro, 2016). The increased rates of these various health disparities for GSM civilians over cisgender heterosexual civilians have been largely attributed to increased vulnerability related to minority stress. Minority stress can be thought of as chronic stress that affects groups of people who experience discrimination, bullying, assault, and marginalization, related to having a minority identity (Meyer, 1995, 2013). The longer the stress continues with ongoing experiences of discrimination and marginalization, the less the individual is able to adapt or tolerate additional stress without a significant impact on various health parameters (Meyer, 2013). This effect may be magnified in GSM military personnel and veterans, particularly those who served either prior to DADT, or after the passage of DADT but prior to its repeal.

Sexual Minority Military Personnel and Veterans

As discussed throughout this book, sexual minority civilians experience a number of health disparities secondary to issues related to access to care, lack of culturally competent providers, and policies that reinforce social stigma, marginalization, and discrimination. Service members and veterans are equally if not at greater risk for similar health disparities, as discussed in the following section.

Depression and Suicide

The rate of depression in GSM civilians is 1.5 times higher than their cisgender heterosexual counterparts and GSM veterans are no different (King et al., 2008). Studies suggest that depression rates are higher in GSM veterans, often linked to concealment of their sexual orientation and/or gender identity while in the service (Cochran, Balsam, Flentje, Malte, & Simpson, 2013). Suicide rates are higher in the veteran population, but there does not appear to be much difference in *recent* suicidal ideation and lifetime suicide attempts between sexual minority and cisgender heterosexual veterans; however, studies have documented a three times higher *lifetime* risk of suicidal ideation among sexual minority veterans when compared to their cisgender heterosexual peers (Blosnich, Mays, & Cochran, 2014). Risk of depression and suicide is therefore an urgent health factor for sexual minority service members and veterans.

Posttraumatic Stress Disorder

PTSD has long been the hallmark mental health injury of military service. Studies suggest that sexual minority veterans have higher rates of PTSD as a group than cisgender heterosexual veterans, and are actually five times more likely to screen positive for PTSD (Cochran et al., 2013). Studies comparing sexual minority female veterans to their cisgender heterosexual counterparts have shown that they experience higher rates of trauma across the lifespan from a variety of causes (e.g., childhood, sexual assault during and after military service, and combat exposure; Mattocks, Sadler, et al., 2013). In a study of 365 cisgender female veterans, 60% of sexual minority women received uninvited sexual attention during military service which included touching, pressure, and remarks, as compared to 49% for heterosexual women. Furthermore, 31% of sexual minority women experienced threat of or actual forced sexual contact during military service, compared to 13% of heterosexual women (Mattocks, Sadler, et al., 2013). In addition to this increased victimization of sexual minority military personnel through military sexual trauma, there is reduced reporting and help seeking because of the potential consequence of being "outed" (Burks, 2011). While the repeal of DADT may affect this dynamic, GSM military personnel may remain less likely to report incidents of sexual assault given the overall lower rates of reporting seen in nonmilitary GSM individuals (Ciarlante & Fountain, 2010). Future research will be necessary to assess if the repeal of DADT does in fact impact reporting.

Tobacco/Substance Use

Cigarette smoking is higher among people currently serving in the military than among the civilian population, and is even higher among people who have been deployed (Poston et al., 2008). While higher rates of cigarette smoking are also found among the general population of sexual minorities, emerging research suggests that the intersectionality of being both a veteran and a sexual minority exacerbates the risks of cigarette use. Namely, sexual minority veterans have been found to have higher rates of smoking when compared to both their nonveteran sexual minority peers and their heterosexual veteran counterparts (Blosnich, Boynes, & Shipherd, 2013; Blosnich & Silenzio, 2013). In addition to smoking, sexual minority veterans have been found to be over twice as likely to report problematic alcohol use and/or to meet full criteria for an alcohol use disorder when compared to their cisgender veteran counterparts (Cochran et al., 2013). Because of the many health consequences of cigarette smoking and excessive alcohol use, future research is needed to better understand and address the alarmingly high rates of smoking and hazardous drinking among GSM service members and veterans, and determine if this is due to intersectional risk (e.g., elevated above the general risk associated with being a GSM individual).

Other Health Disparities

In addition to the previously mentioned mental and behavioral health dispari-ties, sexual minority veterans also face additional disparities related to quality of life and physical health. Overall, what research is available suggests that sexual minority military personnel and veterans face a variety of mental and physical health disparities that are important for providers to be aware of as they work with this population. For example, when compared to their nonveteran sexual minor-ity and/or heterosexual veteran counterparts, sexual minority veterans have been found to have higher rates of overall mental distress, lower life satisfaction, less social support, greater activity limitations due to physical, mental, and/or emo-tional problems, poor physical health, and higher rates of a lifetime diagnosis of asthma (Blosnich, Foynes, & Shipherd, 2013; Blosnich & Silenzio, 2013). Sexual minority veterans are also more likely than their heterosexual veteran peers to forego needed medical care due to cost (Blosnich & Silenzio, 2013).

Gender Minority Military Personnel and Veterans

Recent evidence suggests there are approximately 15,500 transgender individuals serving on active duty or in the Guard/Reserves. Furthermore, it is estimated that approximately 134,000 transgender individuals are veterans or retired from the Guard or Reserves, resulting in an estimated five times the proportion of transgen-der veterans as transgender civilians (Gates & Herman, 2014). Of those transgender persons who have served in the military, it has been estimated that approximately 60% are transgender women and 40% are transgender men (Gates & Herman, 2014). There have been different theoretical conceptualizations to explain the sub-stantially increased representation of transgender individuals in the military. The theory most supported by actual reports, particularly among transgender female service members and veterans, is a desire to immerse oneself in hypermasculine behaviors and cultures in hopes that the deep feelings of gender dysphoria will disappear (Brown, 1988; Brown & Jones, 2016; McDuffie & Brown, 2010).

While the repeal of DADT afforded some protections for sexual minority active duty personnel, it did not extend any protections to gender minority service mem-bers. While military policy was briefly changed in 2016 to allow transgender ser-vice members to openly serve in the military (DoD, 2016), as of the publication of this book these protections were in the process of being rolled back. Implementing policies to protect transgender service members certainly reduces institutional dis-crimination, but it takes much longer to change the culture. Being transgender can almost be seen as being a minority within a minority group. The unique medical needs of transgender persons continues to serve as a means to deny enlistment of transgender persons. Historically, the military argued they could not ensure hormone treatment would be available at some locations and early court rulings argued that gender confirmation surgery was similar to an amputation (leaving the service member "unfit for duty"; DoD, 2011). When President Trump announced his rollback of the policy allowing transgender service members to openly serve in the military in 2017, the cost of providing their medical care was a specific reason cited, and gender-affirming medical care for existing transgender service members was placed in jeopardy. Identifying discriminatory policies offers the opportunity to not only advance equality, but also further understand the health disparities experienced by gender minority service members and veterans (Blosnich et al., 2016).

There is less research on the experiences of gender minority service members and veterans and the health disparities associated with military service; however, the area of research is rapidly growing, with many recent studies beginning to highlight their unique needs and health disparities. For example, descriptive results of a large Internet-based study reveal that many gender minority active duty service members may experience elevated rates of depression (30.9%) and anxiety (18.2%), in addition to knee (23.6%) and back (16.4%) problems (Hill, Bouris, Barnett, & Walker, 2016). In addition, almost half of gender minority service members are currently receiving hormone therapy, representing a unique health consideration for providers caring for this population (Hill et al., 2016). Furthermore, a recent large-scale, case–control study of the mental and medical health outcomes experienced by gender minority veterans receiving services through the VHA revealed a multitude of health disparities (Brown & Jones, 2016). Namely, after adjusting for other demographic factors, when compared to their cisgender peers, gender minority veterans had significantly higher rates of all 10 mental health conditions examined, as well as 16 out of the 17 medical conditions examined (using The International Classification of Diseases, Ninth Revision, Clinical Modification [ICD-9-CM] codes). These disparities included: alcohol abuse, depressive disorders, eating disorders, panic disorder, PTSD, serious mental illness, suicidal ideation/attempt, traumatic brain injury, tobacco use, acute myocardial infarction, benign prostatic hyperplasia, cardiac arrest, cerebral vascular disease, chronic obstructive pulmonary disease, congestive heart failure, diabetes, HIV, hypercholesterolemia, hypertension, ischemic heart disease, obesity, prostate cancer, and renal disease. Gender minority veterans were also more likely to have a service-related disability, to be a combat veteran, to be a victim of military sexual trauma, to have a history of incarceration, and to have previously been homeless (Brown & Jones, 2016).

Emerging research also suggests that suicide is a major health concern among gender minority veterans, with approximately 61% of gender minority veterans reporting a history of suicidal ideation and 11% reporting at least one suicide attempt (McDuffie & Brown, 2010). When compared to the general population of veterans, gender minority veterans have a 20 times higher rate of suicide-related behaviors (i.e., suicidal gestures, plans, and/or attempts; Blosnich, Brown, et al., 2013). Furthermore, an examination of national mortality data from 2000 to 2009 revealed that not only is the crude suicide rate among gender minority veterans higher than the general population, gender minority veterans die by suicide at younger ages than their cisgender veteran peers (Blosnich, Brown, Wojcio, Jones, & Bossarte, 2014). This is consistent with other research highlighting the relatively poorer psychological health and higher rates of mental health service utilization of gender minority veterans (Shipherd, Mizock, Maguen, Green, 2012). Gender minority veterans also utilize VHA services at rates higher than the general population of veterans, with cholesterol, blood pressure, and vision problems being the most commonly reported medical complications treated by the VHA in the past year among gender minority veterans (Shipherd, Mizock, Maguen, Green, 2012). Overall, it appears that gender minorities represent a unique and vulnerable population of military personnel and veterans, and additional research is greatly needed to better understand and address the multitude of health disparities that they appear to face.

▪ DEPARTMENT OF DEFENSE AND VETERANS HEALTH ADMINISTRATION AFTER DADT

The repeal of DADT in 2011 opened the door for both the DoD and the VHA to work toward an inclusive system for service to this country and to meet the health care needs of GSM military personnel and veterans. As DADT did not provide protection for gender minority service members, the military developed a plan to integrate only sexual minority service members after the end of DADT. In October of 2016, the DoD began providing for in-service gender transition and provision of necessary associated medical care and treatment (DoD, 2016). This briefly opened the door for gender minority service members to serve openly while receiving the medical treatment they need to live their true identities and ensuring military readiness and optimization of their potential. Unfortunately, this change is unlikely to remain in place following the announcement in 2017 of the reinstatement of the ban on transgender servicemembers openly serving in the military.

Although GSM veterans may encounter cultural challenges and limited resources within the VHA system, there are frequent opportunities for staff, providers, and leadership to foster the development of a supportive and inclusive environment for these veterans (L. Johnson & Federman, 2013; Sherman et al., 2014). On December 26, 2012, the Principal Deputy Under Secretary for Health and the Deputy Under Secretary for Health Operations and Management delivered a memorandum to all Veterans Administration regional and facility directors asking for three specific initiatives from each site to promote a welcoming and inclusive environment for GSM veterans within their facility. Facilities outlined a number of initiatives that would improve the care of GSM veterans (Sharpe & Uchendu, 2014). Of the initiatives submitted, 29% were to provide GSM-specific trainings to staff and providers, 27% related to policy changes that included inclusive language and protections for GSM veterans and employees, 16% were initiatives to increase awareness of the number of GSM veterans and their health care needs, 7% included strategies to reach out to the local lesbian, gay, bisexual, and transgender (LGBT) community in order to reach GSM veterans who had been receiving care in the community, and 7% were initiatives to create LGBT-specific support groups in their medical centers.

This benchmark movement toward inclusion coincided with the establishment of the Office of Diversity and Inclusion's LGBT Program, which provides federal, employee, and veteran policies and resources to all medical centers (Department of Veterans Affairs, 2012). Each Medical Center was then free to establish services at its facility to meet the needs of GSM veterans and was supported by the Office of Diversity and Inclusion's LGBT Program with education and resources. It also included the development of "LGBT Mental Health Post-Doctoral Fellowships" for doctoral-level psychologists to help meet the growing needs of GSM veterans (Department of Veterans Affairs, 2012). As part of these new initiatives, in 2013 all VA Medical Centers were encouraged to participate in the Human Rights Campaign's LGBT Health Equality Index Survey and as of 2016, 96 out of approximately 114 facilities have achieved LGBT Health Equality Leader status (Human Rights Campaign, 2016). It is unclear, however, how changes in recent political climate will affect these provisions.

In February of 2013 the Department of Veterans Affairs established a directive outlining the care for gender minority veterans (Department of Veterans Affairs, 2013). This directive spelled out specifically what care gender minority veterans could expect to receive as well as providing a directive to all VA staff members. Following the dissemination of this directive, an influx of veterans seeking gender-related health care was observed through the VHA (Kauth et al., 2014). The health care provided for gender minority veterans includes hormone therapy, mental health, preoperative evaluations, and medically necessary postoperative and long-term care following gender confirmation surgery (Department of Veterans Affairs, 2013). Gender confirmation surgery would not, however, be performed or funded by the VHA. This left gender minority veterans seeking care in the community, at their own expense. In an effort to provide specialty care for gender minority veterans in rural areas, the VA utilized its Specialty Care Access Network-Extension for Community Healthcare Outcomes (SCAN ECHO) to train interdisciplinary teams across the country to provide appropriate care to gender minority veterans (Kauth et al., 2015). The program started with four specialty teams located in Loma Linda, California; Boston, Masachussetts; Tucson, Arizona; and Minneapolis, Minnesota. Those sites also serve as expert teams where VA providers can send an e-consult requesting education and treatment recommendations while providing care to gender minority veterans. As with other advancements previously described, it is unclear if these advancements in care will continue to be supported.

In 2016, the VHA mandated that each VA Medical Center identify an "LGBT Clinical Care Coordinator," which appears to have contributed to the development of formalized care programs for GSM veterans (Department of Veterans Affairs, 2016). There are still no specific guidelines for how programs should be established and what care should be provided beyond the specific "LGB and Transgender Care Directives." While each VA Medical Center is different in the services they offer, many offer GSM-specific support groups, GSM mental health services, transgender care, engagement in outreach to their local LGBT community, and provider training. One VA Medical Center developed a model to train providers and test for competency in an effort to identify "LGBT Experts" who demonstrated cultural competency and who could act as a resource to other providers and advocate for the needs of GSM veterans (VA San Diego Health Care System, 2014). Research is lacking as to whether providing a more inclusive health care environment leads to reduction in health disparities among GSM veterans, although in general it is expected that this may lead to increased rates of comfort with and "coming out" to providers as well as reduce delayed access to competent care.

While progress is certainly being made with regard to creating a welcoming and affirming environment in which GSM veterans can receive care, recent research has shown that there is still a strong need for improvement. For example, surveys of VHA mental and medical health providers reveal that many lack formal training on GSM issues and have limited experience providing services to GSM patients (L. Johnson & Federman, 2014; Sherman, Kauth, Shipherd, & Street, 2014b). Furthermore, almost half of a sample of VHA providers indicated a belief that sexual orientation is irrelevant to health care, with providers rarely assessing the sexual orientation of their patients (Sherman, Kauth, Shipherd, & Street, 2014b). Surveys of GSM VHA patients reveal these and other barriers to affirming health care. More specifically, among a sample of GSM veterans receiving care through the VA, the majority indicated that they had not been asked about their gender identity and/or sexual orientation by any of their VA providers (Sherman, Kauth, Shipherd, & Street, 2014a). Furthermore, across studies, many GSM veterans report fears of mistreatment, loss of benefits or disability, and/or denial of VHA services if their providers knew about their sexual orientation and/or gender identity, with many participants perceiving the VA as unwelcoming of GSM veterans (Mattocks et al., 2015; Sherman, Kauth, Shipherd, & Street, 2014a).

Gender minority veterans may face additional barriers to appropriate and affirming health care through the VA. For example, qualitative research suggests that gender minority veterans may experience long delays, greater travel distances, and a significant lack of provider knowledge regarding the provision of transition-related care when attempting to receive these services through the VA health care system (Rosentel, Hill, Lu, & Barnett, 2016). Furthermore, many gender minority veterans report experiencing microaggressions (i.e., being misgendered), harassment, and/or violence due to their gender identity in VA settings (Rosentel et al., 2016).

■ CONCLUSION

In conclusion, GSM military personnel face not only the health disparities that have been demonstrated within the general GSM population, but also increased risk factors associated with their intersecting identities as current or past members of the Armed Forces. At this point, the research focusing on these groups is limited, leaving opportunity for future researchers to further expand on what is known on the health of GSM service members and veterans. It is important to consider the unique experiences these individuals encounter while serving their country and how these experiences shape their overall health over their lifetimes. Notably, gaining further understanding of military systems and the policies that impact service members and veterans can provide a foundation in moving forward with health-specific research for these GSM populations.

ADDITIONAL RESOURCES/REFERENCES

Brown, G. R., & Jones, K. T. (2015). Health correlates of criminal justice involvement in 4,793 transgender veterans. *LGBT Health, 2*(4), 297–305. doi:10.1089/lgbt.2015.0052

Burgess, D., Tran, A., Lee, R., & van Ryn, M. (2007). Effects of perceived discrimination on mental health and mental health services utilization among gay, lesbian, bisexual and transgender persons. *Journal of LGBT Health Research, 3*(4), 1–14. doi:10.1080/15574090802226626

Cianni, V. (2012). Gays in the military: How America thanked me. *Journal of Gay & Lesbian Mental Health, 16,* 322–333. doi:10.1080/19359705.2012.702028

Frank, N. (2013). The president's pleasant surprise: How LGBT advocates ended don't ask, don't tell. *Journal of Homosexuality, 60*(2–3), 159–213. doi:10.1080/00918369.2013.744666

Gates, G. (2005). *Gay Men and Lesbians in the U.S. Military: Estimates from Census 2000.* Los Angeles, CA: Williams Institute, UCLA School of Law. Retrieved from http://williamsinstitute.law.ucla.edu/wp-content/uploads/Gates-GL-Military-Census2000Estimates-Oct-2005.pdf

Monin, J. K., Mota, N., Levy, B., Pachankis, J., & Pietrzak, R. H. (2016). Older age associated with mental health resiliency in sexual minority US veterans. *American Journal of Geriatric Psychiatry.* Advanced online publication. doi:10.1016/j.jagp.2016.09.006.

Price, E., & Limberg, D. (2013). Addressing the mental health needs of gay military veterans: A group counseling approach. *Journal of Military and Government Counseling, 1*(1), 26–39.

Ramirez, M. H., Rogers, S. J., Johnson, H. L., Banks, J., Seay, W. P., Tinsley, B. L., & Grant, A.W. (2013). If we ask, they might tell: Clinical assessment lessons from LGBT military personnel post-DADT. *Journal of Homosexuality, 60*(2–3), 401–418. doi:10.1080/00918369.2013.744931

Roberts, A. L., Austin, S. B., Corliss, H. L., Vandermorris, A. K., & Koenen, K. C., (2010). Pervasive trauma exposure among U.S. sexual orientation minority adults and risk of posttraumatic stress exposure. *American Journal of Public Health, 100*(12), 2433–2424. doi:10.2105/AJPH.2009.168971

Smith, L. N. (2013). Comparison of U.S. gay and heterosexual Veteran Health Services. Master's Thesis, University of Pittsburgh. Retrieved from http://d-scholarship.pitt.edu/id/eprint/18223

Sundevall, F., & Persson, A. (2016). LGBT in the military: Policy development in Sweden 1944–2014. *Sexuality Research and Social Policy, 13*(2), 119–129. doi:10.1007/s13178-015-0217-6

REFERENCES

Anderson, C. W., & Smith, H. R. (1993). Stigma and honor: Gay, lesbian, and bisexual people in the US military. In L. Diamant (Ed.), *Homosexual issues in the workplace* (pp.65–89). Washington, DC: Taylor & Francis.

Blosnich, J. R., Brown, G. R., Shipherd, J. C., Kauth, M., Piegari, R. I., & Bossarte, R. M. (2013). Prevalence of gender identity disorder and suicide risk among transgender veterans utilizing Veterans Health Administration care. *American Journal of Public Health, 103*(10) 27–32. doi:10.2105/AJPH.2013.301507

Blosnich, J. R., Brown, G. R., Wojcio, S., Jones, K. T., & Bossarte, R. M. (2014). Mortality among veterans with transgender-related diagnoses in the Veterans Health Administration, FY2000–2009. *LGBT Health, 1*(4), 269–276. doi:10.1089/lgbt.2014.0050

Blosnich, J. R., Foynes, M. M., & Shipherd, J. C. (2013). Health disparities among sexual minority women veterans. *Journal of Women's Health, 22*(7), 631–636. doi:10.1089/jwh.2012.4214

Blosnich, J. R., Marsiglio, M. C., Gao, S., Gordon, A. J., Shipherd, J. C., Kauth, M.,... Fine, M. J. (2016). Mental health of transgender veterans in US states with and without discrimination and hate crime legal protection. *American Journal of Public Health, 106*(3), 534–540. doi:10.2105/AJPH.2015.302981

Blosnich, J. R., Mays, V. M., & Cochran, S. D. (2014). Suicidality among veterans: Implications of sexual minority status. *American Journal of Public Health, 104*(S4), S535–S537. doi:10.2105/AJPH.2014.302100

Blosnich, J. R., & Silenzio, V. M. (2013). Physical health indicators among lesbian, gay and bisexual U. S. veterans. *Annals of Epidemiology, 23*(7), 448–451. doi:10.1016/j.annepidem.2013.04.009

Brown, G. R. (1988). Transsexuals in the military: Flight into hypermasculinity. *Archives of Sexual Behavior, 17*(6), 527–537.

Brown, G. R., & Jones, K. T. (2016). Mental health and medical health disparities in 5,135 transgender veterans receiving healthcare in the Veterans Health Administration: A case–control study. *LGBT Health, 3*(2), 122–131. doi:10.1089/lgbt.2015.0058

Burks, D. J. (2011) Lesbian, gay and bisexual victimization in the military: An unintended consequence of "Don't Ask, Don't Tell". *American Psychologist, 66*(7), 604–613. doi:10.1037/a0024609

Ciarlante M., & Fountain, K. (2010). *Why it matters: Rethinking victim assistance for lesbian, gay, bisexual, transgender, and queer victims of hate crimes and intimate partner violence.* National Center for Victims of Crime and the National Coalition of Anti-Violence Programs. Retrieved from http://www.victimsofcrime.org/docs/Reports%20and%20Studies/WhyItMatters_LGBTQreport_press.pdf?sfvrsn=0

Cochran, B. N., Balsam, K., Flentje, A., Malte, C. A., & Simpson, T. (2013). Mental health characteristics of sexual minority veterans. *Journal of Homosexuality, 60*, 419–435. doi:10.1080/00918369.2013.744932

Connell, C. (2015). Right to serve or responsibility to protect? Civil rights framing and the DADT repeal. *Boston University Law Review, 95*, 1015–1028. Retrieved from http://www.bu.edu/bulawreview/files/2015/05/CONNELL.pdf

Department of Defense. (2011). Accession processing data collection forms 1304.2. Retrieved from http://www.dtic.mil/whs/directives/corres/pdf/130402p.pdf

Department of Defense. (2016). Military service of transgender service members (DTM 16-005). Retrieved from https://www.defense.gov/Portals/1/features/2016/0616_policy/DTM-16-005.pdf

Department of Veterans Affairs. (2012). Office of Diversity and Inclusion. Retrieved from http://www.diversity.va.gov/programs/lgbt.aspx

Department of Veterans Affairs. (2013). Providing healthcare for transgender and intersex veterans (VHA Directive 2013-003). Retrieved from http://www.va.gov/vhapublications/viewpublication.aspx

Department of Veterans Affairs. (2016). Information bulletin: National Program for Points of Contact for Lesbian, Gay, Bisexual and Transgender (LGBT) Veterans. Retrieved from http://vaww.infoshare.va.gov/site/lgbteducation/siteassess/pages/lgbt-poc/national

Evans, R. (2001). *US military policies concerning homosexuals: Development, implementation and outcomes.* Santa Barbara: The Center for the Study of Sexual Minorities in the Military, University of California at Santa Barbara. Retrieved from http://archive.palmcenter.org/files/active/1/evans1.pdf

Gates, G., & Herman, J. (2014). *Transgender military service in the United States.* Los Angeles, CA: Williams Institute, UCLA School of Law. Retrieved from http://williamsinstitute.law.ucla.edu/wp-content/uploads/Transgender-Military-Service-May-2014.pdf

Goldbach, J. T., & Castro, C. A. (2016). Lesbian, gay, bisexual, and transgender (LGBT) service members: Life after don't ask, don't tell. *Current Psychiatry Reports, 18*(6), 56. doi:10.1007/s11920-016-0695-0

Herek, G. M., Gillis, J. R., & Cogan, J. C. (2009). Internalized stigma among sexual minority adults: Insights from a social psychology perspective. *Journal of Counseling Psychology, 56*(1), 32–43. doi: 10.1037/2376-6972.1.S.18

Hill, B. J., Bouris, A., Barnett, J. T., & Walker, D. (2016). Fit to serve? Exploring mental and physical health and well-being among transgender active-duty service members and veterans in the US Military. *Transgender Health, 1*(1), 4–11. doi:10.1089/trgh.2015.0002

Human Rights Campaign. (2016). *Health Equality Index 2016.* Washington, DC: Author. Retrieved from http://www.hrc.org/hei

Johnson, L., & Federman, E. J. (2013). Pathways and barriers to care for LGBT veterans in the U.S. department of veterans affairs (VA). *Journal of LGBT Issues in Counseling, 7*(3), 218–235. doi:10.1080/15538605.2013.812928

Johnson, L., & Federman, E. J. (2014). Training, experience, and attitudes of VA psychologists regarding LGBT issues: Relation to practice and competence. *Psychology of Sexual Orientation and Gender Diversity, 1*(1), 10–18. doi:10.1037/sgd0000019

Johnson, L., Shipherd, J. Walton, & H. M. (2016). The psychologist's role in the transgender specific care with U.S. veterans. *Psychological Services, 13*(1), 69–76. doi:10.1037/ser0000030

Johnson, W. B., Rosenstein, J. E., Buhrke, R. A., Haldeman, D. C. (2015). After "don't ask don't tell": Competent care of lesbian, gay and bisexual military personnel during the DoD policy transition. *Professional Psychology: Research and Practice, 46*(2), 107–115. doi:10.1037/a0033051

Kane, T. (2006). Who are the recruits?: The demographic characteristics of US Military enlistment, 2003–2005. Retrieved from http://www.heritage.org/research/reports/2006/10/who-are-the-recruits-the-demographic-characteristics-of-us-military-enlistment-2003-2005

Kauth, M. R., & Shipherd, J. C. (2016). Transforming a system: Improving patient-centered care for sexual and gender minority veterans. *LGBT Health, 3*(3), 177–179. doi:10.1089/lgbt.2016.0047

Kauth, M. R., & Shipherd, J. C., Lindsay, J., Blosnich, J. R., Brown, G. R., & Jones, K. T. (2014). Access to care for transgender veterans in the Veterans Health Administration: 2006–2013. *American Journal of Public Health, 104*(S4), S532–S534. doi:10.2105/AJPH.2014.302086

Kauth, M. R., Shipherd, J. C., Lindsay, J.A., Kirsh, S., Knepp, H., & Matza, L. (2015). Teleconsultation and training of VA providers on transgender care: Implementation of a multisite hub system. *Telemedicine and e-Health, 21*(12), 1012–1018. doi:10.1089/tmj2015.0010

King, M., Semlyen, J., Tai, S. S., Killaspy, H., Osborn, D., Popelyuk, D., & Nazareth, I. (2008). A systematic review of mental disorder, suicide, and deliberate self harm in lesbian, gay and bisexual people. *BMC Psychiatry 8*(70). doi:10.1186/1471-244X-8-70

Lutwak, N., Byne, W., Erickson-Schroth, L., Keig, Z., Shipherd, J. C., Mattocks, K. M., & Kauth M. R. (2014). Transgender veterans are inadequately understood by health care providers. *Military Medicine, 179*(5), 483–485. doi:10.7205/MILMED-D-14-00001

Matarazzo, B. B., Barnes, S. M., Pease, J. L., Russell, L. M., Hanson, J. E., Soberay, K. A., & Gutierrez, P. M. (2014). Suicide risk among lesbian, gay, bisexual, and transgender military personnel and veterans: What does the literature tell us? *Suicide and Life-Threatening Behavior, 44*(2), 200–217. doi:10.1111/sltb.12073

Mattocks, K. M., Kauth, M. R., Sandfort, T., Matza, A., Sullivan, J. C., & Shipherd, J. C. (2013). Understanding health-care needs of sexual and gender minority veterans: How targeted research and policy can improve health. *LGBT Health, 1*(1), 30–37. doi:10.1089/lgbt.2013.0003

Mattocks, K. M., Sadler, A., Yano, E. M., Krebs, E. E., Zephyrin, L., Brandt, C.,…Haskell (2013). Sexual victimization, health status, and VA healthcare utilization among lesbian and bisexual OEF/OIF veterans. *Journal of General Internal Medicine, 28*(2), 604–608. doi:10.1007/s11606-013-2357-9

Mattocks, K. M., Sullivan, J. C., Bertrand, C., Kinney, R. L., Sherman, M. D., & Gustason, C. (2015). Perceived stigma, discrimination, and disclosure of sexual orientation among a sample of lesbian veterans receiving care in the Department of Veterans Affairs. *LGBT Health, 2*(2), 147–153. doi:10.1089/lgbt.2014.0131

McDuffie, E., & Brown, G. R. (2010). 70 US veterans with gender identity disturbances: A descriptive study. *International Journal of Transgenderism, 12*(1), 21–30. doi:10.1080/15532731003688962

Meyer, I. H. (1995). Minority stress and mental health in gay men. *Journal of Health and Social Behavior, 36,* 38–56. doi:10.2307/2137286

Meyer, I. H. (2013). Prejudice, social stress, and mental health in lesbian, gay, and bisexual populations: Conceptual issues and research evidence. *Psychology of Sexual Orientation and Gender Diversity, 1*(Suppl.), 3–26. doi:10.1037/2329-0382.1.S.3

Miller, K., & Cray, A. (2013, September). The battles that remain: Military service and LGBT equality. Retrieved from https://www.americanprogress.org/issues/lgbt/reports/2013/09/20/74883/the-battles-that-remain-military-service-and-lgbt-equality

Moradi, B. (2009). Sexual orientation disclosure, concealment, harassment, and military cohesion: Perceptions of LGBT military veterans. *Military Psychology, 21,* 513–533. doi:10.1080/08995600903206453

Poston, W. S. C., Taylor, J. E., Hoffman, K. M., Peterson, A. L., Lando, H. A., Shelton, S., & Haddock, C. K. (2008). Smoking and deployment: Perspectives of junior-enlisted U.S. Air Force and U.S. Army personnel and their supervisors. *Military Medicine, 173*(5), 441–447. doi:10.7205/MILMED.173.5.441

Rosentel, K., Hill, B. J., Lu, C., & Barnett, J. T. (2016). Transgender veterans and the Veterans Health Administration: Exploring the experiences of transgender veterans in the Veterans Affairs healthcare system. *Transgender Health, 1*(1), 108–116. doi:10.1089/trgh.2016.0006

Sears, B., & Mallory, C. (2011). *Documented evidence of employment discrimination & its effects on LGBT people.* Los Angeles, CA: Williams Institute, UCLA School of Law. Retrieved from http://williamsinstitute.law.ucla.edu/wp-content/uploads/Sears-Mallory-Discrimination-July-20111.pdf

Sharpe, V. A., & Uchendu, U. S. (2014). Ensuring appropriate care for LGBT veterans in the Veterans Health Administration. *Hastings Center Report, 44*(5), S53–S55. doi:10.1002/hast.372

Sherman, M. D., Kauth, M. R., Ridener, L., Shipherd, J. C., Bratkovich, K., & Beaulieu, G. (2014). An empirical investigation of challenges and recommendations for welcoming sexual and gender minority veterans into VA care. *Professional Psychology: Research and Practice, 45*(6), 433–442. doi:10.1037/a0034826

Sherman, M. D., Kauth, M. R., Shipherd, J. C., & Street, R. L., Jr. (2014a). Communication between VA providers and sexual and gender minority veterans: A pilot study. *Psychological Services, 11*(2), 235–242. doi:10.1037/a0035840

Sherman, M. D., Kauth, M. R., Shipherd, J. C., & Street, R. L., Jr. (2014b). Provider beliefs and practices about assessing sexual orientation in two veterans health affairs hospitals. *LGBT Health, 1*(3), 185–191. doi:10.1089/lgbt.2014.0008

Shipherd, J. C., Mizock, L., Maguen, S., & Green, K. E. (2012). Male-to-female transgender veterans and VA health care utilization. *International Journal of Sexual Health, 24*(1), 78–87. doi:10.1080/19317611.2011.639440

VA San Diego Healthcare System (2014) Lesbian, gay, bisexual, transgender veterans, VASDHS Certified Providers. Retrieved from http://www.sandiego.va.gov/services/LGBT_Services.asp

CHAPTER **20**

Aging, Resilience, and Health in Gender and Sexual Minority Populations

Lake Dziengel and K. Abel Knochel

This chapter addresses complexities and variations in gender and sexual minority (GSM) populations in relation to aging, and how intersectionality impacts multiple aspects of health through a biopsychosocial-spiritual lens. We examine how risk and resilience can impact overall health and well-being, the distinct differences in age cohorts, protective factors, minority stress, grief and ambiguous loss, supports and the role of caregiving, and conclude with a model for assessment. Specific aspects such as age of coming out or transitioning as well as distinctions within urban and rural settings are included. We further this overall discussion in the context of how minority stress and ageism must be competently assessed and addressed through service provision and training, social policy, and advocacy efforts.

■ AGE COHORTS, DISCRIMINATION, AND DISCLOSURE

Gerontologists have long divided the population of older adults into multiple age cohorts (e.g., Neugarten, 1974). In comparison with the "old-old" (i.e., aged 80 years and older), the "young-old" (i.e., aged 65–79 years) tend to be healthier and more active, possess broader social networks and higher incomes, live independently, and either still work or are recently retired (Metlife Mature Market Institute, 2010).

Social, cultural, and economic factors lead to wide variation within these groups, however. For example, lifelong experiences with oppression mean shorter life expectancies, less financial independence, and poorer health for populations of color and GSM individuals within the young-old age cohort (Fredriksen-Goldsen, et al., 2014; Fredriksen-Goldsen, Kim, Barkan, Muraco, & Hoy-Ellis, 2013; Williams & Mohammed, 2013).

The old-old cohort of sexual minority people largely began to explore their sexual orientation in the 1940s and 1950s, when few positive social outlets were available. They may have passed as heterosexual or been very closeted due to social stigma and fear of violence or law enforcement. Old-old sexual minority people may continue to carry their identity in the way that they learned in earlier adulthood: living as a sexual minority individual without naming it, and socializing with other sexual minority people entirely outside of public view.

The young-old who came out as a sexual minority in the 1970s were more likely to find a culture that (however negatively) at least acknowledged their existence, and may have had access to a gay or lesbian community that socialized in public spaces and actively embraced a collective identity. As older adults, they may continue to be more visibly out about their identity and socialize with other GSM peers in public. These two different ways of surviving and being may clash as these different age cohorts begin to mix in long-term care and other senior spaces.

Because visibility of gender minority populations has only recently begun to advance—and there remains a long way to go—many gender minority older adults may still be beginning to express and transition their gender as they age (Dziengel, 2014). Old-old gender minority people were unlikely to have heard of transgender identities until Christine Jorgensen—largely credited as the first "famous" transgender woman—made headlines in the 1950s for her very public gender confirmation surgery process. Few resources were available to aid in transition and no organized groups existed in the United States. Young-old gender minority people may have found more resources for transitioning in the 1970s, but there were still few social outlets and gender minority people were rarely visible in the public eye. Transgender older adults who transitioned before the 1990s were taught to disappear into mainstream community; this was often a requirement for receiving medical services to transition (Stryker, 2008). As a result, transgender older adults rarely developed social networks with other transgender people (Stryker, 2008).

Many gender minority older adults emerge into their gender identity in retirement or when their children are adults. They may lose important social networks and may not find new ones among gender minority communities, as organized gender minority communities tend to be younger and generational gaps may be similar to those found in mainstream communities (Russell & Bohan, 2005). Gender minority communities and identities have been rapidly evolving over the past couple of decades. An older adult who transitioned before the 1990s may have a different experience and sense of their gender than an older adult who is transitioning now.

Geography and social conservatism come into play in level of outness about sexual orientation for sexual minority older adults. For example, sexual minority people in urban areas were more likely to find an organized, visible community in the 1960s and 1970s or may have been out and activists in the early LGBT movement (Clunis, Fredriksen-Goldsen, Freeman & Nystrom, 2005). Young-old sexual minority people from less urban areas or from conservative regions may not have had access to this and thus their experience and coping style may be more similar to that described for the old-old age cohort.

Many older lesbians who were married were threatened with loss of child custody and lost biological family support when they came out as lesbians and left their marriages (Parks, 1998). Other older lesbians remained in their marriages and did not come out until later in life. Older lesbians who parented had to contend with additional economic, social, and emotional stressors due to homophobia (Parks, 1998). Young-old gay men were impacted by the HIV epidemic in a way unparalleled in other populations. Many witnessed their closest friends and partners grow ill and die in a backdrop of social stigma, lack of adequate medical care, discrimination, and lack of resources. As a result, the social networks of young-old gay men often contain fewer people from their peer groups (Ryan & Gruskin, 2006). These experiences are also an ongoing factor as members of this population access health care (McKinney, 2006).

Unfortunately, stigma remains widespread for many older GSM adults (Fredriksen-Goldsen et al., 2011; Hash & Rogers, 2013), as ageism exists within both the LGBT community and society at large (Averett, Yoon, & Jenkins, 2013). Among gay men, there continues to be an emphasis on a body presentation that is young, thin, and attractive (Schope, 2005). This continued emphasis on young, desirable partners contributes to ongoing ageism (Hash & Rogers, 2013). Similarly, gender minority older adults face transphobia in gay and lesbian communities; this includes transgender men who may have previously identified as part of the lesbian community (Stryker, 2008), and now upon embracing their transgender identity may lose some social support even from within the LGBT community.

Although many older GSM adults report feeling confident about their identity and being satisfied with life, there are still high numbers of older GSM adults who experience distress and fear, particularly if they are single, are not in a partnered/spouse relationship, or have few family and social supports (Kuyper & Fokkema, 2010). This is a particular challenge for this age cohort as gender minority individuals were often more isolated and misunderstood by their cisgender peers, both heterosexual and sexual minority (Fullmer, 2006). While older adults were coming of age in a very critical time of sexual minority oppression, many could "pass" as straight and keep their sexual orientation identities hidden. This was more difficult for persons seeking to express and/or transition their gender minority identity, who faced constant threat of "being found out."

Bisexuality was also not well recognized and remains an area that is not often acknowledged in the same way as gay or lesbian populations (McClellan, 2006). Recognizing that people can have attraction to a variety of genders was not well understood or accepted until quite recently (McClellan, 2006), and the body of research on this population remains limited (see Chapter 16). In the older adult cohort, there was often a dismissive stance against bisexual men and women as being unable to commit to a gay or lesbian identity (Appleby & Anastas, 1998). Bisexual people were often ridiculed or ostracized in gay and lesbian communities if they were in a same-sex relationship and then became involved in an opposite-sex relationship (McClellan, 2006); they faced similar bias in heterosexual communities if they were in an opposite-sex relationship and then became involved in a same-sex relationship (van Wormer, Wells & Boes, 2000). Bisexual older adults may not find acceptance among peer groups of older lesbians or gay men, or because of their past experiences may not even seek such acceptance. Thus, older bisexual persons may have limited social supports and be less likely to reveal their orientation.

It is critical in assessment to discuss the age at which a person began to identify to themselves and then publicly (if ever) as a gender and/or sexual minority because many people may have lived as cisgender heterosexuals only to identify as a member of a GSM group later in life. Others may have internally identified as GSM throughout their lives, but kept it a secret. Some may have attempted to live openly and been subjected to social, legal, and societal oppression. Generationally, GSM older adults experienced and/or witnessed the active psychopathologizing and persecution of people whose sexual orientation or gender identity was considered a sickness (Hash & Rogers, 2013), and GSM individuals continue to face bias from people and systems as they age (Ryan & Guskin, 2006). Research seems to indicate that people who are more self-accepting and comfortable with their sexual orientation and gender identity tend to adjust better to aging as part of the life span (Fullmer, 2006). However, older GSM adults must weigh visibility of their identities against the potential for discrimination, and out and visible GSM older adults may live less openly as their reliance on others and physical vulnerability increase.

■ RESILIENCE

To understand the ways in which older GSM individuals react to the stressors they have faced throughout their lives, it is important to first discuss the concept of resilience. Resilience as a phenomenon is observed in the ability to adapt despite risk factors or adverse situations and other factors that may place a person at greater potential for harm or for a reduction in potential gains (Hill & Gunderson, 2015). Boss (2006) described resilience as a phenomenon in which a person does as well or better in the face of adversity by adapting and continuing to grow over a period of time. Resilience models identify factors that enable resilience, called "protective factors"; these positive assets may "shield individuals from potentially damaging outcomes" (Hill & Gunderson, 2015, p. 233), such as a strong support network or an ability to take actions that enhance personal growth. Some models break factors into further categories. For instance, Cody and Lehmann (2008) discuss assessing predisposing factors, precipitating factors, and perpetuating factors alongside protective factors. Resilience is typically considered a process rather than a specific character trait or ability. It reflects an ongoing ability to effectively adapt and develop skills as needed through various life stages, and may change over time. It is understood as the ongoing means by which people interact with their environment (Bonanno & Burton, 2013). Hill and Gunderson (2015) assert that resilience "must be conceived as comprising a series of specific cognitive, emotional, or behavior events or social transactions" (p. 235).

For GSM people, this includes the ability to assess and navigate social structures in which they are the nondominant group and the ability to adapt to adversity by utilizing effective thinking, emotional regulation, behavioral responses, and social interaction. Such resilience may be reflected by positive interpersonal relationships, including engagement with other GSM persons, maintaining emotional health and outlook, and making use of available community resources (Brotman, Ryan & Cormier, 2003; Dziengel, 2015). For many older GSM adults, discriminatory laws and treatment, including employment law, exclusion from services, and maltreatment at the hands of mental health professionals and other medical providers, have made them cautious about trusting treatment by systems and eroded their ability to express resilience, such as through seeking preventive health care (Brotman et al., 2003; Ryan & Gruskin, 2006). Still, many have persisted and found ways to engage and connect with peers such that resilience could be fostered. Hill and Gunderson (2015) note that psychological functioning for gender minority persons is essentially sound despite additional stressors and adversity.

Meyer (2010) identified three different ways to conceptualize resilience in relation to stress for GSM individuals. First, resilient people may exhibit less stress because they realize they can handle stressors (sense of mastery). Second, highly resilient people have developed internal strength that may make them less susceptible to the forces of stress. Finally, Meyer (2010) found that resilience is its own protective factor, directly protecting both physical and mental health such that stressors are overridden by coping mechanisms. Meyer (2010) acknowledges that resilience may not be as protective for oppressed groups that have inequitable access to resources. For instance, an older transgender woman who faced employment discrimination throughout her working life will still enter old age without financial security and her health will suffer if the medical system discriminates in its care of her.

◼ PROTECTIVE FACTORS AND RISKS

Protective factors are positive aspects in the individual's personality and/or environmental aspects that support ongoing personal growth and adaptation. Some examples of personality-related protective factors include a positive outlook, sense of humor, self-esteem, and motivation (Hill & Gunderson, 2015). In general, protective environmental resources, such as stable employment, stable housing and transportation, and a healthy network of friends or social supports, may be unavailable or limited for many GSM older adults. However, Schope (2005) identified that older lesbians may have stronger ties to social networks, are perhaps more valued by younger lesbians, have increased understanding of feminist thinking, and may feel less pressure to focus on external standards of youth and beauty. Thus, they are more likely to accept aging as a part of life and appear to have stronger self-images than their older gay male counterparts.

Kuyper and Fokkema (2010) determined that a social network is one of the greatest assets in mediating the impacts of living in an oppressive society. Their research on aging sexual minority adults in the Netherlands identified that feelings of loneliness were ameliorated when interventions were focused on increasing social outlets and networks and actively engaging in working to decrease societal oppression. This included the increased need to train providers and caregivers, as participants in their study reported higher levels of loneliness if they perceived caregivers to have negative views about their sexual orientation (Kuyper & Fokkema, 2010).

Maintenance of resilience through protective factors for GSM older adults is essential when events create additional crises and when normative aging starts to impact their quality of life. Yet aging GSM adults also face risks due to direct oppression discussed previously. Efforts need to continue to create environments and services that are welcoming and respectful, as well as proactive, in serving GSM older adults. Accessing inclusive housing, medical services, aging services, and long-term care housing that are competent and prepared to support resilience with a focus on protective factors will support mental and physical health. Education for staff and providers in such settings must be integrated and policies enacted that require appropriate, nonbiased care.

Largely due to lack of training and experience, some significant risk exists in the lack of environmental and social/societal supports for GSM older adults (Morrow, 2001). This may be worse outside of urban areas. Many larger urban areas are developing or have housing communities for older GSM adults with some training for providers, but housing discrimination nationally is not uncommon (Equal Rights Center, 2014). Housing supports are still few and far between, and the price of much of the GSM-specific housing places it out of the reach of most GSM older adults. There is a distinct gap in addressing the housing needs for low-density population areas, such as rural settings (for additional discussion on the health needs of rural GSM populations, see Chapter 18).

Other risk factors for GSM older adults are related to the concerns of mental health stressors, physical health, and substance use. Fredriksen-Goldsen et al. (2011) note that risk levels for obesity, substance abuse, depression, loneliness, and suicide risk are higher among aging sexual minority persons than among their heterosexual peers. This is particularly the case for gender minority older adults, who may also be seeking transition-related physical and mental health care. Resources are limited in terms of the number of providers who are knowledgeable and willing to guide gender minority older adults to safe and affordable treatments (Fredriksen-Goldsen et al., 2011). Further, the desire to maintain privacy and fear of further discrimination by unprofessional providers may cause GSM elders to avoid accessing needed services (Brotman et al., 2003; Fredriksen-Goldsen et al., 2011). Additionally, some therapists still endorse conversion therapy (McGeorge, Carlson & Toomey, 2015), which may increase the likelihood of both experiencing a harmful health care encounter and of avoiding care because of fear of such an encounter. Many GSM elders also have engaged throughout their lives in their own self-care and advocacy, and tended to rely on friends to provide primary care and support (Almack, Seymour & Bellamy, 2010; Muraco & Fredriksen-Goldsen, 2011); therefore, the inherent increased reliance on others, including medical support outside of their constructed support network, may be particularly challenging.

■ SERVICE PROVISION AND TRAINING

The need and demand for GSM-specific aging services, housing, and programming will exist until discrimination (real and anticipated) based on sexual orientation, gender identity, and gender expression ceases to be a part of the lived experience of aging GSM populations. Thus, there is a need to develop a range of mainstream aging services that offer welcoming, nondiscriminatory, and appropriate care to GSM older adults. State-level and national studies of agencies that serve older adults have found that many agencies say that they welcome GSM adults into their programs and that they would like to see more associated training for their staff (Knochel, Quam, & Croghan, 2011; Knochel, Croghan, Moone, & Quam, 2012). Knochel et al. (2012) found that this willingness to receive training on GSM aging issues held true across all regions of the nation. However, agencies also report that GSM clients are underrepresented at their agencies, that providers do not ask an individual's sexual orientation or gender identity, and that they are unclear why their agencies do not attract GSM clients (Knochel et al., 2011, 2012). The silence of the individual staff members leads to poor if not inappropriate service and the likelihood that a client will not return for care if given a choice.

Studies on training in cultural competence and diversity, as well as training aimed at reducing prejudice among providers of aging services, demonstrate effectiveness (Knochel et al., 2012: Leyva, Breshears, & Ringstad, 2014; National Resource Center on LGBT Aging, 2012). Training offered to providers of aging and GSM services across the nation has been found to positively impact providers' understanding of GSM older adults' needs, their compassion toward GSM older adults, their knowledge of how to develop a welcoming, supportive atmosphere, and, in more intensive training, their ability to recognize bias in their organization, program, or service (National Resource Center on LGBT Aging, 2012). These results are mirrored in a study of providers of aging services in central California (Leyva et al., 2014). Knochel, Croghan, Moone, and Quam (2012), too, in their national survey of Area Agencies on Aging (AAAs), found that those agencies that had provided GSM-related training for their staff were more likely to believe in addressing the issues faced by GSM older adults. In addition, Knochel et al. (2012) found that programs that had provided such training were more likely to be approached for services by someone who identifies as a gender or sexual minority, and more likely to offer services targeted to GSM people.

■ GRIEF AND THE IMPACT OF AMBIGUOUS LOSSES

For older adults, grief is an inevitable event. Grief is largely considered a part of normative life development and is generally supported and socially sanctioned. Death of a same-sex partner may not be acknowledged or supported by others, however, as the relationship itself may not have been supported and recognized. For gay men, this is especially punctuated by the early parts of the HIV epidemic in the 1980s and 1990s. Many old-old and young-old adults experienced the deaths of numerous friends and family to HIV. HIV was described as "gay cancer" and health care was provided in an environment of fear and judgment, if it was available at all (Shilts, 1987). Persons in rural areas went largely unserved or needed to seek care in urban areas (Shilts, 1987). The stigma associated with illness carried over into death, including disposition of bodies and funeral arrangements (Shilts, 1987). Thus, people experiencing grief due to an HIV-related death were often not well supported. It remains to be seen how this will affect the grief experiences of this cohort now that they have reached older ages.

Prior to the federalization of same-sex marriage support in *Obergefell v. Hodges* (2015), couples had to determine the best means to protect legal assets and combined property; this varied from state to state before federal marriage protection. This meant seeking legal advice and having wills, advanced health care directives, and funeral planning that allowed a partner to take possession of the body after death. This was not always easy for people to do if they desired anonymity, did not have adequate access to attorneys familiar with same-sex legal issues, or could not afford the financial costs of hiring an attorney. Older sexual minority couples may continue to not wish to publicly/legally acknowledge their relationship through marriage, leaving them vulnerable as they face poorer health and death, and this is an important consideration when providing supportive care to GSM older adults.

In addition to grief, GSM older adults contend with ambiguous losses, or losses that may or may not be related to physical death (Allen, 2007; Dziengel, 2012). These losses are often complex, unresolved or unrecognized, and distinguished by pronounced relationship ambiguity (Boss, 2006). Examples of ambiguous loss include primarily loss of family and friend relationships, but can also be job loss due to discrimination, loss of faith system due to its views on GSM people, or having a sense of a loss of safety in community due to discriminatory laws. Ambiguous losses are contextual and often outside of the person's control. If unrecognized and unaddressed, ambiguous loss can result in ongoing stress. Chronic ambiguity can result in maladaptation to a new circumstance or to a change in roles and norms, difficulties with relationship boundaries, and disrupted family functioning (Boss, 2006).

Ambiguous loss theory takes into context how relationships are affected by a person's absence, presence, or level of engagement (Boss, 1999, 2006). There are two types of ambiguous loss. The first type is when a significant person is physically gone, but psychologically present. Prisoners of War/Missing in Action soldiers, persons disappearing in natural disasters, and kidnapped or runaway youth are all examples of this first type of loss. Without knowing if the person is dead or alive, remaining family members are thrust into chaos, which may then disrupt how they function. For example, norms and roles become unclear and preoccupation with "not knowing" leads to keeping their loved one psychologically "present," potentially decades after the precipitating event. For GSM individuals, being disowned may result in physical absence of people who are important to the individual, yet who remain psychologically present. As people age, these types of ambiguous losses may become more or less salient depending on the presence of other psychosocial supports, and may be more likely to accumulate simply due to more lived experience.

The second type of ambiguous loss is when a person is psychologically gone, but their physical body remains present, such as Alzheimer's, addiction, or traumatic brain injury (Boss, 1999, 2006). Relationships are impacted and people do not know how to respond. For GSM persons, this could be displayed by situations where they continue to interact with family members, but are told they should not bring their partners to family gatherings, or discuss their sexual orientation or gender identity. This could also include a change or withdrawal of acknowledgment, or encouragement and emotional support by key social supports. Some people may have lost friends or close relationships with neighbors, their spiritual community, or even social status at work due to their minority identity (Dziengel, 2012).

Both types of ambiguous loss can occur simultaneously. For some GSM people this may be more prevalent. For example, some family members may continue to engage with the individual physically, but are less emotionally supportive. Others disengage physically, but remain psychologically present and important. Still others remain both physically and psychologically present, but everyone is impacted by ambiguity regarding changed roles and relationships. Boss (2006) described this as "not knowing who is in and out of the family." These ongoing relationships may wax and wane, or change in other ways over time. Thus, the ongoing ambiguity serves as a continual stressor if it goes unrecognized or unacknowledged, and the accumulative stress may particularly impact GSM older adults.

Ambiguous losses can resurface at critical family junctures, such as an elder dying and needing to interact with the family system as a result. GSM older adults may face situations that cause great ambivalence and potential resurfacing of ambiguous losses. With changes in physical health or cognitive functioning, decisions must be made about what kind of supports are desired and whom to include in their lives. A partner's death without clear legal planning may mean needing to interact with a family system that was psychologically and physically absent. As people face end of life, it is not uncommon for people to engage in a life review and have uncomfortable feelings emerge about specific relationships. Feelings such as depression, anger, or guilt may exist. Helping to identify ambiguous losses for what they are can help to normalize the ambivalent feelings, diminish self-reproach, and assist in regaining a sense of equilibrium.

◼ SUPPORTS AND CAREGIVING

The question of caregiving is concerning for many aging GSM persons (Metlife Mature Market Institute, 2010; Quam, Whitford, Dziengel, & Knochel, 2010). As the HIV epidemic emerged, the role of caregiver became more critical as medical systems did not know how to respond appropriately or sensitively to this illness. Many members of the young-old cohort were on the frontlines of developing grassroots advocacy and organizations to address the needs of their peers. For the oldest-old cohort, providing primary care and support was a way of life—a necessity due to the intense stigma and criminalization of same-sex behavior. Weston's (1991) book introduced the concept of "chosen families," and the structures of personal networks that often provide primary supports for GSM persons. However, this perspective and support network may not hold true into old age. Almack, Seymour, and Bellamy (2010) note that in England, a 2008 health study highlighted that discrimination and inequitable treatment are highly probable for sexual minority persons in end-of-life care. Their study focused on types of caregiver relationships and end-of-life care among sexual minority older adults. They found that personal networks may diminish as one ages, and that while "friends were family," there was still a sense of isolation or lack of acknowledgment for these relationships.

Muraco and Fredriksen-Goldsen (2011) also researched informal caregiving for chronically ill older sexual minority adults in the United States and examined how caregiver relationships affected overall care. They interviewed both caregivers and care recipients, who had a variety of illnesses. The caregivers provided everything from instrumental to intimate care needs, and highlighted the ongoing perception of chosen family and friendship networks as critical to providing care for older sexual minority adults. Yet research participants were quite diverse in age, race/ethnicity, and sexual orientation in adopting the role of "family." Caregivers and care recipients alike identified how the relationship was impacted, but most often in a very positive way. While this study had a limited number of participants (36 total), all of the care recipients were receiving care from a friend, many of whom would not be legally able to make decisions without legal documentation. This could create another crisis of sorts in the limitations of involvement as a person's health deteriorates. While caregiving in older age may be expected and desired from one's chosen family and support network, it may also create an expectation that cannot be fully carried out or realized due to complexities of needs or multiple conditions. For older GSM individuals, there remains a greater likelihood that they will desire and/or receive primary caregiving from someone other than a biological family member who may or may not be able to fulfill this role.

■ A MODEL OF ASSESSMENT: THE "P" FACTORS

Another unique consideration when working with GSM older adults is ways in which to competently and supportively assess functioning and needs. One model for assessment that incorporates a more biopsychosocial-spiritual lens examines predisposing, precipitating, perpetuating, and protective factors. This model was designed by Weeresekera in 1993 as a multiperspective model for psychiatric assessment (as cited in Cody & Lehmann, 2008), and extrapolated into a conceptual framework that incorporates the biopsychosocial and person-in-environment perspective (Cody & Lehmann, 2008). We have further extrapolated this model for application in assessment with aging GSM adults (see Table 20.1).

Predisposing factors are preexisting conditions or environmental aspects that result in increased risk, such as economically stressed neighborhoods, family health history (including mental health), or history of abuse and trauma. For GSM people, predisposing factors due to a lifetime of dealing with oppression may include little financial savings, limited family support, and stress-related physical and mental health conditions.

Precipitating factors are specific events or conditions that result in increased stress, such as a medical crisis or the death of a loved one. For GSM older adults, these factors are aggravated by real or anticipated discrimination. For example, a lesbian who joins a bereavement group to grieve the death of her partner may face homophobia from the other group members, or a home health care provider may discriminate against a gay couple by refusing service after learning about their

TABLE 20.1: Factors Assessment Model for Aging GSM Adults

PREDISPOSING	PRECIPITATING
• Economic deprivation/oppression (lifelong) • Social isolation and stigma • Societal oppression: legal and policy • Family health history: predisposed risk • History of abuse/trauma • Medical conditions: long term • Aging-related risks • Lack of family/extended network support • Unacknowledged ambiguous losses due to becoming out as sexual minority or gender transition: loss of family, children, friends	• Job/housing loss/economic crisis • Death or medical illness (partner) • Crisis/medical illness (self) • Death/loss of immediate family or "chosen family" member, pet loss • Discrimination event • Assault or traumatic event (physical) • Need to relocate for work, health care reason (into assisted or transitional living) • Transitioning in gender identity and expression • Unacknowledged event leading to ambiguous loss(es): divorce, child custody, loss of cultural or spiritual affiliation, community
PERPETUATING	**PROTECTIVE**

• Chronic mental health problem
 	
• Lack of adequate income
 	
• Unacknowledged ambiguous losses: legal and policy related
 	
• Lack of adequate community or state-level policies to protect/preserve: assets, employment, housing
 	
• Specific discriminatory laws (public bathroom access, right to refuse services to GSM individuals)
 	
• Institutional and societal oppression: sexual orientation, gender identity, racism: hospital visitation by nonbiological family member
 	
• Limited or lack of resources that are GSM knowledgeable, supportive, and responsive:
  1. Medical care
  2. Housing
  3. Mental Health
  4. Spiritual and/or Religious
  5. Social and Recreational: community centers
	• Network of supportive family, friends
	
	• Ability to adapt to changing life events
	
	• Stable housing: safe, adequate, affordable
	
	• Transportation: safe, adequate, affordable
	
	• Adequate income: economic stability
	
	• Stable and respectful employment
	
	• Supportive colleagues, neighbors
	
	• Educational or intellectual status
	
	• Good physical and mental health
	
	• Adequate social outlets and resources
	
	• Access to supportive and knowledgeable physical and mental health care
	
	• Spiritual resources
	
	• Community/state-level legal and policy protections: support sexual orientation and/or gender identity
	
	• Connected to personal cultural and/or racial community

This table is an extrapolation specifically in application to aging GSM persons.

GSM, gender and sexual minority.

Source: Cody & Lehmann (2008).

relationship. GSM older adults may face additional precipitating factors, such as those related to gender transitioning in older age. A precipitating factor could be a sudden loss of health requiring intervention from outside medical persons or family member caregiving. This could create a crisis if the person has lived independently or has been involved in a significant relationship that they have never disclosed. Bringing in outside caregivers or family members who are not aware of the significance of the relationship could create additional hardship.

Perpetuating factors are what enable a risk to persist, such as inequitable treatment in employment or housing, lack of legal protections, or limited access to social outlets and resources. For instance, a gay couple discriminated against by a home health care provider may not have recourse under the law and they may not be able to locate an alternate provider who will provide unbiased skilled care. The gender minority person who is transitioning in older age and loses key social supports may not be able to locate other gender minority older adults with whom to build new supportive relationships. Perpetuating factors could include having siblings who grew up in the same era and who believe that same-sex orientation is deviant or "not normal." Similarly, if their faith community adheres to strict beliefs regarding same-sex orientation, it may be difficult to manage internal conflict about their faith or they may be reluctant to risk losing their faith community. These kinds of beliefs or ideas as a minority stressor could lead to lowered self-esteem or poor view of the self. Likewise, institutional oppression would be indicated by limited access to resources and care that is specific to the needs of GSM aging persons, including a lack of legal protections and policies, such as specifically addressing the problem of elder abuse in sexual minority populations (Brotman et al., 2003).

As noted earlier, protective factors are positive environmental aspects and/or aspects in the individual's personality that support ongoing personal growth and adaptation. Examples include a healthy social support network, stable employment, good physical health, stable housing and transportation, spiritual supports, education, a positive outlook, sense of humor, self-esteem and motivation, and the ability to utilize resources for support as needed with the understanding that those resources are adequate and available.

In applying this model, we can identify that for the oldest sexual minority cohort and all older gender minority cohorts, assessment for predisposing factors must consider that they grew up in an era of overt discrimination and pathological views of same-sex orientation and transgender identity. To be visibly and verbally "out" as a gender and/or sexual minority person meant risking physical and economic safety, social belonging, the right to parent children, and even personal freedom. Protecting one's self and safety may have often overridden the desire to seek out companionship or friendship. They may have witnessed or experienced maltreatment or abuse.

In assessing overall well-being, predisposing factors identify such things as the history of oppression and lack of adequate income over time, particularly as a person is aging and has more health care needs. Identifying precipitating factors could be thought of as identifying any ambiguous losses that led to increased stress and disequilibrium due to circumstances outside of the person's control. The sudden loss of family or friend relationships because of sexual orientation or gender transition is an external factor. Perpetuating factors might be things such as a person experiencing losses due to lack of legal protections, such as housing due to unmarried status, or loss of a pet due to long-term care facility restrictions. Focusing on protective factors to restore psychological and emotional equilibrium and advocating to affect the perpetuating factors would be crucial steps. Identifying these various factors can provide a multifocal lens that highlights the critical needs of those we are trying to help.

To illustrate this model, please consider the following case study.

■ CASE STUDY

"Terri" (84) and "Carol" (79) have been in a relationship for 30 years, and live in a smaller, urban area. They were both previously married to men: Terri has two adult sons, and Carol has one adult daughter, each from their previous marriages. They began their relationship at ages 54 and 49 years, respectively, citing it was important to them to stay married until their children were older.

Terri and Carol are White and met later in life. They knew each other as neighbors and became friends. Eventually, they realized their friendship included a romantic attraction. They divorced their spouses before starting their relationship. Carol's husband remarried and lives in the same town, but they have minimal contact. Terri's ex-husband moved to a different state and they do not talk. Terri worked as a teacher before retiring 20 years ago. Carol worked in the banking industry as a manager and retired 12 years ago. Neither of them was out at work or with their neighbors. They have a few same-sex female couple friends, and they get together on weekend evenings for dinner or movies. They are financially stable, although they have not legally merged their financial resources. They do not engage at a public level with other gender or sexual minority people other than their closest friends, nor do they attend work events together, such as holiday parties. They have not married.

Their children are married and all live within a 4-hour driving radius. Terri's elder son has two children in college and her younger son has a child who is finishing high school. Carol's daughter has three college-aged children. Neither Terri nor Carol have living parents, but Terri has a younger sister and Carol has an older brother. They have occasional contact with their siblings, usually around family gatherings such as holidays.

Carol's daughter is very accepting of Terri and Carol's relationship, has included Terri in family gatherings, and treats her as a "second mom." She stops by to visit at least once every other week. Terri's children have very limited contact with her and she rarely sees her grandchildren. Terri's children spend holidays with their father, and may call on special occasions, such as her birthday, but she rarely discusses her children. Terri likes to read and volunteers at the public library, while Carol enjoys gardening and bird watching. They state their interests lie in spending time together, going to concerts or art exhibits, walking, and cooking meals together.

They state that "everyone knows" they are in a relationship, but it never was talked about because no one specifically asked. Both state they introduce each other as "my best friend." Terri's family of origin is Catholic, while Carol was raised with very little religious upbringing, stating it wasn't a priority, but with some Christian influences. Terri said she occasionally still goes to Catholic mass by herself and seemed uncomfortable when asked this question.

Terri was recently hospitalized due to a heart attack. She has a long history of alcohol use, and smoked for several years, although she stopped 10 years ago. She needed a by-pass surgery. Carol was also stressed by Terri's hospital stay; it was the first time they had to manage a health crisis. They did not discuss their relationship with medical personnel. However, Carol said she was there every day and sometimes told the staff they were sisters. When asked about her closest relative, Terri cited her older son. He visited once while she was hospitalized and her younger son called after she was discharged home. Carol's daughter visited Terri several times while she was hospitalized. Terri is recovering, but Carol is deeply worried about Terri's stress level and overall health, as well as her safety.

Carol would like to get some legal advice, having gotten a referral from a friend. Terri and Carol have not done an advance health care directive, but they completed their individual wills. They each own half of a side-by-side duplex and have separate living spaces with a connecting front entry. Carol would like to consider selling the duplex to buy a single-level home together. Terri is reluctant to do so, stating she is "fine." Carol also wants to discuss financial planning and their future living situation. Neither is interested in getting legally married, as this feels like a public exposure of their relationship, but Carol believes it is time that they start to be honest with their health care providers. Their friends are very concerned about Terri's health. Like Carol and Terri, they are unwilling to risk the public exposure of legal marriage, but they have gathered legal protections and encourage Terri and Carol to do the same thing.

ANALYZING THE CASE STUDY

What are some potential ambiguous losses?
Identify the predisposing, precipitating, perpetuating, and protective factors.

Ambiguous Losses

For both: A nonacknowledged individual and couple identity by some family members (especially Terri's family); possible loss of identity/role in sibling relationships; loss of authentic relationships with coworkers and neighbors, medical care providers. Possibly with ex-spouses if these relationships seem unfinished or emerge in later life events (such as the eventual death of former spouse).

How does Terri citing her son as "closest relative" emotionally distance Carol?

Terri's relationship with her children: loss of identity as a mother, lack of acknowledgment.
Terri's spiritual faith: conflict seems present.

Predisposing

Social stigma and isolation as an older same-sex couple came out in later life, but grew up with negative social messages—appears to limit public involvement with peer group.

Aging-related risks/chronic health: Terri's heart attack, possibly related to alcohol use and smoking.

Lack of family/strong extended family supports: only visible presence is Carol's daughter.

Precipitating

Terri's heart attack: medical crisis for both of them, causing mental and physical difficulties.

Possible discrimination/active oppression: Carol felt need to be dishonest, Terri's son stepping into role as "closest relative": how does this disenfranchise Carol?

Potential safety concern with housing situation.

Perpetuating

Unacknowledged ambiguous losses: their status as an unmarried same-sex couple may be contributing to stress level.

Legal and financial supports: shared assets are now being examined—concern for Carol.

Potential for ongoing oppression by medical institution: if Carol is not acknowledged as medical decision maker even after doing Advance Health Care Directive.

Terri's relationship with her religious faith: this seems an area of discomfort for her.

Concerns about accessing the appropriate services: dependent upon area of country in which they live, it's a small urban area, but may have limited resources for same-sex couples with regard to housing, community supports as they age.

Protective Factors

Couple for 30 years: have a few close friends and one adult child regularly involved in their lives.

Both seem genuinely concerned for and committed to each other.

Both report some contact with biological families, who may or may not be a source of support.

Stable income and employment history.

Stable housing: may/may not be a safety concern given Terri's health, neither report that it is an unsafe neighborhood.

Have Health Care Access: appear to have insurance and adequate level of care, although may not be sensitive to same-sex couples.

Transportation does not appear to be a concern.

Carol seems to have positive and stable mental health; Terri may have some unresolved emotional or relationship conflicts.

Both seem to have intellectual capability and capacity to problem solve.

Report a variety of interests and hobbies.

Carol remains physically healthy and capable. Also seems interested in accessing more resources.

Terri appears to have some religious faith that may be explored more as a personal strength.

In any case study, it is important to highlight the many strengths and protective factors already in place. Terri and Carol display great care for each other, have been together for more than 30 years, have supportive friends, and demonstrate much resilience in maintaining a home and stable income. They also both seem to be somewhat pragmatic women, and this could be an entry point for discussion as to the impact of the precipitating event: Terri's health crisis. A potential starting point would be to support following up with an attorney to put legal protections in place for health care as well as reviewing decisions about financial assets. Barriers to this could be the overriding social stigma or fear they both experience in a sense of "secretiveness" about their relationship. They may perceive being more open about their relationship as a potential risk for additional losses. Loss of authenticity in their relationship must be measured against what they perceive as additional stressors or losses if they choose to "be/come out" about their relationship (Dziengel, 2015). There are a number of ambiguous losses, primarily for Terri in her relationship with her children and grandchildren, and perhaps her personal faith system. This may best be addressed in a specific support group for older lesbian couples, along with couple's counseling and individual therapy. Adding additional friendship supports will enhance both their individual and couple resiliency. Terri's sense of loss of a close relationship with her children may be deeply ingrained and getting support from other older women who experience similar losses may make it easier for her to also discuss this with Carol and in a therapeutic relationship. It is also recommended that at least one of their primary medical providers be aware of their relationship, or to explore with Terri having Carol and Carol's daughter named on advance health care directives. Again, these may be major shifts in thinking, so approaching such conversations cognitively and focused on problem solving and resilience may be easier than starting with an emotion-focused discussion. Because ambiguous losses are often unresolved and ongoing, Terri may be reluctant to discuss these initially as they may be too painful. Being able to first build a sense of trust in an affirming and caring therapeutic provider will be essential.

■ CONCLUSION

Health needs in older GSM communities are complicated by the ongoing expansion of aging services that largely do not consider the biases and attitudes about GSM elders (Brotman et al., 2003), and concerns continue in the risks of poorer physical and mental health, especially depression (Fredriksen-Goldsen et al., 2012). Brown (2009) identified the "silencing" of GSM aging as a problem not only of mainstream society, but also among researchers and theorists. It is essential that healthcare professionals use a strengths-based approach to better understand and support the needs of aging GSM populations, as well as requiring that geriatric curricula include discussions and skills training on affirming practice with GSM communities. Advocacy at all levels of practice, including policy advocacy at the legislative and organizational level, is crucial. Training of service providers on GSM populations is proven to be helpful in reducing bias and potentially disrespectful behavior, and should be required in all aging service provider settings. Additional training on multiple types of grief and loss related to oppression and stigma is also needed.

We must also continue to research the broad diversity of health needs in the aging community, including physical and mental health, as well as substance use and addictions, access to housing services, economic factors, and explicitly explore differences in sexual orientation and gender identity to enhance the potential for providing appropriate and respectful care. Outreach and intentional, active inclusion of GSM older adult populations will be essential as they may have a higher distrust of providers. Thus, including them in organizational planning of services, and inviting their expertise and ideas such as through committee participation or planning events, can be a critical first step to make sure they feel heard and respected. They can tell us what they need: we must be willing to ask and listen.

▪ REFERENCES

Allen, K. R. (2007). Ambiguous loss after lesbian couples with children break up: A case for same-gender divorce. *Family Relations, 56*(2), 175–183.

Almack, K., Seymour, J., & Bellamy, G. (2010). Exploring the impact of sexual orientation on experiences and concerns about end of life care and on bereavement for lesbian, gay and bisexual older people. *Sociology, 44*(5), 908–924. doi:10.1177/0038038510375739.

Appleby, G. A., & Anastas, J. W. (1998). *Not just a passing phase.* New York, NY: Columbia University Press.

Averett, P., Yoon, I., & Jenkins, C. L. (2013). Older lesbian experiences of homophobia and agism. *Journal of Social Service Research, 39*(1), 3–15.

Bonanno, G. A., & Burton, C. L. (2013). Regulatory flexibility: An individual differences perspective on coping and emotion regulation. *Perspectives on Psychological Science, 8,* 591–612. doi:10.1177/1745691613504116

Boss, P. (1999). *Ambiguous loss: Learning to live with unresolved grief.* Cambridge: MA: Harvard University Press.

Boss, P. (2006). *Loss, trauma and resilience: Therapeutic work with ambiguous loss.* New York, NY: W. W. Norton.

Brotman, S., Ryan, B., & Cormier, R. (2003). The health and social service needs of gay and lesbian elders and their families in Canada. *The Gerontologist, 43*(2), 192–202.

Brown, M. T. (2009). LGBT Aging and rhetorical silence. *Sexuality Research and Social Policy,* 6(4), 65–78.

Clunis, D. M., Fredriksen-Goldsen, K. I., Freeman, P. A., & Nystrom, N. (2005). *Lives of lesbian elders: Looking back, looking forward.* New York, NY: Haworth Press.

Cody, N., & Lehmann, P. (2008). *Theoretical perspectives for direct social work practice: A generalist-eclectic approach* (2nd ed.). New York, NY: Springer Publishing.

Dziengel , L. (2012). Resilience, ambiguous loss and older same sex couples: The Resilience Constellation model. *Journal of Social Service Research , 38*(1), 74–88.

Dziengel, L. (2014). Renaming, reclaiming, renewing the self: Intersections of gender, identity and health care. *Affilia: Journal of Women and Social Work, 29*(1), 105–110. doi:10.1177/0886109913510660

Dziengel, L. (2015). A Be/Coming-out model: Assessing factors of resilience and ambiguity. *Journal of Gay and Lesbian Social Services, 27*(3), 302–325. doi:10.1080/10538720.2015.1053656.

Equal Rights Center (2014). Opening doors: An investigation of barriers to senior housing for same-sex couples. Retrieved from: https://issuu.com/lgbtagingcenter/docs/lgbtseniorhousingreportfinal

Fredriksen-Goldsen, K. I., Cook-Daniels, L., Kim, H. J., Erosheva, E. A., Emlet, C. A., Hoy-Ellis, C. P.,...Muraco, A. (2014). Physical and mental health of transgender older adults: An at-risk and underserved population. *The Gerontologist, 54,* 488–500.

Fredriksen-Goldsen, K. I., Emlet, C. A., Kim, H. J., Muraco, A., Erosheva, E. A., Goldsen, J., & Hoy-Ellis, C. P. (2012). The physical and mental health of lesbian, gay male and bisexual (LGB) older adults: The role of key health indicators and risk and protective factors. *The Gerontologist, 53*(4), 664–675. doi:10.1093/geront/gns123

Fredriksen-Goldsen, K. I., Kim, H. J., Barkan, S. E., Muraco, A., & Hoy-Ellis, C. P. (2013). Health disparities among lesbian, gay male, and bisexual older adults: Results from a population-based study. *American Journal of Public Health, 103*(10), 1802–1809. doi:10.2105/AJPH.2012.301110

Fredriksen-Goldsen, K. I., Kim, H.J., Emlet, C. A., Muraco, A., Erosheva, E. A., Hoy-Ellis, C. P.,...Petry, H. (2011). *The aging and health report: Disparities and resilience among lesbian, gay, bisexual and transgender older adults.* Seattle, WA: Institute for Multigenerational Health.

Fullmer, E. M. (2006). Lesbian, gay, bisexual and transgender aging. In D. F. Morrow & L. Messinger (Eds.), *Sexual orientation & gender expression in social work practice: Working with gay, lesbian, bisexual and transgender people* (pp. 284–303). New York, NY: Columbia University Press.

Hash, K., & Rogers, A. (2013). Clinical practice with older LGBT clients: Overcoming lifelong stigma through strength and resilience. *Journal of Clinical Social Work, 41,* 249–257. doi:10.1007/s10615-013-0437-2.

Hill, C. A., & Gunderson, C. J. (2015). Resilience of lesbian, gay and bisexual individuals in relation to social environment, personal characteristics and emotion regulation strategies. *Psychology of Sexual Orientation and Gender Diversity, 2*(3), 232–252. doi:10.1037/sgd0000129

Knochel, K. A., Croghan, C. F., Moone, R. P., & Quam, J. K. (2012). Training, geography and provision of aging services to lesbian, gay, bisexual, and transgender older adults. *Journal of Gerontological Social Work, 55*(5), 426–443.

Knochel, K. A., Quam, J. K., & Croghan, C. F. (2011). Are old LGBT people well-served? Understanding the perceptions, preparation, and experiences of aging services providers. *Journal of Applied Gerontology, 30*(3), 370–389.

Kuyper, L., & Fokkema, T. (2010). Loneliness among older lesbian, gay and bisexual adults: The role of minority stress. *Archives of Sexual Behavior, 39,* 1171–1180. doi:10.1007/s10508-009-9513-7.

Leyva, V. L., Breshears, E. M., & Ringstad, R. (2014). Assessing the efficacy of LGBT cultural competency training for aging services providers in California's central valley. *Journal of Gerontological Social Work, 57*(2–4), 335–348.

McClellan, D. L. (2006). Bisexual relationships and families. In D. F. Morrow & L. Messinger (Eds.), *Sexual orientation & gender expression in social work practice: Working with gay, lesbian, bisexual and transgender people* (pp. 243–262). New York, NY: Columbia University Press.

McGeorge, C. R., Carlson, T. S., & Toomey, R. B. (2015). An exploration of family therapists' beliefs about the ethics of conversion therapy: The influence of negative beliefs and clinical competence with lesbian, gay and bisexual clients. *Journal of Marital & Family Therapy, 41*(1), 42–56. doi:10.1111/jmf5.12040.

McKinney, R. E. (2006). Gay male relationships and family. In D. F. Morrow & L. Messinger, (Eds.), *Sexual orientation & gender expression in social work practice: Working with gay, lesbian, bisexual and transgender people* (pp. 196–215). New York: Columbia University Press.

MetLife Mature Market Institute. (2010). *Still out, still aging: The MetLife study of lesbian, gay, bisexual and transgender baby boomers.* New York, NY: MetLife Market Institute.

Meyer, I. H. (2010). Identity, stress and resilience in lesbians, gay men and bisexuals of color. *The Counseling Psychologist, 38*(3), 442–454. doi:10.1177/0011000009351601.

Morrow, D. F. (2001). Older gays and lesbians: Surviving a generation of hate. *Journal of Gay and Lesbian Social Services, 13*(1/2), 151–169.

Muraco, A., & Fredriksen-Goldsen, K. (2011). "That's what friend do": Informal caregiving for chronically ill midlife and older lesbian, gay and bisexual adults. *Journal of Social and Personal Relationships, 28*(8), 1073–1092. doi:10.1177/0265407511402419

National Resource Center on LGBT Aging. (2012). Cultural competence training results: July 2011–July 2012. Retrieved from http://www.lgbtagingcenter.org/resources/resource.cfm?r=532

Neugarten, B. L. (1974). Age groups in American society and the rise of the young-old. *The ANNALS of the American Academy of Political and Social Science, 415*(1), 187–198. doi:10.1177/000271627441500114

Obergefell v. Hodges, 135 S.Ct. 2071 (2015).

Parks, C. A. (1998), Lesbian parenthood: A review of the literature. *American Journal of Orthopsychiatry, 68*(3), 376–389. doi: 10.1037/h0080347

Quam, J. K., Whitford, G. S., Dziengel, L. E., & Knochel, K. A. (2010). Exploring the nature of same sex relationships. *Journal of Gerontological Social Work, 53*(8), 702–722. doi:10.1080/01634372.2010.518664

Russell, G.M., & Bohan, J.S. (2005). The gay generation gap: Communicating across the LGBT generational divide. *Angles: The Policy Journal of the Institute for Gay and Lesbian Strategic Studies, 8*(1), 1–7.

Ryan, C., & Gruskin, E. (2006). Health concerns for lesbians, gay men and bisexuals. In D. F. Morrow & L. Messinger (Eds.), *Sexual orientation & gender expression in social work practice: Working with gay, lesbian, bisexual and transgender people* (pp.307–342). New York, NY: Columbia University Press.

Schope, R. D. (2005). Who's afraid of growing old? Gay and lesbian perceptions of aging. *Journal of Gerontological Social Work, 45*(4), 23–39.

Shilts, R. (1987). *And the band played on: Politics, people, and the AIDS epidemic.* New York, NY: St. Martin's Press.

Stryker, S. (2008). *Transgender history.* Berkeley, CA: Seal Press.

van Wormer, K., Wells, J. & Boes, M. (2000). *Social work with lesbians, gays and bisexuals: A strengths perspective.* Needham Heights, MA: Allyn & Bacon.

Weston, K. (1991). *Families we choose: Lesbians, gays and kinship.* New York, NY: Columbia University Press.

Williams, D. R., & Mohammed, S.A. (2013). Racism and health I: Pathways and scientific evidence. *American Behavioral Scientist, 57*(8), 1152–1173.

SECTION **IV**

RECOMMENDATIONS AND FUTURE DIRECTIONS

CHAPTER **21**

Evidence-Based Approaches for Improving Gender and Sexual Minority Health by Reducing Minority Stress

Melvin C. Hampton and John E. Pachankis

Despite many advancements in their social standing in the United States, gender and sexual minority (GSM) populations continue to be disproportionately affected by a wide range of physical and mental health problems, as outlined in previous chapters. This disproportionate burden of negative health outcomes continues despite ongoing structural-level improvements for some GSM groups—for example, the creation of legal marriage protections for same-sex couples in the United States (Liptak, 2015), the removal of homosexuality from the official psychiatric nomenclature (Drescher, 2010), and the lifting by the U.S. Department of Health and Human Services (HHS) of a 33-year-old ban on transitional care for transgender beneficiaries of Medicare and Medicaid services in 2014 (Padula, Heru, & Campbell, 2016). The prevailing framework to explain these ongoing health disparities among GSM individuals and communities is minority stress theory, which builds on both life-course and social-ecological theories of human development and coping (Bronfenbrenner, 1977; Institute of Medicine [IOM], 2011; Meyer, 2003; Pachankis, 2015; Tebbe & Moradi, 2016). Minority stress theory posits that living as a sexual minority in a heterosexist society adversely impacts the day-to-day lives of sexual minorities by generating stress and eroding coping mechanisms for managing stress, ultimately yielding poorer health. Minority stress theory has also been recently extended to frame the adverse health experiences of gender minority individuals in the United States (American Psychological Association [APA], 2015; Hendricks & Testa, 2012; Tebbe & Moradi, 2016) by theorizing that in a cisgender-dominant society, the inability to live as one's authentic gender, or the negative consequences accumulated for doing so, results in increased stress, diminished coping, and poorer health across the life span (Tebbe & Moradi, 2016; White-Hughto, Reisner, & Pachankis, 2015).

Overall, and across GSM groups, minority stress theory hypothesizes that living as a gender or sexual minority in a stigmatizing social context can create a myriad of physical and psychological consequences which, in turn, can predispose GSM individuals and communities to disproportionately higher levels of adverse physical and mental health problems. These include mood disorders, HIV, substance use problems, and potentially certain forms of cancer and cardiac risk via the lack of certain health promotion strategies, such as ceasing tobacco use (Gruskin, Byrne, Atlschuler, & Dibble, 2009). The mechanisms underlying these processes are too numerous to outline individually in this chapter and are largely covered in the preceding chapters in this book; however, it is important to understand the basic processes of their generation in order to explore the evidence-based interventions created in order to address those same processes.

Generally speaking, minority stress theory holds that GSM individuals in the United States experience an increased level of stress due to their ongoing experiences of stigma at various social levels (Meyer, 2003; White-Hughto et al., 2015). These stressors, which originate in the external environment, might, in turn, be internalized by GSM individuals. These stressors potentially undercut health not only because they add to general life stress, but also because minority stress and any internalization effects are often insidious and largely unnoticed. In particular, these stressors tax the body's internal stress systems (McEwen & Gianaros, 2010) while also depleting the cognitive and affective reserves of stigmatized individuals (Richman & Lattanner, 2014) in ways that are not always directly clear to the person experiencing the stressor. Over time, these stressors may contribute to exclusion from or avoidance of specific health promotion strategies and knowledge, such as routine medical care and sufficient access to culturally competent care, out of fear of additional negative experiences (Bränström, Hatzenbuehler, Pachankis, & Link, 2016; White-Hughto, Murchison, Clark, Pachankis, & Reisner, 2016), as well as the development of health-compromising behaviors, such as increased risk-taking behaviors (Pachankis, Hatzenbuehler, Hickson, et al., 2015).

Drawing on research supporting this theoretical framing of GSM health in the United States, clinical interventions have recently emerged to attempt to address not only the underlying negative health consequences of minority stress for GSM individuals, but also the maladaptive coping mechanisms that potentially emerge from these experiences (see Chaudoir, Wang, & Pachankis, in press, for a complete review). The purpose of this chapter is to briefly outline some of the evidence-based health promotion strategies and mental health interventions that have emerged to help GSM individuals cope with and alleviate the adverse consequences of minority stress in their day-to-day lives.

■ EVIDENCE-BASED MINORITY STRESS INTERVENTIONS FOR GENDER AND SEXUAL MINORITY GROUPS

Although evidence-based approaches to promote GSM health may be categorized in a number of ways, interventions may be easily understood according to their intended socioecological level of effecting change. In particular, minority stress–based interventions have sought to intervene on the: (a) individual level, potentially changing intrapsychic experiences, personal behaviors, or socially ingrained biases; (b) interpersonal level, attempting to improve GSM individuals' relationships with others or their assertive responding in stressful interpersonal situations; or (c) structural level, seeking to change the overall social standing or institutional environments that surround GSM individuals. In addition, evidence-based approaches have emerged that attempt to effect change on multiple levels simultaneously. Historically, many of these interventions have focused on reducing HIV risk among sexual minority men and transgender women, given that HIV represents one of the most disparate outcomes affecting these populations in the United States (Centers for Disease Control and Prevention [CDC], 2016a, 2016b). In addition, the evidentiary basis of these interventions varies widely, including everything from case studies up to pre–post designs and randomized controlled trials (RCTs). A comprehensive examination of the entirety of this literature is beyond the scope of this chapter;[1] as such, we include those interventions with the strongest evidence according to their intended level of effecting change, focusing both on interventions that are specifically targeted at improving GSM coping or health, as well as those that seek to reduce bias or discrimination within the heterosexual and cisgender-dominant communities in which GSM individuals live.

Individual-Level Minority Stress Interventions

Minority stress interventions that have sought to effect change on the individual level by directly increasing the well-being of GSM individuals include several brief online interventions, all of which have shown promise for improving psychological functioning among certain subgroups of GSM communities. For example, an expressive writing intervention tested in an RCT with 76 lesbian participants prompted participants to engage in a 20-minute expressive writing exercise three times a week for 2 weeks, or to write about a neutral control topic (Lewis et al., 2005). Results demonstrated that among lesbians who were less "out," expressive writing helped to reduce perceived stress and confusion 2 months after completion of the intervention. A similar RCT of an expressive writing intervention with a similar number of gay men found that men who engaged in the expressive writing intervention reported increased openness about their sexual orientation 3 months after the intervention was completed (Pachankis, & Goldfried, 2010). Furthermore,

---

[1] Of note, in addition to the article by Chaudoir, Wang, and Pachankis (in press), the Centers for Disease Control and Prevention maintains a regularly updated compendium of evidence-based interventions focused specifically on HIV prevention, a number of which are also targeted toward GSM individuals and communities (www.cdc .gov/hiv/research/interventionresearch/compendium/index.html).

men with lower social support prior to the intervention reported the strongest reductions in mental health symptomatology 3 months after the intervention. In addition to expressive writing RCTs delivered online, a multimodule, Internet-based intervention has also been developed to reduce internalized heterosexism among sexual minority individuals (Lin, & Israel, 2012). Findings from an initial trial of this intervention indicated that, compared to controls who completed a similar intervention focused on general stress, those who completed the internalized heterosexism modules reported lower internalized heterosexism scores posttreatment. In all, these interventions show the potential to reach sexual minority individuals using novel technologies, an especially important advantage for promoting GSM health outside of known lesbian, gay, bisexual, and transgender (LGBT) urban epicenters, and support the development of similar interventions designed to meet the needs of gender minority groups.

Interventions to improve GSM health by effecting change on the individual level have also made use of group therapy–based formats. For example, an intervention developed to reduce depressive symptomatology among GSM individuals using group-based cognitive-behavioral therapy (CBT) in which clients were able to directly discuss their experiences of oppression found that participants who completed the 14-week intervention showed decreases in depressive symptoms as well as improved self-esteem (Ross, Doctor, Dimito, Kuehl, & Armstrong, 2008). In addition, these improvements persisted up to 2 months following the completion of the intervention. Another interesting group-based intervention, which specifically targets sexual minority youth in urban high schools, is the Affirmative Supportive Safe and Empowering Talk, or ASSET, intervention (Craig, Austin, & McInroy, 2014). In particular, an analysis of the effectiveness of this intervention with 263 participants across 45 urban schools found that the 8- to 10-week intervention was able to improve both self-esteem and proactive coping among those who completed the intervention. In general, although all of these interventions focus on eliciting change within the person, they also show strong potential for helping GSM individuals to better connect to the world around them in a more positive way by reducing minority stress–created intrapsychic barriers to improved well-being.

In addition to interventions aimed at improving minority stress coping among GSM individuals, some evidence-based individual-level approaches to improving GSM health have directly targeted behaviors that undercut GSM health (e.g., cigarette smoking). For example, the *Last Drag* intervention (Eliason, Dibble, Gordon, & Soliz, 2012) initially emerged among GSM tobacco control professionals in San Francisco to assist GSM individuals to stop smoking. A central component of this group's understanding of the increased rate of tobacco consumption among GSM individuals in the United States was the influence of minority stress (Eliason et al., 2012). As such, the *Last Drag* was developed *by* GSM tobacco interventionists to be delivered *by* GSM tobacco interventionists *for* GSM individuals across sexual orientations and gender identities. An evaluation of this program's effectiveness, using pre- and posttest data collected from 2005 to 2010, indicated that almost 36% of participants had successfully quit smoking 6 months after completing the intervention. Interventions such as this, that focus on discrete health behaviors in an LGBT-affirmative manner, demonstrate how the LGBT community is able to "help itself" address unhealthy behaviors and risk factors, a strategy with an important historical legacy among GSM communities (Shilts, 1987).

In addition to interventions geared toward GSM individuals, previous work to improve GSM health by reducing minority stress has attempted to decrease bias among heterosexual and/or cisgender peers. A strong example of this is the Alien Nation Simulation (Hillman & Martin, 2002; Hodson, Choma, & Costello, 2009). In this program, heterosexual college students were randomly assigned to either an academic lecture on discrimination and homosexuality or an interactive simulation task performed in small groups. The simulation involved students forming a group and then imagining that they had crash-landed on an alien planet, called Aurora, along with 3,000 other students. Participants were informed that residents of this planet lived in same-sex households, used alternative procreation methods, were prohibited from public displays of affection, and were strictly punished for rule violations. The students were then asked to discuss in their small groups how they would adapt to this situation, including if they would adopt the alien culture, attempt to seek out romantic or sexual relationships, and how they would feel about living in such an environment. Small group discussions were then followed by a full group discussion, in which the interventionist compared the experiences discussed in small groups with those of gay men and lesbians. Among the 68 participants involved in the initial trial, Hillman and Martin (2002) found that only those students involved in the simulation task showed a statistically significant reduction in homophobia between their scores 1 week prior to the intervention and 1 week after, while those who participated in the lecture alone showed no significant change. Results from a subsequent replication indicated that participants in the simulation condition reported significantly higher rates of intergroup perspective taking, significantly higher rates of empathy, and significantly more favorable attitudes toward gay men and lesbians than individuals in the control condition, even after adjusting for several key personality differences among participants (Hodson et al., 2009). Similar interventions have made use of theater performances (Iverson & Seher, 2014; Wernick, Dessel, Kulick, & Graham, 2013), as well as film-based educational materials (Ramirez-Valles, Kuhns, & Manjarrez, 2014) to help reduce bias against GSM individuals, as well as people living with HIV/AIDS, among middle school, high school, and college students. Although it is unclear how such changes in perspective might translate into concrete supportive behavior over time, interventions such as these have the potential to reduce minority stress by increasing the number of potential allies in the peer networks of GSM individuals.

Interpersonal-Level Minority Stress Interventions

Another socioecological level of change upon which minority stress interventions have focused includes interpersonal encounters and relationships. For instance, some evidence-based interventions have shown strong promise for improving the interpersonal experiences of GSM individuals within their own families. An example of this is the attachment-based family therapy model for suicidal sexual minority adolescents developed by G. M. Diamond and colleagues (2013). Specifically, this intervention attempted to adapt an empirically informed attachment-based family therapy treatment for adolescents with depressive symptoms (G. S. Diamond, Reis, Diamond, Siqueland, & Isaacs, 2002) for use with suicidal sexual minority adolescents and their families. In particular, this adapted intervention sought to reduce depressive symptoms and suicidality, while also assisting partici- pants to develop a more secure and trusting relationship with their parents. The intervention was delivered over the course of twelve 60-minute therapy sessions that focused on helping sexual minority clients to discuss their relationships with their parents, helping parents to work through their feelings in relation to hav- ing a sexual minority child, and helping both the adolescents and their parents to develop improved communication skills and rapport with each other. Based upon their formative work, G. M. Diamond and colleagues (2013) discovered that a number of these sessions may require meeting with parents alone in order to help them work through their own feelings of shame, disappointment, fear, and anger related to their child's sexual orientation. An initial pilot of this intervention with 10 suicidal sexual minority adolescents demonstrated potential for the interven- tion to reduce suicidal ideation, depressive symptoms, and maternal attachment– related anxiety and avoidance among suicidal adolescents.

Another evidence-based intervention that has sought to improve GSM chil- dren's relationships with their parents is the *Lead with Love* film-based interven- tion (Huebner, Rullo, Thoma, McGarrity, & Mackenzie, 2013). In particular, based on their unpublished data indicating that parents of recently out sexual minority youth often feel unable to access community-level supports to help them better relate to their children, Huebner and colleagues (2013) developed a 35-minute documentary film focused on helping these parents reduce rejecting behavior and increase positive family interactions. In support of this effort, regular and social media campaigns were developed to promote the film, which was placed online for free access (www.leadwithlovefilm.com). Guided by both social-cognitive the- ory (Bandura, 2001) and the transtheoretical model of behavior change (Prochaska & Velicer, 1997), the film includes segments by four ethnically diverse families sharing their experiences of learning to understand their sexual minority child, as well as sections including the perspectives of two psychologists, three religious leaders, and a high school educator. After its first 12 months online, the film was viewed by almost 11,000 individuals. Of these, 1,865 self-identified as parents of sexual minority youth in a brief pretest questionnaire preceding the film. Among parents who viewed the film, roughly 42% completed a post-test questionnaire, with 71.8% indicating they found the film to be "very" or "extremely" helpful, and mothers reporting a statistically significant greater level of assistance from the film than fathers. In addition, parents reported a statistically significant increase in their perceived parental self-efficacy after watching the film. Although limited in its ability to follow up on the subsequent interactions between these parents and their children, interventions such as this show strong promise for reaching a wide audi- ence, while also potentially helping to prevent the adverse consequences of paren- tal rejection on GSM youth later in life (Ryan, Huebner, Diaz, & Sanchez, 2009). Although more empirical tests of interventions focusing on interpersonal change are necessary, the emerging evidence reviewed here points to the importance of assisting families to better support GSM individuals across formative periods of identity development so as to improve later health outcomes.

Structural-Level Minority Stress Interventions

Structural-level interventions represent the broadest type of intervention affecting LGBT communities. Broadly speaking, evidence-based approaches at this level tend to focus on improving GSM persons' experiences within certain institutions, such as medical settings, shifting cultural norms in relation to concrete behavioral risks such as tobacco use or sexually transmitted infections (STIs), or assessing how changes in the social standing or community-level resources of certain GSM groups have impacted specific health promotion behaviors and outcomes. For example, interventions aimed at improving medical provider GSM-specific knowledge and behaviors have recently shown promise for improving access to care for GSM individuals by increasing providers' awareness of potential barriers to care. In one such intervention, Lelutiu-Weinberger and colleagues (2016) tested the impact of a training in New York City geared toward decreasing clinic staff's negative attitudes toward transgender individuals and increasing transgender clinical skills, awareness of transphobic practices, and clinic staff's self-reported readiness to assist transgender clients, as well as fostering a transgender-affirmative clinical environment overall. The researchers delivered three 2-hour transgender-specific trainings across the spectrum of hospital staff, including physicians, registrars, nurses, prevention counselors, social service providers, patient coordinators, administrative staff, security guards, and billing staff. The training was geared to this broad audience in order to reduce the discriminatory experiences that transgender individuals report experiencing across the continuum of care (White-Hughto et al., 2015). Training content specifically addressed transgender-specific care needs as well as guidance for trans-sensitive approaches across hospital settings. Pre- and posttest comparisons found statistically significant increases in acquired clinical skills, a decrease in negative beliefs about transgender individuals, and a trend toward recognizing transphobia 3 months after the completion of the intervention.

Another example of a structural-level approach to improving GSM individuals' experiences of medical settings is the multisite *Healthy Weight in Lesbian and Bisexual Women: Striving for a Healthy Community* program, funded by the HHS Office on Women's Health (Fogel et al., 2016; Ingraham et al., 2016). As part of this intervention, two distinct training programs were developed to decrease minority stress and body-shaming barriers to medical care among larger-bodied lesbian and bisexual women (Ingraham et al., 2016). The two trainings consisted of an academically formatted training for medical students, which incorporated a more traditional medical model of weight management for improved health, and a clinically formatted training for community clinic staff, which culturally adapted the *Healthy at Every Size Model* (Bacon, 2010). This model promotes a weight-neutral approach to health that focuses on intuitive eating and enjoyable movement. Although developed for different audiences (i.e., medical students vs. practicing medical staff), and piloted in different parts of the country, both trainings demonstrated the ability to improve providers' awareness of lesbian and bisexual women's potential avoidance of health care due to body size concerns. And while participants in the academically formatted training reported greater increases in knowledge and understanding of such avoidance, those in the clinically formatted training reported an improved understanding of how to approach discussing possible weight loss with lesbian and bisexual clients. Of note, although both the trainings reviewed here were piloted with smaller samples, similar interventions have been shown to increase positive regard for GSM individuals and communities across medical and educational settings in the United States (Evans, 2002; Finkel, Storaasli, Bandele, & Schaefer, 2003; Hardacker, Rubinstein, Hotton, & Houlberg, 2014; Jaffer et al., 2016).

Other promising evidence-based approaches to improving social structures surrounding GSM communities include public health campaigns aimed at shifting cultural norms in relation to specific behavioral risks for poorer health. For example, the *CRUSH* social branding campaign sought to reduce smoking among GSM bar and nightclub patrons, countering previous social marketing among GSM communities by cigarette companies (Fallin, Neilands, Jordan, & Ling, 2015). Given the historical importance of bars and nightclubs among GSM communities across the United States, this intervention developed a social brand to be implemented in bars and nightclubs, which they named *CRUSH*. This brand was then used to promote a "cute, fresh, and smokefree" lifestyle among GSM bar and nightclub patrons by using popular opinion leaders, such as known DJs, dancers, and models, to create targeted promotional events in which bar patrons participated in interactive games and activities focused on discussing the benefits of a "smokefree lifestyle." The effectiveness of the campaign was assessed using two waves of cross-sectional data, gathered in 2011 and 2012, which included 2,395 individuals surveyed at highly frequented gay bars around Las Vegas. Of those surveyed, 79.2% self-identified with a GSM group. Analyses of these data showed that GSM participants reported overall higher rates of smoking than their heterosexual or cisgender peers. In addition, 53% of those surveyed reported some exposure to the *CRUSH* campaign, including attending *CRUSH* events, going to the brand's Facebook page, or receiving a *CRUSH* mailer to their home, with 86.3% endorsing an awareness and understanding of the campaign's "partying fresh and smokefree" slogan to refer to smoking cessation. Among participants who indicated understanding the campaign's intended purpose, those who endorsed the highest level of exposure to the campaign showed significantly lower odds of smoking. Similar public health campaigns have shown promise for increasing STI testing in San Francisco and Los Angeles (Ahrens et al., 2006; Plant et al., 2010). For example, the *Healthy Penis* campaign in San Francisco created a humorous media campaign in order to raise awareness and testing for syphilis among gay men from 2002 to 2005 (Ahrens et al., 2006). Similar to the above tobacco campaign, two waves of cross-sectional data were collected from 244 participants 6 months after the campaign began and another 150 participants 2.5 years after the campaign began. Analyses showed that 80% and 85% of participants reported exposure to the campaign in each respective wave, with increased awareness of the campaign being significantly related to higher rates of getting tested for syphilis in the

6 months prior to assessment. Overall, campaigns like this show the potential to bolster positive health behaviors among GSM individuals via structural-level, population-resonant public health campaigns designed to be informative rather than judgmental or fear-inducing.

Perhaps the broadest approach to improving GSM health has focused on the implementation of state- and federal-level protections, such as same-sex marriage, anti-bullying policies, and protection from employment discrimination as a means to reduce stigma and improve health. For example, while significant disparities have been shown to exist in employer-sponsored health insurance coverage for same-sex couples in the United States (especially within states previously lacking same-sex marriage protections; Gonzales & Blewett, 2014), research has shown that after the passage of the New York State Marriage Equality Act there was a significant increase in employer-sponsored health insurance usage among men and women in same-sex couples, compared to couples in opposite-sex marriages, as well as a significant decrease in Medicaid usage for men and women in same-sex couples (Gonzales, 2015). Shifts such as this allow more same-sex couples to have access to quality health care without having to navigate the complications of state-sponsored insurance coverage. Same-sex marriage protections were also found to relate to lower psychological distress among same-sex married couples in California after state-level same-sex marriage protections were enacted (Wight, LeBlanc, & Badgett, 2013). Similarly, in Massachusetts, in the 12 months following state legalization of same-sex marriage, medical care visits, mental health care visits, and mental health care costs among gay and bisexual men showed a statistically significant decrease compared to the 12 months prior to the legalization of same-sex marriage, regardless of the marital status of the men included in the analyses (Hatzenbuehler et al., 2012).

Similar to the influence of same-sex marriage protections, anti-bullying policies that are inclusive of sexual orientation have shown strong potential to influence the well-being of sexual minority youth. For example, an exploration of the experiences of teens who participated in the Oregon Healthy Teens survey from 2006 to 2008 found that gay and lesbian teenagers were more than twice as likely to have attempted suicide if they lived in a county that had fewer school districts with anti-bullying policies that included sexual orientation, as compared to those who lived in counties with more school districts that had anti-bullying polices which included sexual orientation (Hatzenbuehler & Keyes, 2013). In addition, sexual minority-inclusive anti-bullying policies were significantly related to a lower risk of suicide attempts among gay and lesbian teenagers even after controlling for peer victimization among those sampled (Hatzenbuehler & Keyes, 2013). More research into the effects of gender minority–specific policies is needed to determine the magnitude of effect within this even more vulnerable population; however, the results among sexual minority youth suggest the effect would likely be strong.

Likewise, state-level antidiscrimination policies that include protections for sexual minorities have been found to be related to higher reported levels of social support, as well as lower levels of internalized homophobia among sexual minority adults (Riggle, Rostosky, & Horne, 2010). Additionally, an analysis of epidemiologic data on alcohol use and other related conditions among noninstitutionalized adults in the United States found that living in states without hate crime legislation inclusive of sexual orientation or protections against employment discrimination based upon sexual orientation predicted a stronger relation between being a sexual minority and suffering from generalized anxiety disorder, posttraumatic stress disorder, as well as dysthymia in the 12 months before assessment (Hatzenbuehler, Keyes, & Hasin, 2009). In all, this research provides a strong evidence base in support of the importance of state- and federal-level protections for GSM health.

Multilevel Minority Stress Interventions

In addition to evidence-based health promotion interventions for GSM individuals that have sought to elicit change on a particular level (i.e., individual, interpersonal, structural), previous interventions have also sought to effect change on multiple levels simultaneously. For example, the *SOMOS* intervention (or "We Are" in English), a culturally based intervention targeted toward Latino gay men in New York City, sought to decrease risk for HIV acquisition among participants while also fostering improved community connections and empowering participants to intervene in their local communities in relation to areas of community concern (Vega, Spieldenner, DeLeon, Nieto, & Stroman, 2011). In particular, this intervention, which ran continuously from 2002 to 2006, consisted of three stages, the first of which involved cohort members participating in five group sessions that focused on family issues, gay identity, homophobia, body image, and sexual practices, respectively. In the second stage, participants were asked to engage in social marketing activities, including creating print media discussions of what they learned in the intervention, as well as giving public presentations at cultural nights in their communities. The third stage of the intervention involved an annual summit, which all of the participants who had participated in the intervention to date could attend. These summits addressed the pressing issues of the local Latino gay community at that time, including topics such as same-sex marriage and immigration, and provided a way for participants to continue to build supportive communities while maintaining their own reduced sexual risk taking as individuals. In total, these three stages of intervention helped participants to decrease their personal risk for HIV, build supportive relationships with other gay Latino men, as well as improve their overall communities via group action and discussion. In particular, pre- and post-test data showed that not only was this intervention successful at decreasing HIV sexual risk taking among those who participated (e.g., the number of sexual partners a participant had in the month prior to assessment), but it also improved participants' self-esteem, coping self-efficacy, and social support 90 days following the intervention. Also, despite the prolonged involvement required of participants, researchers were able to maintain 100% continued participation and follow-up 180 days after the group sessions ended. Two key elements hypothesized to explain this high retention rate include the innovative incentivizing structures used, such as providing culturally linked food at every meeting, as well as the strong social component of the intervention.

Another innovative evidence-based intervention that has focused on effect-ing change on multiple levels simultaneously among gay and bisexual men is the ESTEEM (Effective Skills to Empower Effective Men) intervention (Pachankis, 2014; Pachankis, 2015; Pachankis, Hatzenbuehler, Rendina, Safren, & Parsons, 2015). Specifically, this intervention is a 10-session CBT program adapted to address the underlying effects of minority stress on the multiple, synergistic health conditions affecting gay and bisexual men in the United States (e.g., depression, substance use, HIV risk behavior). Adapted from the Unified Protocol for Transdiagnostic Treatment of Emotional Disorders (Barlow et al., 2010), a cognitive-behavioral intervention that focuses on treating multiple mood disorder symptoms at the level of their shared etiological processes, ESTEEM engages participants in overt discussions of potential minority stress processes, such as increased rejection sen-sitivity related to one's sexual orientation. In addition, ESTEEM helps participants identify early and ongoing minority stress experiences; track cognitive, affective, and behavioral reactions to these experiences; attribute distress to minority stress rather than to personal failings or inadequacies; and enact assertive, approach-oriented behaviors for coping with minority stress. An RCT of ESTEEM with 63 participants showed that, when compared to a waitlist control, participants who had received the intervention reported fewer depressive symptoms, reduced alco-hol consumption, had lower rates of sexual compulsivity, had fewer acts of con-domless anal sex with casual sex partners in the 90 days before the assessment, as well as improved condom use self-efficacy (Pachankis, Hatzenbuehler, Rendina, et al., 2015). Participants also showed statistically significant reductions in gay-related stress, rejection sensitivity, and internalized homophobia from before treat-ment. Similar to *SOMOS*, ESTEEM represents a new model of multilevel minority stress intervention in that it seeks to help participants to understand the impact of minority stress on their own intrapsychic landscape, while also directly assisting them to develop more assertive interpersonal coping skills to improve their inter-personal level of functioning overall. Although both of these interventions focused only on the experiences of cisgender sexual minority men, evidence-based inter-ventions such as *SOMOS* and ESTEEM represent an important transition in think-ing about and intervening upon the effects of minority stress in the lives of other GSM groups. In particular, by simultaneously attempting to improve intrapsychic functioning while paying attention to both the day-to-day social interactions of GSM individuals and the concrete behaviors that may put them at risk for poorer health outcomes over time, interventions such as these show strong promise for maximizing intervention effects while reducing the overall financial expenditures necessary to improve GSM health in the United States.

■ FUTURE DIRECTIONS FOR EVIDENCE-BASED APPROACHES FOR IMPROVING GSM HEALTH BY REDUCING MINORITY STRESS

This chapter has sought to paint a general picture of some of the existing evidence-based approaches for improving the health of GSM groups by reducing minor-ity stress. The field has witnessed a great deal of progress in the development of empirically informed interventions in recent years. Yet some limitations remain for future research to address. In particular, a number of the interventions were tested among relatively small samples. Future research into the efficacy of GSM health promotion interventions should seek to replicate these with larger sample sizes. Larger sample sizes can also afford the necessary statistical power for detecting the mechanisms of change that might underlie intervention efficacy. Similarly, because most of the reviewed interventions use relatively brief follow-up periods, future research would benefit from longer-term prospective study of the efficacy of these interventions over time and across developmental periods. Very few of the reviewed interventions employed RCT designs and those that did employed relatively weak control conditions. Thus, future research should employ strong control conditions when possible, including other existing interventions developed for the general population, in order to provide evidence for the efficacy of interventions specifically developed for GSM populations. Additionally, further research exploring the interactions of minority stress processes with those of racism, classism, intragroup stress, ableism, and other forms of societal stigma is required. Such research and intervention practice will require keen insight into the ways in which minority stress might be exacerbated by forms of stigma-related stress relevant to other stigmatized statuses. For example, a review of the literature on HIV and persons with disabilities found that between 2000 and 2010, on average, only six articles per year were published that explored the intersections of disability and risk for HIV, with little to no attention paid to GSM differences (Groce et al., 2013). Similarly, research regarding the intersections of sexual orientation, race, and gender among GSM women of color has called for a better understanding of how minority women differ in their minority stress experiences from their White male peers (Bowleg, Huang, Brooks, Black, & Burkholder, 2003). In both of these instances, the unique, and potentially additive, impact of minority stress on the health of already stigmatized individuals is strongly needed, so as to then provide an evidence base for effectively intervening on the health conditions disproportionately facing members of these communities.

■ CONCLUSION

As outlined in this chapter, GSM individuals disproportionately experience numerous physical and mental health concerns due to ongoing experiences of minority stress. Evidence-based approaches for improving the health of GSM individuals and communities continue to emerge in order to address these health disparities, with a number of interventions showing strong promise for effectively addressing the adverse effects of minority stress by eliciting change on the individual, interpersonal, and structural level. These interventions, together with future replications of these interventions and new/emerging interventions, will hold the key to helping all members of the various GSM communities in the United States to live healthier lives over time. However, the work of continuing to create, study, and enact these evidence-based approaches to GSM health promotion will require a continued stream of dedicated clinicians, scholars, policy makers, funders, and community members who are able to combine resiliency factors that already exist within these communities into novel and innovative approaches to reducing minority stress over time and across contexts. These individuals will be able to draw upon the knowledge already generated by the GSM health promotion approaches described here to reduce minority stress and the associated health concerns affecting GSM communities across the United States, extending them into new and novel approaches to GSM health promotion. In sum, these opportunities write an exciting new chapter into the health of GSM individuals, a chapter which will continue to identify the necessary resources for GSM groups to empower themselves to promote the sustained health of their communities long into the future.

■ ACKNOWLEDGMENTS

Work on this chapter was supported by Award Numbers T32MH020031, P30MH062294, and R01MH109413 from the National Institute of Mental Health. The content is solely the responsibility of the authors and does not necessarily represent the official views of the National Institute of Mental Health or the National Institutes of Health.

■ REFERENCES

Ahrens, K., Kent, C. K., Montoya, J. A., Rotblatt, H., McCright, J., Kerndt, P., & Klausner, J. D. (2006). Healthy Penis: San Francisco's social marketing campaign to increase syphilis testing among gay and bisexual men. *PLOS Medicine, 3*(12), 2199–2203.

American Psychological Association. (2015). Guidelines for psychological practice with transgender and gender nonconforming people. *American Psychologist, 70*(9), 832–864. doi:10.1037/a0039906

Bacon, L. (2010). *Health at every size: The surprising truth about your weight.* Dallas, TX: BenBella Books.

Bandura, A. (2001). Social cognitive theory of mass communication. *Media Psychology, 3,* 265–298. doi:10.1207/S1532785XMEP0303_03

Barlow, D. H., Farchione, T. J., Fairholme, C. P., Ellard, K. K., Boisseau, C. L., Allen, L. B., & Ehrenreich-May, J. T. (2010). *Unified protocol for transdiagnostic treatment of emotional disorders: Therapist guide.* New York, NY: Oxford University Press.

Bowleg, L., Huang, J., Brooks, K., Black, A., & Burkholder, G. (2003). Triple jeopardy and beyond: Multiple minority stress and resilience among Black lesbians. *Journal of Lesbian Studies, 7*(4), 87–108.

Bränström, R., Hatzenbuehler, M. L., Pachankis, J. E., & Link, B. G. (2016). Sexual orientation disparities in preventable disease: A fundamental cause perspective. *American Journal of Public Health, 106,* 1109–1115. doi:10.2105/AJPH.2016.303051

Bronfenbrenner, U. (1977). *The ecology of human development: Experiments by nature and design.* Cambridge, MA: Harvard University Press.

Centers for Disease Control and Prevention. (2016a). *HIV among gay and bisexual men.* Atlanta, GA: Division of HIV/AIDS Prevention. Retrieved from http://www.cdc.gov/hiv/pdf/group/msm/cdc-hiv-msm.pdf

Centers for Disease Control and Prevention. (2016b). *HIV among transgender people.* Atlanta, GA: Division of HIV/AIDS Prevention. Retrieved from http://www.cdc.gov/hiv/pdf/group/gender/transgender/cdc-hiv-transgender.pdf

Chaudoir, S., Wang, K., & Pachankis, J. E. (in press). What reduces the effect of sexual minority stress on health disparities? Reviewing the intervention toolkit. *Journal of Social Issues.*

Craig, S. L., Austin, A., & McInroy, L. B. (2014). School-based groups to support multiethnic sexual minority youth resiliency: Preliminary effectiveness. *Child and Adolescent Social Work Journal, 31*(1), 87–106.

Diamond, G. M., Diamond, G. S., Levy, S., Closs, C., Ladipo, T., & Siqueland, L. (2013). Attachment-based family therapy for suicidal lesbian, gay, and bisexual adolescents: A treatment development study and open trial with preliminary findings. *Psychology of Sexual Orientation and Gender Diversity, 1*(S), 91–100. doi:10.1037/a0026247

Diamond, G. S., Reis, B. F., Diamond, G. M., Siqueland, L., & Isaacs, L. (2002). Attachment-based family therapy for depressed adolescents: A treatment development study. *Journal of the American Academy of Child & Adolescent Psychiatry, 41*(10), 1190–1193.

Drescher, J. (2010). Queer diagnoses: Parallels and contrasts in the history of homosexuality, gender variance, and the diagnostic and statistical manual. *Archives of Sexual Behavior, 39*, 427–460. doi:10.1007/s10508-009-9531-5

Eliason, M. J., Dibble, S. L., Gordon, R., & Soliz, G. B. (2012). The last drag: An evaluation of an LGBT-specific smoking intervention. *Journal of Homosexuality, 59*, 864–878. doi:10.1080/00918369.2012.694770

Evans, N. J. (2002). The impact of an LGBT Safe Zone project on campus climate. *Journal of College Student Development, 43*(4), 522–539.

Fallin, A., Neilands, T. B., Jordan, J. W., & Ling, P. M. (2015). Social branding to decrease lesbian, gay, bisexual, and transgender young adult smoking. *Nicotine & Tobacco Research, 17*, 983–989. doi:10.1093/ntr/ntu265

Finkel, M. J., Storaasli, R. D., Bandele, A., & Schaefer, V. (2003). Diversity training in graduate school: An exploratory evaluation of the Safe Zone project. *Professional Psychology: Research and Practice, 34*(5), 555–561.

Fogel, S. C., McElroy, J. A., Garbers, S., McDonnell, C., Brooks, J., Eliason, M. J.,… Haynes, S. G. (2016). Program design for healthy weight in lesbian and bisexual women: A ten-city prevention initiative. *Women's Health Issues, 26*(S1), S7–S17. doi:10.1016/j.whi.2015.10.005

Gonzales, G. (2015). Association of the New York State marriage equality act with changes in health insurance coverage. *Journal of the American Medical Association, 314*, 727–728. doi:10.1001/jama.2015.7950

Gonzales, G., & Blewett, L. A. (2014). National and state-specific health insurance disparities for adults in same-sex relationships. *American Journal of Public Health, 104*, e95–e104. doi:10.2105/AJPH.2013.301577

Groce, N. E., Rohleder, P., Eide, A. H., MacLachlan, M., Mall, S., & Swartz, L. (2013). HIV issues and people with disabilities: A review and agenda for research. *Social Science and Medicine, 77*, 31–40. doi:10.1016/j.socscimed.2012.10.024

Gruskin, E. P., Byrne, K. M., Altschuler, A., & Dibble, S. L. (2009). Smoking it all away: Influences of stress, negative emotions, and stigma on lesbian tobacco use. *Journal of LGBT Health Research, 4*(4), 167–179.

Hardacker, C. T., Rubinstein, B., Hotton, A., & Houlberg, M. (2014). Adding silver to the rainbow: The development of the nurses' health education about LGBT elders (HEALE) cultural competency curriculum. *Journal of Nursing Management, 22*(2), 257–266.

Hatzenbuehler, M. L., & Keyes, K. M. (2013). Inclusive anti-bullying policies and reduced risk of suicide attempts in lesbian and gay youth. *Journal of Adolescent Health, 53*(1, Suppl.), S21–S26. doi:10.1016/j.jadohealth.2012.08.010

Hatzenbuehler, M. L., Keyes, K. M., & Hasin, D. S. (2009). State-level policies and psychiatric morbidity in lesbian, gay, and bisexual populations. *American Journal of Public Health, 99*(12), 2275–2281. doi:10.2105/AJPH.2008.153510

Hatzenbuehler, M. L., O'Cleirigh, C., Grasso, C., Mayer, K., Safren, S., & Bradford, J. (2012). Effect of same-sex marriage laws on health care use and expenditures in sexual minority men: A quasi-natural experiment. *American Journal of Public Health, 102*, 285–291. doi:10.2105/AJPH.2011.300382

Hendricks, M. L., & Testa, R. J. (2012). A conceptual framework for clinical work with transgender and gender nonconforming clients: An adaptation of the minority stress model. *Professional Psychology: Research and Practice, 43*, 460–467. doi:10.1037/a0029597

Hillman, J., & Martin, R. A. (2002). Lessons about gay and lesbian lives: A spaceship exercise. *Teaching of Psychology, 29*(4), 308–311.

Hodson, G., Choma, B. L., & Costello, K. (2009). Experiencing alien-nation: Effects of a simulation intervention on attitudes toward homosexuals. *Journal of Experimental Social Psychology, 45*, 974–978. doi:10.1016/j.jesp.2009.02.010

Huebner, D. M., Rullo, J. E., Thoma, B. C., McGarrity, L. A., & Mackenzie, J. (2013). Piloting lead with love: A film-based intervention to improve parents' responses to their lesbian, gay, and bisexual children. *The Journal of Primary Prevention, 34*, 359–369. doi:10.1007/s10935-013-0319-y

Ingraham, N., Magrini, D., Brooks, J., Harbatkin, D., Radix, A., & Haynes, S. G. (2016). Two tailored provider curricula promoting healthy weight in lesbian and bisexual women. *Women's Health Issues, 26*(S1), S36–S42. doi:10.1016/j.whi.2016.04.001

Institute of Medicine. (2011). *The health of lesbian, gay, bisexual, and transgender people: Building a foundation for better understanding.* Washington, DC: National Academies Press.

Iverson, S. V., & Seher, C. (2014). Using theatre to change attitudes toward lesbian, gay, and bisexual students. *Journal of LGBT Youth, 11*(1), 40–61.

Jaffer, M., Ayad, J., Tungol, J. G., MacDonald, R., Dickey, N., & Venters, H. (2016). Improving transgender healthcare in the New York City correctional system. *LGBT Health, 3*(2), 116–121. doi:10.1089/lgbt.2015.0050

Lelutiu-Weinberger, C., Pollard-Thomas, P., Pagano, W., Levitt, N., Lopez, E. I., Golub, S. A., & Radix, A. E. (2016). Implementation and evaluation of a pilot training to improve transgender competency among medical staff in an urban clinic. *Transgender Health, 1*(1), 45–53. doi:10.1089/trgh.2015.0009

Lewis, R. J., Derlega, V. J., Clarke, E. G., Kuang, J. C., Jacobs, A. M., & McElligott, M. D. (2005). An expressive writing intervention to cope with lesbian-related stress: The moderating effects of openness about sexual orientation. *Psychology of Women Quarterly, 29*(2), 149–157.

Lin, Y. J., & Israel, T. (2012). A computer-based intervention to reduce internalized heterosexism in men. *Journal of Counseling Psychology, 59*(3), 458–464.

Liptak, A. (2015, June). Supreme Court ruling makes same-sex marriage a right nationwide. *New York Times.* Retrieved online from http://www.nytimes.com/2015/06/27/us/supreme-court-same-sex-marriage.html?ref=liveblog

McEwen, B. S., & Gianaros, P. J. (2010). Central role of the brain in stress and adaptation: Links to socioeconomic status, health, and disease. *Annals of the New York Academy of Sciences, 1186*, 190–222. doi:10.1111/j.1749-6632.2009.05331.x

Meyer, I. H. (2003). Prejudice, social stress, and mental health in lesbian, gay, and bisexual populations: Conceptual issues and research evidence. *Psychological Bulletin, 129*(5), 674–697.

Pachankis, J. E. (2014). Uncovering clinical principles and techniques to address minority stress, mental health, and related health risks among gay and bisexual men. *Clinical Psychology: Science and Practice, 21*(4), 313–330.

Pachankis, J. E. (2015). A transdiagnostic minority stress treatment approach for gay and bisexual men's syndemic health conditions. *Archives of Sexual Behavior, 44*, 1843–1860. doi:10.1007/s10508-015-0480-x

Pachankis, J. E., & Goldfried, M. R. (2010). Expressive writing for gay-related stress: Psychosocial benefits and mechanisms underlying improvement. *Journal of Consulting and Clinical Psychology, 78*, 98–110. doi:10.1037/a0017580

Pachankis, J. E., Hatzenbuehler, M. L., Hickson, F., Weatherburn, P., Berg, R., Marcus, U., & Schmidt, A. J. (2015). Hidden from health: Structural stigma, sexual orientation concealment, and HIV across 38 countries in the European MSM internet survey. *AIDS, 29,* 1239–1246. doi:10.1097/QAD.0000000000000724

Pachankis, J. E., Hatzenbuehler, M. L., Rendina, H. J., Safren, S. A., & Parsons, J. T. (2015). LGB-affirmative cognitive-behavioral therapy for young adult gay and bisexual men: A randomized controlled trial of a transdiagnostic minority stress approach. *Journal of Consulting and Clinical Psychology, 83*(5), 875–889. doi:10.1037/ccp0000037

Padula, W. V., Heru, S. & Campbell, J. D. (2016). Societal implications of health insurance coverage for medically necessary services in the U.S. transgender population: A cost-effectiveness analysis. *Journal of General Internal Medicine, 31,* 394–401. doi:10.1007/s11606-015-3529-6

Plant, A., Montoya, J. A., Rotblatt, H., Kerndt, P. R., Mall, K. L., Pappas, L. G.,... Klausner, J. D. (2010). Stop the sores: The making and evaluation of a successful social marketing campaign. *Health Promotion Practice, 11,* 23–33. doi:10.1177/1524839907309376

Prochaska, J. O., & Velicer, W. F. (1997). The transtheoretical model of health behavior change. *American Journal of Health Promotion, 12*(1), 38–48.

Ramirez-Valles, J., Kuhns, L. M., & Manjarrez, D. (2014). Tal como somos/just as we are: An educational film to reduce stigma toward gay and bisexual men, transgender individuals, and persons living with HIV/AIDS. *Journal of Health Communication, 19*(4), 478–492.

Richman, L. S., & Lattanner, M. R. (2014). Self-regulatory processes underlying structural stigma and health. *Social Science and Medicine, 103,* 94–100. doi:10.1016/j.socscimed.2013.12.029

Riggle, E. D. B., Rostosky, S. S., & Horne, S. (2010). Does it matter where you live? Nondiscrimination laws and the experiences of LGB residents. *Sexuality Research and Social Policy, 7*(3), 168–175.

Ross, L. E., Doctor, F., Dimito, A., Kuehl, D., & Armstrong, M. S. (2008). Can talking about oppression reduce depression?: Modified CBT group treatment for LGBT people with depression. *Journal of Gay & Lesbian Social Services, 19*(1), 1–15.

Ryan, C., Huebner, D., Diaz, R. M., & Sanchez, J. (2009). Family rejection as a predictor of negative health outcomes in White and Latino lesbian, gay, and bisexual young adults. *Pediatrics, 123,* 346–352. doi:10.1542/peds.2007-3524

Shilts, R. (1987). *And the band played on: Politics, people, and the AIDS epidemic.* New York, NY: St. Martin's Griffin.

Tebbe, E. A., & Moradi, B. (2016). Suicide risk in trans populations: An application of minority stress theory. *Journal of Counseling Psychology 63*(5), 520–533. doi:10.1037/cou0000152

Vega, M. Y., Spieldenner, A. R., DeLeon, D., Nieto, B. X., & Stroman, C. A. (2011). SOMOS: Evaluation of an HIV prevention intervention for Latino gay men. *Health Education Research, 26*(3), 407–418. doi:10.1093/her/cyq068

Wernick, L. J., Dessel, A. B., Kulick, A., & Graham, L. F. (2013). LGBTQQ youth creating change: Developing allies against bullying through performance and dialogue. *Children and Youth Services Review, 35*(9), 1576–1586.

White-Hughto, J. M., Murchison, G. R., Clark, K., Pachankis, J. E., & Reisner, S. L. (2016). Geographic and individual differences in healthcare access for U.S. transgender adults: A multilevel analysis. *LGBT Health, 3*(6), 424–433. doi:10.1089/lgbt.2016.0044

White-Hughto, J. M., Reisner, S. L., & Pachankis, J. E. (2015). Transgender stigma and health: A critical review of stigma determinants, mechanisms, and interventions. *Social Science and Medicine, 147,* 222–231. doi:10.1016/j.socscimed.2015.11.010

Wight, R. G., LeBlanc, A. J., & Badgett, M. V. L. (2013). Same-sex legal marriage and psychological well-being: Findings from the California health interview survey. *American Journal of Public Health, 103,* 339–346. doi:10.2105/AJPH.2012.301113

CHAPTER **22**

Recommendations for Practitioners for Providing Competent Care to Gender and Sexual Minority Individuals

Matthew R. Capriotti and Annesa Flentje

Research on the health and health care needs of gender and sexual minority (GSM) people is burgeoning, in part due to increased awareness of the importance of identifying the health care needs of these long-neglected populations. This increase in knowledge related to GSM health is a critical part of improving the quality of GSM people's health and health care, as noted in the recent Institute of Medicine (IOM, 2011) report on the health of sexual and gender minorities. However, the ability of this growing recognition and associated research to effect meaningful change depends largely on the extent to which practices are actively integrated into clinical practice and health care systems. This chapter considers how practitioners might integrate existing knowledge about GSM health into their clinical work to establish an affirmative context for GSM patients.

■ CULTURAL COMPETENCY IN WORKING WITH GSM PEOPLE

Across disciplines, virtually all contemporary clinical training programs include in their curricula training in "cultural competency," or special skills needed for clinicians to work effectively and compassionately with patients from diverse backgrounds. Diversity and cultural competency can relate to a host of different aspects of identity, including race, ethnicity, socioeconomic status, country of origin, immigration status, able-bodiedness, and sexual orientation and/or gender identity. Historically, cultural competency training has focused on teaching clinicians factual information about cultural practices, beliefs, and norms of minority cultures. More contemporary approaches (e.g., Sue, 1998) take a more process-oriented view, focused on the appreciation of cultural differences at personal, professional, organizational, and societal levels. These approaches place greater emphasis on training clinicians to think critically about how patients' cultural backgrounds and identities impact their life experiences (including their experiences in clinical care). Additionally, strategies toward cultural competence encourage providers to engage in introspection and reflection about their own preconceived notions and biases related to minority groups, and to monitor the ways in which these influence their clinical practice (for more on this shift in ideology, refer to literature regarding "cultural humility"). Learning specific information about minority group culture is seen as a necessary component of cultural competence, but insufficient per se to operate as a culturally competent clinician. For the purposes of this chapter, we draw on these approaches to provide practical recommendations for providers to deliver competent care to GSM individuals. Thorough discussions on the theories that ground this work can be found elsewhere (e.g., Sue, 1998).

Because cultural competence requires a clinician to think and act in sophisticated ways across a variety of settings and interactions, it is not possible to enumerate specific prescriptions for each scenario that may arise. Rather, a general framework toward providing competent care, in combination with categorical recommendations, may be best suited in guiding clinicians toward providing competent care. Here, we build upon this foundation by discussing five guiding principles for clinicians working with GSM patients, as well as a number of more specific, actionable recommendations.

Guiding Principles for Competent Care of Gender and Sexual Minorities

1. Competent care affirms all sexualities and genders as valid, important, and nonpathological.

   Historically, Western medicine and other institutions have regarded nonheterosexual and noncisgender identities as inferior and pathological. For instance, the American Psychiatric Association (APA) classified homosexuality as a mental illness until 1973, and it was not until 2013 that their diagnostic system moved toward depathologizing transgender identities (APA, 1973, 2013). Similarly, the World Health Organization's International Classification of Diseases (ICD) system declassified homosexuality as a mental disorder in 1990, but its current (10th) version still contains numerous mental health diagnostic codes specific to GSM people (e.g., F64.0 Transsexualism; F64.1 Dual Role Transvestism), the validity of which has been strongly challenged of late (Cochran et al., 2014).

Given high historical levels of institutional and societal discrimination (Hatzenbuehler, McLaughlin, Keyes, & Hasin, 2010), providers should expect that GSM patients presenting in clinical settings will have experienced personal and/or institutional discrimination. Because past experiences color future expectations and perceptions (Aday & Andersen, 1974), clinical environments that are merely nondiscriminatory (i.e., one free of overt discrimination against GSM people) may still evoke discomfort for GSM patients in ways that impede clinical care (see Sue, 1998, for a discussion of the importance of cultural competence at the organizational level).

Given this context, instead of maintaining a nondiscriminatory setting, it is recommended that practitioners adopt an *affirmative* stance toward sexual orientation and gender identity, which actively signals that different sexual orientations and gender identities are held as equally worthy and valid. Validating the equal worth of GSM identities occurs on two levels: direct and functional. Direct validation refers to attitudes and beliefs expressed by providers, such as providers directly stating that they value patients of diverse sexual orientations. For example, a clinician may want to state overtly something that they admire or respect about nonheterosexual sexual orientations. Functional validation refers to implicit forms of valuing and supporting by a clinician, such as appropriately inquiring about sexual orientation and gender identity while avoiding statements that unintentionally alienate or marginalize GSM individuals (i.e., microaggressions; Nadal, 2013).

2. Competent care appreciates institutional and societal context.

Providing competent care should include an acknowledgment and appreciation of the institutional and societal context experienced by the client. Though providers may be aware that anti-GSM discrimination and stigma experienced from *individuals* surrounding a patient can impact their emotional well-being, recent research shows that these influences can also have detrimental effects when enacted by *institutions*. In one example, an epidemiologic study found that institutional discrimination against sexual minorities, in this case the adoption of legislation banning same-sex marriage, was directly associated with increased prevalence of mental health problems among sexual minority people, including a 248% increase in anxiety disorders among sexual minority people (Hatzenbuehler et al., 2010). Similarly, when considering the physical health and well-being of sexual minority people, sexual minority people living in locations with high levels of anti-GSM attitudes had shorter life expectancies, estimated at approximately 12 fewer years, than those living in locations with lower levels of anti-GSM attitudes (Hatzenbuehler et al., 2014). Taken together, it is clear that the societal environment can have significant impacts on the physical and mental health of GSM people.

With the above in mind, it is important to evaluate how the clinical environment may also impact GSM patients. This can include asking clients about ways in which they may have been impacted by institutional contexts. In order to be competent, providers need to stay abreast of issues that may impact GSM individuals. For instance, providers living in areas where there are governmental policies that restrict nondiscrimination policies may want to query their patients about how they may have been impacted by these policies. Similarly, providers may want to consider how patients' cultural context, community, or religion may have impacted their experience and/ or their beliefs about their health. For instance, a patient from a religious context which sees a nonheterosexual identity as evidence of spiritual defect may also view their health problem as tied into that spiritual defect.

3. Competent providers recognize themselves as fallible and biased, catch mistakes, attend to ruptures, and check in with patients.

A first step in providing competent care is having a better understanding of our own personal biases, or the lens through which we see the world (Sue, 1998). All providers, regardless of how strongly they strive to affirm patients of diverse backgrounds, have their own biases that can affect their interactions with patients. The goal of competent care is not to be a person without biases, as this is functionally impossible, but rather for clinicians to work toward bringing their biases into awareness, monitoring when biases arise in the course of their professional work, and actively working to overcome potentially detrimental sequelae of these biases. Said more simply: culturally competent care is not about "being perfect," but rather in committing one's self to an active practice of becoming more culturally aware and skilled in working with diverse individuals. Based on the setting of their practice, providers may work toward this goal through professional development trainings, exposure to literature and art created by diverse individuals, personal reflection, and/or peer consultation.

Despite the best intentions and efforts to provide optimal care to GSM individuals, most providers will still, on occasion, inadvertently make incorrect assumptions, commit microaggressions (unintended alienations of patients), or, at the very least, make statements that do not sit well with patients. When these things happen, competent providers will notice their mistake, acknowledge their role in the situation, express openness to learn to provide better care, and listen to patients' input to understand their experience. For example, even the most well-intentioned provider may mistakenly misgender a patient (e.g., refer to a patient as male when they prefer female or neutral pronouns). The competent provider will identify this mistake, apologize to the patient, and then work to repair the relationship. Repair comes in many forms but may occur through a conversation, for instance, by saying, "I am sorry that I misspoke just now. You prefer male pronouns and I called you 'she.' I hope that this doesn't harm our relationship and I will try to do better in the future. It is really important to me to honor your preference because that is part of me providing you with good care."

4. Competent care recognizes patients as unique individuals.

Across disciplines, clinicians attempt to integrate the idiosyncratic experience of their patients with universal knowledge about behavioral and biological principles common to all humans. Culture-specific issues (here, related to sexual orientation and gender identity) regard the ways in which cultural group membership *may* impact a patient's health. In training curricula, these questions are sometimes addressed by providing aggregate data on the "average" health status of minority group members. For instance, medical students may learn that lesbian women are more likely to be obese than heterosexual women, and mental health professionals may learn that suicide is more common in gay men than heterosexual men. These aggregate data have important implications for public health policy and research, and can also aid clinicians in screening demographically at-risk populations. However, in clinical work with GSM individuals and other minorities, clinicians must not use knowledge of demographic correlates of disease to supplant thorough clinical assessment.

In a similar fashion, clinicians should consider differences in identity among patients who belong to a common sexual or gender minority group. For instance, consider two bisexually identified women: The first is single, has no children, has many GSM friends, is "out" to her family and coworkers, predominantly dates women, and sometimes finds herself physically attracted to men. The second woman has been married to a man for 20 years and has two biological children with him; sexually, she is monogamous with her husband and only "out" as bisexual to him, though she still is attracted to and fantasizes about other women, and had a number of sexual encounters with women before her current marriage. These two patients are likely to have very different experiences of their sexual orientation, with some shared aspects. A clinician could not accurately apply a single, monolithic view of what "being bisexual" means to these two women. Rather, it is here more appropriate to take an open stance by *exploring* aspects of bisexual identity with these patients, rather than applying a single set of labels, expectations, and heuristics based on their bisexual identity.

5. Competent care appreciates intersectionality of GSM identity and other identities.

All humans are a product of complex backgrounds and carry multifaceted identities. Though this statement may appear a simple truism at first blush, it has important implications for constructing an affirming environment and providing appropriate care for patients, including GSM patients. One issue related to this topic regards the intersection of sexual orientation and gender identity with other identities. For instance, many sexual minority men of any cultural background face challenges related to reconciling their sexual orientation with heteronormative ideals of masculinity. However, the precise nature of these challenges will differ based on intersections with other factors, such as the patient's race/ethnicity. That is, sexual minority Latinos may live in a social context rife with traditional cultural norms of *machismo, marianismo,* and *caballerismo* (Morales, 1996), whereas African American men may be more likely to encounter different (though overlapping) norms related to Black masculinity (Abreu, Goodyear, Campos, & Newcomb, 2000). Non-Latino, White sexual minority men can confront parallel challenges as they navigate diverse masculine ideals within "majority" culture and/or their own ethnic background groups (e.g., Irish, Italian, and Eastern European). The culturally competent clinician will explore such intersectionalities between GSM status and other cultural variables in an *individualized* way that involves actively exploring these topics without assuming that a particular cultural norm affects all members of a minority group equally. As it relates to the above, this means that different sexual minority Latino men will have different perspectives on masculine ideals such as *machismo* and *caballerismo* as they relate to their own lives.

It is also important to note that individuals may be impacted by multiple cultural identities, which may send, at times, conflicting messages. For instance, a woman with both Middle Eastern and Northern European backgrounds may receive distinct messages from these different identities (e.g., about independence, emotional expression, and the role of men and women in the family). Another important area of intersection regards the coexistence of sexual orientation and gender identity. Providers should understand that a person may have both gender minority *and* sexual minority identities, and should query both. Furthermore, providers will want to try to understand the interplay of these identities. Patients who identify as both a sexual minority and a gender minority may experience one identity as more central than the other in general, or may experience both as central and overlapping. Providers should query both sexual orientation and gender identity, and should be prepared to provide affirmative approaches for both intersecting identities.

RECOMMENDATIONS FOR ADDRESSING HEALTH DISPARITIES

We believe the most effective path to creating an inclusive, affirmative environment for GSM patients is to take a patient-centered approach. This allows for a more comprehensive view of the GSM patient's experience and allows for consideration of changes that may be made outside of the patient–provider interaction. In taking this approach, providers should consider taking action at the levels of the institution, provider, and individual person or patient.

Institutional Level: Setting a Context of Affirmation

When patients see a health care provider, they navigate a series of processes before the "core" of their visit. For instance, when searching for a primary care provider, patients may browse referral listings, insurance provider lists, provider websites, and/or other resources. The first visit begins with registration paperwork, consent and insurance forms, screening by an allied provider, all before they even meet the intended care provider. The nature of this process has at least two important implications for the present discussion. First, it means that a person-centered approach begins with recommendations toward establishing an affirmative and supportive context prior to the clinical encounter itself. Second, it means that establishing a GSM-affirmative care environment requires training all employees who may interact with patients in the course of this care. This, of course, includes clinical providers, but also support personnel such as front desk staff, billing coordinators, and other administrators.

Recommendation 1: Make GSM Inclusion Visually Salient

Like all patients, GSM individuals are motivated to seek care most appropriate for them. Providers can signal that they embrace caring for GSM people by reflecting this in their materials for patients and other supporting documents (e.g., advertising, websites, and informational materials). An obvious opportunity for this includes explicitly stating on a practice's website that providers welcome GSM individuals and have a history of working with them. Office spaces may include "pride" imagery and signage directly indicating celebration of LGBT communities (e.g., a rainbow flag). Providers may also consider how they "brand" their practice in less overt ways. Many office websites and office spaces depict images of people that are taken to symbolize patient care. Affirmation and support of GSM people can be expressed by simply including GSM individuals in these depictions. For example, a pediatrician's website may include a stock photo image of a child playing while being watched by her two moms. Similarly, an orthopedist's office may include images of GSM athletes along with other athletes. These changes do not require the addition of an out-of-place token of GSM support, but rather an effort to give GSM people their due portrayal as visible and valued individuals.

Considerations about exactly how to project an inclusive clinical environment may be nuanced and vary by clinical setting and geographic region. For instance, a child/adolescent psychologist whose waiting area is adorned with many colorful displays of families and children of different backgrounds may easily incorporate a "safe space" sign or photos of families headed by same-gender parents. However, this kind of addition may seem somewhat out of place in a dermatologist's relatively austere waiting room. In all, we encourage providers to take stock of ways that they can nonverbally communicate celebration of GSM individuals in a manner that fits with their own clinical setting.

Recommendation 2: Modify Paperwork to be GSM-Inclusive

Patients seeking medical care complete a significant amount of paperwork for medical and legal purposes. As part of this, individuals provide demographic and clinical information about themselves and their families. In our experience, some providers are less deliberate about how their paperwork asks about this information than how they themselves ask about these topics during clinical interview. Nonetheless, patients may still be impacted by noninclusive or disaffirming language in a provider's paperwork. After all, the patient's experience completing this paperwork is most often their "first taste" of answering questions about themselves under the care of the provider. Thus, we recommend that clinicians carefully review and modify paperwork to ensure that it is appropriate for GSM individuals.

First and foremost, paperwork should *ask* about sexual orientation and gender identity. Inquiring about these aspects of identity in a proactive way is a core and foundational piece of establishing an inclusive environment of care. Many medical providers and researchers simply do not include sexual orientation or gender identity (beyond binary male/female) in demographic surveys, which leads to widespread "invisibility" of GSM groups in medical research and policy (Heck, Mirabito, LeMaire, Livingston, & Flentje, 2016; IOM, 2013). Thus, simply recognizing the diversity in people's sexual orientation and gender identity provides an important demonstration of affirmation.

Of course, when paperwork enquires about sexual orientation and gender identity, it should do so using appropriate and contemporary terminology. Within the area of sexual orientation, this means including options for the most common identities (gay, lesbian, and bisexual), as well as opportunities for patients to provide other identities. Some organizations choose to include a long, nearly exhaustive list of identities, though we recommend always providing a free-response option, as even the most comprehensive lists quickly become outdated, given the rapid rate of social change around sexual orientation in current times.

When asking about gender identity, we believe particular sensitivity is warranted, as most gender minority people have extensive experiences with erasure, invalidation, and disrespect around their gender. Questions should be designed to capture a variety of noncisgender and nonbinary identities, while also collecting information needed for care. We recommend that paperwork include two separate questions about gender, one assessing an individual's gender identity and another querying the sex they were assigned at birth (i.e., on their birth certificate). To be clear, the function of asking the latter question is to obtain an accurate history (so as to inform care for the patient), and *not* to negate their current gender identity. We recommend that the question about gender identity appear first and include binary options (i.e., male and female), "transgender," and a free-response space for other identities. This approach allows for inclusion not only of cisgender and trans-identified individuals, but also of individuals who do not fully identify as cisgender but do not view themselves as transgender. By explicitly listing a nonbinary identity (i.e., transgender), this wording communicates recognition of the validity of genders outside of the traditional male/female dichotomy. This is considered preferable to arrangements that list only "male," "female," and "other." To query what sex a patient was assigned at birth, a question might read, "What sex were you assigned on your birth certificate?" This avoids problems associated with asking about one's "sex at birth" (e.g., for intersex people, this can be inappropriate) or "biological sex" (many transgender people have always experienced their current gender and therefore consider it to be their biologically determined one). The two-step method described above has been recommended by several researchers in this area (e.g., Sausa, Sevelius, Keatley, Iñiguez, & Reyes, 2009; The GenIUSS Group, 2014), but as research in this area is rapidly evolving, providers may want to apprise themselves of the most up-to-date methods.

To further establish an affirmative environment for gender minority people, we encourage providers to provide an option for patients to indicate their preferred pronouns and names on demographic forms. Though the most commonly used pronouns are traditional masculine (he/him/his), feminine (she/her/hers), and gender-neutral (they/them/their) sets, providers should be aware that a variety of other gender-neutral pronouns are used (e.g., xe/xem/xis). Use of these pronouns has evolved rapidly over the past several years and varies by generation and geographical location. When a patient prefers pronouns with which a provider is not familiar, we recommend that the provider simply ask the patient how these are pronounced. We recommend also including a space for patients to list a preferred name. This can be a great aid in creating an affirmative environment for transgender people who are transitioning and have a preferred first name (gender-neutral or associated with their self-identified gender) that they go by in daily life. Incidentally, this can also help build rapport with non-GSM patients who prefer to be called by a nickname rather than their legal name (e.g., a "Dylan James Smith" who prefers to be called "D. J.").

Provider-Level Recommendations for Interactions With All Patients

Just as the above recommendations involve modifying the experience of all patients to enhance that of GSM patients, providers may adapt the way they interact with all patients (GSM or not) toward creating a more inclusive environment. These efforts can set an affirmative tone and form a foundation for GSM patients to feel comfortable discussing these aspects of their identity with a provider.

Recommendation 3: Use Affirmative and Inclusive Language in All Communications

As discussed earlier, using language that reflects an appreciation for GSM identities is a critical aspect of expressing affirmation. Like all of us, health care providers have been socialized in a world rife with heteronormativity and cisnormativity. These cultural norms produce a tendency to "automatically" speak in a way that assumes involved parties have a heterosexual and cisgender identity. It is important to note that these tendencies are not necessarily reflective of personal prejudice against GSM people (Röndahl, Innala, & Carlsson, 2006) and may even be present in the speech of GSM people. Thus, providers must make an active effort to monitor their language use in clinical interactions, and not fall into the pitfall of assuming that their positive/affirmative views of GSM people automatically lead them to affirmative communications.

A common example of disaffirming language involves presuming the gender of one's romantic partner. For example, if a male patient indicates he is married, a provider may immediately follow up by asking questions about his "wife." Instead, the provider should inquire about this patient's "spouse" until their gender is clarified in conversation. With unmarried patients, a provider might ask if they are "in a committed relationship," "dating anyone," or "have a partner." Similarly, when working with families, a provider might inquire about a patient's "parents" or "caregivers" rather than "mother and father." This wording is inclusive not only of same-gender parenting couples, but also of other patients with various types of family constellations (e.g., grandparents and foster parents), which may or may not include GSM individuals.

Typically, affirmative language begins with using open-ended questions, so that patients can provide the relevant information about their history and background. As an example, imagine providing care for a gay cisgender man. Many assumptions may be incorrectly made about this man's parenting status. Some providers may assume that this man has no children or, if he does have children, they are from a previous opposite-sex relationship. In fact, there are many pathways to parenting among same-sex male couples, including, but not limited to, shared parenting with one or more other adults, foster parenting, adoption, a known or unknown surrogate, or a known or unknown egg donor with surrogacy (see Chapter 7 for more details on family planning among same-sex couples). Therefore, providers are advised to ask open-ended questions about parenting status, such as "Are you a parent to any children?" or "Families are created in many different ways, can you tell me more about your family?" Parenting status is only one of the many background areas that providers may wish to approach with open-ended questions; others may include social support systems, family relationships, and reproductive health.

Recommendation 4: Openly, Proactively Express Your GSM-Affirmative Stance

While using inclusive language and paperwork are important first steps, providers can best build alliances and trust with their patients by outwardly expressing an affirmative stance. Take a moment and think about a health care provider you felt was really in your court and had your best interests in mind. Perhaps that provider shared your views. Perhaps you and they shared a common aspect of identity, and this increased your trust in them. If they were "different" from you in some important way(s), how did they show you that they were truly concerned about your health and well-being? Making a patient feel cared for often involves letting them know that you are truly interested in them. One way to do this is on an individual level, though you can also express affirmations for the patient's community, or the greater LGBT community.

To begin with, let's explore a clinical example. Alan, a 40-year-old transgender man, comes to see Dr. Jones for an initial visit in her clinic, but remains unsure if Dr. Jones is the right provider for him. Dr. Jones has never had a transgender patient in her practice before. She is careful to use open-ended questions in her assessment with Alan, finds out that he prefers male pronouns, and carefully documents his health needs. Alan leaves thinking, "That Dr. Jones is OK. Well, much better than Dr. Farley from before who was always calling me a 'her' and using my old name!" After the first visit, Alan is still somewhat guarded, however, as he has had numerous experiences with providers who behaved in an unfriendly, or at the least, uncomfortable manner toward him. After Alan leaves his first visit, Dr. Jones decides that she ought to do some research to make sure that she is providing optimal care, as well as consult with a colleague who is extremely experienced in providing care for transgender men. In Dr. Jones's second meeting with Alan, she lets him know that she appreciates Alan coming to see her, as she understands he may have previously had providers who did not provide him with the best care. Dr. Jones tells Alan that she wants to make sure she provides him with excellent care. She also lets Alan know she has done some research to make sure that she is providing the best medication regimen possible, which will neither interfere with his current medications nor jeopardize his use of hormones in the future. Alan leaves the appointment significantly reassured, noting that Dr. Jones has done more background work than previous providers.

Alternatively, providers can take the approach of expressing affirmations for the community. One can do this through working as a community ally, advocating for rights for GSM individuals, or directly by expressing affirmations for the community. For example, in the example above, Dr. Jones took the tack of making it clear to Alan that she wanted to provide excellent care. Dr. Jones could have also taken an extra step of expressing an affirmation for the transgender community. For example, she could have commented on her respect for the courage that transgender individuals have in taking the often-difficult steps to honor their authentic selves. This is taking an additional step in affirmation.

Recommendation 5: Thoroughly Discuss Confidentiality and Privacy Policies

While most patients of any background are concerned about privacy of their clinical information, this issue may be particularly important for GSM patients, given long-standing histories with societal discrimination and anti-GSM stigma. Many GSM individuals may be "out" to some people in their lives, but not others, often including family members. Additionally, in many jurisdictions, antidiscrimination laws do not cover sexual orientation and gender identity, such that being "outed" may carry risk of losing one's job and/or housing. These and other concerns combine to make privacy tantamount in providing clinical care for GSM people.

From a provider standpoint, the issue of privacy may seem quite simple. If one follows ethical and legal parameters of confidentiality, there are extremely few conditions under which a provider would disclose information about a patient's sexual orientation or gender identity without consent. Of course, we recommend that providers, first and foremost, strictly follow guidelines for confidentiality and privacy as set forth by legal codes and their profession's ethical standards. Yet, beyond maintaining best practices around confidentiality, providers may create a more comfortable environment for GSM individuals by proactively discussing confidentiality with patients during their initial interview.

In some clinical contexts (e.g., outpatient mental health services), it is standard practice for a clinician and patient to discuss confidentiality policies in the first session. Clinicians who provide these services will have a brief "speech" about confidentiality they give to all patients, explaining what that confidentiality means, as well as discussing the limits of confidentiality. In other clinical contexts, there is greater variability in the extent to which confidentiality and privacy policies are actively discussed face-to-face, above and beyond information conveyed in preappointment paperwork. We encourage providers in all settings to discuss confidentiality with their patients; this is consistent with best clinical practice in general, and it gives patients an opportunity to ask questions they may have around their privacy. Of course, the nature and depth of this discussion will vary based on clinical context, but even a cursory overview can allay many patients' concerns while providing a jumping-off point for a more in-depth conversation when patients have further questions and/or concerns.

Although patient information is generally held confidential, certain clinical situations engender special limitations around confidentiality that warrant discussion.

For instance, information disclosed by a minor patient to a provider may, in turn, be disclosed to the patient's parents or guardians. Patients may be at high risk for a medical or behavioral emergency (e.g., suicide), in which case confidentiality may be broken to keep the patient safe or allow designated individuals to make care decisions. In these sorts of situations, we recommend that providers explicitly discuss relevant limits of confidentiality with patients at the onset of their treatment relationship. We recommend that providers specifically discuss what would (and would not) be disclosed to specific individuals in these situations. Often, this conversation serves to clarify the degree to which information about sensitive information is protected. For instance, in doing psychotherapy with a sexual minority adolescent experiencing suicidal urges, it would be clarified that, although the therapist would discuss suicidal urges, plans, and behaviors with the parent, the therapist would not disclose information about the adolescent's sexual orientation. In areas where confidentiality is "gray," this degree of specificity is helpful both in clarifying expectations and in allaying patient concerns.

Person-Specific Level: Understanding the Individual GSM Patient

The task of exploring the direct relevance of sexual orientation and gender identity to an individual patient's health may be seen as the sine qua non of GSM competence. In order to provide competent care, the clinician must *both* establish a GSM-friendly context *and* work sensitively and effectively with individual patients around the intersection of their health with sexual orientation and gender identity. The following three recommendations concern both the "what" and "how" skills providers must employ to accurately frame patients' presenting concerns in the context of sexual orientation and gender identity.

Recommendation 6: Conceptualize GSM Patients' Experiences Through a Systematic Framework That Accounts for Variability Among Individuals

Group research studies show that GSM individuals experience certain discriminatory and stressful life events at higher rates than non-GSM individuals. These include rejection by family and peers, social ostracism, and sexual and physical victimization (Dank, Lachman, Zweig, & Yahner, 2014; Katz-Wise & Hyde, 2012; Mays & Cochran, 2001, Rothman, Exner, & Baughman, 2011). Other studies have found that GSM people are on average more likely to exhibit more mental health problems such as anxiety, depression, and substance use (for reviews, see King et al., 2008; Meyer, 2013; and various chapters in this text). At the same time, this body of research, in fact, indicates that the majority of GSM people do *not* have any mental health disorders; many GSM people experience extremely high quality of life, thrive in the face of adversity, and draw strength and resilience from various sources. Clearly, the health and life experiences of GSM people are not monolithic. We believe it is critical that providers view the diverse experiences of GSM people within a consistent and coherent framework, thus allowing for a rational, cause-and-effect framework in case formulation.

The minority stress model (Meyer, 1995, 2013) is one popular and empirically supported framework that provides a systematic view of factors that lead to poor adjustment and health outcomes in minority individuals, including GSM individuals. Though originally developed as a model of mental health outcomes in sexual minority individuals (Meyer, 1995, 2013), the minority stress model has been extended to explain physical health outcomes (Lick, Durson, & Johnson, 2013) and to include gender minority individuals (Hendricks & Testa, 2012). Briefly, this model suggests that minority status is not directly linked to poor health outcomes in a causal fashion; rather, it holds that the stress associated with one's minority status can greatly influence health. That is, poor health outcomes are seen as primarily influenced by experiences of rejection and stigma (including overt discrimination, exposure to negative societal views about GSM people, familial rejection, stress related to concealing one's identity, and others). In contrast, GSM individuals who experience positive, supportive reactions and/or have excellent social support to help cope with minority stress would be at lower risk for poor outcomes (Russell, Ryan, Toomey, Diaz, & Sanchez, 2011; Ryan, Huebner, Diaz, & Sanchez, 2009). Still, it is crucial to note that even individuals whose friends, families, and communities are highly supportive may still experience significant minority stress from societal sources (e.g., anti-GSM media; anti-GSM legislation), which may be detrimental to their psychosocial functioning (Hatzenbuehler et al., 2010). Simply put, the minority stress model sees the *context* in which one exists as a minority individual as strongly mediating the link between minority status and health, and thus may be a useful model for understanding a patient's context. Despite its usefulness as one systematic framework, the minority stress model may not apply to all patients; individual differences should be considered.

Recommendation 7: Query History of GSM-Related Stressors With an Interested and Inquisitive Stance

Importantly, the minority stress model provides clinicians with a cohesive framework for clinical thinking. This view suggests that providers not merely assume that an individual patient is likely to experience poor health because they are GSM per se. Rather, it suggests that clinicians must assess the individual's *experience* of being a GSM person to evaluate risk. To do so appropriately, we recommend that providers broach this topic from an inquisitive, open stance with patients who self-identify as a gender and/or sexual minority person. For instance, a primary care provider screening for depression might say something like, "I see you marked on your paperwork that you are gay. A lot of gay people find that the world has been pretty unkind to them…they might experience a lot of concerns about what people will think of them, or they might also have been discriminated against or harassed directly. This kind of stress can be really hard to deal with. What have your experiences been with these kinds of things?" This kind of setup indicates that the provider would view a wide range of experiences and views as valid, important, and real, increasing comfort on the part of the patient. For the clinician, discussing this topic in this fashion is likely to provide useful information toward assessing the patient's social history and risk for current behavioral health problems.

In clinical contexts where psychological distress and social relationships are particularly germane to the patient's presenting problem (e.g., mental health services and substance use treatment), clinicians may also assess specific domains that commonly contribute to minority stress. In addition to asking about experiences with harassment and anti-GSM discrimination, we recommend that clinicians discuss issues related to identity disclosure (i.e., "coming out") and concealment with GSM patients. Though these two behaviors may seem like "different sides of the same coin," recent empirical research with sexual minority individuals indicates that they represent two independent aspects of how people live their lives (Meidlinger & Hope, 2014), and each should be assessed independently in patient–provider conversations about outness. Multiple studies converge to suggest that actively concealing or hiding one's sexual orientation is correlated with increased psychological distress (Meidlinger & Hope, 2014; Schrimshaw, Siegel, Downing, & Parsons, 2013). However, research does *not* clearly suggest that individuals who are more "out" experience better mental health on the whole; in fact, several studies have found sexual orientation disclosure to be unrelated to mental health (Meidlinger & Hope, 2014; Schrimshaw et al., 2013), or even related to poorer mental health (Pachankis, Cochran, & Mays, 2015). It is important to note that concealment and disclosure processes are different for gender minority people than for sexual minority individuals, and little research has examined the contributions of each to the health and well-being of gender minority individuals; thus, we must be cautious to assume that the same patterns apply to transgender and other gender minority people.

Finally, clinicians are likely to be most effective in working with GSM patients when they recognize that GSM people are diverse, and that there can be significant differences both within and between GSM subgroups. For instance, transgender individuals often report experiencing rejection and discrimination from cisgender sexual minority people. Similarly, bisexual individuals, or those with fluid sexual orientations, may experience anti-bi sentiment from other sexual minorities. Similarly, within a specific subgroup, there can be distinctive racial or ethnic subgroups, or subgroups that are centered around specific preferences.

Recommendation 8: Consider the Relationship Between GSM-Related Issues and Presenting Complaints

As discussed earlier, GSM people may experience minority-related stress that is significantly related to their presenting complaints. However, it is just as important for clinicians to realize that GSM clients most often seek care for problems that are *not* functionally related to their sexual orientation or gender identity. We believe that avoiding assumptions about links between GSM status and clinical problems is just as critical a component of providing affirmative care as recognizing challenges faced by GSM patients. Thus, GSM-affirmative clinicians are faced with a balancing act of sorts; they must consider possible linkages between sexual orientation and gender identity and a client's presenting problem, without assuming that a significant relationship exists.

For instance, consider a psychologist, Dr. Eaton, assessing Shawna, a 32-year-old lesbian woman of Irish-American background, who presents to therapy for depression. Both Shawna and Dr. Eaton live in a rural area where most residents espouse conservative views. Shawna lives with her wife, Beth, a White, cisgender woman, and their 6-year-old daughter, Hope. Dr. Eaton has gay and lesbian family members, does advocacy work with a nearby LGBTQ center, and keeps up on political issues that affect GSM people. As Dr. Eaton is a strong ally and is attuned to GSM issues, he recognizes that sexual minority people in this area are likely to experience very high levels of stigma, discrimination, and even harassment. During the interview, the clinician finds himself thinking "Well of course! I'd be depressed if I had to deal with all of that hate that she must have to face! This town is full of closed-minded people!" Dr. Eaton spends much of their first few sessions beyond the intake asking Shawna about her experience as a lesbian woman living in a rural town, expressing effusive support and admiration for sexual minority people. Shawna discusses how she experienced a fair amount of anti-lesbian discrimination and some harassment as a teenager and young adult, but she notes that these occurrences are rare of late. She notes that a few classmates' parents don't seem to want to have Hope over for playdates, but Shawna says she is not sure if this is because her parents are in a same-sex partnership, and reports not being very bothered by this, as both she and Hope have many friends.

Shawna feels relieved to have a provider who is an ally to GSM people. However, she begins to grow concerned with Dr. Eaton's focus on her sexual orientation. Shawna feels her current depression is due mostly to recently increased workload at her job, fighting with her sister over how to handle their recently deceased parents' estate, and flare-ups of her chronic low back pain. Although she has mentioned each of these factors to Dr. Eaton, the psychologist seems to be asking more questions about Shawna's being lesbian than about the factors Shawna feels are driving her depression. Meanwhile, Dr. Eaton feels he is doing his due diligence to fully explore issues related to Shawna's sexual orientation, as he surmises that few other mental health providers in the region would be so knowledgeable. After three sessions, Shawna grows frustrated at not "feeling heard," becomes pessimistic about the therapy's chances of success, and stops coming to therapy.

In the above example, Dr. Eaton's efforts to create an affirmative context for care backfire, and he unwittingly winds up providing ineffective services to Shawna. Said another way, Dr. Eaton clung to his initial clinical hypothesis (that minority stress was contributing greatly to Shawna's depression) and, in doing so, failed to develop more accurate hypotheses (Shawna's depression was due to work stress, family conflict, and chronic pain). In this case, it is important to note that it was Dr. Eaton's assumption that sexual orientation was a primary issue for Shawna that led to Dr. Eaton providing suboptimal care. By more closely examining his own biases in his work with Shawna, Dr. Eaton may have been able to "catch" that he was focusing largely on only one possible explanation for her depression and neglecting other plausible clinical hypotheses.

In contrast, providers may also inadvertently assume a null relation between patients' GSM identity and their presenting complaint, when, in fact, one exists. This may be more common in certain areas of health care where discussion of social and lifestyle issues is generally limited. Though providers working in these contexts may not be "forced" to integrate social and lifestyle factors broadly into their thinking, factors such as sexual orientation and gender identity may indeed be relevant. For instance, consider the case of Juan, a 26-year-old gay Latino man who has been living in a large city in the Midwestern United States since college. He is gainfully employed and has private medical and dental insurance. Shortly after moving to the city, Juan started taking Truvada for HIV prevention (i.e., pre-exposure prophylaxis [PrEP]) in consultation with his primary care doctor. Juan went for a routine dental visit and, on intake paperwork, marked that he was HIV negative and taking Truvada. His dentist, having never heard of Truvada being used as PrEP, asked him smugly, "*How* can you be HIV negative if you're taking *that* medication? I know what that's for, you know!" Juan calmly reiterated his HIV status, told the dentist that he had tested negative for HIV last month in a routine checkup, and briefly described how Truvada can be used for PrEP. The dentist replied with a puzzled look and hurriedly asked him "Why can't you just use condoms?"; he proceeded to begin the cleaning before Juan could respond, with a heavy tension in the air.

Feeling defeated by this experience, Juan decided not to return to this particular dentist when his next routine appointment approached. When he thought about scheduling an appointment with a new dentist, he found himself thinking of this negative experience, feeling angry, and, ultimately, not following through on making the appointment. This cycle repeated for 2 years until recently, when Juan began to notice that his gums bled heavily when he brushed his teeth. Now, he goes to a new dentist, Dr. Smith, as a new patient for a routine cleaning. Dr. Smith is more knowledgeable about HIV prevention than Juan's previous dentist, and matter-of-factly notes that Juan is taking PrEP when he reviews the intake paperwork. However, Dr. Smith is astounded that this young man has gone so long without routine dental care, despite having the material means to do so. He begins to counsel Juan extensively, with a hint of condescension, about the dangers of skipping routine dental visits. At no point does Dr. Smith query Juan's reasons for not seeking care sooner; rather, he operates on the assumption that Juan was "just lazy" or "didn't think it mattered," as he feels some of his other young male patients believe. Juan politely nods as Dr. Smith explains this to him, but picks up on the dentist's negative attitude toward him, and again feels uncomfortable.

In the above example, Juan's reason for seeking care was not directly tied to his sexual orientation, but he did indeed have a negative prior experience around being a gay man taking PrEP. Dr. Smith might have learned about this by asking Juan, in an open-ended and nonjudgmental way, about his reasons for not getting care sooner. For instance, he might have said, "So it's been 2 years since your last cleaning. I see a lot of different patients who wait this long (or longer) to get their teeth cleaned. This can be for all kind of reasons; some people don't have the means to pay for it; some people have had bad experiences at the dentist before in the past; some people hate the way the instruments feel in their mouth; and some people simply just forget or put it off. What would you say are the reasons that you're coming in now, rather than sooner?" This would have provided Juan an opportunity to recount his negative experience with his last dentist and, in turn, provided Dr. Smith an appropriate context to express an affirmative stance toward

GSM people, likely putting Juan at ease. It is worth noting that this process would not have required Dr. Smith to begin by asking specifically about whether Juan's sexual orientation impacted his dental care; rather, this could have been accomplished by simply inquiring broadly about reasons for delaying care.

■ CONCLUSION

Sexual orientation and gender identity are complex topics that intersect with patient–provider interactions in myriad ways. This chapter has outlined the clinical implications of some of these interactions. This may provide a foundation for providers to consider how they might refine their clinical approach, both to create a more inclusive environment broadly and to provide improved care to GSM patients specifically. As we have stated, providing competent care to GSM individuals requires providers not only to adopt specific practices, but also to take an active, ongoing, and reflective view of their own interactions with patients. We hope that providers will combine these considerations with ongoing self-reflection, formal professional development, and practical learning to move toward providing inclusive, affirmative, and clinically optimal care for GSM individuals.

■ REFERENCES

Abreu, J. M., Goodyear, R. K., Campos, A., & Newcomb, D. (2000). Ethnic belonging and traditional masculinity ideology among African Americans, European Americans, and Latinos. *Psychology of Men and Masculinity, 1*, 75–86. doi:10.1037/1524-9220.1.2.75

Aday, L. A., & Andersen, R. A. (1974). A framework for the study of access to medical care. *Health Services Research, 9*(3), 208–220.

American Psychiatric Association. (1973). *Diagnostic and statistical manual of mental disorders* (3rd ed.). Washington, DC: Author.

American Psychiatric Association. (2013). *Diagnostic and statistical manual of mental disorders* (5th ed.). Arlington, VA: American Psychiatric Publishing.

Cochran, S. D., Drescher, J., Kismodi, E., Giami, A., Garcia-Moreno, C., Attala, E.,…Reed, G. M. (2014). Proposed declassification of disease categories related to sexual orientation in the International Statistical Classification of Diseases and Related Health Problems (ICD-11). *Bulletin of the World Health Organization, 92*, 672–679. doi:10.2471/BLT.14.135541

Dank, M. D., Lachman, P., Zweig, J. M., & Yahner, J. (2014). Dating violence experiences of lesbian, gay, bisexual, and transgender youth. *Journal of Youth and Adolescence, 43*, 846–857. doi:10.1007/s10964-013-9975-8

Hatzenbuehler, M. L., Bellatorre, A., Lee, Y., Finch, B. K., Muennig, P., & Fiscella, K. (2014). Structural stigma and all-cause mortality in sexual minority populations. *Social Science & Medicine, 103*, 33–41. doi:10.1016/j.socscimed.2013.06.005

Hatzenbuehler, M. L., McLaughlin, K. A., Keyes, K. M., & Hasin, D. S. (2010). The impact of institutional discrimination on psychiatric disorders in lesbian, gay, and bisexual populations: A prospective study. *American Journal of Public Health, 100*, 452–459. doi:10.2105/AJPH.2009.168815

Heck, N. C., Mirabito, L. A., LeMaire, K., Livingston, N. C., Flentje, A. (2016). Omitted data in randomized controlled trials for anxiety and depression: A systematic review of the inclusion of sexual orientation and gender identity. *Journal of Consulting and Clinical Psychology, 85*(1), 72–76. Advanced online publication. doi:10.1037/ccp0000123

Hendricks, M. L., & Testa, R. J. (2012). A conceptual framework for clinical work with transgender and gender nonconforming clients: An adaptation of the Minority Stress Model. *Professional Psychology: Research and Practice, 43*, 460–487. doi:10.1037/a0029597

Institute of Medicine. (2011). *The health of lesbian, gay, bisexual, and transgender people: Building a foundation for better understanding.* Washington, DC: National Academy of Sciences.

Institute of Medicine, Board on the Health of Select Populations. (2013). *Collecting sexual orientation and gender identity data in electronic health records: Workshop summary.* Washington, DC: National Academies Press. Retrieved from http://www.ncbi.nlm .nih.gov/books/NBK154075

Katz-Wise, S. L., & Hyde, J. S. (2012). Victimization experiences of lesbian, gay, and bisexual individuals: A meta-analysis. *Journal of Sex Research, 49*, 142–167. doi:10.1080/ 00224499.2011.637247

King, M., Semlyen, J., Tai, S. S., Killaspy, H., Osborn, D., Popelyuk, D., & Nazareth, I. A. (2008). Systematic review of mental disorder, suicide, and deliberate self harm in lesbian, gay and bisexual people. *BMC Psychiatry, 8*. doi:10.1186/1471-244X-8-70

Lick, D. J., Durson, L. E., & Johnson, K. L. (2013). Minority stress and physical health among sexual minorities. *Perspectives on Psychological Science, 8*, 521–548. doi:10.1177/ 1745691613497965

Mays, V. M., & Cochran, S. D. (2001). Mental health correlates of perceived discrimination among lesbian, gay, and bisexual adults in the United States. *American Journal of Public Health, 91*, 1869–1876. doi:10.1080/00224499.2011.637247

Meidlinger, P. C., & Hope, D. A. (2014). Differentiating disclosure and concealment in measurement of outness for sexual minorities: The Nebraska Outness Scale. *Psychology of Sexual Orientation and Gender Diversity, 1*, 489–497. doi:10.1037/sgd0000080

Meyer, I. H. (1995). Minority stress and mental health in gay men. *Journal of Health and Social Behavior, 36*, 38–56. doi:10.2307/2137286

Meyer, I. H. (2013). Prejudice, social stress, and mental health in lesbian, gay, and bisexual populations: Conceptual issues and research evidence. *Psychology of Sexual Orientation and Gender Diversity, 1*, 3–26. doi:10.1037/2329-0382.1.S.3

Morales, E. S. (1996). Gender roles among Latino gay and bisexual men: Implications for family and couple relationship. In J. Laird & R. J. Green (Eds.), *Lesbians and gays in couples and families* (pp. 272–297). San Francisco, CA: Jossey-Bass.

Nadal, K. L. (2013). *That's so gay! Microaggressions and the lesbian, gay, bisexual, and transgender community.* Washington, DC: American Psychological Association.

Pachankis, J. E., Cochran, S. D., & Mays, V. M. (2015). The mental health of sexual minority adults in and out of the closet: A population-based study. *Journal of Consulting and Clinical Psychology, 83*, 890–901. doi:10.1037/ccp0000047

Röndahl, G., Innala, S., & Carlsson, M. (2006). Heterosexual assumptions in verbal and nonverbal communication in nursing. *Journal of Advanced Nursing, 56*, 373–381. doi:10.1111/ j.1365-2648.2006.04018.x

Rothman, E. F., Exner, D., & Baughman, A. L. (2011). The prevalence of sexual assault against people who identify as gay, lesbian, or bisexual in the United States: A systematic review. *Trauma, Violence, and Abuse, 12*, 55–66. doi:10.1177/1524838010390707

Russell, S. T., Ryan, C., Toomey, R. B., Diaz, R. M., & Sanchez, J. (2011). Lesbian, gay, bisexual, and transgender adolescent school victimization: Implications for young adult health and adjustment. *Journal of School Health, 81*, 223–230. doi:10.1111/ j.1746-1561.2011.00583.x

Ryan, C., Huebner, D., Diaz, R. M., & Sanchez, J. (2009). Family rejection as a predictor of negative health outcomes in White and Latino lesbian, gay, and bisexual young adults. *Pediatrics, 123*, 346–352. doi:10.1542/peds.2007-3524

Sausa, L. A., Sevelius, J., Keatley, J., Iñiguez, J. R., & Reyes, M. (2009). *Policy recommendations for inclusive data collection of trans people in HIV prevention, care & services.*

San Francisco: Center of Excellence for Transgender HIV Prevention, University of California, San Francisco. Retrieved from http://transhealth.ucsf.edu/tcoe?page=lib-data-collection

Schrimshaw, E. W., Siegel, K., Downing, M. J., & Parsons, J. T. (2013). Disclosure and concealment of sexual orientation and the mental health of non-gay-identified, behaviorally bisexual men. *Journal of Consulting and Clinical Psychology, 81*, 141–153. doi:10.1037/a0031272

Sue, S. (1998). In search of cultural competence in psychotherapy and counseling. *American Psychologist, 53*(4), 440–448.

The GenIUSS Group. (2014). Best practices for asking questions to identify transgender and other gender minority respondents on population-based surveys. J. L. Herman (Ed.). Los Angeles, CA: Williams Institute. Retrieved from https://williamsinstitute.law.ucla.edu/wp-content/uploads/geniuss-report-sep-2014.pdf

CHAPTER **23**

Future Directions in Gender and Sexual Minority Health Research

K. Bryant Smalley, Jacob C. Warren, and K. Nikki Barefoot

We hope that the preceding chapters have provided a comprehensive and informative view of the current state of gender and sexual minority (GSM) health research, and have helped to frame both the challenges and the opportunities in advancing the field. The chapters immediately before this have already summarized the recommendations for practitioners—both preventive and clinical. In this concluding chapter, therefore, we focus on some of the ongoing considerations necessary in achieving health equity for GSM populations.

■ RESPONSIBLE REPORTING OF FINDINGS

As the field continues to grow, the importance of responsibly reporting research findings will become more critical than ever. In the early years of the AIDS pandemic, findings of elevated prevalence of HIV and AIDS within sexual minority men were quickly twisted into "proof" of underlying biases and prejudices that may have in turn perpetuated those biases (Halkitis, 2012; Herek & Glunt, 1988; Herek et al., 1998). While this was potentially unavoidable, scientists learned of the importance of responsibly reporting findings related to the lesbian, gay, bisexual, and transgender (LGBT) community. For example, in our own previous work, findings have indicated a higher level of alcohol use among individuals who score highly on measures of gay community attachment. As scientists, it is incumbent upon us all to be precise in the reporting of those results. Taken out of context, they could easily be interpreted as suggesting that involvement with the gay community is a risk factor for alcohol use. On deeper examination, however, it becomes clear that it is a function of the measure used—many measures of LGBT community involvement specifically ask questions about frequency of patronage of LGBT bars and clubs, and naturally individuals who frequent bars and clubs of any kind would be expected to in turn also be more likely to report alcohol use.

Similarly, it is important to be thoughtful with wording related to risks. Throughout this text, we have repeatedly referred to the elevated risk of several outcomes, such as suicide, among gender minority individuals. When stating results such as these, it is important to not unintentionally semantically associate these outcomes with being a gender or sexual minority—for instance, in the case of suicide among transgender men and women the consensus is not that being transgender in turn increases the risk of suicide, but rather that the experiences of stigmatization, discrimination, and transphobia encountered by transgender individuals elevate the risk of suicide. While the distinction may seem academic to some, it is important to correctly identify the true underlying factor at play—there is no evidence that gender minority individuals are inherently more prone to suicide, while there is overwhelming evidence that gender minority individuals are dramatically more susceptible to discrimination and prejudice than even their sexual minority counterparts, and such experiences are well-recognized risk factors for suicide. Thus, we recommend always considering the broader context of risk behaviors and interpreting results precisely, as well as considering how results may be misunderstood or taken out of context without appropriate wording.

■ FUNDING

Recent years have thankfully shown a continued expansion of funding opportunities available for the field of GSM health research and outreach. Funders, including federal and foundation, are increasingly recognizing the importance of examining the overall health and wellness of GSM people. For some new funding agencies such as the Patient-Centered Outcomes Research Institute (PCORI), the health of GSM groups has even been integrated into their foundational missions. While the gains from this work will be years in the making, it represents an essential step in understanding and improving the health of the population.

In perhaps the most exciting development in the area of GSM health research in recent years, in late 2016, the National Institutes of Health (NIH) officially designated the GSM population as a health disparity population. This designation officially recognizes the unique dynamics of health for the population, and underscores the need for specific investigation of not only the group as a whole, but also of subgroups within the broader population. This designation opens the door for many additional funding streams within NIH, and officially federally recognizes the field of GSM health as critical to "[advancing] the health of all Americans" (Pérez-Stable, 2016). In combination with the work of NIH's Sexual and Gender

Minority Research Office (SGMRO), there is the true potential for a landmark swell of research to improve the health of GSM groups.

RESEARCH NEEDS

As the opportunity to expand GSM health research becomes a reality, there are a number of areas that will be critical lines of inquiry to successfully move the entire field forward. These include: (a) conducting subgroup investigations and cross-group comparisons; (b) focusing on the role of intersectionality and minority health; (c) recognizing the role of geography in health; (d) developing an understanding of aging and caretaking within the LGBT community; and (e) determining what community-driven health priorities are.

One of the most important considerations for the advancement of GSM health research is the fundamental recognition of the diversity of the LGBT community. As discussed throughout this text, the need for the umbrella term *GSM* stems from the remarkable spectrum of identities existing outside that of the cisgender, heterosexual majority. Up until only recently, subgroup investigations and cross-group comparisons—for example, contrasting the health needs of gay men to those of bisexual men—were nearly nonexistent. The pressures, barriers, and opportunities that each distinct subgroup faces can vary substantially, having a quite different effect both on outcomes and on the suitability of certain intervention strategies. As research continues to develop, separately examining needs and underlying dynamics will reveal how to more effectively meet the needs of each group. Similarly, conducting cross-group comparisons can help to elucidate potential differences in comparison to the non-LGBT community that are masked by differences across those groups that cancel each other out in GSM to non-GSM comparisons. As an example, if a study compares the overall LGBT community to the non-LGBT community, it might find no difference in outcomes related to, for instance, heart disease (hypothetically). However, cross-group analyses may reveal that while gay men have lower risk for heart disease than heterosexual men, lesbians may have increased risk. When combined in a single analysis, this effect may be entirely washed out and lead to an erroneous conclusion that heart disease rates are not in fact elevated within the GSM population. When considering the extreme difference in lived experiences of, say, a transgender heterosexual man and a cisgender bisexual woman, it is intuitive that the relevant factors and outcomes will be different. However, for the most part, the field has continued to collapse groups together. This is particularly the case for research involving gender minority individuals, who are typically collapsed entirely into one comparison group. This type of approach ignores the clear differences between transgender men and transgender women, not to mention the rest of the gender minority spectrum. Research that is specifically designed and powered to investigate cross-group differences is highly needed.

Another critical area of research is investigating the impact of racial/ethnic minority status and associated intersectionalities. The field of health disparities itself was initially predicated on the stark differences in health associated with being a member of a racial and/or ethnic minority group, and it comes as no surprise that early research presented previously in this text reveals that individuals who are members of both a racial/ethnic minority group and a gender/sexual minority group are at an even more elevated risk for negative health outcomes. However, research is frequently not designed or powered to specifically investigate these within-group differences (i.e., powered to sufficiently contrast not only gay men to lesbians, but also to contrast racial/ethnic minority lesbians to nonminority lesbians). There is a rich field of research within health disparities to support this line of inquiry, and robust methodologies available, and there is a need for both funders and researchers to consider the importance of race and ethnicity within GSM health. Although methodologically challenging, incorporating non-GSM comparison groups is essential in fully measuring the impact of intersectionality—that is, there is a strong need to power studies to not only compare specific racial/ethnic minority GSM groups to nonminority GSM groups, but also have simultaneous comparison groups of racial/ethnic minority non-GSM groups and nonminority non-GSM groups. Fully understanding the effects of other intersectionalities (e.g., age and veteran status) will require similar approaches.

An additional component of intersectionality and multiple identities relates to geographic location. The role of geography in health is well established, with inner cities, suburbs, rural areas, and regions (e.g., northeast vs. southeast United States) all having demonstrable variations in not only health outcomes, but also the underlying factors at play in establishing and maintaining health (e.g., provider availability and insurance coverage). Because the field of GSM health is currently challenged in its ability to achieve representative samples (discussed in more detail later in this chapter), the importance of considering region and rurality becomes even more pronounced. As discussed earlier in the text, not only does residing in a rural area enhance many of the health risks faced by GSM individuals, it also presents unique challenges to even being able to conduct research in this area. Similarly, certain geographical locations have become "go-to" destinations for GSM research (e.g., San Francisco and New York), largely due to higher concentration of GSM individuals within those locations. While this has been a function of necessity, it is critical to expand out the locales in which GSM health research takes place in order to ensure the full diversity of experiences of GSM individuals is represented. This will require the development of new recruitment and engagement methodologies to ensure a more diverse group is engaged in research, and funding to support such methodological investigation is strongly needed.

As with all of health research, the aging of the population cannot be ignored. While discussed in detail within Chapter 20, it is important to again underscore that society is currently facing an unprecedented explosion in the number of outwardly identified GSM older adults that will only continue to grow. This raises first-of-their-kind questions about the role of caregiving within the LGBT community, the ability of same-sex partners to receive adequate support in end-of-life decision making, challenges in identifying same-sex friendly retirement communities and nursing homes, the unique age-related outcomes that may have disparate outcomes within the LGBT community (e.g., Alzheimer's), and so on. The simple fact of the matter is that the field is in its extreme infancy, and to ensure we are fully able to meet the needs of the aging population, specific inquiry into the needs of aging GSM individuals is critical.

Finally, and potentially most importantly, there is a substantial need to support projects investigating community-driven priorities and concerns. The traditional, investigator-driven model of health research is important; however, for a population that has received so little historical research focus, an elegant, efficient, and effective method to meet unknown needs is to have those needs identified by the community itself. Community-driven methods such as community-based participatory research have emerged as some of the most successful methods of engaging health disparity populations in disparities-elimination research (Berge, Mendenhall, & Doherty, 2009; Israel, Schulz, Parker, & Becker, 1998; Wallerstein & Duran, 2006, 2010). By bringing a community's voice to the forefront of research within that particular community, insights can be gained that external, investigator-driven projects often cannot mimic, and the targets and goals of the research being conducted are inherently more person-centered. For a historically disenfranchised group such as GSM individuals, there is tremendous power in going straight to the source to ask about what issues are most relevant to them, and collaboratively building strategies to specifically address those priorities.

ON THE HORIZON

As the field becomes both more recognized and more robust, there are current and upcoming developments that will have a substantial impact on the field. The unprecedented progress made in social acceptance and inclusion of the community in recent years is inspiring. While substantial progress continues to be needed, the trajectory is very promising. As acceptance and inclusion continue to grow, and more legal rights are guaranteed to the GSM population, it will be interesting to see the impact in mitigating some of the negative consequences associated with minority stress. Similarly, developments in methodologies and data capturing hold much promise for advancing the field. The development and promulgation of the two-step gender identity assessment process (querying gender assigned at birth and gender most identified with) will allow for more robust examinations of the health of gender minority individuals. Another development with broad implications is the issuance in New York of the first-ever birth certificate designating an individual as intersex (Segal, 2017)—if this becomes standard across the nation, this will allow for unprecedented documentation of prevalence essential in building a foundation of intersex research.

Finally, the federal support behind inclusion of an assessment of sexual orientation and gender identity within medical records—while controversial—would prove landmark in the documentation of health needs. While originally, as of 2018 medical providers were to be required to assess both the sexual orientation and gender identity of their patients to achieve "meaningful use" designation for electronic health records, and similar assessments were slated to be required for Medicare and Medicaid patients (U.S. Department of Health and Human Services, Centers for Medicare and Medicaid Services, 2015), as of the publication of this text the status of these previously enacted recommendations and guidelines is uncertain due to changes in the political climate. Were the original guidelines to be implemented, the potential to provide previously unavailable levels of data regarding GSM health would be game-changing, as secondary chart reviews, national registries, and claims data would then be available. The importance of these data cannot be overstated—for the first time ever, there would be the ability to collect nationally representative data regarding GSM health.

This potential change is not without controversy, however, both inside and outside the LGBT community. The rule change was originally delayed until 2018 in order to allow time for providers to become culturally competent in assessing very sensitive personal information (Human Rights Campaign, 2015); however, it is unclear to what extent the availability of competency training has been ensured, and the overall future of the rule change is currently uncertain. Further, concerns regarding a potential increase in health care discrimination due to disclosure have not been adequately considered—as discussed throughout this book, health care discrimination is a real and present concern for GSM populations, and by effectively legislating disclosure, individuals who would not otherwise disclose may end up doing so (believing their provider is affirming, when in fact they may not be). From a privacy standpoint, there are understandable concerns regarding adequate protection of information that, if disclosed, could legally result in employment termination and other consequences due to the lack of federal non-discrimination legislation. As a result, individuals may not feel comfortable disclosing this information even to affirming providers, instead either not disclosing at all or reporting a heterosexual, cisgender identity. If sexual orientation and/or gender identity is clinically relevant to the presenting concern, this could inadvertently lead to suboptimal care being provided, as the provider will believe (based on what is perceived to be evidence) that the patient is not a gender and/or sexual minority. From a research methodology standpoint, the data generated from intake forms could be biased, particularly in minority and rural communities, as increased stigma in those communities could lead to underreporting of GSM status, which could in turn lead to erroneous conclusions generated from the associated data. Despite these concerns and potential limitations, however, it is clear that this shift would bring about a revolution in the availability of data regarding GSM health.

■ CONCLUSION

In conclusion, there is tremendous work being done to understand and advance the health of GSM individuals. The field itself is in an exciting stage of development, and it is clear that its future is full of promise and potential. There are certainly challenges to overcome to not only achieve health equity, but also to promote the overall health and well-being of the LGBT community, but these challenges present countless opportunities for researchers, clinicians, and communities to make a true difference in the health of the nation.

■ REFERENCES

Berge, J. M., Mendenhall, T. J., & Doherty, W. J. (2009). Using community-based partici-patory research (CBPR) to target health disparities in families. *Family Relations, 58*(4), 475–488.

Halkitis, P. N. (2012, April). Discrimination and homophobia fuel the HIV epidemic in gay and bisexual men. *Psychology and AIDS Exchange Newsletter*. Retrieved from http://www.apa.org/pi/aids/resources/exchange/2012/04/discrimination-homophobia.aspx

Herek, G. M., & Glunt, E. K. (1988). An epidemic of stigma: Public reactions to AIDS. *American Psychologist, 43*(11), 886–891. doi:10.1037/0003-066X.43.11.886

Herek, G. M., Mitnick, L., Burris, S., Chesney, M., Devine, P., Fullilove, M. T.,…Sweeney, T. (1998). Workshop report: AIDS and stigma: A conceptual framework and research agenda. *AIDS and Public Policy Journal, 13*(1), 36–47.

Human Rights Campaign. (2015, October). HHS to include sexual orientation & gender identity in Meaningful Use of Electronic Health Program. Retrieved from http://www.hrc.org/blog/hhs-to-include-sexual-orientation-gender-identity-in-meaningful-use-of-elec

Israel, B. A., Schulz, A. J., Parker, E. A., & Becker, A. B. (1998). Review of community-based research: Assessing partnership approaches to improve public health. *Annual Review of Public Health, 19*, 173–202.

Pérez-Stable, E. J. (2016, October). *Director's message: Sexual and gender minorities formally designated as a health disparity population for research purposes*. National Institute on Minority Health and Health Disparities, National Institutes of Health. Retrieved from https://www.nimhd.nih.gov/about/directors-corner/message.html

Segal, C. (2017, January). Nation's first known 'intersex' birth certificate issued in New York City. *PBS NewsHour*. Retrieved from http://www.pbs.org/newshour/rundown/new-york-city-issues-nations-first-birth-certificate-marked-intersex

U.S. Department of Health and Human Services, Centers for Medicare and Medicaid Services. (2015). Medicare and Medicaid Programs; Electronic Health Record Incentive Program—Stage 3 and modifications to Meaningful Use in 2015 through 2017. Retrieved from https://www.federalregister.gov/documents/2015/10/16/2015-25595/medicare-and-medicaid-programs-electronic-health-record-incentive-program-stage-3-and-modifications

Wallerstein, N. B., & Duran, B. (2006). Using community-based participatory research to address health disparities. *Health Promotion Practice, 7*(3), 312–323.

Wallerstein, N., & Duran, B. (2010). Community-based participatory research contributions to intervention research: The intersection of science and practice to improve health equity. *American Journal of Public Health, 100* (Suppl. 1), S40–S46.

INDEX